Lyttle's Mental Health and Disorder

THIRD EDITION

Edited by

Tony Thompson
MA BEd(Hons) RMN RNMH DipN(Lond)
CertEd RNT
Director of Practice Development
Ashworth Hospital Authority
Ashworth Centre
Liverpool, UK

Peter Mathias
BSc MA MSc PhD
Manager of City and Guilds Affinity
London, UK

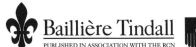

Baillière Tindall
PUBLISHED IN ASSOCIATION WITH THE RCN

Royal College
of Nursing

EDINBURGH LONDON NEW YORK PHILADELPHIA
ST LOUIS SYDNEY TORONTO 2000

BAILLIÈRE TINDALL
An imprint of Harcourt Publishers Limited

© Harcourt Publishers Limited 2000

✤ is a registered trademark of Harcourt Publishers Limited

First edition 1986
Second edition 1994
Third edition 2000

0 7020 2449 X

British Library Cataloguing in Publication Data
A catalogue record for this book is available from the British Library

Library of Congress Cataloging in Publication Data
A catalog record for this book is available from the Library of Congress

Note
Medical knowledge is constantly changing. As new information
becomes available, changes in treatment, procedures, equipment and the
use of drugs become necessary. The editors and the publishers have
taken care to ensure that the information given in this text is accurate
and up to date. However, readers are strongly advised to confirm that
the information, especially with regard to drug usage, complies with the
latest legislation and standards of practice.

The
publisher's
policy is to use
**paper manufactured
from sustainable forests**

Printed in China

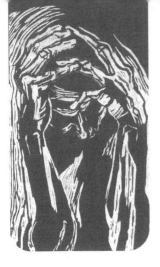

Contents

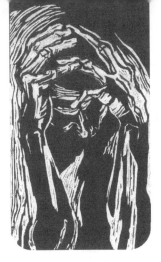

Contributors

Fran Aiken RMN RGN SCM RNT CertEd BA MSc
Lecturer/Practitioner, The Ashworth Centre, Ashworth Hospital, Maghull, Merseyside, UK

Carol Baxter PhD MSc RGN RM RHV DN FETC
Professor of Nursing, School of Health, Biological and Environmental Sciences, Middlesex University, London, UK

Clancy Borastero RMN SRN RCNT ENB 770
Lecturer Practitioner, The Ashworth Centre, Ashworth Hospital, Maghull, Merseyside, UK

Judy Boxer RMN CQSW MA
Senior Lecturer Mental Health Nursing, School of Health and Social Care, Sheffield Hallam University, Collegiate Campus, Sheffield, UK

Mike Dudley BA(Hons) RMN ENB650
Training Coordinator, Community Health Sheffield NHS Trust, Sheffield, UK

David Duffy BA(Hons) MSc RMN CertHSM
Professional Head of Nursing, Mental Health Services of Salford NHS Trust, Prestwich, Manchester, UK

Kieran Fahy RMN CPN(Cert) BSc(Hons)
Lecturer Practitioner, Tameside Community Rehabilitation Team, Wilshaw House, Ashton-Under-Lyme, UK

Antoine P Farine MSc BA RGN RCNT RNT DipN
(Part A & B) CertEd BTTA
Specialist Leader, Biological Sciences, School of Nursing, Undergraduate Division, Faculty of Medicine and Health Sciences, University of Nottingham, Queens Medical Centre, Nottingham, UK

Chahid E Fourali PhD MA DipCP LICENCE
Research Adviser, City and Guilds of London Institute, London, UK

Dr Robert C Gibb MBChB MRCPsych CTL
Consultant Forensic Psychiatrist, The State Hospital, Carstairs, UK

Les Jennings RNMH RMN BSc(Hons) MSc
PostGradDiploma Counselling
Lecturer/Practitioner, Ashworth Centre, Ashworth Hospital, Maghull, Liverpool, UK

F Clifford Johnson RMN SRN RNT STD
Formerly Education Officer, English National Board for Nursing, Midwifery and Health Visiting, UK

Christine A Kirk MB BChir FRCPsych
Consultant Psychiatrist for the Elderly, Bootham Park Hospital, York, UK

Gary F McCulloch BA RMN DipHP
Senior Health Promotion Specialist, Sheffield Health Authority Sheffield, UK

Dr Gary J D Macpherson BA(Hons) MPhil AFBPsS
DClin Psychol CPsychol
Clinical and Forensic Pyschologist, The Douglas Inch Centre, Glasgow, UK

Sue Marshall RGN BA(Hons) MPhil
Clinical Psychologist, Edward Street Day
Hospital, West Bromwich, UK

Peter Mathias BSc MA MSc PhD
General Manager, City and Guilds Affinity,
London, UK

Pete Melia MA BA(Hons) RMN FETC
Clinical Manager, Personality Disorder Services,
Ashworth Hospital, Liverpool, UK

Tony Moran RNMH RMN
Ward Manager, Ashworth Special Hospital,
Maghull, Liverpool, UK

Mike Musker RMN DPSN BA(Hons) MSc PGDE
Ward Manager, Tennyson Ward (Intensive Care
Unit), Ashworth Hospital Authority, Maghull,
Liverpool, UK

Aru Narayanasamy RGN RMN BA MSc CertEd RNT
CFP Curriculum Coordinator/Honorary Nurse
Adviser (Transcultural Health Care),
University of Nottingham, Queens Medical
Centre, Nottingham, UK

Karen Rea MA BA(Hons) RNMH DPSN RNT CertEd
Lecturer Practitioner, Ashworth Centre, Maghull,
Liverpool, UK

Julie M Repper RGN RMN BA(Hons) MPhil
Research Student, University of Manchester,

School of Nursing, Midwifery and Health
Visiting, Manchester, UK

Lynne D Smith RMN RGN DipNurse(Lond) CertEd(FE)
RNT Cert SocialResearchMethodology
Freelance Teacher and Consultant in Nursing
Practice, Stafford, UK

Patrick Sullivan RMN DipN(Lond) BSc(Hons) MSocSc
FAETC
Locality Manager, Southern Derbyshire Mental
Health NHS Trust, Kingsway Hospital, Derby,
UK

Tony Thompson MA BEd(Hons) RMN RNMH
DipN(Lond) CertEd RNT
Director of Practice Development, The Ashworth
Centre, Maghull, Liverpool, UK

Robert Tunmore MA PeDipEd BSc(Hons) RMN RGN
IPD Cert
Academic Co-ordinator and Principal Lecturer,
Institute of Health Studies, Faculty of Human
Sciences, University of Plymouth, Plymouth, UK

Colin P Vose MA BA(Hons) PGCE RMN
Mental Health Strategy Co-ordinator, Merseyside
NHS Education and Training Consortium,
Mossley Hill Hospital, Liverpool, UK

Enid E Wright BSc(Econ) Diploma AppliedSocialStudies
Formerly Policy Analyst, CCETSW, London, UK

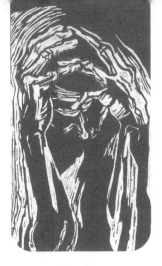

Introduction

This edition owes its style and inspiration to the author of the first edition, Jack Lyttle. There is a need for interprofessional collaboration, which has been reinforced many times throughout the life of the first and second editions of the book and which is particularly evident today. Psychiatric care delivered by any of the agencies, but particularly nursing and social work, has undoubtedly travelled a long way since the first edition. However, there continues to be a variety of views about the best way to address the predicament of people who have mental health problems and who are sometimes disabled by the response of society to these problems.

The chapters in this edition illustrate this variety and are the contemporary perceptions of highly experienced people committed to the development of knowledge and practice in psychiatric care. Most of the chapters integrate and promote understanding and insights from a variety of disciplines in their efforts to lay the foundations for high standards of intervention.

It is particularly poignant that in 1986 Jack identified in his preface that uncritical adherence to the medical model of mental disorder had largely been replaced by broader social perspectives incorporating a skills-orientated approach to care. Now it is possible to see a return to a more paternalistic or controlling view of mental disorder as the services struggle to base their work on scientific evidence and at the same time respond with humanistic concern to those who require mental health support.

The single ambition of any contemporary text-book must be to assist in the provision of guidance that will support practitioners in delivering systems of care that are sensitive and responsive to the needs of the patient or client. Public safety and security for people who display mental disorders are extremely important, and some of the failures of the systems in the past have now brought mental health care into an arena that recognizes the need for specialist expertise. Aspects of delivery such as accurate and strong clinical leadership, risk assessment, medication management programmes and rational care planning processes feature in most policy statements and are to be found throughout this current volume.

The editors and most authors have taken the view that the reader would welcome a whole system approach to services that are either established or are likely to be put in place in the forthcoming years. There are concerns about the standards of care provided for clients and patients, particularly those who require ongoing inpatient facilities. These concerns revolve around safety, security, dignity and proper access to therapeutic interventions. Whilst the focus of mental health policy has been in recent years associated with deinstitutionalization this has brought its own problems when service users are presented with a severe illness and with associated social care needs. It is a fact that the complexity of the care that patients require is far greater than it was in the past and it is essential that clinical skills of a high order are available and that proper governance of the professions who hold those skills takes place. These concerns are reflected throughout the following chapters, which are arranged in four parts:

I Understanding mental health, disorder and illness
II Interventions in mental health practice
III Challenges for service delivery
IV Issues for practitioners

It is timely that the national service frameworks for mental health are now being disseminated. This sets a comprehensive change agenda that is intended to drive quality upwards and eliminate inconsistencies within the present services. It is a credit that the central administration of government now recognizes that all aspects of mental health have to be thought about and covered if we are to expect practitioners and managers to offer well-coordinated services. The services of the future will embrace health promotion, assessment and diagnosis, treatment, rehabilitation and care in primary and specialist provision. Effective services will require the development of interprofessional and collaborative ventures by specialists and the various agencies likely to be involved.

It is now recognized that mental health services face critical challenges and therefore the framework that all professionals should be working to should be based on standards associated with evidence of effectiveness. The frameworks, which were developed by external reference groups, require that performance will be assessed through a number of national milestones and the basis of this will be that mental health systems have to be integrated into all local delivery organizations.

The learning and development agenda created by the national service frameworks, and the need to build capacity and capability in service and professional organizations and in individual practitioners will mean that ways will have to be found to share good practice. The frameworks and the national standards will require recruitment of additional staff who are properly trained and will also require rethinking of the mix of skills available to the patient or client. The future workforce will have to focus on functional aspects of providing a high standard of care within a framework that has seven key components or standards including the following:

◆ Standard one puts an emphasis on mental health promotion and the need to counter and eliminate the discrimination and social exclusion associated with mental health problems.

◆ Standard two puts a focus on primary care, which means that individuals who contact primary health care teams should have their mental health needs identified and properly assessed and addressed through effective treatments, including a referral to specialist services and further assessment and intervention if it is thought to be required.

◆ Standard three is an exhortation for systems to be available to ensure that those individuals with common, frequently occurring mental health problems will be able to make contact around the clock with local services that can provide adequate care.

◆ Standard four is a requirement that people who are on a care programme receive care that optimizes engagement, prevents or anticipates crisis and therefore reduces risk. In the future it is the aim that such individuals will have a copy of a written care plan which includes the action to be taken in a crisis by the user, their carers and those professionals charged with coordinating their care. The plan will also advise general practitioners how they should respond if someone who presents with a problem needs additional help.

◆ Standard five is a demand that all service users who are assessed as requiring a period of care away from their home should have timely access to an appropriate hospital bed, or an alternative place. Such a place will be in the least restrictive environment consistent with the need to protect them and the public and be as close as possible to where they live. A copy of a written aftercare plan agreed on discharge should accompany the patient; this sets out the care and rehabilitation to be provided, identifies the care coordinator and specifies the action to be taken in a crisis.

◆ Standard six highlights the needs of those people who care for service users and identifies that they should have an assessment of their caring, physical and mental health needs repeated on at least an annual basis. They should also have a written care plan which is offered to them and implemented in discussion with them.

◆ Lastly standard seven highlights the need for prevention of suicide. This important standard is intended to promote mental health for all and incorporates all of the other standards. In addition it supports the need for local prison staff to be assisted in preventing suicides amongst prisoners. Further, it ensures that staff are competent to assess the risk of suicide amongst individuals at greatest risk and encourages the development of local systems for suicide audit in order that lessons can be learned and subsequent action taken.

This is the first time in a number of decades when people who provide mental health services have a national benchmark against which their own services can be measured. The frameworks are not couched in rhetoric and they acknowledge the difficulties in recruiting and retraining adequate numbers of staff in this important area of service delivery. The framework probably offers the best introduction that we can have to this current edition as it asserts that the provision of good quality mental health services can be achieved only with close partnership between all the relevant agencies.

We would like to thank Jacqueline Curthoys, Jane Shanks and Karen Gilmour of Harcourt Health Sciences for the very considerable help, encouragement and support they gave to the production of this book. We also wish to express our gratitude to the authors for the effort and creativity they have given so readily and generously. Thank you.

Liverpool   Tony Thompson
London   Peter Mathias
2000

Part I
Understanding mental health, disorder and illness

The first chapter of this part introduces different models, perspectives and ways of looking at mental health, disorder and illness. The physical, psychological and social perspectives it examines are echoed and reinforced in the remainder of the part. Disturbances of feeling (affect), behaviour and thinking (cognition) are described and analysed in a series of three chapters that explore the interaction of biopsychosocial factors in more detail. Other chapters emphasize the need for practitioners and others to take a multidimensional approach to mental health and illness and to apply it in understanding the experience of people in disturbance, distress and illness.

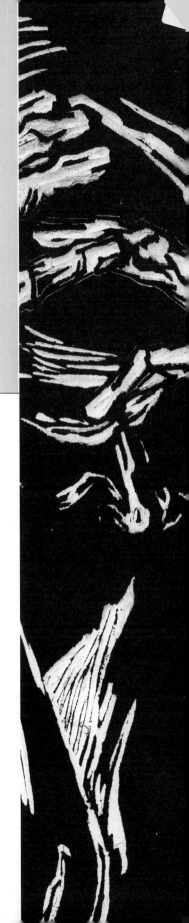

Chapter One

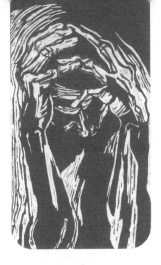

A common language of classification and understanding

Robert C Gibb   Gary JD Macpherson

AIMS

- ◆ To understand the differences between normality, disease and illness
- ◆ To seek a definition for abnormality
- ◆ To explore the psychosis–neurosis dichotomy
- ◆ To review classificatory systems within mental health practice
- ◆ To understand medical, psychological and social models of causation
- ◆ To recognize vulnerability and risk factors for the development of mental disorder
- ◆ To introduce nursing diagnostic systems

KEY ISSUES

Normality and abnormality

ICD-10 and DSM-IV diagnostic categories

Causation

Syndrome, aetiology and treatment

Medical model

Psychodynamic, behavioural and cognitive models

Predisposing, precipitating and perpetuating factors

Self-actualization

NANDA

Health and Sickness are not essentially different, as the ancient physicians and some practitioners even today suppose. One must not make of them distinct principles or entities. In fact, there are only differences in degree between these two kinds of existence.
Friedrich Nietzsche 1888

INTRODUCTION

This chapter could be subheaded 'Towards an integrative approach to mental health practice'. Most lay people believe that the principal therapeutic avenue in modern mental health practice is via 'talking about problems'. The lay person is also aware of the influence of physical factors in mental health, mainly as a result of less commonly used practices such as electroconvulsive therapy (ECT). It is important from the outset that the reader keeps in mind the involvement of physical, psychological and social factors in the topics discussed in the following pages.

Spectrum of illness including classification

Normality, disease and illness

What does it mean to say that a person is 'ill'? What is understood by the term 'normality' and how does it differ from the terms 'disease' and 'illness'? How does someone become ill? How can this be changed? These are important questions for the mental health practitioner.

We can define abnormality in a number of ways:

1. deviation from statistical norms
2. deviation from social norms
3. maladaptive behaviours
4. personal or subjective distress.

1 **Statistical norms.** Literally, the word *abnormal* means 'away from the norm'. In a statistical sense, an individual who is 8 feet tall is considered to be abnormal. In other words, the individual's height is beyond that accepted as normal. They are *abnormally* tall. The same notion of statistical abnormality also applies to intelligence. An excep-

tionally intelligent individual or a 5-year-old child prodigy might both be considered as statistically abnormal. Of course, it might be positively advantageous to be 8 feet tall or highly intelligent, but in a statistical sense both are abnormal. We therefore cannot rely on statistical methods alone in defining abnormality.

2 **Social norms.** Every society has certain standards of acceptable behaviour. Behaviour that deviates from society's notion of normal behaviour is often considered to be abnormal. As above, such behaviour might also be classified as statistically abnormal. However, we clearly encounter problems when we apply a statistical notion of abnormality in terms of societal norms. First, the passage of time alters what we consider to be normal behaviour within the same society. This might be considered as the generation gap. Secondly, each society has its own definitions of normal and acceptable behaviour. Therefore, in examining abnormality, we should look beyond the concept of what is believed to be socially normal behaviour.

3 **Behaviours.** There have always existed people who have been singled out by the rest of the community as odd or bizarre as a consequence of their maladaptive behaviour. There are certain mental states and behaviours that have adverse effects on the individual or society, although this may not always be the case. People may experience delusions of grandeur or a manic state of mind that they do not wish to alter, although practitioners may see it in individuals' best interests to treat them. Some mental states and behaviours interfere with the individual concerned (for example, individuals with anxiety disorder who are afraid to travel on buses, or drug users who are damaging their health by injecting). Other states and behaviours interfere with society (for example, paranoid individuals who plot to assassinate political figures or individuals whose personality makes them behave aggressively towards others). These behaviours would be considered abnormal through the criterion of maladaptiveness. People who are diagnosed as mentally ill do not always support this idea, far less that they are in need of treatment.

4 Feelings of distress. Our last criterion considers an individual's personal or subjective feelings of abnormality. It should be clear to practitioners that many individuals diagnosed as mentally ill experience anguish, despair and feelings of hopelessness. This may be immediately apparent to those involved in their care. In other cases it may be less obvious to the observing practitioner, for example the agoraphobic man who cannot leave the house, the elderly lady suffering from feelings of panic who tries desperately to control herself in the face of impending doom, or the depressed teenager who suffers from insomnia or poverty of appetite. Sometimes the practitioner will discover that a person is distressed only from the latter's subjective report.

It should be clear from the above description that none of the criteria alone is sufficient to satisfy a complete description or understanding of abnormality. What we can do, however, is to use these criteria in combination to help us to understand abnormality and mental disorder. We shall discuss formal diagnostic procedures later in the chapter.

From a practitioner's perspective, the term 'normality' means simply the absence of abnormality. The terms 'disease' and 'illness' have been used in medical text as being distinct from 'health' or 'normality'. This separation can be particularly helpful when conceptualizing physical diseases such as tuberculosis. For instance, if individuals are not infected then they are in a 'normal' physical state. However, if they are infected by the tuberculosis bacterium, then they are said to be suffering from a 'disease'.

Although this 'way of seeing things' is most useful in branches of physical medicine, it is less so in areas of mental health practice. For instance, when does the experience of fear or anxiety (a clinical state of apprehension, tension and worry) become pathological, and when is it just an exaggeration of a 'normal' experience? For example, in the past fear developed to allow human beings to escape from danger. Some authors have therefore suggested that there exists a continuum ranging from normality at one end through to disease at the other end. An extension of this is the concept of the dimensional approach to diagnosis.

In modern psychiatric practice clinicians will commonly come across formal syndromal classificatory systems. Those most commonly used will be referred to later in this chapter. Such systems describe clusters of symptoms, which when they occur together confer a formal diagnosis. The term 'diagnosis' comes from the Greek word *gnosis*, which means to recognize, nosology being the branch of medicine involved in the classification of disease.

Disorders such as personality disorders and anxiety states seem to fit the continuum model better, whereas those such as dementia and schizophrenia seem to fit better into the disease entity model. However, there are critics of both models, and some have even suggested that both can co-exist in the same disorder!

Psychosis and neurosis

In traditional psychiatric text, the terms 'neurosis' and 'psychosis' are commonly found. Let us first consider *neurosis*. Individuals suffering from neurotic disorders, by and large, were believed to retain insight into their everyday thoughts and functioning. They could, however, experience intermittent or constant anxiety or depression. For example, an individual suffering from a phobia about dogs behaved irrationally and was filled with terror in the presence of such animals. The essential element of neurotic disorders was that they were experienced by so-called 'normal' individuals. Often they were seen as less severe disorders that were readily understood. Unlike psychotic individuals, sufferers themselves might be the first to admit that their fears or beliefs had no basis in reality.

Consider people suffering from obsessive–compulsive disorder. They may experience persistent and intrusive thoughts (obsessions) about their personal cleanliness. In order to decrease the level of anxiety that these thoughts cause, they may wash their hands many hundreds of times (compulsions). Such thoughts and behaviours at their most extreme may be so unusual that they appear to the observer to be evidence that the person is mentally ill. Unlike those suffering from a psychotic condition, individuals may have a considerable degree of insight into their condition, and may indeed be the first to admit that these thoughts are senseless. The individuals concerned may continue to be able to function in society despite their considerable handicap. To the mental health practitioner, neurotic disorders are characterized generally by anxiety, personal unhappiness and maladaptive behaviours.

Psychosis was a term used to describe disorders such as schizophrenia and manic depression, where the symptoms experienced by the sufferer were not like those that a normal person would experience. An individual with psychosis may experience a severe impairment of mental functioning including disturbed perceptions, poverty of language, disrupted thought processes and emotional dysfunction. The individuals concerned may think that they are Christ, or of alien origin, and can weave a coherent *modus vivendi* around such a belief. Alternatively they may be experiencing hallucinatory phenomena or maintain persecutory delusional beliefs, as well as many other abnormalities of mental state.

This neurosis–psychosis dichotomy is further compounded by subdividing psychosis into *organic* and *functional*. The practitioner may consider organic psychosis to be closest to the field of physical medicine. The disorders subsumed under this category are clearly related to physical factors. For example, organic brain syndromes such as acute or chronic (alcoholic) poisoning, traumatic brain injuries or Alzheimer's disease may cause a disruption in a person's mental state and social functioning, and consequently produce a range of bizarre observable behaviours.

Traditionally these categories, along with *personality disorders*, were placed into a diagnostic hierarchy (Fig. 1.1). In this, diagnoses were based on produced symptoms or phenomena, and organized into syndromes. If the patient presented with symptoms from different categories, then the category further down the hierarchy would be subsumed by the category above it. In practical terms this would mean that if you had symptoms of both an anxiety disorder and a schizophrenic disorder, then only the schizophrenic disorder would be diagnosed as it belonged to a higher category in the hierarchical system.

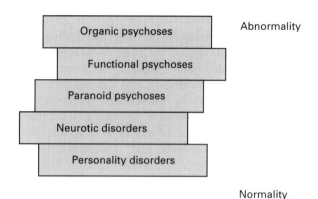

Fig. 1.1 A traditional hierarchy.

Classificatory systems

Although the use of the terms neurosis and psychosis have fallen relatively out of favour, they did help early practitioners structure their approach towards classifying and treating mental illness. One of the major criticisms of the neurosis–psychosis dichotomy was that many of the neurotic symptoms could be found in psychotic disorders, and neurotic disorders could have an equally severe impact on personal functioning. It was also suggested that in psychosis individuals lost insight into their being psychiatrically disordered, but this was in practice an artificial divide as loss of insight was often incomplete. Further criticism was levelled at the broad nature of the terms used, with some diagnostic categories being difficult to place.

As a result the use of the terms psychosis and neurosis has been greatly reduced in recent classificatory systems. In the United States the terms have been practically abolished, although have been retained to a limited extent in the classificatory system most frequently used in the United Kingdom. In the latter, the term psychosis is most commonly employed when describing severe mental disorders where hallucinations or delusions are present.

From a United Kingdom perspective, there are two diagnostic systems that are referred to most frequently. These have arisen out of practitioners' attempts to achieve more precision in their diagnostic methods allowing more accurate communication between mental health professionals. The International classification of diseases 10th revision (ICD-10 1992), developed by the World Health Organization, is the main system used in the United Kingdom. The Diagnostic and statistical manual, now in its fourth revision (DSM-IV 1994) and developed by the American Psychiatric Association (APA), is referred to frequently in psychiatric literature, although is not commonly used in clinical practice in the United Kingdom. Both classificatory systems use slightly different terms to describe broadly similar concepts. In fact, in developing the ICD-10, collaborators from the APA were involved in contributing to the genesis of the ICD diagnostic categories, to enable the two systems to be compatible where possible.

DSM was the first of the two systems to use a multiaxial system. This system attempts to classify disorders using both aetiology and symptomatology. A classificatory system based on aetiology relies on a clear understanding of the cause of the disorder, which is often not possible. Aetiologically based diagnostic systems have been used traditionally in psychodynamic circles, particularly in the USA. In the United Kingdom and Europe, diagnostic classification has more often been based on the individual's symptom cluster or phenomena. The attempt in DSM to bring in the best features of both phenomenological and psychodynamic diagnostic systems allowed a more holistic understanding of the individual's difficulties resulting from the psychiatric disorder. In DSM-IV, five axes are used:

◆ axis I refers to the psychiatric diagnosis itself
◆ axis II refers to any specific developmental or personality disorder
◆ axis III refers to any important concurrent physical factors
◆ axis IV refers to any relevant social stressors
◆ axis V refers to the degree of effect of the disorder on adaptive functioning.

ICD-10 has chosen to continue with the use of an uniaxial system. Those involved in the development of ICD-10 believed that the drawback of a multiaxial system was its complexity.

DSM also introduced the concept of operational criteria. These were diagnostic criteria that, when present in an individual, would lead the clinician to employ that particular diagnostic category.

Critics of DSM believe that this approach is too rigid and inflexible, and that the ICD system with its descriptive approach is more in keeping with clinical practice. In ICD-10, although operational criteria are employed only in the research version, guidelines leading to confident diagnosis are given in the standard version. In both diagnostic systems, the term 'disorder' is used rather than the term 'illness' or 'disease'. Box 1.1 highlights some of these issues.

Any classification system has its advantages and disadvantages. Criticisms of classificatory systems, especially from the so-called antipsychiatry movement, state that few of the diagnostic categories have any aetiological validity. The critics go on to say that the diagnostic labels cannot always be found to fit the presentation of the individual, are perjorative and label socially deviant behaviour as illness. They suggest that the terms employed are metaphors for behaviour that does not conform to societal norms, employed by agents of social control (i.e. mental health workers). Such views may be particularly attractive when clinicians use diagnostic terms such as alcohol dependence and personality disorder. However, they would also include terms such as schizophrenia in their criticism. These critics would state that studies of such concepts as schizophrenia have never come up with consistent clusters of symptoms, nor has a consistent biological underpinning been found. An international pilot study of schizophrenia carried out in nine different countries throughout the world (World Health Organization 1973) found a wider use of this diagnostic label in the old USSR. One interpretation of this finding was that political dissidents and social activists were being conveniently removed from society into psychiatric institutions using this label as justification.

Similarly the high incidence of second generation individuals of Afro-Caribbean descent admitted to hospital with the diagnostic label of schizophrenia (Harrison et al 1988) has been put forward as evidence of the invalidity of this diagnosis and the ease with which such terms can be abused. This finding has complex causes and is not replicated in other minority groups within British society.

Box 1.1   A comparison of ICD-10 and DSM-IV

ICD-10
Generalized anxiety disorder
The essential feature is anxiety, which is generalized and persistent, but not restricted to or even strongly predominating in any particular environmental circumstances (i.e. it is 'free floating'). As in other anxiety disorders the dominant symptoms are highly variable, but complaints of continuous feelings of nervousness, trembling, muscular tension, sweating, light-headedness, palpitations, dizziness and epigastric discomfort are common. Fears that the sufferer or a relative will shortly become ill or have an accident are often expressed, together with a variety of other worries and foreboding. This disorder is more common in women, and often related to chronic environmental stress. Its course is variable but tends to be fluctuating and chronic.

Diagnostic guidelines
The sufferer must have primary symptoms of anxiety most days for at least several weeks at a time and usually for several months. These symptoms should usually involve elements of:
(a) apprehension (worries about future misfortunes, feeling 'on edge', difficulty in concentrating, etc.)
(b) motor tension (restless fidgeting, tension headaches, trembling, inability to relax) and
(c) autonomic overactivity (light-headedness, sweating, tachycardia or tachypnoea, epigastric discomfort, dizziness, dry mouth, etc.).

In children, frequent need for reassurance and recurrent somatic complaints may be prominent.

The transient appearance (for a few days at a time) of other symptoms, particularly depression, does not rule out generalized anxiety disorder as the main diagnosis, but the sufferer must not meet the full criteria for depressive episode (F32. -), phobic anxiety disorder (F40. -), panic disorder (F41.0), or obsessive–compulsive disorder (F42. -).
   Includes: anxiety neurosis
                   anxiety reaction
                   anxiety state
   Excludes: neurasthenia (F48.0)

DSM-IV
Diagnostic criteria for generalized anxiety disorder
A Excessive anxiety and worry (apprehensive expectation), occurring more days than not for at least 6 months, about a number of events or activities (such as work or school performance).
B The person finds it difficult to control the worry.
C The anxiety and worry are associated with three of the following:
   (1) restlessness or feeling keyed up or on edge
   (2) being easily fatigued
   (3) difficulty concentrating or mind going blank
   (4) irritability
   (5) muscle tension
   (6) sleep disturbance (difficulty falling or staying asleep, or restless unsatisfying sleep).
D The focus of the anxiety and worry is not confined to features of an axis I disorder, e.g. the anxiety or worry is not about having a panic attack (as in panic disorder), being embarrassed in public (as in social phobia), being contaminated (as in obsessive–compulsive disorder), being away from home or close relatives (as in separation anxiety disorder), gaining weight (as in anorexia nervosa), having multiple physical complaints (as in somatization disorder), or having a serious illness (as in hypochondriasis), and the anxiety and worry do not occur exclusively during post-traumatic stress disorder.
E The anxiety, worry or physical symptoms cause clinically significant distress or impairment in social, occupational or other important areas of functioning.
F The disturbance is not due to the direct physiological effects of a substance (e.g. a drug of abuse, a medication) or of a general medical condition (e.g. hyperthyroidism) and does not occur exclusively during a mood disorder, a psychotic disorder, or a pervasive developmental disorder.

Finally homosexuality appeared in diagnostic classification in the past, presumably owing to its unacceptability to some sections of society. This is no longer included in either ICD-10 or DSM-IV.

Some criticisms may be justified, but in other cases the diagnostic groupings reflect the current level of understanding of psychiatric aetiology, rather than providing evidence that diagnostic classificatory systems be scrapped. There are many examples of diagnostic concepts in other health fields where debates exist over diagnostic cut-off points, with variable clusters of symptoms or unknown aetiological factors. Hypertension is one such example but few would argue that this is a useless or unhelpful concept. In any case, in classificatory systems the diagnostic categories used are frequently being revised to take new understanding into consideration.

Major reasons for retaining classificatory systems are:

◆ They help to understand clusters of symptoms as distinct diagnostic entities.
◆ This facilitates research into the aetiology of the specific disorders, allowing redefinition.
◆ The concepts allow effective communication between professionals where everyone is speaking 'a common language'.
◆ They help development of management plans and prognostic indicators.

Systems and causation

Because of the historical prominence of the medical profession within mental health practice, much of the early interest has been shown in relevant aetiological factors of a medical or physical nature. However, this has not been to the total exclusion of looking at psychological or social factors. The work of Freud at the beginning of the twentieth century examining psychological and developmental factors involved in the production of psychiatric symptoms is well known (Freud 1957). Similarly, early work looking at important social factors has been carried out by psychiatrists, for example Birley (Brown & Birley 1968).

Since the advent of a multidisciplinary approach to mental health practice, non-medical ways of viewing mental disorder have been brought much more sharply into focus. There are three main models, namely the *physical*, *psychological* and *social* models. Although they appear to view mental health issues from different perspectives, it is important to emphasize that they are all different ways of looking at the *same* disorder. Thus it is important when attempting to understand any psychiatric disorder that the practitioner employs all three models, using an integrative approach.

Physical/Medical

What is meant by the 'medical model'? In simple terms this model explains illness as a physical malfunction, such as a chemical or anatomical defect. Loss of memory or speech production, difficulties in the area of social skills and everyday abilities, or a decrease in someone's ability to adapt to new situations are viewed by the medical model as primarily a result of a physical abnormality or one in the production of neurotransmitters (brain chemicals).

Therefore in its simplest form it refers to the belief that there is a putative physical cause for the disorder being examined. These physical causes can be separated into *acquired* and *non-acquired*. Acquired causes would include, for instance, head injuries, cerebral infection and substance misuse/drug ingestion. Non-acquired would include genetic causes, electrical wave changes such as those that occur in epilepsy, or alterations in endogenous neurotransmitters (the brain's own chemical transmitters). Thus a medical approach to treatment may emphasize a chemical therapy or medication to counteract such deficits in neurotransmitters.

The medical model makes certain assumptions about health and illness. It can be viewed as a three-stage model.

syndrome → *aetiology* → *treatment*

As we have seen above, a co-occurrence of symptoms may be defined as a *syndrome*. The practitioner using the medical model would then look for the cause or *aetiology* of the syndrome. This potentially could be done on a number of levels, such as recording the person's genetic make-up, or examining the individual's brain chemistry for any abnormality. However, given the practical limitations of current technology to test these variables and in light of current knowledge of the relative importance of these particular variables, this approach is unable to give accurate enough information. Therefore a phenomenological approach is more commonly employed in order to group together the relevant symptoms into a syndrome. It is hoped that specific phenomena, such as an hallucination, can be shown to correspond to an abnormality of a specific part of the brain. Once the syndrome is recognized, and the aetiology determined, a biological treatment might be used to restore someone's mental health.

Some mental health practitioners have been criticized for using this model religiously to the exclusion of other models. In response to this criticism, the practitioners would defend themselves by stating that the interaction of psychological and social factors is reducible to the physical (e.g. social difficulties lead to stress, which in turn can lead to changes in brain neurotransmitters). This is sometimes referred to as reductionism.

Psychological/Psychodynamic

Probably the most well-known mental health professional has been Sigmund Freud. His original and controversial work led to the development of the psychoanalytical school and the practice of psychodynamic psychotherapy. Since Freud's work in the early part of the twentieth century his ideas have been refined and added to by many writers, although fundamental principles remain (Freud 1957). Freud postulated that an individual was born with innate energy (libido), which required modification to make it consonant with everyday living. The individual passes through certain pre-programmed psychosexual developmental stages in childhood, the success of this passage having a major bearing on future mental health.

Freud separated mental life into three categories: the *unconscious*, the *preconscious* and the *conscious*. This classification was termed the *topographical model*. Most practitioners will be aware of the conscious aspects of mental experience, and

the preconscious (that part of experience that is readily brought to consciousness if required). The unconscious (that which is normally unavailable to the conscious mind) often manifests itself through slips of the tongue and dreams, as well as in psychiatric dysfunction such as conversion and anxiety disorders.

Freud constructed a comprehensive theory for the different levels of intrapsychic functioning. This has been referred to as the *structural theory*; it divides the psyche into the *superego* (the conscience based on parental and societal standards), the *id* (instinctual drives and urges) and the *ego* (censorship and defence mechanisms). The defence mechanisms inherent in the ego (such as denial, projection and reaction formation) allow the instinctual drives of the id to be modified in a manner that is consonant with everyday living. Neo-Freudian authors such as Jung, Klein and Eriksson and many others have developed psychodynamic thinking further, but discussion of their theories is outside the scope of this chapter.

Psychodynamic theories introduced the role of psychological factors in health and illness, and the possibility of psychotherapeutic treatment for a person's distress. However, some critics have suggested that such theories have problems in their proof and are indifferent to scientific method (Eysenck 1952). Since then, psychodynamic research has continued to attempt to identify the effective parts of dynamic interventions.

Developing alongside psychodynamic theory have been behavioural and cognitive approaches to the understanding and treatment of mental disorder. The foundations of these latter approaches stem from a single movement that dominated academic psychology for many decades – *behaviourism* (Watson 1914). This model derives many of its principles from animal learning, deduced through laboratory research and experiment. It makes three assumptions:

◆ Healthy behaviour and abnormality are *learned* from past experience. Illness is seen as learning of maladaptive habits.
◆ We can find out which aspects of a person's behaviour are maladaptive through *hypothesis testing*.

◆ A practitioner can replace maladaptive habits with *adaptive* behaviours.

To use our above example of dog phobia, we can see the value of a behavioural approach to understanding mental health problems. Someone suffering from a dog phobia (a fear that is greatly out of proportion to any real danger), for example, may have had an unpleasant childhood experience involving being growled at or bitten by a dog. This in turn produced a fear at even the sight of a dog in the distance, despite the fact that dogs are generally not dangerous. According to the behaviourist view the symptom *is* the disorder, and is not indicative of an underlying disease process, but rather is a result of maladaptive learning.

Behaviourism was extended further, most notably by B. F. Skinner (1969), who developed the concept of behaviour modification. This is based on the analysis of how the frequency of behaviours may be affected by their consequences and the setting in which the behaviours occur. A *positive reinforcer* is an event that increases the likelihood that a behaviour will occur again. In essence, a positive reinforcer rewards behaviour. A *negative reinforcer* is an event whose removal increases the likelihood of a behaviour occurring again. A *punisher* is an event that decreases the reoccurrence of a behaviour.

Fundamentally, the behavioural approach to abnormality emphasizes that maladaptive behaviours, such as phobias, anxiety, depression, are *learned* and can thus be unlearned. In this respect it can be considered *antimentalist*—that is, mental events, feelings and thoughts are not valid targets to change because they cannot be observed directly.

Critics challenged the behaviourist's premise that behaviour alone was sufficient to explain how an individual relates to the world. They noted that individuals with mental health problems not only behaved in maladaptive ways, but also held unrealistic or irrational beliefs, expectations and thoughts. Thus a *cognitive* approach to mental health began to become influential (Beck 1976).

Essentially, the cognitive school contends that individuals' ways of thinking or belief system influence their behaviour. For example, individuals suffering from depression may report thoughts that they are worthless as a person, that their situation is hopeless and that the world is against them. In turn, they may become increasingly passive and unwilling to engage in any meaningful behaviour. Their opportunity to prove themselves as worthy is further reduced, and such individuals may become increasingly low in their mood. (Cognitive and behavioural therapeutic techniques for this will be discussed in a later chapter of this book.)

Social

And finally there is the social model. Proponents of this model draw attention to the impact of factors within persons' social environment such as social status, social support, isolation and poverty on mental health. Authors such as Holmes & Rahe (1967) suggested that any *change* in life circumstances, whether positive or negative, can lead to stress, with negative effects on psychological well-being. As one might expect, these authors rate that life events such as a bereavement or death have more impact than going on holiday or a change of residence. The authors quantified the impact of social change in *life change units*. For instance, the death of a spouse received 100 units whereas going on vacation received 13 units, taking into account the relative impact of these events. They postulated that the more life change units individuals were exposed to the greater the likelihood they had of developing mental health problems.

Social status has frequently been found to be linked with both medical and psychiatric disorders. The Black report (DHSS 1980) highlighted the effect of social class on medical morbidity. Black found that the risk of death was twice as high in social class V as opposed to social class I. This study used the five occupational categories (detailed below) as defined in the Office of Population Censuses and Surveys, which have since been superseded:

I — professional, higher managerial

II — intermediate

III — skilled manual, routine non-manual

IV — partly skilled
V — unskilled.

There have been many studies showing a link between social class and psychiatric disorder. For instance, schizophrenia has been found to be increased in lower socioeconomic groups. As early as 1939, Farris & Dunham found a higher incidence of schizophrenia in urban and inner city areas of Chicago compared with rural areas, with an increased incidence in lower social classes. It has been hypothesized that being in a socially disadvantaged position is itself instrumental in leading to the development of schizophrenia. Opponents of this *breeder hypothesis*, however, have suggested that this finding is an effect of downward social drift in those whose lives have been devastated by schizophrenia. It may be that both explanations have some merit. Certainly, most readers will be only too aware that social disadvantage affects mental state, with the consequent development of depression and anxiety.

Social isolation is felt to be important in a number of psychiatric disorders, such as schizophrenia (Hare 1956), depression, stress and suicidal behaviour (Durkheim 1897). Similar debates rage about whether the causative factor is isolation itself, or whether the isolation is consequent on the development of the particular disorder. Certainly the presence of a social confidante or organized social support system can have a major impact on the psychological well-being of individuals, as well as helping to prevent further relapse in their condition.

Vulnerability and risk factors

Any given disorder can be examined using the three models referred to in the previous section. Another way of categorizing mental health problems is using factors important in the production or maintenance of the disorder. These are commonly referred to as:

◆ *predisposing or vulnerability factors*—those parts of the individual's physical, psychological or social make-up that lead to an increased vulnerability to the disorder in question

◆ *precipitating factors*—factors that directly bring on the manifestation of the disorder
◆ *maintaining factors*—once the individual has developed a specific disorder, then these factors maintain its production.

These three factors interact with each other with a degree of overlap. It is possible to subdivide each factor into medical, psychological and social components. For example, a life event such as bereavement may act as a precipitant. The impact of this and the resultant production of stress will be heavily influenced by social support and psychological hardiness. The effect of this stress and subsequent development of psychiatric disorder will be greatly influenced by the biological make-up of the individual concerned. In other words, individuals exposed to the same life events may not develop the same degree of stress and, even if they do, might be able to deal with it better. Even if psychological or social ways of dealing with the stress are not developed, the latter still may not lead to the production of a psychiatric disorder because of the individual's physical constitution.

At this point, we will examine how these factors work in clinical practice using the example of depression.

Predisposing or vulnerability factors

Medical. Research has shown that there is a genetic predisposition or loading to the development of depression (McGuffin & Katz 1989). Expressed another way, this means that first degree relatives of depressives have at least twice the risk of developing depression than do those in the general population. A genetic component has been further supported by studies showing that identical twins are more likely both to have a history of depression, compared with non-identical twins (McGuffin, Katz & Rutherford 1991). That is not to say that it is inevitable that biologically predisposed individuals will develop depression, but rather that there is an increased chance that they will develop the disorder.

Acquired abnormalities predisposing to the development of depression may also be important and include neurological damage. Brain damage to the left hemisphere due, for example, to a stroke results in depression more often than does damage to the right hemisphere. In total, around 25% of those who have had strokes develop a major depressive disorder in the acute phase (Robinson et al 1986). Lesions in the frontal lobes of the brain in particular can produce depression.

Research has drawn attention to the fact that depression is twice as high amongst women than amongst men. It may be that biological reasons account for this finding, such as differing chemical enzyme activity or genetic proneness. Also, if there is a valid phenomenon of premenstrual depression then, at any given time, one-quarter of any adult female sample will be within a week of menstruating, but no men will, for obvious reasons. As a result this may influence the numbers of women reporting depressed mood at any given time. Finally the increased numbers of women with depression may be explained by women being more willing to express depressive symptoms, and more ready to seek out treatment, than men.

Psychological. The role of personality traits has long been considered as contributing to a person's vulnerability towards depression. Post-Freudian theorists have considered the depressive personality to be characterized by an excessive dependence on others for self-esteem. In simple terms, they could be considered 'love addicts' who require a constant flow of attention and demonstrations of love in an effort to relieve their own feelings of worthlessness.

Melanie Klein (Mitchell 1986) described 'the depressive position'—a stage that all infants had to progress through in their first year of life. This stage followed what she termed 'the paranoid schizoid position'. Klein believed that failure to pass through this stage successfully led to clinical depression at a later stage.

The importance of cognitive factors in predisposing an individual towards depression has been emphasized by Beck in his *cognitive theory of depression* (Beck 1976). This model postulates that depressed individuals' thinking patterns are characterized by a cognitive triad of negative thoughts about the self, their ongoing experience, and their view of the future. They may misinterpret minor, unrelated experiences as indicative of

their poor coping ability, which are impassable barriers leading to continued hopelessness.

Another model concerning vulnerability towards depression is the *learned helplessness model*, which is based on findings from animal experiments (Seligman 1981). This model suggests that depression results from an individual's expectation that bad events will inevitably occur and that nothing can be done to prevent them. In essence, individuals who learn that their responding is futile come to expect this to be the case in future situations.

Social. There is growing evidence that we live in an age of melancholia (Seligman 1975). Epidemiological studies show that the chances of developing a depressive episode of clinical proportions throughout one's lifetime are around 1 in 10 (Boyd & Weissman 1982). The most commonly quoted study looking at socially determined vulnerability factors within depressed individuals is that of Brown & Harris (1978). They looked at a community-based sample of depressed women in south-east London, and found four vulnerability factors within this group: loss of a mother before the age of 11, having three or more children at home below the age of 14, the lack of a confiding relationship and lack of employment.

In addition, social isolation can be a predisposing factor to the development of depression, the so-called *anomie*, which was so well described by Durkheim (1897) in his description of factors predisposing to suicidal behaviour. As suggested earlier it may be that social isolation is an effect rather than a cause, and therefore could be subsumed under maintaining factors instead. Low social class similarly could predispose to depression by leading to lack of finance, poor accommodation and a resultant lack of opportunity in this materialistic society.

We are not suggesting that these social factors *cause* depression, but rather that they contribute to and increase the risk of developing depression, which is the individual's response to coping with adverse circumstances.

Precipitating factors

Medical. A number of physical factors can precipitate depression. Most people are aware of the 'low' feeling immediately following a viral infection. Although not directly proven, it has been postulated that viral illnesses such as influenza and hepatitis A can precipitate depressive episodes.

Endocrine disorders such as hypothyroidism, Cushing's syndrome and hypo- and hyperparathyroidism have also been implicated, mediating their effect through hormonal imbalance. Individuals suffering from cancer, especially of lung or pancreas, may also develop depression as a result. These processes may act through an effect on neurotransmitters or by leading to physical dysequilibrium and general malaise.

Finally it may be that ingestion of substances such as alcohol, illicit drugs and prescribed drugs (e.g. steroids, beta blockers) may precipitate depression. Illicit drugs are especially important nowadays given the effects of 3,4-methylenedioxyamphetamine (MDMA or 'Ecstasy'), cocaine and amphetamines on neurotransmitter pathways and mood.

Psychological. We have highlighted above the influence of cognitions and explanatory style as vulnerability factors in depression. The cognitive model emphasizes five thinking processes that lead individuals to perceive events negatively. These cognitive processes are called systematic *errors in logic*. The first, *arbitrary inference*, refers to drawing a conclusion where there is little or no evidence to support it—for example, thinking that friends no longer care about you because they did not send a birthday card. A second, *selective abstraction*, involves focusing on one insignificant detail at the expense of more important features. To illustrate, an author failed to see that his written work was both entertaining in style and content. He focused almost entirely on one spelling mistake as indicative that he was careless, and consequently thought of himself as a useless writer. *Overgeneralization* is a third error in logic. This refers to drawing a global conclusion about personal worth on the basis of a single event. For instance, a student who failed one exam thought, 'I will never pass another exam again'. *Magnification* and *minimization* are further errors in evaluation; positive events are minimized and

negative events are exaggerated out of all proportion. Finally, *personalization* refers to taking personal responsibility for negative events. For example, a depressed individual took the blame for a neighbour's car accident because she had not warned him that there was ice on the road that morning. We can see that it is often the interpretation of an event, rather than the event itself, that can precede a period of depression. Essentially, a negative event may activate an individual's negatively biased thoughts and perceptions.

Freud (1917) brought to our attention the important role of loss in the production of depression. Depression, for instance, could occur after a bereavement, although of course it is not an inevitable sequelae after major losses. Freud attempted to clarify the distinction between depression and normal grief, and highlighted the inward turning of anger related to such losses.

Social. Depressive episodes are often preceded by a negative life event. The loss of a job, a marital separation or the death of a loved one are common precipitants of depressed mood, and a typical clinical finding is that individuals who become depressed show an excess of such losses compared with those without depression. One point of optimism, however, is that not all losses bring on depression. Only 10% of those who have experienced a significant loss develop depression afterwards (Paykel 1974). The majority of individuals *do not* become depressed after major life events. As we have seen above, Brown & Harris (1978) proposed several factors to explain the importance of social vulnerability. Therefore we might propose *invulnerability* factors, such as an intimate relationship, part-time or full-time employment, and fewer than three children still at home, as helping to prevent the occurrence of depression.

Maintaining factors

Medical. Common physical treatments used in the treatment of the depressed individual include drug treatments. Less commonly in severe depression is the use of ECT. If the wrong type of medication or inadequate dosage is given then this may lead to a continuation of depressive symptomatology, despite individuals believing that they are being adequately treated. Continued substance misuse may be another reason for poor treatment response, despite seemingly adequate pharmacological therapy.

It is important that if one is treating a depressive disorder to diagnose and treat it as such. Depression can be missed, as it commonly masquerades as other disorders such as chronic pain, eating disorders or general malaise. Medical treatment should be started when appropriate, rather than continuing with non-medical treatments, as the administration of the wrong treatment can lead to a maintenance of the original disorder. This is particularly important in a disorder such as

depression with a suicide rate of anything up to 15% in its most severe form (Coryell & Winokur 1982). A pharmacological treatment in combination with a cognitive approach has been shown to be an effective treatment strategy in the treatment of depression (Hollon et al 1992).

Psychological. The above examples of errors in logic can point the clinician to schema that underlie negative thoughts. *Schema* refer to rigid assumptions, attitudes or personal rules that are often characteristic of depressive thinking patterns. Depressed individuals may make excessive use of such directives as 'should' or 'always', which leads to them setting unrealistic goals for

CASE STUDY

A 32-year-old woman, Ms X, presents to her general practitioner (GP) complaining of depressed mood over the last 6 months. During that time she had gone off her food and lost 10 kg in weight. On further interviewing her sleep is disrupted—she finds it difficult to get off to sleep (initial insomnia), taking 1–3 hours. She tosses and turns, worrying over her role as a mother, financial difficulties (debts of £1000 mainly through unpaid credit) and her ability to function as a wife. Over the last month she has been waking up at 6 a.m. and can't get back to sleep, and generally lacks energy. She has stopped going out with her one close confidante (an old schoolfriend) on regular social pursuits. She has begun to question her religious faith and withdrawn from church. She has lost interest in sexual intercourse with her husband, her last intercourse being 9 months ago. She feels generally hopeless, guilty and worthless with recent suicidal ideation. She feels unable to fulfil her role as mother—and has withdrawn from caring for her 1-year-old child (her child is generally healthy but has been crying more than usual). She has begun to use alcohol to improve her self-esteem and help her insomnia.

In childhood she is said to have been vulnerable. Her mother died when she was 9 years of age, having been knocked down by a car whilst Ms X was accompanying her. Following this she was

brought up by her father. She spent most summers with her maternal aunt who lived 100 km from the family home. Her father is said to have been a heavy alcohol abuser at weekends—he was also a hard-working man who worked as a foreman on a building site. Her father was never violent towards her, but was unable to play with her to any great degree. She states that throughout her childhood she was always pondering on the negative aspects of life and generally saw things in black and white. She was put down by her peers at school, who told her that she was ugly and unintelligent.

In her family history, her mother was said to be highly strung, and her paternal grandmother had a nervous breakdown. Her older brother is said to be a jolly, generous man who 'loves his drink' and is always in debt. Her father is said to have favoured her brother and always supported her brother financially.

Recent worries related to her husband (a middle manager) spending more time outside the family home (the couple live in a semidetached house with a large mortgage). He spends two nights out per week on average and says that he is at the golf club or with friends on a social venture. He has asked her to join him and get a baby-sitter, but she feels unable to do so. She worries that he may be having an affair but has no positive evidence for this.

themselves and finding difficulty in considering an alternative perspective to their problem circumstances. These rigid rules maintain depression and should be the focus of a cognitive approach to treatment (Fennell 1989).

Social. If social factors are determined as being of importance in the genesis of the depressive symptomatology, it is important to alleviate these if at all possible. However, this is extremely difficult in an increasingly alienating society with a poorly developed social conscience. Without means at the individual's disposal to rectify the depressogenic sociological factors, the depression will be maintained.

The case study on page 15 illustrates the interaction of the preceding factors.

Major psychiatric categories

As the main diagnostic classificatory system currently used in the United Kingdom is the ICD-10, psychiatric categories from this will be referred to in this section. ICD-10 separates the diagnostic syndromes into 11 categories. A brief description of each will be provided. (Practitioners who wish further information should refer to the full manual published by the World Health Organization.)

◆ *Organic including symptomatic and mental disorders*—this category includes disorders that are the result of trauma to the brain, or a result of degenerative diseases of the nervous system, or the effect of toxic substances (excluding alcohol and illicit drugs) on the brain. The disorders may also be secondary to systemic disorders affecting other organs or systems throughout the body. It includes a number of different types of dementing disorder, memory disorders, deliriums and other mental and personality disorders consequent to the organic precipitant.

◆ *Mental and behavioural disorders due to psychoactive substance abuse*—this category consists of disorders resultant on the excessive and problematic use of alcohol, barbiturates, amphetamines and other illicit substances that alter mental functioning and behaviour. It includes acute intoxication, dependence syndrome and with-drawal states, in addition to psychotic and memory disorders secondary to the precipitant.

◆ *Schizophrenia, schizotypal and delusional disorders*—this is a group of disorders characterized by marked impairment of reality, disturbances of thought and perception, and bizarre behaviour. This section includes schizophrenia, schizotypal disorder, schizoaffective disorders (including symptoms of both a mood disorder and schizophrenia) and persistent delusional disorders, as well as acute and transient psychotic disorders.

◆ *Mood (affective) disorders*—this category includes disturbances of normal mood that are non-persistent including depression (depressive episode), abnormal elation (manic episode), or swings between the two (bipolar affective disorder). It also includes persistent mood disorders (e.g. cyclothymia and dysthymia), which are viewed as mood disturbances present for many years but not fulfilling the criteria for major mood disorders such as mania or depression.

◆ *Neurotic, stress-related and somatoform disorders*—these disorders have been grouped together mainly because of their historical links with neurosis, and their putative psychological causes. Many of these have also been formulated using physical and social models to explain their aetiology. They include phobic anxiety disorders, other anxiety disorders (including panic disorder), obsessive–compulsive disorder and dissociative (conversion) disorder. The diagnosis grouping of somatoform disorders includes physical symptoms, which are believed to have a psychological cause.

◆ *Behavioural syndromes associated with physiological and physical factors*—this category includes a mixed bag of syndromes with a preponderance of physical symptoms. It includes eating disorders, non-organic sleep disorders, sexual dysfunction (not caused by organic disorder or disease) and abuse of non-dependence-producing substances (such as laxatives, painkillers, steroids and hormones).

◆ *Disorders of personality and behaviour*—these consist of deeply ingrained and long-standing pervasive patterns of maladaptive behaviours and cognitions that constitute immature and inappropriate ways of problem solving or coping. The personality disorders are long lasting and are a function of faulty or deviant personality development. The category contains a number of personality subgroups including schizoid, dissocial and histrionic. There is overlap between individual personality subtypes. The category also includes disorders of sexual preference and habit, and impulse disorders such as pathological gambling.

◆ *Mental retardation*—historically these developmental disorders have been described using a number of nosological terms such as mental handicap, subnormality and the current term of learning disability. There is no attempt to define this group using aetiology, and it is broken down using measured IQ as a guide into mild, moderate and severe subgroups. It is important to note that level of disability is not only determined by ability on IQ tests but also encompasses a much wider spectrum of abilities including social functioning.

◆ *Disorders of psychological development*— these disorders lead to a less global damaging effect on the individual's function with more clearly defined dysfunction. However, this is not to say that they lead to any less severe impairment and many can be quite devastating to the individual affected. In this category are included specific developmental disorders of speech and language and scholastic skills and pervasive disorders (such as autism).

◆ *Behavioural and emotional disorders with onset usually in childhood and adolescence*—these disorders are of most relevance to the practitioner working within the area of child and adolescent mental health. This category includes disorders such as hyperkinetic disorders (childhood hyperactivity), conduct disorders and emotional disorders with onset specific to childhood, amongst others.

Nursing diagnostic systems

Criticisms of the medical syndromal classificatory systems have been alluded to previously. In response to reservations about the applicability of these diagnostic categories in psychiatric nursing practice, members of the nursing profession have begun to develop their own classificatory systems. These systems attempt to construct diagnostic terms for the clinical issues of relevance to nurses, enabling them to communicate with one another using a common language. It is intended that such systems will be regularly reviewed and updated, incorporating up to date knowledge. From the authors' experience few mental health nurses in the United Kingdom have used nursing diagnostic systems and many are only vaguely aware of their existence. If such systems are to become of use in everyday practice, there needs to be a major educational drive in their application.

The North American Nursing Diagnoses Association (NANDA) incorporated Maslow's 'hierarchy of needs' (Fig. 1.2) system alongside psychodynamic, existential and humanistic thinking when developing their diagnostic criteria. Their approach attempts to take a holistic view looking at the individual as a whole person, rather than independently studying parts of the individual's personality or behaviour. Maslow (1968) proposed that the human had a number of basic and fundamental needs, which were hierarchical in nature. At the bottom of the hierarchy, basic or instinctual needs such as hunger and thirst needed to be fulfilled before higher, less powerful needs. The next level included spiritual needs, and a longing for affection and self-esteem. The highest need according to Maslow is that of self-actualization, and should be what all humans attempt to strive for to attain full health. This can be understood as the fulfilment of the person's potential.

The NANDA diagnostic categories are summarized in Nursing diagnosis and process in psychiatric mental health nursing by MacFarland, Wasli & Gerety (1992). This book also includes

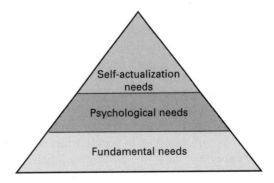

Fig. 1.2 A triangle.

sections on nursing interventions and major psychiatric disorders. Each nursing diagnostic category includes descriptions under the headings: (1) definition, (2) general principles, (3) related factors, (4) defining characteristics, (5) principles of nursing assessment, (6) patient outcomes and nursing interventions and (7) evaluation/outcome criteria, each of which is explored in some detail. Some of the diagnostic categories are very similar to medically equivalent diagnoses, for example anxiety (mild, moderate, severe, extreme/panic) and depression. Others, however, have no equivalent medical diagnostic partner, for example self-esteem disturbance, powerlessness and alteration of family processes.

A similar venture was undertaken by the American Nursing Association (ANA), who set up a task force to look at the issue of nursing diagnosis, following the publication of the document Nursing: a social policy statement. According to the ANA, the phenomena of primary concern to those working within the area of psychiatric and mental health nursing practice are human responses to actual or potential health problems. It is human responses to the physical, cognitive, emotional, social, family and cultural responses that the diagnostic system primarily addresses. The ANA have attempted to develop a system that works in a complementary fashion alongside medical classificatory systems such as DSM-IV or ICD-10.

SUMMARY

Critics have suggested that the use of differing diagnostic models leads to unnecessary complications muddying the waters, leading to diagnostic chaos, interdisciplinary rivalry and worst of all a lack of clarity in the way forward in evaluating and treating mental health problems. It is the authors' opinion that there is a place for aspects of many of the systems involved. However, these systems should be set against a background of cross-disciplinary collaboration in what is ultimately the most important task of all professionals: the improvement in all spheres of their clients' functioning.

> ## DISCUSSION QUESTIONS
>
> 1. When would an understanding of the terms 'normality' and 'abnormality' be useful in clinical practice?
> 2. Do you think one of the above-described models (i.e. physical, psychological or social) should hold precedence?
> 3. Do you think that there has been too much focus placed on physical aetiological factors in mental health practice?
> 4. Do you think that there is a requirement for a nursing diagnostic system in addition to DSM-IV and ICD-10?
> 5. How could you facilitate other practitioners in the use of an integrated approach to their practice?

There have been many criticisms against the adoption of formal diagnostic systems. However, the need for these continues allowing better communication between professionals and research into aetiology and treatment to develop. Such systems should not be viewed, in our opinion, in a sceptical manner. Many clients using mental health services want to be able to discuss issues such as diagnosis and prognosis. They do not want to feel isolated in an individualized non-diagnosis-based approach to their difficulties, as such an approach may deny that their abnormal and sometimes frightening experiences are shared with others and amenable to modern treatment.

REFERENCES

American Nurses Association 1980 Nursing: a social policy statement. MO, Kansas City

Beck A T 1976 Cognitive therapy and the emotional disorders. International Universities Press, New York

Boyd J H, Weissman M M 1982 Epidemiology. In: Paykel E S (ed) Handbook of affective disorders. Churchill Livingstone, New York, pp 109–125

Brown G M, Birley J L T 1968 Crisis and life change at the onset of schizophrenia. Journal of Health and Social Behaviour 9:203–204

Brown G M, Harris T O 1978 Social origins of

FURTHER READING

Brown D, Pedder J 1979 Introduction to psychotherapy—an outline of psychodynamic principles and practice. Tavistock, London
Good introductory textbook looking at psychodynamic principles.

Laing R D 1990 The divided self: an existential study in sanity and madness. Penguin, London
Seminal book looking at schizoid personality and schizophrenia from non-biological perspective.

MacFarland G K, Wasli E L, Gerety E K 1992 Nursing diagnosis and process in psychiatric mental health nursing, 2nd edn. J P Lippincott, Philadelphia
Contains nursing diagnostic categories and discusses philosophy behind developing a separate nursing system.

Sims A 1995 Symptoms in the mind: an introduction to descriptive psychopathology, 2nd edn. W B Saunders, London
Book describing phenomenology that underpins the ICD-10 and DSM-IV systems.

Szasz T 1961 The myth of mental illness. Hoeber Harper, New York
Seminal book suggesting that so-called psychiatric disorders may be metaphors for individuals who do not fit rather than being underpinned by biological processes.

depression: a study of psychiatric disorder in women. Tavistock, London

Coryell W, Winokur G 1982 Course and outcome. In: Paykel E S (ed) Handbook of affective disorders. Churchill Livingstone, New York, pp 93–106

DHSS (Department of Health and Social Security) 1980 Inequalities in health: report of a research working group. HMSO, London

DSM-IV (Diagnostic and Statistical Manual of Mental Disorders—4th edn) 1994 American Psychiatric Association, Washington DC

Durkheim E 1897 Suicide: a study in sociology (transl Spaulding J A, Simpson G) 1952 Routledge Kegan Paul, London

Eysenck H J 1952 The effects of psychotherapy: an evaluation. Journal of Consultative Psychology 16:319

Farris R E L, Dunham H W 1939 Mental disorders in urban areas. Chicago University Press, Chicago

Fennell M J V 1989 Depression. In: Hawton K, Salkovskis P, Kirk J, Clark D (eds) Cognitive behaviour therapy for psychiatric problems: a practical guide. Oxford Medical Publications, Oxford

Freud S 1917 Mourning and melancholia. The standard edition of the complete psychological works, vol 14. Hogarth Press, London, pp 243–258

Freud S 1957 Introductory lectures on psychoanalysis. The standard edition of the complete psychological works, vol 15. Hogarth Press, London

Hare E H 1956 Family setting and the urban distribution of schizophrenia. Journal of Mental Science 102:753–760

Harrison G, Owens D, Holton A, Neilson D, Boot D 1988 A prospective study of severe mental disorder in Afro-Caribbean patients. Psychological Medicine 18:643–657

Hollon S, Du Rubresi R, Evans M et al 1992 Cognitive therapy and pharmacotherapy for depression. Singly and in combination. Archives of General Psychiatry 49:774–781

Holmes T H, Rahe R H 1967 The Social Adjustment Rating Scale. Journal of Psychosomatic Research 11:213–218

ICD-10 (International classification of mental and behavioural disorders, 10th edn) 1992. World Health Organization, Geneva

MacFarland G K, Wasli E L, Gerety E K 1992 Nursing diagnosis and process in psychiatric mental health nursing, 2nd edn. J P Lippincott, Philadelphia

McGuffin P, Katz R 1989 The genetics of depression and manic–depressive disorder. British Journal of Psychiatry 155:294

McGuffin P, Katz R, Rutherford J 1991 Nature, nurture and depression: a twin study. Psychological Medicine 21:329

Maslow A R 1968 Towards a psychology of being. Van Nostrand, New York

Mitchell J (Ed) 1986 The selected Melanie Klein. Penguin, Harmondsworth

Nietzsche F 1888 The will to power. Translated by Kaufmann W, Hollingdale R J 1967 Vintage, New York

Paykel E S 1974 Recent life events and clinical depression. In: Gunderson E K E, Rahe R H (eds) Life stress and illness. Thomas, Springfield Ill, pp 134–163

Robinson R G, Lipsey J R, Rao K, Price T R 1986 Two year longitudinal study of post stroke mood disorders: comparison of acute onset with delayed onset depression. American Journal of Psychiatry 143:1238

Seligman M E P 1975 Helplessness. Freeman, San Francisco CA

Seligman M E P 1981 A learned helplessness point of view. In: Rehm L P (ed) Behaviour therapy for depression. Academic Press, New York, pp 123–141

Skinner B F 1969 Contingencies of reinforcement. International Universities Press, New York

Watson J B 1914 Behaviour: an introduction to comparative psychology. Holt, Rinehart & Winston, London

World Health Organization 1973 Report of the international pilot study of schizophrenia, vol. 1. World Health Organization, Geneva

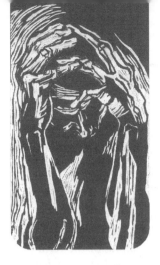

Chapter Two

The nature of health and the effects of disorder

Lynne D Smith

 AIMS

- ◆ To contrast professional organization of care and treatment with the manner in which health and ill health are experienced and exteriorized by people
- ◆ To highlight the possible repercussions of a single health problem upon the individual as a whole being
- ◆ To relate the above to the person experiencing mental health problems
- ◆ To explore the implications of this for treatment and care
- ◆ To explore issues surrounding the prevalence of mental disorder

KEY ISSUES

Role of specialization

Integrated human functioning

Extended human functioning

Interconnectedness of affect, behaviour and cognition

The personal nature of our mental health

Incidence of mental disorder

INTRODUCTION

Professionals have been taken along the route of specialization. They are provided with a generic background of study and then invited by the relevant authorizing body to focus in on a more defined and discrete area for enhanced practice. This applies whether that professional is a lawyer, who may specialize in corporate law or personal injury cases for example, a teacher, who may opt to teach 5 or 15 year olds, and subjects as diverse as mathematics or a foreign language, or a junior doctor, eventually choosing medicine or surgery, obstetrics or psychiatry from many specialist areas available after completing the basic course of study. Nurses are no different. We specialize in the care of the child, or the adult, experiencing the effects of a learning disability or a mental disorder.

On the whole, it is easy to imagine the potential benefits to both client and practitioner of this arrangement. The client receives the attention of a skilled and expert individual, who in turn has had the advantage of being able to concentrate on one specific area of attention, rather than try to be all things to all people and attain competence in all areas of the entire field. The latter would be impossible, and therefore the situation operating is clearly the most advantageous and efficient to all concerned.

The only seeming disadvantage is that we may require to seek additional expertise from a second expert practitioner when specific needs are complicated and recognized as beyond the scope of one individual. An example may be that of when, having been significantly physically damaged in a road traffic accident and seeking assistance with a claim for compensation, we decide it is time to make a will. We would probably need to seek advice from a second solicitor specializing in wills and testaments to do this.

AN ANOMALY—HEALTH AND DISORDER

The problem, however, for health care professionals is that people do not function in discrete and

separate compartments and in no field is this more obvious than that relating to mental disorder.

Human beings are integrated units. Each comes as a total package of feelings, thoughts and behaviours wrapped in a waterproof skin, which encompasses the various organs and their supportive structures necessary for survival. Take away the 'feelings, thoughts and behaviour' bit of the conglomeration and the individual, whilst surviving, will not be living in the meaning of the term that you and I take it to mean. To live is to feel, to breathe, eat, excrete and sleep. These physiological functions are vital, but they alone do not make up the living, sentient human being.

Within many aspects of health care, the wider concept of human health and comfort may safely be allocated a secondary importance, as the experience of the health problem is relatively short lived and the repercussions are not expected or perceived to be dramatic. Individuals with broken legs are given appropriate treatment to repair the damage. They may be unable to drive for a few weeks, not be able to work or socialize for that time, receive a reduced income, or indeed no income during their incapacity, etc., etc., but these repercussions are frequently able to be accommodated without too much long term difficulty.

The potential difficulties surrounding a woman who has to undergo radical surgery for breast cancer, for example arising from reduced life expectancy and changed body image, would hopefully be recognized prior to treatment and attention to these aspects would be an integral part of total care. This extended care would be deemed necessary because of the significance of repercussions upon other aspects of life. One would expect that networks would have been forged and referral to other necessary experts would be almost automatic in the planning and carrying out of treatment.

MENTAL HEALTH AND DISORDER

Our specialist area of study *has* to concentrate on the whole individual as a matter of course, because within mental health we are able to see that a problem in one sphere of functioning has a knock-on effect on all other spheres.

If you are feeling low, there is a greater or lesser effect upon your behaviour; for example, you may eat more or less than usual, sleep more or less soundly, or for more or less time than usual, move around less, sit down more, go out less, socialize less, desire more or less sex than usual—all sorts of behaviours may be affected, according to just how low you are feeling.

Similarly, when low, you may find that particular thoughts preoccupy you, that where other things come to mind they are very negative, instances which merely reinforce how stupid or inadequate you are feeling. Memories evoked may be negative, too, with other past incidences remembered to consolidate this low mood. You may hear only those comments around you that support this current mood and misinterpret positive elements and statements to add further fuel to the fire. You may doubt your competence and lose confidence in your everyday activities and contacts.

Whilst apparently a grossly embellished example, and whilst accepting the fact that not one of us would accept ever feeling these repercussions— or would we?—the principle is clear to see. A stone, or problem, thrown in the pool of mental health will create some disturbance of the water across the entire pool. Maintaining the analogy, it does not matter how big the stone or the precise point within the pool that the stone is thrown, there will be ripples that will affect the entire smooth surface of the pool.

Take any example you care to. This interconnection between all three spheres of activity cannot be isolated.

◆ Persistent sleep difficulties may engender mood changes of irritability, poor concentration and attention levels, reduced learning and retrieval, and clumsiness in an increasingly accident prone individual.

◆ Misuse of alcohol may engender mood changes—perhaps depression, anxiety or anger— preoccupation with using alcohol, increasing time and energy spent in acquiring and using the substance, and sleep and eating disturbances.

◆ Obsessive, intruding thoughts may provoke ritualistic patterns of behaviour, and will engender greater anxiety, feelings of guilt or anger.

Human affect (that is our moods, feelings and emotions), human behaviours (for example, eating and drinking, sleeping and moving), and human cognition (the faculties of, for example, thinking, remembering and perceiving the world around us), are inextricably linked.

Much like the picture produced by a completed jigsaw puzzle, all individual pieces have to be the correct size, shape and colouring to interlock with all others to produce the completed whole (Fig. 2.1). One piece incorrectly placed, or a piece from another jigsaw inadvertently used, will prevent the desired product being achieved. The interplay of the individual parts to form the corporate whole is clear to see. There is no room for compartmentalization within mental health care.

THE SPHERE OF INDIVIDUAL INFLUENCE

The situation becomes compounded when the individual experiencing mental health problems is unable to recognize this fact. Such people, quite

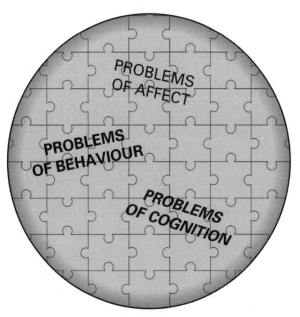

Fig. 2.1 Aggregation of problems to provide a diagnosis.

understandably, may see only that others are determined to thwart their every action, argue their every utterance and generally deny everything that the individual understands as real.

Few health care professionals besides those involved within this area of care will find that they have to treat and care for individuals who are completely antagonistic to their every move and action. The law recognizes this situation and seeks to protect both the client and the professional where it occurs. Individuals' mental health status is their sole business as long as it does not interfere with others—thus acknowledging the fact that individuals are not islands, that they do live within a greater society where there are expectations and norms to be observed.

People are an integral part of a wider world, like it or not. We have families, and live in communities, which are a part of that society. We cannot totally escape that world around us, no matter how much we attempt to be self-sufficient or desire to live like a hermit. There are rules and regulations to be observed and sanctions to be applied to those that flout or break such sanctions. There are roles, norms and expectations that moderate and modify our behaviours to prevent total breakdown of cooperative living. Our mental health status will affect our ability to meet the demands made upon us by everyday living.

This second jigsaw, depicted in Figure 2.2, serves to remind the professional that when we assess needs, and treat, care for and subsequently evaluate progress made within the activities and strategies to restore health, the total functioning of the client is under scrutiny. Something in our life has predisposed us to, or precipitated, the onset of current difficulties. Something within this second jigsaw is creating the disrupted picture being viewed, which we call mental illness or mental disorder.

We may have a predisposition to mood disorder that is precipitated by a series of traumatic life events, or our lifestyle may heap more serious stressors upon us than we can hope to manage effectively at a single moment in time. We may experience negative relationships with those we love and who are supposed, in an ideal world, to love and support us as individuals, which create

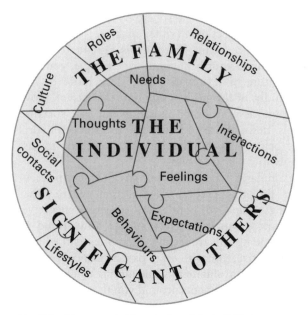

Fig. 2.2 The extended functioning of the individual.

insecurity, lack of confidence and feelings of inadequacy and guilt. Somewhere in this extended jigsaw is the key to the individual's current difficulties with life and living.

Any assessment, treatment and care schedule designed to assist the individual that does not include the facets within this extended jigsaw is merely scraping the surface of the problems experienced, and applying adhesive plaster to the superficial signs of ill health. It merely stores up the problem for management at a later time, when more and more of the true extent of the problem surfaces.

CONTINUING CONSIDERATIONS

In embarrassment or shame, many of our clients may fail to tell us all of the difficulties that they are experiencing, or the true nature of those difficulties, and therefore full assistance may not be possible at the onset of the professional relationship. A less than satisfactory outcome for some clients, with a continuation of the problems that provoked the initial consultation, or a re-emergence of problems, only superficially contained or covered by treatment and care delivered, may create the need or opportunity for clients to share more fundamental or previously unconnected areas of unhappiness or dissatisfaction in their lives.

The trusting, confidential relationship required to facilitate this sharing of intimate and often intensely uncomfortable material takes time to develop. It requires consistency of personnel and approach, a genuine comfort in the approach used, and in the personality of the nurse or therapist assisting the client. These aspects alone generate problems for both clients and professionals. Rejection may be a difficult process to instigate or face, and the professionals should make it clear to the client at the outset, that, because this relationship is so fundamental to the healing process, they will not take it personally should the client prefer to work with someone else.

Returning to the previous example of the individual with a broken leg, there is little that is threatening about the information that has to be shared to achieve a cure. Clients may not admit that they were, for example, swinging from the bedroom chandelier before falling and sustaining the injury, but the substitution of 'fixing a light bulb' is sufficiently close to the truth to inform the orthopaedic surgeon of the anticipated nature of the fracture, and the amount of soft tissue damage likely to be encountered, and therefore indicate the most appropriate intervention to be used to repair the damage done, to the greatest benefit to the client's mobility in the future. In the field of mental health care, however, were such clients not to share the fact that, for example, the only way they had found to achieve a satisfactory sexual arousal was to swing from a chandelier, we would have great difficulty in assisting them overcome their problems.

Mental health care is all about exposure—exposure of ourselves, our innermost secrets and fears—to the scrutiny of others, who may quite easily think we are 'odd', 'abnormal', 'sick' or 'weird' or any of the epithets or pejorative terms used in our society to describe the 'different' amongst us.

Those processes that go on in the privacy of our own head, and are only rendered somewhat more concrete for others to see and examine via our behaviours and interactions with others, are intensely personal to us. It can be observed that we tend to guard the face that we present to the world at large, reserving exteriorization of the real, relatively unadulterated people we are only to those closest to us. To test this statement consider for a few moments, across the range of your relatives, friends and acquaintances, just who knows you best and most accurately. The sensitivity of this necessary exposure of our personality and traits, warts and all, should not be dismissed lightly.

Within this context of personal, 'head-bound' functions, we are none of us sure as to whether we are like everyone else. We think, but do we think as others think, making the same sort of connections as others do, worrying about the same sort of things that others worry about, and placing the same levels of emphasis on similar things? We know that we walk like others, using our limbs to effect locomotion, and, whilst we may not look so smooth, elegant or controlled as some, we fit into the range that society would accept as 'normal'—in other words, we would not be stared at or commented on as we walked down a street, under most circumstances.

But these head-bound functions, these feelings, thoughts, memories, motivations and behaviours, are hard to compare in everyday life because of the fact that few of us show our real selves much of the time. Whether we feel that we will be rejected if the reality is seen in totality, or that others will ridicule us or take advantage of us, we 'drip-feed' information about ourselves to a rate in keeping with others' need to know. Within mental health care scenarios we are probably exteriorizing these head-bound functions more completely and honestly than we have ever done before—and at a time when we are feeling at our most vulnerable!

RESTORATION OF HEALTH

Mental disorder is complex to manage. Successful outcomes for the client require competent and skilled personnel who remember that they have to attend to whole people within their specific frameworks of living. Restoration of health demands sensitive interactions to generate the basis for a comfortable exchange of the information required to assist in problem identification and problem solving. It requires tact and diplomacy on the part of health care professionals, a knowledge of timing and when to leave an issue alone for the present. It requires trust, time and space for clients, who need to expose these hidden facets of their functioning, and patient perseverance on the part of all concerned, because this is not as simple and clear cut as the fractured femur. There are many ways to assist individuals experiencing mental disorder. We have to find those strategies—and people—which suit them, their personalities and particular needs for care because, in this area of health care, their individuality is paramount.

But is restoration of health our actual goal? The pat answer comes back, 'But yes, of course!'. That, however, can never be the reality. Return to our second jigsaw. Something of that configuration made the individual ill. We may not be able to take away the cause of that ill health, but to assist clients' long term health we have to proffer alternative strategies for managing that configuration in a manner more satisfying to them, not necessarily to the partners or the families, or the professionals involved, but to them. A different picture is likely to emerge from our jigsaw puzzle and, whilst it may only be an alteration in the colour shading, both clients and those involved with them must be prepared for a completely different scene to result from the individuals' own direction as to what they need to make their lives better for them. Clients and no one else must set the pace and the agenda to be followed. If they don't, if they feel that the proceedings are out of step with their needs, they are likely to assert their good health and deny their need for further assistance, or simply not to turn up for the next appointment.

This other critical difference in caring for the mentally disordered must similarly guide professionals. Intervention must be to clients' pace and their direction, for they must be able to see the advantages to be gained in embarking on what may be a protracted period of personal discomfort and change.

THE EXTENT OF THE PROBLEM

It would seem an appropriate juncture to explore the incidence of mental disorder, in order to clarify just how rare or common a phenomenon this is. Table 2.1 gives us a clear picture of the salient facts—or does it?

The International classification of diseases, ninth edition (ICD-9 1992), which was current in the years quoted, is utilized in Table 2.1 to compare and contrast various facts about each group of disorders. The 'facts' relating to mental disorders are highlighted for ease of referral. Let us now examine these more closely.

Column 1 in the table identifies the numbers of people, per hundred of the population, experiencing the effects of long-standing illness. The figure (V) for mental disorders can only relate to those people who have come to the attention of the statisticians—that is, those who have sought help or been co-opted into the health services by others, having been deemed mentally ill under legislation. It cannot, however, include those who have significant mental health problems but who are able to continue to meet their responsibilities and commitments, and who never come into contact with the health services. Similarly, it cannot include those individuals who, aware of the impact of their mental health problems on their life, seek assistance via non-NHS therapists of a wide number of disciplines, including alternative therapies. Private mental health units, because of the nature of the 'business' and the threat of competition, do not publish their statistics regarding uptake of facilities, either on an outpatient or on a residential basis. There is no definite figure therefore relating to the number of people experiencing long term mental illness.

The figures in column 2 relate only to certified incapacity, and therefore do not take into account any of the days taken without the need of a certificate. Those days when individuals roll over in bed when an alarm sounds, thinking 'I can't face it today', and switch off and snuggle down again, are not accounted for in this column. Neither are the instances when individuals phone in sick complaining of a 'migraine', 'backache', 'stomach ache' or 'diarrhoea from a bad curry last

Table 2.1 Statistics from the International classification of diseases, ninth edition, for England and Wales

Chapter	Chapter headings	Long-standing illness 1989 (1) (rate per 100)	Days of certified incapacity by cause 1990/1 (2) (%)	Patients consulting in general practice 1991/2 (3) (rate per 100)	Inpatient cases 1992/3 (4) (%)	Deaths 1992 (%)
I	Infectious and parasitic diseases	0.2	0.7	14.0	1.2	0.5
II	Neoplasms	0.8	1.5	2.4	8.9	26.1
III	Endocrine and immunity disorders	2.5	2.9	3.8	1.3	1.9
IV	Diseases of blood	0.4	0.3	1.0	1.2	0.4
V	**Mental disorders**	**1.8**	**18.2**	**7.3**	**3.2**	**2.3**
VI	Diseases of the nervous system	2.4	7.0	17.3	5.3	2.1
VII	Diseases of the circulatory system	7.3	20.00	9.3	8.9	45.6
VIII	Diseases of the respiratory system	6.7	7.7	30.7	6.2	10.8
IX	Diseases of the digestive system	3.2	2.8	8.7	9.6	3.4
X	Diseases of the genitourinary system	1.3	1.4	11.3	8.2	1.0
XI	Complications of pregnancy	—	0.7	1.1	11.7	0.0
XII	Diseases of the skin	1.6	0.6	14.6	1.9	0.2
XIII	Diseases of the musculoskeletal system	11.6	26.4	15.2	5.4	1.0
XIV	Congenital anomalies	—	0.3	0.5	1.1	0.3
XV	Perinatal period	—	—	0.1	2.0	0.0
XVI	Signs, symptoms and ill-defined conditions	—	3.9	15.1	7.1	0.9
XVII	Injury and poisoning	—	5.6	13.9	7.0	3.0
XVII	Supplementary classification	0.1	—	33.5	9.8	0.0
	Total		100	78.0	100	100

From Charlton & Murphy 1997 (New Earnings Survey, Office for National Statistics © Crown Copyright 1999).

night' rather than admitting that they are stressed, depressed or anxious, whether it be about their work or about some other aspect of their life.

Column **3** relates the number of general practitioner (GP) consultations, but is this figure inclusive of the many times clients may attend complaining of all sorts of vague aches and pains before doctors realize that there is a mental health problem at the root of the visits, which clients either do not recognize or find great difficulty in verbalizing?

In research relating to GP recognition and subsequent diagnosis of mental illness, both in this country and in the United States of America, more than 50% of individuals presenting to their family doctors complained of physical ailments, which significantly influenced the diagnosis made. When Goldberg & Huxley (1980) studied the incidence of mental disorder they assessed that, of a general population of 1000, 250 people would be experiencing mental health distress, that 230 of these would visit the GP and that 140 would be identified as in need of assistance. For the vast majority of these people, this was given in the form of tranquillizer and antidepressant medication, with only 17 being referred on to specialist services. Of these 17, six would require inpatient care. The levels of consultation were relatively high and yet the degree of recognition of the specific problem was only around 60%.

Comparison between the GP diagnosis and that of an experienced psychiatrist revealed an overemphasis on somatic complaints and an underemphasis on depression (Goldberg 1984, Mann,

Jenkins & Belsey 1981). Beaber & Rodney (1984) found a great reluctance to record a psychological basis for somatic complaints, and surveys using strict operational criteria consistently reveal that some 25–30% of people presenting to GPs do so with predominantly mental health symptomatology and yet detection and diagnosis show a 10% lower level of recording.

So, can we rely on these tabulated figures for GP consultations? Further study is needed in the light of continuing education and awareness of the presentation of mental disorder to assess the level of GP consultation.

Column **4** shows the number of inpatient cases; however, the fact that the type of service provision in this field is predominantly community based suggests that these are merely a tip of an iceberg. The figures give us little insight into the actual incidence of mental disorder, and merely indicates the number of people considered to be of sufficient danger to themselves or others to warrant removal from the home situation for a period of more than a day. Even in this regard, however, we have little idea of the numbers admitted to alternative centres for mental health care, and so these figures are further flawed.

With regard to the final column, which indicates the number of deaths directly attributable to mental disorder, the picture is similarly less than clear. To begin with, the ICD figures for suicide are collated within Chapter XVII, Injury and poisoning, and do not appear separately. Whilst the World Health Organization produce data relating to suicide (Fig. 2.3) across a number of countries, the apparently low figure for England of 6.2 relates only to those sad situations where individuals are known to have intended to take their own lives. There are, however, also instances where the presence of the intention, the motivation to commit suicide, cannot be adjudged as certain, and therefore these figures must be considered dubious, too. The footnote 'England rate for suicide plus undetermined injury is 8.9 for 1996' does not help— 'undetermined injury' may include a wide variety of causes of mortality.

To add to the confusion, many drug-related deaths are likely to be classified in a different ICD chapter; for example, alcoholic cardiomyopathy, a

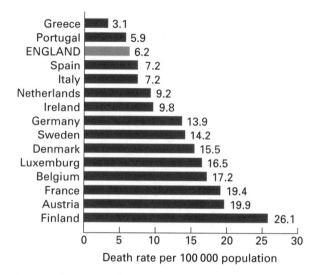

Data are for 1996, definitions of suicide will vary between countries (see Glossary and Technical note). England rate for suicide plus undetermined injury is 8.9 for 1996.

Fig. 2.3 World Health Organization figures on death rates from suicide: England has one of the lowest rates in the European Union (from DOH 1997. Crown copyright material is reproduced with the permission of the Controller of Her Majesty's Stationery Office).

complication of alcohol misuse in which there is degeneration of the heart muscle, which directly causes death, is likely to be collated within Chapter VII, diseases of the circulatory system.

Studies that seek to quantify the prevalence of specific disorders are as accurate as they are able to be, when one considers that all, to some extent or other, rely on the willingness of individuals to expose the true nature of their thoughts, feelings and emotions and/or to seek assistance from a recognized source that collates statistics. So much, too, is dependent upon the age group. For example, in their survey Meltzer et al (1995) identified that, up to the age of 54 years, the proportion of women reporting neurotic disorders was higher than that in men, some 20% in contrast to 13%. Between the ages of 55 and 64 years, however, the differences seemed to disappear, with a proportion for both groups of around 13%. The health care professional needs to research the specific areas of relevance to their practice, thereby ensuring that information retrieved is the most up to date available, for the specific client's or group of clients' needs.

Within this generalized introduction to the subject of mental disorders, it is sufficient to explore the restrictions and difficulties generated merely by the question, 'How many people suffer from mental disorders?'.

SUMMARY

It has been asserted in this chapter that the individual cannot be separated into 'body' and 'mind' sections for our comfort and ease, and that individuals and their families and significant others as well as their environment are all integral to health. This needs to be recognized and accepted, for as a mental health nurse or associated professional, you are as likely to be assisting with the mental health sequelae surrounding the experience of cancer of the breast as you are to be assisting the client experiencing schizophrenia. The effects of poverty and unemployment on mental health are just as devastating to the individual as are those relating to post-traumatic stress disorder. You will be helping all sorts of people, with all sorts of problems, due to all sorts of biochemical, social and environmental predispositions or precipitating causes.

We can only fundamentally help when we know as much as we can about clients and their extended sphere of functioning, and include aspects of care to address or redress situations detrimental to health. We are aware of the intensely personal nature of much of the information we need to know, and of strategies to ameliorate this.

Similarly, it has been asserted that problems associated with mental illness occur within the spheres of affect, behaviour and cognition, and that a problem in one of those spheres will create problems in the others.

Problems + Problems + Problems of → Diagnosis
of affect   of behaviour   cognition

Examples have been provided to illustrate this assertion, and the further activities found at the end of this chapter are offered as a further demonstration of both assertions.

Finally, the incidence of mental disorder within the population as a whole has been explored, using available statistics. In recognition of the reasons why these official statistics are less than the whole story in regard to mental illness, it must be concluded that those clients who do seek the help of a professional or self-help group are the tip of what may be an iceberg of enormous proportions.

Remembering all that has been stated in the above, the next step in the logical progression through the study of mental disorder is to explore those functions of affect, behaviour and cognition and the problems associated with each, which may indicate mental disorder.

FURTHER ACTIVITIES

With the first jigsaw in mind, talk to clients and spend time in relationship-making activities. Try to elicit what their problems are, and why they have sought assistance. Examine the way in which each domain—affect, behaviour and cognition—has been affected.

Using the second jigsaw to guide your discussion, discuss with your clients the manner in which these problems have affected their extended living and functioning.

Read the newspapers. What do they tell us about who develops mental disorders and the types of problem encountered?

REFERENCES

Beaber R J, Rodney W M 1984 Underdiagnosis of hypochondriasis in family practice. Psychodynamics 25:39–46

DOH 1997 Death rates from suicide: England one of the best records in the European Union. WHO Copenhagen, as analysed by Dept of Health, Statistical Division 2, Office of National Statistics Data, London

Goldberg D 1984 The recognition of psychiatric illness by non-psychiatrists. Australian and New Zealand Journal of Psychiatry 18:128–133

Goldberg D, Huxley P 1980 Mental illness in the community. Tavistock, London

ICD-9 (International classification of mental and behavioural disorders, 9th edn) 1992. World Health Organization, Geneva

Mann A H, Jenkins R, Belsey E 1981 The twelve month outcome of patients with neurotic illness in general practice. Psychological Medicine 11:535–550

Meltzer H, Gill B, Petticrew M, Hinds K 1995 OPCS surveys of psychiatric morbidity in Great Britain, report 1: The prevalence of psychiatric morbidity among adults living in private households. HMSO, London

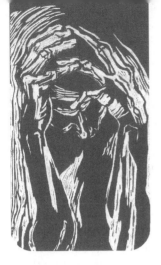

Chapter Three

Affect and emotion

F Clifford Johnson   Lynne D Smith

AIMS

- ◆ To review the basis of the experience of human emotion
- ◆ To formularize a continuum of the emotional responses associated with healthy living
- ◆ To determine the characteristics of the variety of human emotions
- ◆ To identify anomalies in the above that may indicate the presence of mental health problems

KEY ISSUES

Physiology

Role of higher cognitive function

Analysis of each emotion

Content, duration, quality and appropriacy

Verbal and non-verbal cues to determine problem

Depression

Elation

Apathy

Blunting

Lability

Inappropriacy

INTRODUCTION

Emotional feelings and responses are an integral and all-pervasive aspect of daily life. From the moment of wakening to the last one before sleeping, the individual is constantly bombarded with mood-altering stimuli, which, in turn, colour and influence thoughts, perceptions and behaviours.

An example may be of value:

'Good morning, and here is the 8 o'clock news from your local independent radio station.'

'Six people died and 18 others were seriously injured in a multiple pile-up on the motorway this morning. A police spokesman at the scene said that drivers had ignored warnings of freezing fog and had been driving well in excess of speed limits advised. The injured are being treated at the City Infirmary.'

'200 more jobs are to be lost with the closure of Bainbridges Tiling Company. This brings total job losses in the area in the last month to 2500.'

'There is to be a further 0.5% interest rate reduction. Major building societies have reported record receipts from savers, who are ignoring Government calls to spend their way out of the recession.'

'On the international front, sporadic fighting between Serbs and Bosnians continues to prevent United Nations relief forces' efforts to provide urgent food and medical supplies to the besieged town of Sarajevo.'

'In Somalia, local militia have agreed a ceasefire, enabling United Nations forces to reach feeding centres in the north of the country. Aid workers believe supplies will have no significant impact on death rates for several weeks.'

'Arms reduction talks continue today and both superpower spokespersons believe an agreement is imminent.'

'And now the weather. Temperatures will remain low—in the region of 4°C for the remainder of the day. Fog will continue to be a major hazard to drivers. A low of 2°C is expected overnight.'

The feelings evoked by the morning news may be various in nature. There may be a great sadness

that so many people were killed and injured on the motorway, but also anger, at the senselessness of such an accident, and the stupidity of those driving too fast in such appalling road conditions. There may be fear and anxiety for the safety of a loved one, who was expected to be travelling on that stretch of the road at about that time of the morning, or a sigh of relief breathed that one's own car is still safely tucked up in the garage, out of harm's way. The news of more job losses in the area is likely to engender sadness for those involved and an anxious concern for any specific acquaintance who is to be affected. Should a partner or close member(s) of the family be amongst those being given redundancies, the emotion experienced may be one of despair, with fears for future security. Of course, there is great news for home-owners, with a half of 1% reduction in the interest rate. It may bring a feeling of relief— almost joy—to those struggling to make the monthly repayments, but for those who have already experienced the repossession of their home and the break up of the family unit, there may be anger and bitterness that reductions are coming too late to be of help to them. Some will be indifferent, or apathetic, to the news, with half a percentage point not being significant enough to get excited about one way or the other. Of course those people who don't have mortgages may experience resentment, at what are effectively 'rent reductions' for home owners whilst the actual rent payers never get any relief.

The international headlines may again evoke both anger and sadness. The hatred, greed and wanton disregard for human life and suffering inherent in war may engender feelings of despair for the state and progress of civilized society. The knowledge that some people in the world are cold, hungry, hurt or in fear for their continuing safety may provoke feelings of guilt in individuals who are sitting toasting their feet by the fire and enjoying breakfast. Feelings of shame and embarrassment may be associated with impotency or a previous lack of willingness to do more to assist the starving in the world. There may be feelings of frustration towards the powerful people in the world who appear to be loathe or slow in stepping in to prevent such carnage, or anger that innocent, uninvolved people have been sent to a place by a government who, they believe, has no right to interfere, no matter what is happening. There may be disgust felt towards countries who spend years arming different factions and militia, and then expect applause for reducing the risk of damage to their own people by agreeing to destroy their own weapons.

Of course, there may be no such acute emotional response to any of the news items. The individual may have become so accustomed to hearing such distressing news that he or she fails to be stimulated by it, absorbing details and yet experiencing no qualitative feeling as a response. For some, the weather forecast will provoke the strongest reaction, as they envisage the day's planned activities severely curtailed or made extremely difficult by the continuing foggy conditions.

'That concludes the news report and, with the time coming up to 3 minutes past 8, we ask you to drive safely and have a nice day!'

It is not, however, the end of the emotional content for the day. Whether the individual's taste is for the popular music of the day or something a little more timeless and classical in nature, the potential is there for a change of mood. It is not only music, of course, that can evoke or engender emotion and mood in this way. There are artists, poets, scriptwriters and authors who spend a lifetime trying to stimulate people to pleasurable feelings and moods. The theme parks of the nation charge an entrance fee to individuals for the use of the rides and amusements. Often people are terrified but really enjoy the experience. Similarly, people wallow in the floods of tears evoked by a sad film or book, and some gain genuine pleasure from being scared to death by a horror story. The 'arts' rely on such emotions to sell the product for if a book bores the reader, there is the likelihood that the story will neither be finished nor recommended to friends and certainly the reader will not buy any more of that author's work.

Everyday life creates emotional rollercoasters for the individual. The pleasures associated with touching the fingers of a newborn baby and

admiring its wonderful perfection; of wandering unhurriedly by the river or seashore within an environment of peace, tranquillity and absence of demands upon self; or the success associated with the attainment of a hard-fought objective, may be experiences of emotional significance for some. The fears and anxieties associated with any potential or actual threat to well-being, no matter the biopsychosocial factor generating such fears, have been experienced by everyone. Anger is a frequent response to the behaviour exhibited by others and sadness and unhappiness may be experienced as a result of the argument which resulted from one's own anger. Remorse and guilt may be exteriorized in trying to compensate for verbal damage—or worse—inherent in any disagreement, or pain may be deep seated and too intense to eradicate. Emotions and moods are an integral part of life and living, a daily occurrence and something unavoidable for the vast majority of the population. So, what are these moods and emotions? How do they arise and how are they exteriorized?

DEFINING TERMINOLOGY

There is a tendency to use the terms 'emotion', 'affect' and 'mood' interchangeably. However, there are differences between them and, whilst overlap may be a feature, it may at times be important to differentiate between the concepts.

The term 'emotion' relates to those consciously perceived feelings and their manifestations which occur in response to external stimuli (Campbell 1989). For example:

'I feel anxious and apprehensive. My mouth is always dry and my heart races uncontrollably. My hands are sweating and yet I'm cold'.

'I'm happy—I feel fit and well, lively and enthusiastic—everything's going well'.

'I'm so angry, my blood's boiling and I really can't think about anything else'.

'Affect' is the term reserved for the experience of the emotion plus the drive energies that are presumed to generate the conscious and unconscious feelings associated with it. It is the subjective, personal, fluctuating aspect of the individual's experience and relates to the here and now; not the past observations made (Campbell 1989). Examples may help:

> 'I've tried so hard to be everything she wanted me to be. I've tried to be a good husband; I've worked hard and we have a nice home and two lovely kids. Now she says she's leaving me and I'm worried that she means it. I feel anxious and apprehensive. My mouth is always dry and my heart races uncontrollably. My hands are sweating and yet I'm cold'.

> 'I'm successful. I have everything I've always wanted and needed. I feel safe, secure and fulfilled. I'm happy; I feel fit and well, lively and enthusiastic—everything's going well'.

> 'How dare he belittle me in front of everyone. He made me look stupid and incompetent—and it was his error not mine. He's always treating me like this. I'm so angry; my blood's boiling and I really can't think about anything else'.

The differences between the three are of relevance, for individuals may report that, whilst they have been depressed for quite some time (mood), they now really have gone beyond this point. They do not care for anyone or anything; they are totally apathetic (affect), disinterested in life and living. They believe themselves beyond feeling (emotion) and their world is dark and drab. These are important elements within individuals' descriptions of this experience, for whilst they feel apathy, they are likely to be too disinterested to take their own lives. When they feel despair, however, with thoughts associated with the pointlessness of life and being better off dead, they may be motivated to self-harm and present therefore as at greater risk and in need of modified care and attention. The nurse needs to be posing appropriate questions to elicit important details of the individual's current experience to be of most value in the care process, and to enable judgements to be made in relation to the efficacy of health care.

The focus of concentration in this chapter will, therefore, be on affect and emotion, on the premise that mood may be elicited by appropriate questioning, where affect and emotion rely on accurate observations being made to elicit those appropriate questions. In analysing one, it is hoped to provide insight into the successful exploration of the other.

THE BASIS OF EMOTION

In any analysis of the theoretical perspectives applied to emotion, it would be inconceivable not to include the words of William James (1842–1910), the American psychologist, who made the first real attempt to link the experience of emotions with physiological function. In his work What is emotion? published in 1884, James analysed the role of emotion in life:

> Conceive yourself, if possible, suddenly stripped of all the emotion with which your world now inspires you and try to imagine it as it exists, purely by itself, without your favourable or unfavourable, hopeful or apprehensive comment. It will be almost impossible for you to realise such a condition of negativity and deadness. No one portion of the universe would then have importance beyond another; and the whole collection of its things and series of its events would be without significance, character, expression or perspective. Whatever of value, interest or meaning our respective worlds may appear imbued with are thus pure gifts of the spectator's mind.

James' work centred around the *order of events* that occur within the emotional state. Utilizing the ideas of a Danish psychologist, Carl Lange, he proposed what has become known as the James–Lange theory of emotions. The theory asserts that the overt responses and bodily changes associated with an emotion *precede* the conscious feelings accompanying the stimuli. The feelings of fear or rage were viewed as the awareness of the inner and outer changes created by the stimuli. An example may be useful:

> We feel sorry because we cry, angry because we strike, afraid because we tremble.
> James 1884

For James, the physical sensations *were* the emotion. He asserted that each emotional experience was the result of its own specific set of physiological activities and hence emotions were perceived as discrete entities, unlike each other, psychologically and physiologically speaking.

In 1927, Walter Cannon's studies cast doubts upon the James–Lange theory, for he 'proved' erroneous the assumptions of discrete physiological activities occurring within each emotion. Cannon discovered that the same pattern of physiological arousal accompanies a number of different emotions. To cast further doubt upon the theory, Cannon, in experiments on dogs and cats, severed the sympathetic nerves that James had considered to arouse the body changes preceding the emotional awareness. The animals were unaware, therefore, of physiological reaction because none was possible, and yet they demonstrated the expressions and emotions appropriate to the stimuli presented. Cannon asserted that emotional feelings do not depend upon the receipt of sensations arising from within the body, turning attention back to the brain.

As a result of his studies, Cannon constructed an alternative explanation for emotion, which was later modified by Phillip Bard, and became known as the Cannon–Bard theory. In essence, the theory asserts that a *simultaneous reaction* from both psychological experience and also physiological reaction to the stimuli is necessary to produce emotion. The individual facing an emotionally arousing event is subject to nerve impulses passing to the thalamus, where they split into two; half travelling on to the cerebral cortex and the other half to the hypothalamus. Those impulses arriving at the cortex produce the subjective experience of anger, fear, joy, etc., whilst the hypothalamus initiates the physiological changes associated with the feeling.

In 1937, James Papez proved that no specific brain centre assumed responsibility for emotional experience as Cannon had asserted. Instead, the anatomist suggested that a 'stream of feeling' and a 'stream of movement' provided a circuit—the Papez circuit—of relay stations via which sensations travelled and merged to create emotion. Papez believed the 'stream of thought' to relay sensations through the thalamus to the major

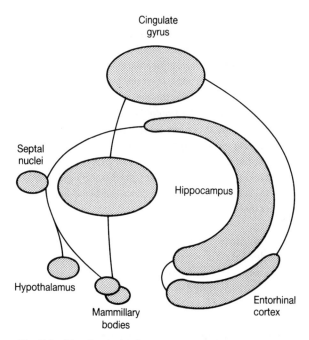

Fig. 3.1 The Papez circuit.

areas of the cortex, whilst the 'stream of movement' involved impulse transmission through the thalamus to the corpus striatum. Papez (1937) believed that as a result of the merging of the two streams 'sensory expectations ... receive their emotional colouring' (see Fig. 3.1).

The work of Papez provided the foundation for today's knowledge relating to the neuroanatomy of emotion. The structures that he referred to became known as the Papez circuit, and are included within the area referred to today as the limbic system. However, in addition to those limbic stuctures it is now known that areas of the brainstem—the reticular formation, the locus coeruleus or 'blue area' of the pons, and the substantia nigra of the midbrain—plus the frontal lobes of the cerebral cortex and the autonomic nervous system, are all involved within emotion generated (Tortora & Anagnostakos 1984). Exactly how they function remains a matter, largely, of guesswork and inference but it is believed that:

When faced with an event that requires mobilization, a twofold response occurs. Impulses are transmitted along neural pathways from the sensory receptor, via the reticular system and the thalamus, to the cortex. Motor responses required are initiated immediately, but in the meantime impulses pass, via the neural connections, from the thalamus to the hypothalamus and, via the amygdala and hippocampus, to the frontal lobe of the cortex. The arousal of all structures provokes the initiation of automatic nervous system mechanism, and an effect is elicited within 1 to 2 seconds of perception of the provoking event. By this point, the pituitary gland is activated and provides assistance via blood-borne hormonal influences.

Neuroanatomy and physiology are dealt with in considerably more detail in other chapters and hence no further attention will be awarded to the subject at this juncture.

INTENSITY OF EMOTION

Previous reference has been made to Cannon's (1927) experiments with cats and dogs, where sympathetic nerve fibres had been severed and yet expressions and emotions displayed were appropriate to the stimuli presented. Whilst this may have proved the case in animal studies, there is some dispute of the fact with regard to humans.

A great deal of anecdotal evidence—often based upon the impressions of physicians—existed to suggest that no alteration in the capacity for experiencing intense emotion occurred in those individuals unfortunate enough to have severed their spinal cord in accidents. George Hohmann (1966), himself a victim of spinal cord injury, compared the emotional reactions of individuals with varying levels and sites of cord injury, reported before and after their injuries. He found a diminution in the intensity of their emotions and that individuals with injuries high on the spinal cord reported the greatest difference in the before and after emotional experience. The higher the damage, the less visceral sensation the person is able to feel. Individuals reported that the 'heat' had gone out of emotion and that feelings were more 'mental' than whole body experiences.

Whilst able to 'react' emotionally, the individuals did not 'feel' emotional.

> *'It's a sort of cold anger. Sometimes I act angry when I see some injustice. I yell and cuss and raise hell, because if you don't do it sometimes, I've learned people will take advantage of you; but it doesn't have the heat to it that it used to.'*

> *'I say I'm afraid, like when I'm going into a real stiff exam at school, but I don't really feel afraid, not all tense and shaky with the hollow feeling in my stomach, like I used to.'*
> Hohmann 1966

Whilst the reporting of remembered emotions and comparing them with current emotional experiences is not particularly objective as a method of scientific study, Jasmos & Hakmiller (1975) provided a less subjective but similar analysis. Men with spinal cord damage were presented with photographs of both clothed and nude women, and asked to imagine being alone with each woman. Thoughts and feelings reported were analysed in relation to expressed emotion, and results demonstrated that those individuals with higher spinal lesions reported less sexual excitement than those with lower-sited injuries. In 1985, Lowe & Carroll repeated Hohmann's original study and found no evidence of diminution of emotional intensity in paraplegic subjects. The role of feedback from the autonomic nervous system in the experience of emotion is therefore still an area of dispute, so many years after the studies of James (1884) and Cannon (1927).

PHYSIOLOGICAL DIFFERENTIATION OF EMOTION

Again, Walter Cannon (1927) asserted, only one pattern of autonomic arousal occurs in response to a wide number of emotional stimuli. More recent studies by Ax (1953), in which he was able to reliably evoke emotions of fear and anger in his subjects, reported differing patterns of peripheral physiological activity for each of the two emotions elicited.

More recently, Ekman, Levenson & Frierson (1983) demonstrated distinct autonomic patterns of activity for each of six emotions—surprise, sadness, anger, fear, disgust and happiness. Whilst actor subjects held an emotional expression for 10 seconds, heart rate, skin temperature and other indicators of autonomic arousal were recorded by researchers. Results showed that the heart rate experienced during the emotions of anger, fear and sadness was higher than that related to the more positively judged emotions of happiness, surprise or disgust. In anger, skin temperature was higher than shown in fear or sadness, and hence a fine differentiation of emotional states is seen via autonomic nervous system patterns of arousal. However, there is a general belief that such differences identified cannot be totally responsible for differentiation of an individual's emotional experiences. Cognitive appraisal of the presenting stimuli has been considered a potential factor in this differentiation for some years.

EMOTION AND COGNITION

In 1924, Gregorio Marañon published a largely anecdotal study on emotions, which centres on the subjective reports of a group of individuals to whom he had administered adrenaline (epinephrine) by injection. About one-third of the subjects reported an experience 'something like' an emotional state, 'as if' something exciting were about to happen or 'as if' they were afraid. The remaining subjects reported that whilst they had experienced no emotion, they felt symptoms associated with arousal. In later discussions with the group members who had reported the 'as if' emotional experiences, Marañon talked with them about emotionally significant events experienced in the recent past. He reported the exteriorization of the full emotional response in regard to these events—the 'as if' status had disappeared.

Utilizing Marañon's work and other available evidence, Stanley Schachter (1971) theorized that, in order for an emotion to be experienced, both cognitive evaluation and physiological arousal must be available to the individual. In a widely cited experiment, Schachter & Singer (1962) administered a placebo—a saline injection—to control subjects whilst subjects were given adrenaline. Both groups were informed that the substance given was a vitamin preparation, but then subjects from both groups were, in essence, treated in one of three ways. Some were informed—without naming the drug—of the physiological effects of adrenaline and warned of feelings such as palpitations, tremors, etc. A second group was given no information and a third group were misinformed. Each subject was then placed in a room with another person, who, whilst claiming also to be an experimental subject, was in fact a 'stooge' and part of the experimental team. Some confederates assumed a euphoric type of behaviour, whilst others were irritable and feigned increasing anger, until they left the room, totally 'enraged'. Researchers made observations via a one-way mirror and also questioned subjects about their experience. Correctly informed adrenaline-injected subjects reported the least effect to the stooge's behaviour, whilst misinformed subjects, experiencing physiological symptoms unlike those they had been informed to expect, were most affected by the confederate's antics. This latter group mirrored the behaviour exhibited by the stooge and also reported feelings of great happiness or intense anger, according to the behaviour exteriorized by the stooge. Individuals given no information after the injection showed behaviour of neither excess, but responses were seen to be in the middle band of a no-reaction/excessive-reaction continuum.

Schachter & Singer (1962) appeared to prove their hypothesis, namely that an emotion is jointly determined by cognitive appraisal and physiological arousal, and that arousal would be interpreted as non-emotional where subjects had received the correct information with regard to the effects of adrenaline. They asserted that those subjects who had either been misinformed or uninformed would experience an arousal for which they could not find a reason, and therefore that they would seek an explanation for their behaviour in the context provided by the stooge. For those given a placebo, the social context on its own—that is, the stooge's behaviour—would not generate emotion. Whilst many criticisms have been levelled at Schachter & Singer's interpretation of results, replications of the study since by Erdman & Janke (1978) have produced a broad agreement with regard to the basic assertion that it is a combination of physiological and cognitive factors that produces the experience of emotion.

George Mandler (1982) asserts the importance of a sense of control with the cognitive analysis of the event evoking emotional experiences and certainly one may be able to differentiate the emotions inherent within two different situations:

1. during a ride on a rollercoaster or other theme park amusement, the individual feels the support beneath him, in the form of the rail, fall away suddenly
2. whilst sitting in an aeroplane at the start of a holiday, the plane suddenly drops in an air pocket.

The cause of the arousal is similar in each scenario, and due to a release from the effects of gravity. In the former example, the reader has *chosen* to ride the rollercoaster and is able to anticipate some of the sensations that may be experienced. He has a sense of control therefore. However, in the second scenario there are feelings of *helplessness* and fear in response to the lack of control over the situation experienced. Two different emotions are perceived, in response to a similar stimulus, where, in essence, a sense of control is the only real variable. Mandler argues that there is an *interruption of ongoing behaviour and thought*, which serves as a trigger for appraisal processes to analyse the exact nature of the interruption. Whilst autonomic activity is also triggered at this interruption, Mandler believes that it is the nature of the situation, as determined by cognitive appraisal, that determines the quality of the experience.

AN ANALYSIS OF THE EMOTIONS

Emotion is a derivative of the Latin word, '*movere*', meaning to move or to stir, and certainly some sources may consider an emotion to be defined variously as 'a state of agitation'; 'disturbance of equilibrium'; or 'an intense random and disorganized response to a stimulus' (Sperling 1960). Roget's Thesaurus (1982) lists dozens of states, all purported to be emotions and it is possible to spend hours attempting to decide which are actually emotions. Wise people have already addressed the subject and have created much dispute and argument in the process.

Two approaches have been taken in relation to the identification of the specific nature of emotions. One theory assumes that there are a relatively small number of *primary* emotions and that each of these is associated with a specific event which triggers its arousal. For example, Plutchik (1980) identified eight emotions and their triggers which, he observed, were evident universally within every human culture and throughout the animal world.

Emotion	Trigger
Grief (sorrow)	Loss
Fear	Threat
Anger	Impediment
Joy	Potential partner
Trust	Group membership
Disgust	Unpleasant stimulus
Anticipation	New territory
Surprise	Sudden novel experience

Certainly studies by Ekman (1982), Izard (1984) and others would support the universal recognition of facial expressions associated with happiness, anger, disgust, sadness and a combined notion of fear and surprise and there tends to be support for a theory in which, initially at least, emotional reactions occur without cognitive appraisal. Zajonc (1984) and Ekman & Oster (1982) argue for such 'ontogenetic primacy' of emotion over cognitive appraisal, suggesting the newly born infant's facial expression of disgust in response to a nasty taste, as an example. Whilst cognitive elaboration may ensue as part of the development process, Zajonc believed it likely that these universally recognized emotional reactions may be linked reflexly to the perception of a limited range of stimuli.

The role of cognitive appraisal within emotional development is also threatened via the experiments by individuals such as Garcia & Rusinak (1980) who demonstrated that successful conditioning (classical conditioning) can occur, even when the unconditional stimulus is administered—and has its effect—under anaesthesia. Animals demonstrated nausea when presented with food that had been utilized as a conditioned stimulus, even though the nausea-provoking agent had been presented and had its effect during anaesthesia. Animals were able to respond adversely to a stimulus at an unconscious level and, therefore, without cognitive appraisal.

A second approach, taken by Roseman (1979) and others, asserts that it is the cognitive appraisal of a situation or event that generates the emotion and that if, for example, an experience is desired and occurs, the emotion felt will be one of joy. However, if the event is dreaded (i.e. not desired) and it occurs, the emotion experienced will be one of distress. There are four potential emotional experiences available from the differing combinations of these two elements:

Selection of emotion

	Desired	Undesirable
Occurring	Happiness	Distress
Not occurring	Sadness	Relief

After Roseman 1979

The approach asserts that there is a myriad of such aspects taken into consideration within any situation or event prior to the arousal of any specific emotion. 'Selection' of emotion appropriate to any event is, therefore, a little like manipulating a 'Rubik's cube', with the various elements combining to form an overall picture or response.

THE INFLUENCE OF AFFECT ON COGNITIVE PROCESSES

Whilst discussions will continue in relation to the relative role of cognition in the nature of the emotion experienced, there would seem little doubt that affect—the current emotional experience including drives—influences cognitive processes, and particularly memory.

Bower (1981) believes that each emotion occupies a specific node or niche within memory and is linked with the memories of specific events or experiences during which that emotion was aroused. 'Affect nodes' are connected to all other nodes in a sort of semantic network, facilitating the spread of any activation of one node through others nearby. Bower believes that it is by such means that selective retrieval of congruent memories occurs during an emotion, with nodes in semantic memory being activated, thus eliciting associated memories of a similar emotional quality and nature to that currently being experienced.

Whether ·or not the above explanation is the 'correct' one, we cannot say but we are aware that the emotional state of an individual is not the sole factor at work in relation to memory processes. The retrieval of material would appear to be dependent both upon the emotion currently experienced and on the affective content of material to be retrieved. Individuals in a positive mood show a tendency to retrieve positive memories, whilst negative mood subjects tend towards negative past event material. It has long been recognized that individuals who are experiencing a depressed mood will recall sad life episodes in excess of those recalled by control subjects and, indeed, Beck (1974) suggests these biased cognitive processes play an important part in both causing and maintaining a depressive episode. Studies by Johnson et al (1983) have found that depressed subjects recalled more tasks associated with failure, or lack of project completion, than did the non-depressed control group.

Blaney (1986), in a review of many such studies, suggests that such mood congruence is a genuine occurrence, but that, whilst all point in a similar direction, the specifics of whether a depressed individual actually recalls *more* negative events or *fewer* positive ones is dependent upon the study format utilized and therefore not clear. Certainly it would be of interest—and value—to ascertain at which level within the lowering of mood, such congruence comes into effect. Should a specific threshold need to be reached to see its occurrence, intervention at such point may prevent the adverse effects of biased cognitive processes described previously by Beck (1974).

The effects of emotion on thinking processes are well known. When too anxious, the individual 'can't think straight' and finds attention and concentration difficult. Feeling 'too happy'—if there can be such a state!—may evoke disinterest in routine events and activities preferring 'to go with the flow'. Sadness and anger are similarly pervasive, causing preoccupation of thoughts and reducing levels and quality of performance. Hebb (1972) suggested a relationship between the level of arousal and efficiency of performance, and that this differs with each task or behaviour (Fig. 3.2).

It is suggested that a mild level of arousal will evoke an alert interest in a current event or situation, whilst intense emotional feelings will disrupt thoughts and behaviours and, hence, reduce effectiveness of performance. Of course, the nature of the task will be significant in regard to the degree of disruption experienced, for many 'routine' aspects of life may be performed quite adequately whilst thoughts are preoccupied elsewhere. Complex tasks requiring attention and reasoning to achieve completion would be significantly

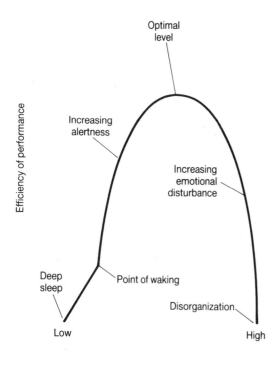

Fig. 3.2 Relationship between the level of arousal and efficiency of performance.

impaired. Selye's (1956) work in relation to the potentially damaging effect of prolonged, intense emotional arousal on body systems and general health is well known and lies at the heart of theories of psychosomiasis (the relationship between stress and illness).

RECOGNIZING EMOTION

It is valuable to be aware of the nature of emotion, the manner in which it is evoked and of the body's mechanisms that are involved in the experience. It is of importance, too, to have an understanding of the various perspectives applied to the experience of an emotion and the factors that may influence that experience. The effect of emotion and mood on the processes involved in cognition and performance is a necessary part of overall management of emotion in everyday life and the mental health nurse must recognize the prevailing mood of an individual and elicit the current affect operating.

One may observe individuals and conclude within a fraction of a minute that they are happy, sad, angry, hurt or embarrassed. The clues are easy to see. Happy individuals wear a smile, have sparkling eyes and are bouncy and lively in their movements, showing energy and vitality. The sad person wears an 'unhappy face', eyes are dull (maybe full of tears) and often directed towards the floor. There is little movement, the individual often preferring to sit huddled in a chair, and where movement is observed it is slow, heavy and deliberate. Anger finds expression in expansive movements, the individual utilizing an increased amount of space to perform sharp and sudden activities. Facial expression is characteristically 'like thunder', with skin red and warm from the exercise and eyes wide open and acute in their observations. The pale, tearful face of the individual who feels hurt, bottom lip trembling as he or she cowers from the source of the emotion, and the red-faced fidgety individual standing with head hung low are all characteristic behaviours associated with specific affective experiences. The mental health nurse's observations are important but equally vital is the recognition of what is seen.

An increased activity in the eyes of individuals who are depressed, with apparently surreptitious observations of the movement of others within the environment, may just indicate their increasing interest in life and elevation of depressed mood. However, in the absence of other cues, it is more likely that they may be awaiting an opportunity to slip quietly away, whether to harm themselves, absent themselves from the care facility, or merely withdraw from therapeutic interventions. The smile that does not reach the eyes, the hollow, forced laugh and the 'miraculous cure' evinced by the individual as 'But I feel much better nurse, really!' are shams and the care worker needs to be aware of their potential.

The mental health nurse not only has to observe and recognize cues available, but also needs to analyse their meanings both as individual pieces of information and within the overview of all available data. Only by these activities may an accurate insight into an individual's affect be gained, prompting effective exploration towards total assessment of need.

PROBLEMS OF EMOTION

There should be little need to affirm the 'normality' of emotional expression but one should be aware of the potential problems associated with somatic disease. Selye (1956) identified the 'general adaptation syndrome', a physiological degeneration of body tissues as a direct result of intense and prolonged emotion, and therefore the relevance of psychosocially directed care within overall health plans for many individuals should be the norm. Coronary artery disease, hypertension, migraine, ulcerative bowel conditions and many other somatic disorders may be precipitated or exacerbated by such prolonged emotional experience and hence warrant the mental health nurse's attention and expertise.

In addition to being implicated within causation and maintenance of somatic dysfunction, problems of an emotional nature may be seen as sequelae in a wide variety of experiences of somatic ill health. Depressed mood and anxiety feelings may, quite naturally, be evoked where individuals feel

their life or lifestyle is threatened in any way and may be prolonged. The same is true for partners and family members involved within the experience. On occasions reactions may be severe with loss of contact with reality, perceptual disturbances and delusional ideation, and those caring for such individuals need to be aware of such strong mental health responses.

Emotional problems may form an integral part of an individual's somatic disease/dysfunction complaints and may indeed prompt medical assistance being sought. Endocrine glands, presumably because of their direct role in the generation of emotion, are particularly prone to emotional symptomatology. In Addison's disease (primary adrenal insufficiency) for example, what would normally be considered a minor problem may evoke a *catastrophic reaction* with the individual rapidly bursting into tears, extremely sad and anxious in mood. Phaeochromocytoma, a neoplasm of the adrenal medulla, may cause individuals to experience the 'as if' feelings discussed within Marañon's (1924) adrenaline tests, being edgy, nervous, tremulous and anticipatory of something about to happen. Anxious, apprehensive feelings are commonly experienced by individuals who have hyperthyroidism (thyrotoxicosis) whilst those experiencing the reverse, hypothyroidism (myxoedema), may complain of always feeling low, emotionally lethargic and disinterested in surroundings.

Neurological disorders may create emotional problems for the individual. Within multiple sclerosis (MS), for example, *emotional lability*, where emotions are uncontrolled and mobile, and hence unpredictable, may be a feature, as may an unwarranted and excessive level of optimism and happiness, termed *euphoria*. Parkinson's disease may show emotional detachment and *anhedonia*, that is, the inability to feel pleasure. Some, indeed, experience an 'on–off' syndrome, where pronounced changes in affect occur, being anxious or depressed when 'off' and aroused and elated when 'on'. This may be a feature of prolonged treatment. Similarly, according to position and extent, cerebral neoplasia and trauma may engender similar problems of mood and emotion for the client. The brief overview above suggests the extreme importance of a thorough physical examination prior to any diagnosis of a primary mental health problem being made. Indeed, the client's health history is of great importance since a variety of medications may similarly create problems, including certain antibiotic, cardiovascular-acting and steroid preparations, and should therefore be excluded as causative agents.

Within mental health care, individuals may be seen to experience a variety of different problems associated with emotion. *Depression*, a lowering of mood and profound sadness, may be a problem for many, but to be considered 'pathological', that is, in need of treatment, certain characteristics tend to be associated with the experience. Whilst frequently a response to a traumatic life event, it may be that the mood is lowered for no apparent reason. The individual may then be seen to have relinquished contact with reality and also be experiencing a variety of perceptual and thought-related problems. Where contact with reality is maintained, depressed mood may have been of an excessive depth, in relation to the nature of the precipitating event, or may be of a prolonged duration. Such depression will always feature some degree of physical disinterest and self-neglect on the part of the individual and therefore somatic health may suffer. Self-harm and injury to others may be behaviours exhibited during the individual's experience of lowered mood.

Elevated mood, in the form of *elation* or where it is of a lower level, *euphoria*, may also be experienced and is problematical where it arises when not justifiable in relation to the individual's circumstances. Hold on reality is tenuous initially as mood begins to rise and is subsequently lost. Such elation or euphoria is accompanied by some degree of complete psychomotor acceleration and hence presents other problems for both client and carer.

Anxiety may be seen as a response to any threat, whether potential, actual or imagined. Some individuals experience a generalized feeling of apprehension and fear which they are unable to attribute to any specific focus. This is termed '*free-floating anxiety*'. However, where anxiety experienced is both disproportionate and produced in response to a threat recognized by the individual

as not a genuine danger to well-being, the anxiety is termed *phobic*.

A lack of anxiety in some individuals may give rise to concern, for '*la belle indifférence*' represents a markedly less than expected level of distress and concern exhibited by someone experiencing somatic symptomatology. Their apparent unconcern in relation to motor or sensory manifestations is a classical sign in the diagnostic category known as '*conversion disorders*'. The physiological symptomatology occurs in the absence of a physical disorder. Instead, symptoms are a symbolic representation of psychic conflicts, for example, an individual who has difficulty acknowledging the traumas associated with an event witnessed, may express this conflict in the form of 'blindness', which exists for the individual and yet has no physical basis. The somatic problem may present less trauma to the individual than that associated with acknowledging the psychic conflict.

Guilt may be problematical where it is misplaced; for example, survivors of traumatic events who feel guilt because of their survival when others have died, or where it becomes excessive, creating incapacitating tensions that interfere with life and living. Equally problematical is the inability to feel guilt or remorse following antisocial activities or conduct, which is characteristic of individuals who lack insight into reality and also of some personality limitations.

Apathy represents a loss of interest and drive, and may be seen in combination with many other problems. It may be associated with severely depressed mood, for example, in post-traumatic stress responses and organic brain damage. When witnessed in conjunction with a lack of insight, thought and perceptual problems, diagnostic labels of 'schizophrenia' or 'schizoaffective disorder' may be applied.

Lability of mood has been referred to above in relation to somatic dysfunction as rapid changes of mood, either in the absence of an appropriate stimulus or in response to very minor stimulation. Moods are mobile and unpredictable, and this problem is commonly witnessed in the care of individuals experiencing organic impairment. When extreme, it may be referred to as *emotional incontinence* and that less rapid, more persistent mood swing which may be experienced is termed *cyclothymia*.

Blunted affect refers to emotional expression that appears in response to stimuli and yet lacks 'body'. It is neutral, flat and shallow and the normal range of emotional expression is restricted and lacking. *Incongruity* or *inappropriacy of affect* describes emotional responses that are out of keeping with the prevailing events or circumstances. A commonly quoted example is that of giggling at a funeral. Both emotional blunting and incongruity are associated with a lack of insight, and thought and perceptual problems.

Psychoactive substance *abuse* and *dependence* tend to be associated with the extremes of mood. Depression and anhedonia are commonly associated with the use of alcohol, amphetamines (and similarly acting sympathomimetics), cannabis and cocaine. Euphoria tends to feature in the use and dependence associated with phencyclidine (and similarly acting arylcyclohexylamines) and with sedatives, hypnotics and anxiolytic preparations. Opioids are usually similarly euphoric in effect, although on occasions supplemental substances may be added, either to enhance the 'high' or to counteract any depressive effect experienced.

Intoxication may elicit other problems of mood. Where alcohol is the causative substance euphoria, depression and emotional lability may be observed. In amphetamine intoxication, anxiety and apprehension may occur and with cannabis, euphoria, inappropriacy, anxiety and panic attacks may feature. Cocaine intoxication may provoke euphoria and anxiety and hallucinogens often create anxiety and depression. All psychoactive substances will create some degree of mood problem. *Withdrawal* from use will create similar problems, depression, anxiety and irritability all being common. Delirium, a state of altered consciousness, disorientation and confusion, is characteristic of acute and subacute organic reaction and may be a feature of both use and withdrawal of psychoactive preparations. Alcohol, amphetamines, cocaine and phencyclidine are examples of potential causes of delirium states, and emotional disturbances are very common in such scenarios. Anxiety, fear, depression, irritability, anger, euphoria and apathy may all occur.

Some substances, notably hallucinogens and phencyclidine, are specifically associated with a mood disorder. In either instance it may be difficult to ascertain whether mood disorder precipitated substance utilization—that is, the substance was taken to elevate mood, but depression was only exacerbated by its use—or whether the mood disturbance is a direct result of preparation usage. Most commonly, depression and anxiety are the problems experienced, and only rarely elation.

There are other problems associated with emotion that are often overlooked because they have not acquired psychiatric terminology. These are frequently experienced by individuals who fall through the mental health safety net one way or another, either because they keep their emotions to themselves and on a very tight rein, or because their response to such emotions is considered within the parameters of 'normal' behaviours.

Whilst many may not be as cynical as George Bernard Shaw when he said 'Love is a gross exaggeration of the difference between one person and everybody else' or Benjamin Disraeli who believed 'The magic of first love is our ignorance that it can never end' it has to be admitted that love is a major preoccupation for many and an integral part of life for most. Romantic love is the stuff of films, novels and poetry, and yet it is not the only focus of love feelings experienced within life and living. Think of parental love and its problems, which may be many and varied. Loving children too much, and trying to shelter them from the world, and being unable to love children at all, and eliciting an almost blatant disregard for their health and well-being, are two extremes of a continuum, and a happy medium somewhere in between may be hard for some to find. Neither overprotectiveness nor neglect is of benefit to the developing youngster, but the parent who vacilates between the two extremes is even worse for the child's mental health prognosis.

Problems may similarly arise in the situation where parental love replaces a previous love-based relationship with a partner. The child(ren) form the focus of existence for one or both parents, preventing care between equals and that symbiotic love represented by a partnership. Difficulties present for all involved in situations where parental love somehow becomes distorted and assumes a heterosexual basis. Sexual abuse is a subject increasingly explored and reported by the media and will no doubt elicit continuing study over the next decade and beyond. The problems of physical and emotional abuse, too, are areas of difficulty that are well publicized, as is filial violence: that is, violence perpetrated by a child upon a parent. All evoke major biopsychosocial traumas.

There are problems, too, associated with the parent who cannot 'let go' of an adult child. This is the parent who is unable to make the transition from protector and provider to friend. It is the parent who is unable to (or experiences great difficulty) allow the child to develop new, lasting relationships outside of the family of origin and who often provokes guilt in the offspring in relation to 'having no further use' for the parent, who is 'obviously in the way'. Such parents may resent any attention that is not directed towards themselves, or any activity in which they have not been included as an automatic right. The 'unreasonable' expectations of such parents may create significant problems for their children's relationships and adult roles.

Romantic love must be considered problematical for many—if not most—of the population at some time within their lifespan. There are those who find themselves sacrificing self, own needs and aspirations to 'please' a partner who has been elevated to 'god' status. In addition there are those who expect too much of a partner and can never find someone sufficiently selfless to suit, and individuals who really do not expect another to love them, because they are so 'worthless', that is, lacking in confidence. Some have problems exteriorizing their love for another, whilst others will 'fall in love' all the time. Many may in fact be 'in love with being in love', desperately seeking someone to fulfil the idealistic dreams and images promulgated regarding romantic love. Whether the rescued or the rescuer, romantic love is envisaged by most as an integral and expected part of life, hence the roaring trade in dating agencies and 'introduction' services.

Sibling love may, for some, be non-existent, creating severe family discord and occasionally intense guilt within the individual. There may conversely be a prolonged or excessive dependence upon siblings to meet one's own needs, which may continue into adult life. Responsibility for an individual's health, happiness and achievements in life may be firmly placed on another's shoulders rather than being assumed by oneself, and that someone may be anyone, parent, sibling, partner or child. It may be that a relationship within the family of origin *always* assumes a higher priority than those with a partner and one's own children and again may create significant discord and resentment.

Altruism—love experienced towards fellow man—again may be non-existent at one extreme and excessive at the other. Individuals who demonstrate a total disregard or disinterest in the effects of their behaviour upon others, for example, business persons who will tread on anyone to get whatever it is they desire, joy-riders who steal cars without thought for either the owners or anyone who may happen to get in their way, gun-runners who arm one or both sides in a conflict, generating financial gain at the expense of lost lives and maimed bodies, have no care for their fellow man. The individual who sacrifices self, own needs and aspirations within a total absorption of assisting others, whilst profoundly altruistic, may be missing out on a great deal of personal growth and development inherent in a 'well-balanced' life of partnerships—some equal, others not so equal—of giving *and* receiving, of being valued, valuing others and self, and all of the other experiences available within the lifespan.

There are those whose love for a spiritual god, of whatever nature and characteristics, assumes obsessional proportions, whilst others 'worship' material goods, which acquire a value above that of people. There may be a love of animals and pets, which, again, may supersede that awarded to humans, for all sorts of reasons. For many, love may provide an area of considerable difficulty.

It would be inconceivable to mention love without mentioning hate and hatred, which may so often cripple the emotional lives of individuals and prevent attainment towards reaching their potential of 'being', feeling and experiencing other emotions. The emotion itself is often a very understandable response—the possible hatred of the Jews for the Nazi concentration camps and gas-chambers, that of an innocent victim towards the perpetrator of a terrorist bombing or that of parents towards the individual who molested or murdered their child—and one with which everyone would empathize. Such hatred has to be managed and dealt with, to prevent the individuals from falling victim to the event or occurrence, or from continuing to be victims for the rest of their lives. To be totally preoccupied with seeking revenge, asserting the 'truth' of a situation or hurting others to compensate for the hurt and pain experienced by self, is damaging to the mental health of the individuals themselves and those who come into contact with them. It alters the perspectives applied to life and living and prevents maximization of opportunities available, or potentially available, for life, living, personal happiness and peace of mind.

There are individuals whose fear of life and living inhibits their experiences, creating continual unease and distress. Such fears may relate to almost anything in life, for example, being afraid to try, afraid to fail or afraid to succeed. Some may be terrified of showing their true self, for fear of rejection and 'not suiting' individuals who have no real significance in their existence. Others are afraid to find out about themselves, their likes, dislikes, needs, drives, emotions, for fear of having to face what may be traumatic revelations. There are people who are physically or emotionally afraid of loved ones, or who conversely enjoy the terror that they are capable of evoking or instilling in others. This lack of self-esteem, worth and confidence, or conversely, that lack of value, or trust and faith, in others, in comparison to self, cripples the individual emotionally.

Guilt feelings may be similarly problematical for an individual. Shame and self-loathing as a result of some action or omission on one's own part, whether actual, inferred, imagined, potential or exaggerated, may be persistent or intermittent in nature. Such feelings may evoke avoidance of situations or relationships that characterized the original problem, or a continuous placing of oneself in similar positions, whether compensatory in nature or as a form of punishment. There are those whose skill in life appears to be evoking guilt in others, perhaps to detract from their own responsibility in a situation or just as a means of achieving one's own ends. Again, there is a need to explore the emotion, come to terms with issues and feelings, and move on in life.

We have almost avoided the mention of anger as a response within this section, mainly for the reason that anger would be a relatively 'normal' reaction in biopsychosocial traumas. However, problems do occur for many individuals who may never approach mental health care services, and these merit identification. Just as with hatred and guilt feelings, some individuals always carry anger around with them, preventing the full experience of life. It may be a reaction to many events and circumstances—feelings of 'not being good enough' as a child and hence spending a lifetime proving parents wrong in their beliefs, is one such example. Being angry at a loved one's desertion, or at one's treatment at the hands of society, or an employer, are others. Some individuals find anger to be their predominant reaction in many situations and this may represent the individual's defensiveness and anticipation of attack by others, or blame being apportioned to them in other spheres of life. Lack of verbal fluency may predispose to violence and aggressive acts where anger or frustration features. Certainly, the prime focus of anger may be either self or some vulnerable loved one—a parent, a partner or a child—or society at large via antisocial acts.

SUMMARY

A brief analysis of problems that may be observed within both individuals and society in general has been presented. When not publicized too loudly or broadly, in the main, people are left alone with their emotional distress. However, where antisocial activities result from feelings—a parent shoots the driver responsible for an accident that killed his child, a deserted wife repeatedly drives over the body of her husband's mistress, or a battered wife sets fire to her husband while he sleeps—society, often in the form of legal action, pays attention to the problems that have long exerted their detrimental influence.

DISCUSSION QUESTIONS

1. Reflect upon the ways that you would recognize that a close friend was feeling low, anxious or guilty. Would these feelings be evident to others around, or does much of your ability to interpret these feelings stem from the nature of your relationship?

   If this closeness of relationship is important, what are the repercussions of this upon client–nurse interactions, and the value or otherwise of significant family involvement within care?

2. Nurses frequently need to control the exteriorization of their own emotions. How do you currently, or how do you plan to, compensate for this need to defer or delay ventilation of your feelings? Who will assist you, and how may your expressed feelings affect that individual?

3. Select a client from the group you are currently caring for, and ask for his or her cooperation in your studies. The diagnosis of the client is not important here; it is crucial however that you have built some degree of trusting relationship with the person, and that person is willing to explore his or her feelings with you. Assess the client's affect, mood and feelings. Explore how these have and are affecting daily functioning and perceptions of the future. Determine, with the client, those aspects of care and treatment felt by the client to most in tune with needs, and those found to be less valuable or comfortable to deal with.

   Record your findings as appropriate or report them to the supervising nurse for information or action.

   Plan and conduct a follow-up meeting with the client to ascertain movement from this baseline, with the client and the supervising nurse.

Problems of emotion may be seen in a variety of shades and degrees and like all mental health problems, do not exist in isolation from problems associated with cognition and behaviour. A prob-lem experienced in one domain will, of necessity, infringe upon the others and Chapter 6 will be seen to demonstrate this interaction.

REFERENCES

Ax A F 1953 The physiological differentiation between fear and anger in humans. Psychomotor Medicine 15:433–442

Beck A T 1974 The development of depression: a cognitive model. In: Friedman R J, Katz M M (eds) The psychology of depression. Winston, Washington

Blaney P 1986 Affect and memory: a review. Psychological Bulletin 99(2):229–246

Bower G H 1981 Mood and memory. American Psychologist 36:129–148

Campbell R J 1989 Psychiatric dictionary, 5th edn. Oxford University Press, Oxford

Cannon W B 1927 The James–Lange theory of emotion: a critical examination and an alternative theory. American Journal of Psychology 39:106–124

Ekman P 1982 Emotion in the human face, 2nd edn. Cambridge University Press, Cambridge

Ekman P, Oster H 1982 Review and prospect. In: Ekman P (ed) Emotion in the human face, 2nd edn. Cambridge University Press, Cambridge

Ekman P, Levenson R W, Frierson W V 1983 Autonomic nervous system activity distinguishes among emotions. Science 221:1208–1210

Erdman G, Janke W 1978 Interaction between physiological and cognitive determinants of emotions: experimental studies on Schachter's theory of emotions. Biological Psychology 6:61–74

Garcia J, Rusinak K W 1980 What the nose learns from the mouth. In: Muller-Schwarze D, Silverstein R M (eds) Chemical signals. Plenum, New York

Hebb D O 1972 Textbook of psychology, 3rd edn. W B Saunders, Philadelphia

Hohmann G W 1966 Some effects of spinal cord lesions on experienced emotional feelings. Psychophysiology 3:143–156

Izard C E 1984 Emotion–cognition relationships and human development. In: Izard C E, Kagan J, Zajonc R B (eds) Emotions, cognition and behaviour. Cambridge University Press, Cambridge

James W 1884 What is emotion? Mind 9:188–204

Jasmos T M, Hakmiller K L 1975 Some effects of lesion level and emotional cues on affective expression in spinal cord patients. Psychological Reports 37:859–870

FURTHER READING

Brain W R 1985 Brain's diseases of the nervous system. University Press Oxford, Oxford

Lishman W A 1978 Organic psychiatry: the psychological consequences of cerebral disorder. Blackwell Scientific, Oxford
Excellent texts, providing detailed analysis and discussion on organic neurological disease. The mental health professional needs to have a greater knowledge and understanding of the overlaps and dividing line between symptomatology which may be assumed to be of psychological origin. For me, they consistently raise the questions, 'Why do neurologists treat some clients and psychiatrists treat others? Where is the dividing line?'

Hinchliffe S. Montague S 1988 Physiology for nursing practice. Baillière Tindall, London

Hinwood B 1993 A textbook of science for the health professions, 2nd edn. Chapman & Hall, London
These texts generate the sound background knowledge required to understand and predict the way that the body and brain work. They provide the baseline for the detailed neurology that is necessary to an understanding of the manner in which the individual interacts with its individual parts, and with the outside world. This knowledge facilitates questions being asked as to the aetiology of mental illness rather than an automatic acceptance of 'psychological' causation for every symptom.

Roth I (ed) 1990 Introduction to psychology, vols 1 and 2. Laurence Erlbaum Associates in conjunction with the Open University, Milton Keynes
A readable text which offers insights into the parameters and developments in the world of psychology, and the accepted links with psychiatry. This text provides that baseline knowledge required to delve deeper into the theoretical and practical perspectives applied for so long to the mentally ill, and to generate questions in the analytical mind as to where we go from here.

All other texts used within Chapters 3, 4 and 5 are used to expand knowledge and analysis of that knowledge of specific areas of function of mental ill health. Each is a reader friendly book, identifying the knowledge and theories surrounding the subject and an analysis of all of this within care and treatment of clients. Each is a milestone in its own right, and whilst in every instance the world has moved on since publication, these texts provide that baseline understanding for each subject served.

Johnson J E, Petzel T P, Hartney M N, Morgan L M 1983 Recall and importance ratings of completed and uncompleted tasks as a function of depression. Cognitive Therapy and Research 7:51–56

Lowe J, Carroll D 1985 The effects of spinal injury on the intensity of emotional experience. British Journal of Clinical Psychology 24:135–136

Mandler G 1982 Mind and emotion. Norton, New York

Marañon G 1924 Contribution to the study of the role of adrenaline in emotion. Revue Francaise d'Endocrinologie 2:301–325

Papez J W 1937 A proposed mechanism of emotion. Archives of Neurology and Psychiatry 38:725–744

Plutchik R 1980 A general psychoevolutionary theory of emotion. In: Plutchik R, Kellerman H (eds) Emotion: theory, research and experience, vol 1. Academic Press, New York

Roget P 1982 Roget's thesaurus of English words and phrases. Longman, Harlow

Roseman I 1979 Cognitive aspects of emotion and emotional behaviour. 87th annual convention of the American Psychological Association, New York, September 1979

Schachter S 1971 Some extraordinary facts about obese humans and rats. American Psychologist 26:129–144

Schachter S, Singer J E 1962 Cognitive, social and physiological determinants of emotional state. Psychological Review 69:379–399

Seyle H 1956 The stress of life. McGraw-Hill, New York

Sperling G 1960 The information available in brief visual presentations. Psychological Monographs 74(11):498

Tortora G J, Anagnostakos N P 1984 Principles of anatomy and psychology. Harper & Row, New York

Zajonc R B 1984 On the primacy of affect. American Psychologist 39(2):117–123

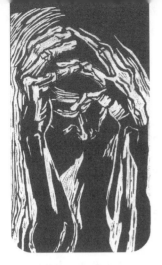

Chapter Four

Behaviour

F Clifford Johnson   Lynne D Smith

AIMS

- ◆ To explore the concept of behaviour and innate influencing factors
- ◆ To discuss selected aspects of behaviour; the norms, expectations and characteristics associated with:
  1 movement
  2 eating
  3 sleeping
- ◆ To determine potential problems which may indicate mental health assistance is required

KEY ISSUES

Definitions
Innate body rhythms
Paralysis, paresis, rigidity
Overactivity/stereotyping, etc.
Starvation, bingeing, compensation
Insomnia, nightmares and terrors
Withdrawal, compensation

BEHAVIOUR AND MOVEMENT—NORMS AND PROBLEMS

INTRODUCTION

After man's emergence as truly man, the same sort of thing continued to happen, but with an important difference. Man's evolution is not biological but psychosocial: it operates by the mechanism of cultural tradition, which involves the cumulative self-reproduction and self-variation of mental activities and their products. Accordingly, major steps in the human phase of evolution are achieved by breakthroughs to new dominant patterns of mental organization, of knowledge, ideas and beliefs— ideological instead of physiological or biological organization.

The words above are those of the twentieth-century biologist, Julian Huxley (1958). Having evolved to the degree whereby locomotion could be achieved on two legs, rather than four, where objects could be manipulated as tools and weapons, thereby providing an advantage over many other species of the animal kingdom, and language could be utilized to share 'innovations' and observations, human physiological transformation was completed. A by-product of the increased interaction and control over the environment was the gradual development of an enlarged and more advanced cerebral cortex, which became incorporated into genetic coding and which continued to be perpetuated via the 'survival of the fittest' and the destruction of less able competition. The effects of environmental stimuli on the basic brain provided at birth are explored in Chapter 5 on cognition. Learning and experiencing the environment may be seen to be of the utmost importance in achieving potential function and abilities. Certainly it may be that limitations on performance are merely self-imposed or socially induced, and that the potential is almost limitless where the environment is appropriate and conducive to learning. As society, its systems and structures, its rules and norms are made by

people and 'ideological instead of physiological or biological' (Huxley 1958), we may be only part-way along the path towards full emancipation from our animal origins. How far along the path may be inferred from the following discussion.

HUMAN NATURE OR ANIMAL INSTINCT?

Today, in a world of advanced technology and increasingly sophisticated methods of investigation and analysis, it is possible to confirm that we are indeed basically animal plus a highly developed cortex. The remainder of the human brain and its structures show very little difference, in situation or function, to those of 'lesser species'. The subcortical centres of grey matter elicit remarkable similarities, particularly the thalamus and hypothalamus, which, whilst regulating the autonomic nervous system and, to some degree, metabolic and endocrine activities, also, and importantly in the following discussions, play the major role in emotional and instinctual life, adding the affective elements to feelings. The thalamus, for example, possesses nuclei within its internal core, and the projections from these nuclei extend through the medial and basal telencephalon. Stimulation of these structures, in animals, is seen to create disturbances of feeding, fighting, pain avoidance, mating and nurturing behaviours. The hypothalamus is associated with temperature regulation, cardiovascular and endocrine activities but, in addition, appears to accommodate the mechanisms relating to certain drives, for example, hunger and thirst. The role of the hypothalamus within the exteriorization of behaviours associated with the docility–rage continuum, and within sleep, is similarly demonstrable and the relevance of thalamic and hypothalamic activity within each behaviour will be discussed in more detail within the appropriate sections of this chapter. Limbic influences are similarly brought to bear upon motor activity via connections between the basal ganglia and the areas generating emotion. The roles and effects of various neurotransmitters, discussed by Farine in Chapter 11, provide an integral aspect of the study of behaviour and its influences: there is little difference at this point between the human brain and that of other animals.

Role of the cerebral cortex

In turning attention towards the cerebral cortex, it may be remembered that it is, essentially, the ultimate destination of data collected via the sensory receptors and organs. Its continual interaction with subcortical centres is elicited via the phenomena of perception arousing emotion, and, conversely, emotion focusing attention and therefore perception. Cortical regions are linked via association pathways and by this process, crude and raw perceptual experiences are transformed into meaningful information, with the addition of memories of previous experiences and learning. At the point at which all relevant data have been evoked, including those which relate to the current degree of angularity of joints and the relative tension of body muscles, the sensorimotor cortex activates the specific motor changes necessary to achieve rapid motor responses to information received. It is the cortex that discriminates between the perceptions emanating from internal and external environments, initiating and supporting responses to some stimuli, whilst concurrently inhibiting potential activities and reactions to others. With a highly developed cortex comes the potential to demonstrate a greater ability to discriminate between a wider range of somatosensory stimuli and their increased associations, plus an increased number of possible reactions are available from which to select an appropriate response. Thus our advantage over competitors within the remainder of the animal kingdom is, in theory, tremendous.

The evolutionary development of the frontal lobe of the cerebral cortex must, however, be our greatest advantage. Its role and value within social behaviour is well demonstrated in the following story:

In 1848, Phineas Gage was a hardworking, dependable and well-liked, 25-year-old foreman on a railway construction. An explosion of the site blew a thirteen pound metal rod through the front of his skull, causing extensive bifrontal lobe damage.

Although surviving this horrendous accident, Phineas demonstrated a marked change in behaviour and personality. He was described as 'fitful, irreverent, indulging at times in the greatest profanity … manifesting little deference for his fellows, impatient of restraint or advice when it conflicts with his desires, at times pertinaciously obstinate, yet capricious and vacillatory, devising many plans of future operations, which are no sooner arranged than they are abandoned'.

Phineas experienced no pain in relation to the accident and indeed spent some time with P. T. Barnum's circus, exhibiting himself as a freak along with the offending rod.
Harlow 1848

There are direct neural projections from the thalamus to the frontal lobe and therefore a connection between emotion and innate behaviour and the higher functions related to judgement, reasoning, the development of intellectual resources and the pursuit of long term goals. The frontal lobe assists in the demonstration of socially aware behaviour, tact, sensitivity and self-control—it is the 'policeman' moderating animal instincts.

From the above, it may be seen that the 'model' is that of 'animal' with the significant additions of judgement, the ability to plan ahead and work towards deferred gratification, and an emphasis on behaviour conducive to group acceptance.

AN INFLUENTIAL HERITAGE

Though basically animal, we have the higher cognitive powers necessary to interact to our advantage with the environment and control—within reason—our behaviour. It is observed, for example, that we may override some of our defence-oriented reflex actions when perceived to be beneficial to us:

Imagine, that knowing the pantry is bare, you stop off on the way home from work to pick up fish and chips, or a take-away. By the time home is in sight, the meal is not feeling too warm and so, you put the meal on a plate in the oven to heat it up. Ten minutes later and presumably warm enough to eat with enjoyment, the meal is taken out of the oven, and despite the use of a cloth, the heat of the plate burns your fingers. Do you drop the plate? Not if it can be helped—it represents the only food in the house and the thought of scraping it off the floor into the bin would be more than a hungry stomach could condone. The instinct to release the plate and let it smash, food and all, is countermanded as evinced by the 'juggling act' undertaken in order to transfer the hot plate to a suitable surface. The pain in the fingers and hands is reduced to the greatest extent possible by the intermittent grasp of the plate achieved by the juggling act, but it remains the overwhelming priority of the moment to deposit the meal safely.

You will be aware, however, of situations and events when you were unable to control your own innate behaviours, which may have evoked feelings ranging in intensity from mild disappointment to intense anger directed at self. Wanting specifically to stay up late to watch a particular TV film and waking up only to find the credits rolling may be a 'mild' example. Losing control in a situation in which it is deemed important to maintain it, whether in the form of shedding tears or inflicting pain on someone, either verbally or physically, may provide another instance.

We need to be aware of the fact that there are biological influences which exert so subtle an effect upon general functioning, and hence behaviour, that the individual may not appreciate their existence. These influences may, in part, account for fluctuations in performance and are, in effect, rhythms adapted to the earth's cycles, and nature's norms. If we look at a garden, the rhythms of plants and flowers may be observable. The snowdrop *knows* when it is time for it to raise itself from the confines of the earth, as does every other bulb, shrub and tree in the garden. Daffodils are not evident in the long summer days and delphiniums are not naturally seen in the border in the depths of winter or early springtime. It is known that some species of birds migrate to warmer climates for the winter and, in the forest, some animals hibernate at that time. Salmon will find their way back to their birthplace in time to lay their eggs and then immediately die. How do frogs know when to spawn and tortoises to wake up

from hibernation? The answer is that all possess in-built, genetically coded rhythms, which, whilst influenced by environmental conditions, are evoked automatically and at around the same time of the year and reflect a long evolutionary patterning of behaviour, designed to prevent disruption by weather vagaries.

There are three observable and natural rhythms that influence activities. Some garden flowers open their flowers in the day and close them at night, synchronized with the day/night–light/dark cycle of the day. Removed from the garden environment and placed in a dark cupboard, plants such as the heliotrope will continue to open and close their leaves in tune with the day/night cycle outside. It is not, therefore, stimulated directly by the amount of light and its pattern of opening and closing must be integral to plant structure. This is an example of a *circadian rhythm*, named from two Latin words, *circa* = about and *dies* = a day; rhythms that occur on an approximately daily basis.

In the human being, the sleep–wake cycle is the most visible of the circadian rhythms, but there are a hundred or so such cycles, many of which appear to be coordinated with sleep and wakefulness. Temperature, for example, is seen to rise and fall over the 24-hour period, with its peak in the afternoon and its low—about 1 to 1.5°C lower—between 2.00 a.m. and 5.00 a.m. Urinary output is also governed by a circadian rhythm, as the antidiuretic hormone, produced by the posterior pituitary lobe, demonstrates a rise and fall in blood concentration levels, being lowest during the night. Cortisol, secreted by the adrenal cortex, peaks in humans just before dawn to prepare for the day's energy expenditure, whilst in nocturnal animals, that peak is seen in the early evening.

Infradian rhythms (*infra* = below, *dies* = day) occur at a rate lower than once a day, that is, are seen in a cycle of longer than 24 hours' duration. Animal hibernation is an example as, once each year, there is a prolonged inactive period, during which the body temperature of the animal drops significantly. The annual migration of birds follows an infradian rhythm, as does the return of the salmon to its birthing grounds. The stag grows antlers in the spring and summer for use as weapons of horn in the fight with other stags for possession of the does of the herd in the rutting season. The antler growth signifies the rising levels of the testosterone cycle and once rutting is over and hormone levels drop, the horns are lost to be replaced the following spring.

Within humans, the female menstrual cycle follows an infradian rhythm. Neurons within the preoptic portion of the hypothalamus initiate the cycle via the release of gonadotrophin-releasing hormone (GRH) which acts directly upon the anterior pituitary, stimulating it to produce two hormones in a precise pattern of secretion. Initially, follicle-stimulating hormone (FSH) is released and acts upon the hollow ball, or follicle, within the ovary that contains the ovum. Development of this follicle is accompanied by its release of oestrogen in increasing amounts, which reduces further secretion of the FSH by the pituitary gland, and prompts it, instead, to release high levels of luteinizing hormone (LH). Luteinizing hormone provokes a rupture in the follicle wall and release of the mature ovum. The process of *ovulation* is complete within a period of 10–14 days, and, during this period of the cycle, the lining of the uterus regenerates, beginning the gradual development of the endometrium.

The remainder of the follicle is transformed into the corpus luteum, which secretes progesterone under the influence of LH. Progesterone has two effects, for it increases the blood supply to the uterus, facilitating further development of the endometrium, in preparation for implantation of the fertilized ovum, and also signals the pituitary gland to reduce production of LH. Where the egg remains unfertilized, levels of progesterone fall as the corpus luteum begins to degenerate, and this loss of hormonal support causes a reduction in blood supply to the endometrium, which ultimately leads to its death and evacuation as menstrual flow. Following fertilization, the corpus luteum continues to produce oestrogen and progesterone for approximately 3 months, when the placenta takes over the function.

Seasonal affective disorder (SAD) is of interest here, for whilst most individuals feel a little less energetic and enthusiastic as winter months approach, this is usually a subtle change accompanied by a similar slight lowering of mood. However, it has been noted that, in areas near or above the Arctic Circle in Scandinavia, there is a higher rate of suicide in winter than in summer. The phenomenon is not solely restricted to Scandinavia, for some individuals find that a significant depressed mood coincides with the onset of winter, only to lift with the arrival of spring. Wehr and his colleagues (1979) reasoned that provision of artificial sunlight during the dark winter days may relieve lowered mood and therefore experimented with full spectrum fluorescent lamps. By bathing the individual in bright white light for a few hours each day to supplement exposure to natural light, depressed mood was relieved quite dramatically for some within a couple of days of treatment commencing. Perhaps this is indicative of a period within the human evolutionary history when the species hibernated in winter!

There is a third type of rhythm demonstrable, that is, one that occurs more frequently than once each day. *Ultradian rhythms* (*ultra* = beyond, *dies* = day) are most easily discussed within the context of the human for several hormones are secreted into circulation episodically and over the 24-hour period evince an ultradian rhythm. The problems experienced by Mitch Heller provide a useful example:

CASE STUDY

An American engineer, avid hockey player and all-round sports enthusiast, Mitch was involved in a road traffic accident in August 1978, and sustained a minor blow to the head. Within a month of the bump, Mitch noticed that his desire for sexual intercourse was waning and that his body and facial hair seemed to be disappearing. His general practitioner suspected damage to the hypothalamus and referred him to William Crowley, an expert in the specialty (Crowley et al 1980).

A defect in hypothalamic secretion of gonadotrophin-releasing hormone (GRH), which in men, in exactly the same mechanism as women, prompts the pituitary gland to release sex hormones. In men these hormones act upon the testes, facilitating both sperm manufacture and secretion of testosterone, which provides male characteristics including the sex urge. GRH had been successfully produced artificially and was therefore available for treatment.

Ernst Knobil and his team (1988) at the University of Pittsburgh had discovered, in studies of monkeys, that the hypothalamus releases GRH rhythmically, in short sharp bursts. This knowledge was utilized by Crowley in Mitch's treatment, for a needle was permanently inserted into Mitch's abdomen, attached to an automatic syringe and pump worn on his belt. A timing device made it possible to deliver injections of GRH at 2-hourly intervals throughout the day and night, in exactly the same way as nature would have organized it, or as Crowley himself stated, 'Only by administering the hypothalamic message in a pulsatile fashion could the normal physiology and normal endocrine conversation of the hypothalamus, pituitary and gonads be mimicked'.

Whilst initially hating the injections and associated paraphernalia, by the end of the first week, Mitch hardly noticed them. His desire for sex quickly returned, along with the hair on his chest, and within 6 months of the treatment commencing, Mitch and his wife, Debbie, were expecting their first baby.

Another similarly subtle ultradian rhythm is occurring in approximately 90-minute cycles in the human throughout the day and night, as demonstrated by electroencephalographic (EEG) recordings of brain activity. Human alertness and cognitive performance appear to follow this same cycle, with verbal and spatial matching tasks eliciting differing levels of competency and accuracy at different points of the cycle (Lavie & Kripke 1975). As we will discuss later within this chapter, this 90-minute cycle has long been known in relation to the sleep hours, but largely was unrecognized in relation to daytime activity.

MOTIVATION

Campbell (1989) in his excellent definition of the term 'behaviour' includes the phrases:

—the manner in which anything acts or operates. With regard to the human being, usually regards to the action of the individual as a unit. He may be, and ordinarily is, acting in response to some given organ or impulse, but it is his general reaction that gives rise to the concept of behaviour.

People are driven towards particular behaviours because of a desire or need and as such are motivated. But what motivates us? We believe that the basic initiators of behaviour may be divided into two main categories—*personal survival* and *progenitive* (or perpetuating the species).

For personal survival, people need internal homeostasis and a degree of environmental control. We need a constant amount of water to operate normal functions and, as those functions include respiration, micturition, defaecation and perspiration as methods of waste product removal, fluid intake is a necessary drive. Growth, repair and general activities of living utilize energy and this is only sourced by continual food intake of appropriate materials. The body's machinery and processes are designed to work within a particular narrow range of temperatures and therefore control of body heat is an important drive to behaviour. To actively achieve homeostasis, movement is a necessity. People must similarly protect themselves from the hazards of the environment and the power of movement is again an essential characteristic for this. During evolution humans have discovered the values of affiliation with others of our kind, for there is not only a greater degree of safety from predators by this, but also a valuable pool of sexual partners, to facilitate dissemination of superior genes, and in addition assistance is available to gather and produce food. Humans are at their most vulnerable in the dark, when there is no artificial light available. As sleep fulfils necessary functions apart from merely resting organs, the ideal time to use was the hours of darkness, and therefore humans are by nature, nocturnally inactive. Similarly aggression is an instinct that motivates behaviour, for via such actions, the individual is able to defend self—and dependants—from harm and ensure a reliable supply of food.

This brings us to progenitor instincts. There is little value in achieving survival of one generation, if there is no second generation to ensure the continuation of the species. Sexual reproduction is the method through which that further generation is ensured and sexual behaviour is therefore an instinct, designed to maintain the race. It is likewise necessary to protect and nurture offspring until sufficiently mature to function as a self-sufficient unit, and therefore humans possess the drive towards nurturing behaviour.

MOVEMENT

Although a detailed analysis of motor functioning is not within the remit of this chapter, a brief reminder of its basic characteristics is necessary.

Basically, the system comprises of an information 'originator' within the motor cortex of the brain, a series of pathways, formed by motor nerves, and action 'effectors', in the form of muscles. Simplistically, an impulse arises in the motor cortex, as a response to a sensory input, which then travels to the appropriate muscle causing contraction of that muscle and therefore movement.

With exceptions such as those provided by the eyeball and the tongue, the majority of the muscles in the body link two bones across a common joint, and, when activated by a motor nerve, contraction causes shortening and bulking of the muscle and movement of the end of the bone, farthest away from the body, towards the body. Each muscle that moves a bone in one direction, like this, has an opposing muscle that pulls in the opposite direction, thus facilitating standing erect and steady, against the effects of gravity and also graduation of the degree of contraction required to effect the desired movement.

A motor nerve, when activated, releases a neurotransmitter, acetylcholine, into specialized receptor sites at the junction with the muscle tissue, thus facilitating passage of the impulse to that tissue. Any one muscle fibre is controlled by only one motor neuron, but one motor neuron may control numerous muscle fibres via branches in the axon depending on the fine or coarse nature of movements necessary. The muscle fibres of the thigh, for example, may have one neuron for every hundred or so fibres, whereas the movements of the eye are evinced by one neuron for every three muscle fibres. The larger the axon branch serving an area, the larger the muscle served, so for example those controlling the fine muscle movements of the fingers are proportionally smaller than those controlling the biceps of the forearm. The motor neurons, axons and muscles which they control are referred to as *motor units*. The fact that such muscles usually move on volition renders this type of movement *voluntary* in nature, thus differentiating between this and *reflex movement*. Motor neurons that originate in the motor cortex and terminate at a synapse, with a short connecting neuron in the spinal cord, or at cranial nerve nuclei, are termed *upper motor neurons*. Those that actually terminate in the skeletal muscle are referred to as *lower motor neurons*.

Reflex movement is involuntary and protective in function. Humans have the ability to override such reflexes at times. Reflex activities are achieved via spinal cord command, in conjunction with assistance from local sensory receptors. *Proprioceptors*, tiny sensors within muscle and tendon tissue, monitor the position and tension evident within these tissues and relay that information via the spinal cord to higher, cortical motor centres. Thus the cortex is always aware of the precise current degree of angularity, muscle and tendon tension relating to body joints, and has a knowledge therefore of the degree of movement necessary in order to achieve new positioning. In reflex movement, activity is generated via the spinal cord and the higher centres are informed with some slight delay of the need for action, thus it may be observed that the painful finger has already been removed from the hot plate before cognitive awareness has occurred. Pain activates sensory fibres which carry the impulse to the spinal cord. In turn spinal motor neurons are activated directly and impulses for movement are evoked. Muscle activity occurs and flexion of the joint removes the painful area away from the stimulus provoking the response. To maintain equilibrium, a counter-balancing manoeuvre is evoked, so that, for example, if you should firmly plant a foot on a pin during walking, as the injured foot is removed by flexion of muscles, the muscles of the opposite leg—which was up in the air, in the process of taking the next step—extend to compensate for the imbalance. *Crossed extension*, or this opposing movement of the limbs, is achieved as the sensory fibre of the injured limb interacts with the spinal motor neuron which controls the opposite limb, as well as its own effector. Therefore cross-innervation within the spinal cord provides for reciprocal muscle control, and balance is achieved during both normal and emergency muscular activity, with synchronized arm and leg movements made automatically.

The motor cortex is, of course, the originator of voluntary movement, and this is arranged as a strip in each cerebral hemisphere, adjacent to those relating to somatosensory function. The neurons in both the motor and sensory areas are organized in patterns of column-like, vertical structures and form a *functional column*. You may recall the disproportionate amount of space devoted to different surfaces of the body in relation to the somatosensory cortex and the misshapen little person, or *homunculus*, which represents this allocation of sensory neurons. The motor cortex is entirely different in its organization, with motor columns required to achieve specific joint positions rather than actually activate muscles. The knowledge of the *status quo*, that is, the current joint, muscle and tendon positions, is already available to the motor cortex via proprioceptor communication. The motor column is thought to be responsible for all muscles acting upon a particular joint and that an impulse to move is actually a command to assume a specific joint position, which all related muscles effect, rather than being an instruction to the various individual muscles to assume different degrees of contraction.

Some cortical motor neurons, the *Betz cells*, communicate directly with motor cells of the spinal cord and their axons amalgamate to form a large bundle of nerve fibres, termed the *pyramidal tract*. On the descending path towards the spinal cord, the pyramidal tract arising from the right motor cortex and that from the left, cross over each other, the *decussation of the pyramids*, so that the right pyramidal tract is seen to control movement of the left side of the body and vice versa. Also on this downward journey to the spinal cord, many axons produce spurs, or collaterals, to connect with other brain structures, for example the red nucleus of the reticular formation, the basal ganglia and thalamus.

Extrapyramidal motor control is the term generally utilized to describe the influences upon motor activity of other brain structures, the most important of which are the *basal ganglia* (Fig. 4.1).

1. The basal ganglia are paired masses of grey matter in each cerebral hemisphere.
2. The largest of these is formed by the corpus striatum.
3. The corpus striatum may be anatomically divided into:
   (a) The caudate nucleus, thought to control large, subconscious movements, for example, swinging the arms whilst walking.
   In conjunction with:
   (b) The putamen (and the cortex) controlled patterns of movement are attained.
   (c) The globus pallidus, controls muscle tone and hence positioning of the body for complex movement. (The putamen and globus pallidus together form the lentiform nucleus.)
4. The claustrum, a thin sliver of grey matter, lateral to the putamen, and the amygdaloid nucleus are, on occasion, considered to be a part of the basal ganglia.
5. The subthalamic nucleus is thought to control walking and perhaps rhythmic movements.
6. The substantia nigra, comprising of dopamine-transmitting neurons which provide its colour, is necessary for smooth operation of the motor system, including the cortex, spinal cord and subcortical motivational control.
7. Potential functions of the basal ganglia are moderated, and therefore held in check, by the cerebrum.

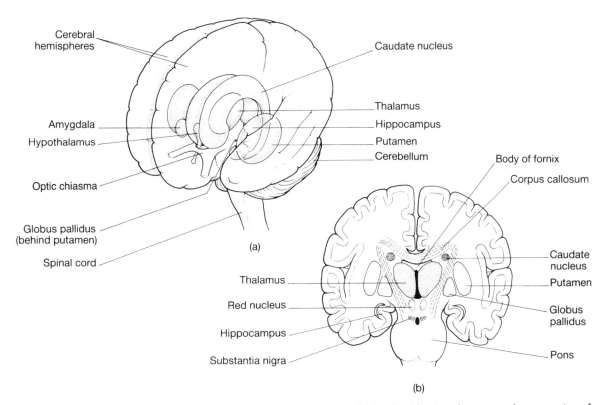

Fig. 4.1 Basal ganglia of the brain: (a) position of basal ganglia in the brain; (b) basal ganglia viewed in a coronal cross-section of the brain (from Hinchliff & Montague 1988).

The final area of significance for review in this section is that provided by the cerebellum, the large portion of tissue tucked underneath the cerebrum at the rear of the brain. It is attached to the brainstem by three pairs of fibre bundles, called the *cerebellar peduncles*, the *inferior* connecting it with the medulla, the *medial* with the pons and the *superior* to the midbrain. The grey matter on the surface of the cerebellum falls into fine, parallel ridges called *folia*, which, whilst increasing the surface area to accommodate an increased number of neurons, in the same manner as the convolutions or gyri of the cerebrum, are far less prominent. The white matter of the nerve fibres beneath the cerebellar cortex resembles the branches of a tree and hence are termed *arbor vitae*. The *cerebellar nuclei* are small masses of neuronal tissue positioned deep within the white matter, just as the basal ganglia are subcortical to the cerebrum, and again like the cerebrum, the gross appearance of the cerebellum is of two hemispheres.

You may recall that, via proprioception, the motor cortex is made aware of the position of one joint in relation to all others and therefore is aware of changes necessary for continuing voluntary movement. Impulses generated by the motor cortex pass to the pons and midbrain and thence via the medial and superior peduncles to the cerebellum. Subconscious impulses generated in response by the cerebellum pass via the inferior cerebellar peduncles to the medulla and spinal cord, and out to the muscles which will effect the voluntary movement desired. By inhibiting contraction of the opposing muscles, and stimulating the effector muscle to contract, smooth coordinated movement is achieved.

The cerebellum has connections with the inner ear and therefore is called into action when equilibrium is disturbed by the body leaning to the left or right. Impulses are initiated as a response by the cerebellum, causing contraction of appropriate muscles and restoration of balance. The area similarly controls postural muscles and therefore maintains muscle tone.

All areas are required to be fully functioning for voluntary movement and for the defensive reflex activities to be performed. Proprioception is necessary for current knowledge of position, and therefore passage of impulses to the somatosensory cortex and an intact somatosensory cortex are a must. Transfer to the motor cortex plus the desire for particular movement activities provoke new instructions being sent via healthy motor neurons to skeletal muscles. Parallel and integrated modification via the basal ganglia and cerebellum provide smooth, coordinated, balanced and polished movement (Hinchliff & Montague 1988).

Of course, movement is influenced by so many factors, for example, by cognitive appraisal of a situation, by the emotional component of experiencing events within the environment, including interactions with others, and current motivation. Movement should, however, be goal directed, and therefore purposeful, synchronized and flowing.

PROBLEMS OF MOVEMENT

It is appropriate to start this section with an analysis of the degree of movement exhibited, ranging on a continuum of no movement to hyperactivity and you may be able to identify those aspects which might fall within healthy behaviour.

Many have experienced the phenomenon of being 'unable to move a muscle' and of remaining totally immobile for a period extending from a brief moment of time to several minutes. Conscious and aware but unable to move, perhaps because of shock, surprise or fear, such immobility is a well-known feature. You will no doubt be aware, however, of individuals who, whilst also conscious and aware, and despite a cognitive desire or intention to move are quite unable to achieve this because of some degree of *paralysis* being evident.

Paralysis

Paralysis simply infers a loss of power over muscle contraction and is a common manifestation of neurological problems. It may be exhibited as a total loss, or by a weakness, a *paresis*, and may be classified according to the extent of the affected area, for example, as *monoplegia*, a paralysis of one limb, *hemiplegia*, a loss of power to one side of the body, *paraplegia*, a loss of function in both lower limbs, or *quadriplegia*, where all four limbs are affected. Problems related to a paralysis of one side of the face plus paralysis of the opposite side of the body are occasionally seen and termed *alternate hemiplegia*, but all are indicative of a lesion within the central nervous system, the level of paralysis observable being indicative of the site of damage. You may have first hand personal or professional knowledge of individuals experiencing hemiplegia associated with *cardiovascular accidents* (or strokes) or of individuals who have sustained damage to the cervical cord during a road traffic accident and are sadly paralysed from this point down. Both are unfortunately a common enough occurrence, and as paralysis is usually accompanied by loss of sensation to that area, the sequelae are obviously profound for the individuals and their carers. Damage does not have to be of a central nervous system source, for a *peripheral nerve injury* may be sustained, resulting in the loss of contractile ability of one muscle of a group. This is an important distinguishing characteristic of the injury in regard to those paralyses seen within mental health care as will be demonstrated.

Some individuals may be predisposed to paralysis of skeletal muscle and a concomitant disturbance in the functioning of the body's smooth muscles, for example, cardiac and gut muscles, due to *hypokalaemia*, a depletion of potassium, necessary, amongst other functions, for the regulation of neuromuscular excitability and stimulation, and for nerve impulse transmission. Individuals who exteriorize a deficiency of potassium intake or an excessive loss, via prolonged vomiting and diarrhoea (including the individual experiencing problems of anorexia nervosa and bulimia), or use of diuretics or corticosteriod preparations are at risk. Muscle weakness, loss of tone and reflexes, and numbness gradually progress to paralysis of arms, legs and respiratory muscles if untreated. Simultaneously, diminished peristalsis within the gastrointestinal tract (a para-lytic ileus) is demonstrated, with nausea, vomit-ing, abdominal distension and loss of bowel sounds and activity, and cardiac arrhythmias and increased sensitivity to digitalis may be seen.

Earlier we indicated that the *extent* of the paral-ysis is indicative of the site of the causative lesion, but the *type* of paralysis is also of significance. It may, for example, demonstrate retained reflex movements, exaggerated reflexes and hypertonici-ty (spasticity). This type of paralysis shows that damage is to the area of the cerebral cortex or pyramidal tracts and is termed therefore an *upper motor neuron lesion* or *spastic paralysis*. Injury lower down the pathway, in either the nuclei of cranial nerves, in the anterior columns of the spinal cord or the subsequent axons to the periph-ery, results in flaccidity because the reflex arc has been interrupted and therefore there is no reflex innervation or response. This represents a *lower motor neuron lesion* or *flaccid paralysis*.

All of the above is of great significance not only to the individual experiencing the paralysis, who, it must be remembered, will have added problems to contend with besides the paralysis which result from the nature of the specific problem, but also for his carers and the professional within mental health services. Paralysis may be a feature of presentation where a deviation in mental health status is suspected and therefore differentiation between organic and psychogenic causation is necessary. Paralysis may be, for example, the major problem for an individual who has recently experienced one or more profound life stressors, such as unemployment, divorce or retirement. It may be seen to develop within a 3-month period of the event and is usually resolved within 6 months, and may be one of many features which become diagnosed as an *adjustment disorder*, causing impairment of social or occupational functioning and demonstrating an excessive reac-tion, above that considered expected or 'accept-able'. Similarly paralysis may be a problem where the diagnosis is one of *conversion disorder*, when the symptom is said to represent an expression or psychological conflict or need, and is associated with two elements of advantage. The first, or *pri-mary gain*, keeps the conflict away from conscious awareness as, for example, a 'paralysed arm' will preclude the need for concern regarding a poten-tial exteriorization of anger and damage to a loved one. The *secondary gain* may facilitate avoidance of an unpleasant activity and may evoke support from a previously or potentially hostile environ-ment, and, again, an example may be provided by an individual who develops paraplegia, and whose wife therefore decides not to leave him for another man because of his inability to care for himself. The relative lack of concern regarding the prob-lem—la belle indifference—may be suggestive of the nature of the symptom, but may also be exhib-ited by the stoic, but seriously ill, individual. Paralysis may also be seen in *somatization disor-ders*, where there is a persistent belief that one is 'sick' or has a specific physical complaint, and yet where medical opinion finds no evidence in sup-port of this.

Since the 'paralyses' seen within mental health care correspond with the individual's subcon-scious ideas regarding the way the body works and performs, there are usually discrepancies in the area of distribution of the paralysis in compar-ison to that caused by an organic lesion, and symptomatology described is often physiologically impossible. Often when the individual attempts to move the 'affected' limb, as well as a strong prime-mover muscle contraction, a simultaneous con-traction of the antagonistic muscle may be exhibited, thereby preventing any movement tak-ing place. Such antagonistic contraction would not be evident when a 'true' paralysis exists and effort evokes little contraction of the prime mover at all. 'Hysterical paralysis' sufferers may exhibit a great expenditure of effort in their attempt to move the offending limb but with little result. The paralysis may appear flaccid or spastic, or there may be no disturbance of tone. Reflexes may be difficult to elicit but, when demonstrated, may be exaggerated or inconsistent, and are never dimin-ished. Contractures and muscle wasting are rarely evident, except in situations where the problem has been exhibited for months or years. Even then, however, improvement may be achieved by electri-cal stimulation of antagonistic muscles, or under the influence of anaesthetic drugs.

You will no doubt recognize situations and circumstances where movement is possible but where individuals remain motionless and probably the best examples to be offered here are those that evince a total disregard or disinterest in the environment and that may occur for a variety of reasons. Deep thought and reflection is the commonest cause elicited for such behaviour within the general population, there being an intense concentration on some particular aspect of life and living which represents a challenge, problem or area of curiosity.

A reduced motor activity level is observable in those individuals experiencing a *malfunction of the thyroid gland*, which results in insufficient secretion of its hormone, thyroxine. In the child, it is associated with a failure to achieve physical and cognitive milestones and a characteristic presentation of a limp, inactive, puffy and coarse-featured infant, the tongue often appearing too large for the mouth. The adult shows apathy, fatigue and the sequelae of decreased cellular metabolism, in addition to severely reduced activity levels. The latter may be considered as depressed or demonstrating the prodromal signs of organic impairment, on occasions, rather than being somatically dysfunctioning.

Similarly, a reduced level of activity is associated with *Addison's disease* (primary adrenal insufficiency) and with the exteriorization of a lowered ability to cope with everyday stressors, tearfulness at the least cause, and the extreme fatigue and listlessness experienced, again may provoke thoughts of psychosocial rather than somatic health problems. Irritability, impaired cognitive performance, and anorexia may compound the picture but the bronze/brown pigmented areas that develop on skin exposed to sunlight or friction is classically indicative of Addison's disease.

In mental health care, some individuals may experience extreme motor retardation, despite an intact motor system. The individual, for example, whose mood is *severely depressed* may appear as mute and motionless or, alternatively, exhibit a much reduced level of motor activity. *Catatonic stupor*, eliciting an almost total lack of reactivity to the environment, and a drastic reduction in spontaneous movement or activity, is a characteristic associated with a specific variation of the 'schizophrenia' group of syndromes. It may include features of *negativism*, in a passive resistance to being moved, *rigidity, posturing*, where an often bizarre position is voluntarily assumed and maintained for prolonged periods, and *waxy flexibility*, where limbs may be moulded by an observer into any position which will then be held by the individual for an indeterminable length of time. It appears that the individual's muscles do not feel fatigue in these postures assumed, or that such fatigue does not intrude upon conscious awareness. In many 'diagnostic classifications', where depressed mood is a feature, for example, *organic mood syndrome, phencyclidine mood disorder* and *primary dementia* of the *Alzheimer type with depression*, such catatonic behaviour may be evidenced in various degrees and shades.

Agitation

Accelerated motor activity may indicate that the mentally healthy individual is happy and optimistic, or terribly pressurized and rushed to achieve a goal. Sometimes a person may have so many priorities and stressors that this accelerated level of activity is unproductive, as there is a flitting to and from different targets with little being achieved. The anxiety levels may concomitantly rise, with the consistent failure to attain goals. Again, agitated behaviour may accompany both anxious and depressed moods, the individual finding difficulty in sitting still and settling to a specific task, needing to be mobile, active and occupied. Whether anticipating a pleasant or dreaded event, agitation may be a feature, and motor acceleration, a possibility.

A similar picture of agitation may be exhibited by those individuals who have a neoplastic mass of the adrenal medulla—a *phaeochromocytoma*. Its production of excessive amounts of adrenaline and noradrenaline causes hypertension, hyperglycaemia and hypermetabolism and therefore symptoms such as nausea, vomiting, air hunger, palpitations, nervousness, tremor and weakness are prominent. A severe and pounding headache, sweating, pallor, pupil dilation and tachycardia complete a picture that could be that of anxiety. It is, however, a gradually increasing phenomenon, initially lasting for minutes, at most for hours. It is rarely of a continual nature. It is a problem, though relatively rare, that needs to be borne in mind by professionals.

Similarly *hyperthyroidism*, an excessive production of the thyroid hormone, may elicit agitated and hyperactive movement levels. The increased metabolic rate evoked by hypersecretion again provides a picture of nervousness, apprehension, irritability and restlessness, and may be indicative of an anxiety-type reaction. Gastrointestinal symptoms, palpitations and shortness of breath are frequent features too, but an elevated sleeping pulse rate may be the observation that rings an alarm bell. The protrusion of the eyeballs (exophthalmos) and enlargement of the thyroid gland shown within textbook pictures may not always be evident or dramatic enough for a stranger to notice, and may have been so insidious in onset as to go relatively unnoticed by the family.

Within mental health care, the prime example of hyperactivity must be that experienced by the individual labelled as *'bipolar mood disorder—manic episode'*. The accelerated motor activity reflects the concomitant acceleration of cognitive processes, thought being rapid and transient, attention span severely limited, speech incoherent and circumstantial, and perceptions heightened. Social inhibitions are lost, and therefore there is a lack of insight into the implications of, what may be considered, grossly antisocial or meddling behaviour. Those individuals previously referred to as potentially experiencing catatonic stupor, its associated posture-related problems and negativistic demonstrations, may similarly experience a *catatonic excitement* (or frenzy), where motor activity is highly accelerated, purposeless and apparently not influenced by external stimuli. The transition from a stuporosed state to one of excitement, and vice versa, may be rapid and without warning, and may therefore evoke safety concerns in relation to the individual, other clients and carers. Whilst a potential problem in regards to any client evincing a lack of insight and accompanying hallucinatory and delusional experiences, it is more common in those where an organic aetiology is absent.

Agitation, in the form of pacing activities, a continual wringing of hands, pulling of clothes or playing with hair, is associated with individuals who feel tense and 'on edge'. You may hear the term utilized to describe varying degrees of restlessness accompanied by an excessive or increased motor activity, in a wide variety of individuals seeking mental health or assistance. The depressed or anxious person, those expressing phobic or intrusive thoughts, individuals experiencing problems associated with psychoactive substance use and those exhibiting problems provoked by organic impairment may all elicit such a problem.

MOVEMENT AND MENTAL DISORDERS

We mentioned within the last section the *rigidity* associated with catatonic behaviours and it may therefore be appropriate to consider other examples of the phenomenon, which may again provoke thought in regard to 'differential diagnosis'.

CASE STUDY

George was in his late 60s and had been an inpatient for many years. The various 'treatment' regimes utilized over those years, in efforts to ameliorate or eradicate mental health symptoms displayed, had achieved very little, for George continued to exhibit bizarre delusions and hallucinations, stereotyped and excited behaviour and the most dramatic catatonic posturing and posing features imaginable. Everyone in the hospital knew George, for, during medical and nurse education programmes, he would be identified as a valuable example of the various phenomena.

When, one morning, George 'refused' to bend in the middle and sit up for breakfast, no one really thought it significant. Similarly when George vomited some dark brown granular fluid it was put down to his regular excursions into the ward bins and to eating cigarette tobacco. George did, however, not seem quite himself—the pallor of his skin was nothing so unusual but the cold, clammy sweating was and, whilst he didn't groan or appear to be in discomfort, his features seemed pinched and taut.

The morning saw no improvement and the doctor, doing his daily visits, was asked to see him. George was promptly diagnosed as suffering from peritonitis, and sent to the general hospital following commencement of intravenous fluid administration and nasogastric intubation. Laparotomy revealed a perforated duodenal ulcer, and, though seriously ill for some days, George made a full recovery.

People receiving mental health care may become somatically ill just like anyone else and yet, at times, symptomatology exhibited is assumed to be a 'part of the mental condition'. In George's instance—and many others—objective analysis and reflection of problems observed may just be a life-saver. The *board-like rigidity of abdominal muscles*, accompanied by 'coffee ground' vomit (*haematemesis*), clinical shock and pain are classical signs of irritation of the contents of the abdomen by some foreign substance and is usually indicative of a 'leak' from some part of the gastrointestinal tract. Observation by carers becomes even more important when an individual's ability to communicate and insight into reality are impaired by mental health problems.

Spasms

Painful spasms (*trismus*) leading to rigidity of the jaw and the distortion of facial muscles are the initial indicator of *tetanus*, the invasion of the nervous system by *Clostridium tetani*, a bacillus that gains entry through an open wound, and is found in soil and the faecal material of both animals and humans. Whilst less commonly seen in this country in these days of prophylactic immunization, the all-encompassing and progressive muscle rigidity that results in cessation of respiratory function and the back arching off the bed (*opisthotonos*) is one of those experiences never to be forgotten. The spasms increase in frequency and severity for about 10 days but may be controlled with tranquillizers/sedatives and muscle relaxants. Human tetanus immunoglobulin and antibiotics are also administered and tracheostomy may be necessary. The spasms are associated with any sort of stimulation—noise, touch, movement—and therefore gentle handling and good communication prior to any attention given is the order of the day.

Rigidity

The *decerebrate*, or *decorticate rigidity* seen following the rupture of a cerebral aneurysm and severe haemorrhage into the subarachnoid space also provides a classical picture. The person is moribund and unresponsive. The adduction of the arms, flexion of arms, wrists and fingers, extension and internal rotation of lower limbs and plantar flexion exhibited is the result of interruption of the corticospinal tract, usually in the midbrain or pons. Such aneurysms are frequently asymptomatic until rupture occurs, which is often associated with psychological stress or physical strain and which produces sudden severe headache, nausea and vomiting and, in some instances, loss of consciousness. The decerebrate rigidity referred to signifies an extensive bleed and carries a poor prognosis, but many individuals with lesser bleeds will demonstrate *nuchal rigidity*, where the neck is stiff and attempts towards flexion provoke pain. A similar neck rigidity, to which flexion is resisted, is observable in individuals who suffer meningitis.

Hypoparathyroidism

Hypoparathyroidism, resulting in a fall in plasma calcium levels with a concomitant rise in phosphate concentration, will result in *tetany*, and demonstrate an increased excitability of nerves, pins and needle sensations (*paraesthesia*) and muscle spasm. *Carpopedal spasms*—flexion of the metacarpophalangeal joints and extension of the interphalangeal joints of the thumb and fingers—in adults and, more commonly, *laryngeal spasm* in children, are common findings. Hypoparathyroidism is frequently a complication of thyroidectomy, when parathyroid glands are removed along with a portion of an overactive thyroid. It may, however, be an idiopathic problem and a wide variety of mental health disturbances are associated with hypoparathyroidism. Robinson, Kallberg & Crowley (1954) reported the case of a 51-year-old woman who presented with status epilepticus, developed dementia-like symptoms and only 10 days after admission began to demonstrate signs of parathyroid deficiency. Fourman et al (1967) studied 33 individuals, all of whom had previously undergone thyroidectomy, and whose mental health diagnoses were related to anxiety and panic attacks or depression. A quarter of the population studied showed calcium levels at the 'low end of normal' and yet no other indicators of parathormone problems were exhibited. Calcium citrate tablets were found to produce a significant amelioration in symptomatology, particularly in relation to lowered mood and poor appetite. Whilst more rare, schizophrenia and bipolar mood disorder, mixed, have also been presenting features of this endocrine problem and Denko & Kaelbling (1962) on discovering several clients similarly mislabelled as 'mentally retarded', suggest that serum calcium levels should be investigated as a routine on admission to facilities for those with learning disabilities. We repeat the plea in relation to individuals 'apparently' experiencing mental health problems.

Alkalosis/alkalaemia

The carpopedal spasms of tetany are a feature of any situation in which a rise in pH (the acid–alkaline continuum) of plasma is provoked, that is, an *alkalosis*, or *alkalaemia*. Severe vomiting, a depletion of potassium and burns may all be causative of a *metabolic alkalaemia*, whilst hyperventilation may engender *respiratory alkalaemia*. This is, of course, of great interest to those working within the sphere of mental health care, for the individual experiencing problems associated with generalized anxiety or panic attacks, or indeed any diagnostic category in which anxiety presents as a major feature, may exhibit hyperventilation and therefore potentially may be prone to tetany and

carpopedal spasms. Hyperthyroidism and fever may similarly provoke hyperventilation, as may certain central nervous system lesions—cerebrovacsular accidents, subarachnoid haemorrhage and meningitis.

Parkinsonism

The rigidity associated with Parkinsonism is again 'classical'. It affects both small and large muscles of the limbs, trunk and neck and agonists and antagonists equally. It may be unilateral, is unaffected by emotion and is found to persist during sleep. Limbs resist passive extension, the so-called *lead pipe rigidity*, and the combination of rigidity plus tremor demonstrates the *cogwheel rigidity*, best elicited by grasping the individual's hand, as in a hand shake, and alternately pronating and supinating the hand. As Parkinsonism is evoked by a variety of problems including neuroleptic drug administration, it may be valuable to shake hands with that individual on a regular basis, in an attempt to elicit minor changes in function. Parkinsonism tends to creep up on carers, who see the individual regularly and hence may not notice prodromal indicators of a problem.

Mannerisms

Voluntary movement is, by design, purposeful, smooth and coordinated but yet again there are exceptions to the rule. Many, if not most, people exhibit habitual movements and characteristic mannerisms which are apparently purposeless—and perhaps an irritant—to an onlooker and yet which are utilized on a more or less regular and even predictable basis. The automatic adjustment of spectacles when one is expected to make some reply to a statement from another individual, pulling an earlobe or earring during conversation, clearing the throat on cue, or twiddling a piece of hair, may all be habits that have been acquired. In the past the movement may have provided great value—comfort as felt by the thumb-sucking child, a focus of attention in an awkward or uncomfortable situation, such as playing with a loose thread on a hem, or as a relief of inner tension or anxiety, by, for example, sorting, straightening, lining up or generally tidying the immediate environment. The habit may have been found to be a valuable preparation for ensuing activities, for by clearing the throat prior to speaking it may prevent the necessity during speech and hence becomes habitual. Similarly a mannerism may provide useful thinking time and have acceptably covered slight hesitations in communication and so become integral or automatic in certain situations. Many classes—and not just those of children and early adolescents—have a mimic, who will entertain his peers in the breaktimes, or behind teacher's back, by imitating that individual's mannerisms and some manage to earn a very successful living at it. Mannerisms tend to be an individual's 'trademark' and hence are integral to behaviour.

Stereotyped movement

Mannerisms may be seen in an exaggerated form in several situations, for example, when an individual becomes pressurized or hassled, but when the patterned responses become a monotonously and frequently performed aspect of behaviour, the term *stereotyped movement* may be applied. This may be seen in the form of a single, or group, of actions or in the assumption of an unusual posture or position which may be maintained long after muscle fatigue would normally have forced cessation of the activity.

Stereotypic blindism may be associated with people who are congenitally blind. Activities such as head rocking, pressing the eyeballs, directing the eyes towards strong lights and exaggerated 'smelling' of objects or people, may all be utilized by an individual to create or increase sensory stimulation. On occasions, individuals may, knowing their propensity to self-injury during such activities, assume self-restraining characteristics, for example, keeping hands in pockets or inside a shirt or other clothing, and thereby assume another stereotyped activity.

Non-functional and apparently purposeless activities such as headbanging, body rocking, slapping, biting or picking movements, may be exhibited by individuals who have serious learning difficulties and profound multiple handicaps. The

diagnosis of *stereotypy/habit disorder* relates to a wide number and variety of intentional and repetitive movements, which may include teeth grinding (bruxism), air swallowing (aerophagia), breath holding and hyperventilation, all in a rhythmic fashion. *Pervasive developmental disorders*, the best known being that of *autistic disorder*, are diagnostic categories utilized to describe children whose development within spheres of reciprocal social interaction, verbal and non-verbal communication skills and imaginative activity are severely and qualitively impaired. Children with such problems demonstrate motor and verbal stereotypies. Hand clapping and peculiar hand movements, such as flapping, body rocking, dipping and swaying actions and repetitious sniffing and smelling of objects or feeling of textures may all be examples of stereotypies seen.

On occasions, stereotype motor activities may be seen to enable individuals experiencing the sequelae of progressive organic impairment to cope with everyday life and living activities. *Over orderliness* may be utilized to compensate for perceived deficits in intellectual organization, emotional control or social awareness, as the individual demonstrates a rigid adherence to routine and repeated checking activities. *Perseveration*, the repetition of a recent movement, despite the individual's efforts towards production of a new movement and *literative* phenomena, as endless repetition of words or phrases (*echolalia*) may therefore be a feature in the presentation of many individuals seeking assistance.

Stereotyped movements of the mouth and tongue, and sorting and piling manoeuvres are seen in situations where amphetamines or cocaine intoxication is creating problems for the individual and repetitive motor activities and grimacing are similarly a feature of phencyclidine intoxication. The face pulling in 'catatonic–schizophrenia' may include the lips being thrust forwards like an animal's snout (schnauzkramp), and is accompanied by bizarre and excited stereotyped movements. The shorter duration 'schizophreniform disorder' may elicit similar characteristics as may manic episodes of mood disorders, and, whilst all may begin as an expression of emotional tension, or have a special and complex, almost magical, significance, they tend to become habitual and be produced automatically. The *compulsive* element of obsessive–compulsive behaviour differs somewhat in that the continued performance of ritualistic, stereotyped behaviour relieves the tensions and anxieties experienced and is therefore purposeful and intentionally conducted or initiated.

Tremors

Tremors are also something that you may have personal, or previous professional, experience of.

Her hands trembled and her knees shook, her legs feeling weak and powerless as he approached her. She could almost hear her racing heart as it thumped, in an effort to escape the ribcage which confined it …

The stuff that 'Mills and Boon' paperbacks are made of or an 'encounter in the Mummy's tomb'? Suffice to say, people experience a tremor when angry, afraid or anxious, or alternatively when excited or full of anticipation for a pleasurable event. Tremor may be an integral part of any emotion and, just to destroy completely the romantic associations which may have been provoked by the above example, we will reveal that a tremor represents a rhythmic and repetitive movement induced by alternating contractions of antagonistic muscle groups. Three variations of tremor are clearly distinguishable, the *rest tremor* is more pronounced at rest, the *intention tremor* worse on initiation of voluntary movement and the *postural tremor* is exaggerated, for example, when limbs are outstretched.

Rest tremor is a characteristic of *Parkinsonism*, with Parkinson's disease reflecting just one cause of the clinical picture demonstrated. Parkinsonism may be drug induced (neuroleptics), a sequela of encephalitis or arteriosclerotic changes, or may be the result of repeated head trauma, for example, as in boxing. It may be seen following anoxia and carbon monoxide poisoning, as well as many other events. The rest tremor of Parkinsonism is *coarse*, and demonstrates a characteristic 'pill-rolling' action as the thumb moves across the fingers. It is the result of interference with, or

degeneration of, the dopaminergic neurons in the substantia nigra and is accompanied by *bradykinesia*, a slowness in initiating and executing movement, including facial muscles and those related to speech production, and *rigidity*. The tremor of Parkinsonism is more resistant to amelioration by medication than the bradykinesia and rigidity experienced.

Intention tremor is associated with cerebellar lesions—tumours, aneurysms, abscesses, etc.—and is therefore often accompanied by *ataxia, dysarthria, nystagmus* and *dysdiadochokinesis* (poor, rapid alternating movements). Multiple sclerosis (MS) is one of the best examples of a 'discrete' somatic problem associated with such lesions, as the degeneration of the myelin sheath and resultant secondary destruction of axons, whilst scattered throughout the brain and spinal cord, are more common around the sites of the lateral ventricles and cerebellum. In response to destruction, glial cells proliferate and lymphocytes and macrophage cells infiltrate the tissues, the subsequent scar tissue being microscopically visible in the affected brain by translucent plaque distribution. The neurological manifestions associated with multiple sclerosis are multifocal and relapsing in nature, providing serially gained evidence of the lesions produced, rather than an immediately obvious, visible diagnosis.

Early symptoms of oculomotor function (diplopia or nystagmus), lesion of the long sensory and/or motor tracts of the cord (paraesthesia or spastic paraparesis) and cerebellar involvement (ataxia and intention tremor) may settle in weeks or months, leaving no or little residual disability. Further attacks may bring new symptoms or exacerbate pre-existing ones, with relapses and remissions demonstrating a variable course. Most frequently, a progressive and accumulatory picture develops and the individual experiences multiple handicaps. A slight intellectual impairment has been elicited, as in Surridge's (1969) study, particularly in relation to memory for recent events when it is often accompanied by confabulation, perseveration and dysphasia. Non-verbal reasoning abilities seemed similarly impaired along with general intellectual efficiency. Mood disturbances are also a common problem, with both depressed and elevated affect seen. Often depression is an early, and understandable, feature, whilst euphoria is more common as the lesions progress. Koenig (1968) described seven individuals who had presented and were diagnosed as having dementia, with relatively silent neurological manifestations. Careful neurological investigation had elicited the disseminated central nervous system lesions of MS and Koenig therefore suggested that silent MS may be a commoner cause of organic impairment than had previously been assumed or recognized. We will return to this point later.

Postural tremor is relatively more commonly seen than either rest or intention tremor, and may arise as a result of a variety of problems. Transmission, for example, of an autosomal dominant gene may elicit tremor of the arms and head in an individual of any age within an affected family. *Benign essential tremor* is rarely progressive, but may be suppressed by moderate amounts of alcohol or, in about one-third of individuals, by propranolol or primidone medication. Similarly, *Wilson's disease* or *hepatolenticular degeneration*, transmitted via an autosomal recessive gene, is a problem associated with metabolism of copper and may present as a hepatic dysfunction (40%), a neurological disorder (40%) or a mental health-related behavioural disorder (20%) (Bearn 1972). Jaundice, liver and spleen enlargement (hepatosplenomegaly), ascites and ankle oedema may all develop, and rupture of oesophageal varicies (dilated veins in collateral circulation at the oesophagogastric junction, 'haemorrhoids' in the oesophagus) may result in haematemesis. Neurologically, tremor may be one of several manifestations—rigidity, athetoid writhing movements and dystonic postures of the limbs. The tremor may be seen as a 'flapping' movement of the wrists, or a 'wing-beating' motion when arms are abducted and elbows flexed. The facial expression is stiff and the mouth is open and bears a rigid smile. Seizures, paralyses and disturbances in consciousness are not uncommon. A severe change in personality characteristics, hallucinations, delusional ideation, euphoria and catatonia and fatuous silliness have all been noted in relation to Wilson's disease. Whilst a rare condition,

Scheinberg, Sternlieb & Richman (1968) found that more than one-quarter of the 49 individuals studied demonstrated mental health-related problems as the first indicator of a dysfunction. Walker (1969) identified that all 12 of the people he studied had similarly developed mental health status deviations primarily and had been treated with drugs, electroplexy and psychotherapy.

Some early cognitive impairment, minor speech difficulties or distractibility provided the only evidence of neurological dysfunction in these individuals who had been categorized as school phobic, behaviour problem, personality disorder, depression, hysteria, schizophrenia and mental retardation. Eye examination, utilizing a slit lamp, will reveal the *Kayser–Fleischer ring*, a brown or greyish-green circle at the margin of the cornea that may be visible to the naked eye. No Kayser–Fleischer ring—no Wilson's disease, and as treatment may significantly improve the individual's health status, and as symptom-free siblings may respond well to prophylactic attention, slit-lamp examination would seem to be a sensible inclusion in client examination. Postural tremor may arise, therefore, from genetic transmission.

It may similarly be demonstrated due to metabolic dysfunctions, for example, where carbon dioxide retention (*hypercapnia*) is a problem, as in respiratory disease, respiratory muscle disease, left ventricular heart failure and brainstem lesions. Yet again the 'flapping tremor', previously described, is evident. Coarse tremor is a feature of other metabolic dysfunction, such as that associated with liver failure, when it may be referred to as *liver flap*.

Postural tremor may be exhibited as an exaggerated physiological mechanism associated with thyrotoxicosis, where as in anxious individuals, a *fine finger tremor* is witnessed. Perhaps attention may usefully be directed at this point to the indicators that may ring a warning bell and evoke concerns towards a diagnosis of thyroid problems rather than purely psychosocial aetiology. Any sensitivity to heat and an individual's expressed preference for cold conditions and environments should ring that bell. Similarly the appetite of the 'thyrotoxic' individual is characteristically increased and yet there is a concomitant steady weight loss evident. The individual experiencing anxiety, when complaining of weight loss, typically complains of a poor appetite and reduced intake of food to boot. Some people are equally likely to put on weight when anxious, via 'comfort eating' and in this instance, thyrotoxicosis is not a differential diagnosis which evokes concern. A simple blood test may ascertain a certain diagnosis where suspicions are raised.

The fine finger tremor of anxiety is often accompanied by complaints of disordered sensation—numbness (*anaesthesia*) and pins and needles (*paraesthesia*)—and by muscle tension and restlessness. Similarly, tremors may find exteriorization within somatically orientated mental health problems, for example, in *conversion* and *somatoform disorders*, where motor symptomatology associated with anaesthesias, paraesthesias, paralyses and coordination disturbances are frequent foci of attention. Tremors are a common experience in psychoactive substance intoxication and withdrawal with, for example, those individuals withdrawing from alcohol and sedatives, hypnotics and anxiolytic substances demonstrating a coarse tremor of hands, eyelids and tongue, as well as, on occasions, myoclonic jerks. Intoxication frequently produces tremor, incoordination and an unsteady gait.

Tics

Tics are involuntary in nature, and may be described as sudden, rapid, recurrent though non-rhythmic, stereotyped movements, or vocalizations. Simple tics, such as eye blinking, neck jerking, coughing and grunting may be seen in childhood, and are always exacerbated by stress and greatly diminished during sleep. Tics may appear and disappear almost overnight for some, although any recurrence is always associated with stress. On occasions, multiple tics are seen and whilst at times these may revolve around the facial area, whole head, torso and limb involvement may also be a problem. Where more than one tic is evident, these may appear simultaneously, sequentially or randomly, and whilst some individuals may become adept at suppressing them for varying lengths of time, they are eventually irresistible.

Children and young adolescents affected are frequently seen to be 'uncomfortable' with themselves and social situations, and this may obviously lead to depressed mood.

Tourette's disorder is probably the best known of the pathological categories seen and involves multiple motor and one, or more, vocal tics which may appear simultaneously or at different points along the course of development. They are manifest several times a day, most days, and whilst typically affecting the head area, may also involve the rest of the body. The vocal tics may resemble barks, grunts, yelps, sniffs or words, and *coprolalia* (uttering obscene words) may be a problem for approximately one-third of all sufferers. Lesser extremes of the Tourette disorder may be seen in some who demonstrate motor or vocal tics but not both, which may be referred to as a *chronic motor or vocal tic*, and where the duration of the problem is seen to be of less than 12 months, a *transient tic disorder* may be diagnosed.

Myoclonus is an involuntary, unexpected and sudden jerk of a muscle, or part of a muscle, and you may have experience of the phenomenon when dropping off to sleep at night. However, as well as being an innocent and benign occurrence, myoclonus may be indicative of serious somatic health problems. It may be seen, for example, in childhood as *benign essential myoclonus*, when it is associated with an autosomal dominant genetic inheritance. Similarly it may be indicative of encephalopathy in response to a variety of metabolic disorders, for example, lysosomal storage enzyme deficits, and focal myoclonic jerks may herald viral myelitis. Both single and multiple myoclonic jerks are associated with epilepsy, and, as epilepsy should be regarded as a symptom rather than as a specific dysfunction or entity in its own right, myoclonus may be associated with somatic health problems ranging in aetiology from trauma to space-occupying lesions, encephalitis to syphilis, hypo- and hyperglycaemia to hypo/hypernatraemia, and from liver to renal disease. Drugs may precipitate seizures, phenothiazines, tricyclics and cocaine may all be culpable, and similarly withdrawal from alcohol, sedatives, hypnotics and anxiolytic preparations may provoke myoclonus and seizures. There is, however, a rare epilepsy that is associated with inheritance via an autosomal recessive gene. The *myoclonic epilepsy of Unverricht* comprises of increasingly frequent myoclonic jerks and a severe and progressive dementia. The link between epilepsy and myoclonus is well recognized.

Human variant *Creutzfeldt–Jakob disease* (CJD) has been brought to public attention via the problems of 'mad cow disease' or *bovine spongiform encephalopathy* (BSE). A progressive organic deterioration in which the grey matter of the brain degenerates and assumes a spongy appearance, the aetiology is one of a slow viral nature. Survival usually appears to be of a period not exceeding two years' duration, the individual sinking into a coma for several weeks prior to death. Myoclonic jerks and epilepsy are frequent features, and may be accompanied by spasticity, progressive paralysis or choreoathetoid movements. Speech may be impaired, with dysarthria and dysphasia, and cortical degeneration may provoke blindness. Neurological features vary considerably and are dependent, of course, upon structures involved. Progressive intellectual and neurological deterioration, with, on occasions, auditory hallucinations and delusional ideation demonstrated, leads to a profound dementia, spastic paralysis and severe emaciation.

The similarities between Creutzfeldt–Jakob disease, Kuru and 'scrapie' have long since been linked. *Kuru* is a dementia, restricted to the Fore tribe of New Guinea and, again, the sequelae of a transmissible agent, although genetic predisposition and a 'taste', in the past, for cannibalism may also have a role in transmission. *Scrapie* is a degenerative brain disease of sheep and is also the agent discovered in some forms of Creutzfeldt–Jakob disease. All result in this spongy appearance of the brain and therefore are, in the present climate, worthy of further investigation, via, for example, the work of Beck and his colleagues (Beck et al 1966, 1969a,b). Links between scrapie and BSE are already confirmed, with aetiology of the latter firmly laid on feeding affected cows with infected sheep offal. Concern for human health must be raised in this regard.

Of course tics and myoclonus must be differentiated from a wide number of involuntary and

more complex patterns of movement, for example, *choreiform movements*, which tend to be irregular, random, non-repetitive dance-like movements. These are semipurposive and involve muscle groups of the face, limbs or trunk and, as in Huntington's disease, which is inherited via an autosomal dominant gene, may begin as small tics or mannerisms, which are easily disguised, but progress to involve the whole body. That associated with an inflammatory encephalitis, Sydenham's chorea (or St Vitus' dance), may be seen to resolve slowly over several months but may recur at a later date. *Athetosis*, a slow writhing movement of fingers, hands and arms, is associated with damage to the putamen and globus pallidus and *hemiballismus*, characterized by sudden, forceful, violent and flailing movements of one side of the body, and commonly affecting proximal muscles of the limbs, is associated with subthalamic nucleus damage. It is, on occasions, a feature following cerebrovascular accident, particularly in elderly diabetic individuals and usually subsides within months of the lesion. *Dystonia* describes distressing, painful and involuntary muscular contractions which may commonly be associated with the ocular, facial, neck, lingual and spinal muscles and more rarely the limbs. *Dystonia musculorum deformans* describes a generalized torsion dystonia, of unknown aetiology and yet with an apparently genetic basis in some instances, which is severe and progressively crippling. Anoxia or jaundice at birth may create a similar problem, as may tumours and infarctions of the basal ganglia. Cerebral pathology is known therefore to cause such problems, and the *oculogyric crises* and *spasmodic torticollis* occasionally seen following neuroleptic administration would appear to support such a view. However, there continues to be some dispute as to the organic versus psychogenic causation of several dystonias, including spasmodic torticollis, writer's cramp and blepharospasm.

Akathisia is similarly a problem associated with involuntary movement and again with neuroleptic use. The individual complains of an inability to stand or sit still and rocks, paces, shifts from foot to foot or taps his feet continuously, feeling 'tightened up and out of control'. This purposeless limb movement may be accompanied by myoclonus and a coarse tremor.

Tardive or *orofacial dyskinesia* represents another extrapyramidal side-effect of neuroleptic use. It occurs in 1–2% of individuals administered such preparations for a year or more, though this risk is seen to increase in a variety of situations, for example, with increasing age (elderly women are said to be most at risk), increasing dosage and administration period, where there is underlying cerebral pathology and with anticholinergic medication, which may exacerbate existing, or expose latent, symptomatology. It may be seen to be reversible in only one-third of presentations (Appleby & Forshaw 1990). Problems experienced by the individual include involuntary chewing, mouth and jaw movements, and grimacing. Mild choreiform movements of the extremities, shoulder shrugging and rocking actions may also be evident. An early, prodromal, indicator of the problem is the individuals' inability to stick out (extrude) their tongue and keep it there for a minute or two. On occasions, a *tardive dystonia* or *tardive Tourette's syndrome* have also been exhibited in relation to neuroleptic use.

Ataxia

You may recall the previously identified need for proprioceptive information via skeletal muscles and tendons to facilitate kinaesthetic knowledge, that is, where and in what position limbs are currently in relation to the rest of the body position. *Ataxia* is the term used to describe a loss of that proprioceptive sense, with the result that there is a lack of coordination of muscle action between the extremities and the head and trunk. Individuals are not quite sure of their position and are unable therefore to judge or control skeletal movements. The cerebellum, which receives all information concerning this orientation and is therefore crucial in coordination of such activities, may be elicited as the site of a lesion which evokes ataxia. The 'finger to nose' test is failed and a characteristic gait of staggering, reeling, erratic steps, with perhaps a deviation to one side is seen. This *cerebellar gait* is also characterized by the vigorous projection of the legs forwards and the forceful slapping

of the feet on to the floor. If truncal ataxia is seen to be worse when the individual's eyes are closed, the lesion is in the dorsal columns, the spinocerebellar tracts, rather than the cerebellum. *Friedreich's ataxia*, one of the commonest hereditary diseases of the nervous system, is also one of the commonest spinocerebellar ataxias seen. It is inherited via an autosomal recessive or, rarely, sex-linked gene, and with an onset typically in childhood or the teenage years, it may be mistaken for the 'normal' clumsy, incoordinated motor behaviour of youth. Spinocerebellar tracts degenerate, so that the original unsteadiness of gait progresses to the broad-based, lurching action associated with cerebellar dysfunction. Dysarthria, nystagmus and dysdiadochokinesis are all accompanying features. Myocardial involvement and optic atrophy may occur and characteristic deformities of musculature as *kyphoscoliosis*, a forward and lateral curvature of the spine and *pes cava*, a shortened, inverted, high arched foot with clawed toes, may precede neurological symptomatology.

Wernicke–Korsakoff's syndrome, often incorrectly solely linked with alcohol abuse, is in fact the result of a thiamine (vitamin B_1) deficiency of a variety of causes—dietary deficiency, pernicious anaemia, carcinoma of the stomach as well as alcohol-related problems. The problems demonstrated are the sequelae of tiny haemorrhages, particularly in the area surrounding the ventricles of the brain, with cell loss and subsequent glial and vascular proliferation. The *staggering gait* is accompanied by ataxia, demonstrated as the inability to stand upright and steady without support and on occasions by an inability to walk heel to toe, as along a straight line. These tests are of course utilized to assess an individual's capability to drive in relation to alcohol ingestion, indicating that intoxication will elicit similar, though temporary, features. Wernicke's encephalopathy is considered as the acute reaction to the causative factor and an emergency situation, whilst Korsakoff's is considered to be the stage of permanent damage. They represent two points on the same continuum, and may both elicit, therefore, confusion, nystagmus and eye muscle weakness or paralysis (*ophthalmoplegia*). The latter, due to third nerve lesion, shows an outward deviation of the eyeball and a dilated pupil, which is unresponsive to light and accommodation. *Ptosis*, a drooping of the upper lids, is also evident.

The *high-stepping gait* indicative of the *sensory ataxia* of *tabes dorsalis*, due to neurosyphilis, demonstrates the effect on coordination of degeneration of the ascending fibres. The individual describes the sensation of 'walking on cotton wool', with extreme skin hypersensitivity, paraesthesia in the legs and feet and severe, sharp, episodic stabbing pains in the legs that may extend to the trunk as girdle pains.

Whilst mentioning the specific gaits associated with ataxia, it is worth nothing the characteristic *small-stepped gait* of *multi-infarct dementia*, the shuffling, flexed trunk, *festinant gait* of Parkinsonism and the *scissor gait* associated with spasticity of the lower limbs, where one leg is placed directly in front of the other and where thighs and legs are abducted, the knees rubbing with each step. The amount of information available by mere observation of the manner in which an individual walks into a room can be astounding.

Apraxia

We feel obliged to refer to one more phenomenon prior to closure of this section on movement and its related problems, and this relates to *apraxia*, the inability to execute purposive coordinated movement despite intact sensory and motor function and the desire to perform that movement. The association cortex of the parietal lobes, and particularly that of the non-dominant hemisphere, is responsible for an awareness of the body and the relationship between objects in the environment. Lesions within the non-dominant hemisphere lead to *constructional apraxia*, a defect in assembling or drawing items and *dressing apraxia*, where the individual is unable to get limbs into garments or clothing over the head. *Ideomotor apraxia*, an inability to perform a series of coordinated movements despite an understanding of the request preceding it, is a feature of dominant parietal lobe lesion. *Gait apraxia* may be the explanation for a gait disorder when each of the separate components required for walking is found to be intact. It is seen to be a problem where lesions affect bilateral frontal lobes or posterior temporal lobe regions. *Ideational apraxia* finds the individual 'unaware' of the coordinated actions necessary to achieve a task, for example, taking a match from a closed box of matches and striking it. The concepts of the required acts and the planning of the act both appear disturbed. It is always bilateral, usually a lesion of the dominant hemisphere and most frequently of parietal or temporal lobe origin. Apraxias are more often evident where damage is diffuse rather than localized and therefore cognitive and intellectual functioning is frequently impaired.

SUMMARY

We have outlined some of the problems associated with movement and provided examples of these problems within both somatic and mental health care specialties. There are very fine dividing lines at times between the two fields and frequently incorrect diagnosis is a potential. Clients have been admitted to mental health and learning disability care facilities when somatic health care was necessary and examples of somatic care being offered or instigated where problems are of a predominantly psychosocial origin abound. It is, therefore, of vital importance that the health care worker, regardless of the specialty service provided, has an awareness of what is on the 'other side' of that fine dividing line and is therefore competent to ask appropriate questions of the client, based upon that knowledge and the observations made. It is imperative that entrance into mental health orientated services does not evoke an assumption that problems exteriorized or experienced are automatically psychogenic in origin. Investigation may prove a somatic basis for the symptomatology, which may be eradicated or ameliorated with appropriate care and treatment. Similarly the individual with a history of psychosocial problems and mental health care *can* become physically ill in the same way as any other member of society and that any alteration in functioning is worthy of further exploration. Remember George!

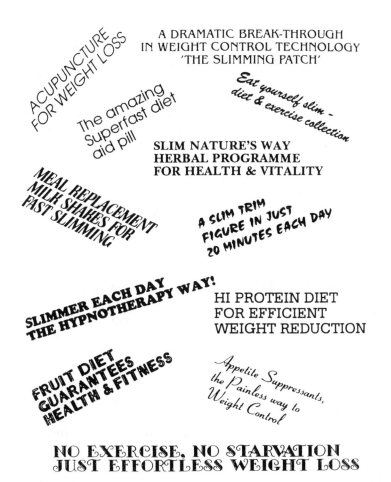

A DRAMATIC BREAK-THROUGH
IN WEIGHT CONTROL TECHNOLOGY
'THE SLIMMING PATCH'

ACUPUNCTURE FOR WEIGHT LOSS

The amazing Superfast diet aid pill

Eat yourself slim - diet & exercise collection

SLIM NATURE'S WAY
HERBAL PROGRAMME
FOR HEALTH & VITALITY

MEAL REPLACEMENT MILK SHAKES FOR FAST SLIMMING

A SLIM TRIM FIGURE IN JUST 20 MINUTES EACH DAY

SLIMMER EACH DAY THE HYPNOTHERAPY WAY!

HI PROTEIN DIET
FOR EFFICIENT
WEIGHT REDUCTION

FRUIT DIET GUARANTEES HEALTH & FITNESS

Appetite Suppressants, the Painless way to Weight Control

NO EXERCISE, NO STARVATION
JUST EFFORTLESS WEIGHT LOSS

Fig. 4.2 Typical dieting slogans.

EATING

INTRODUCTION

Millions of pounds every year are spent on slimming products and everywhere one looks, advertisements suggest products that will assist the individual, 'as part of a calorie controlled diet' to lose weight, more or less quickly, to have a 'fabulous physique in just 20 minutes a day' to produce a 'slimmer, more attractive youthful you' (Fig. 4.2). It is official, however, that some of the population *are* overweight and, if you were to secrete yourself in any large chemist store and note the number of slimming products purchased, it would be assumed that the figure must be a high

one. One of the targets included in The health of the nation (DOH 1992), indeed is the goal:

To reduce the percentages of men and women aged 16–64 who are obese by at least 25% for men and at least 33% for women by the year 2005 ...

So, it would seem that the diet-preparation manufacturers are set for a boom time over the next 10 years or so—or are they? The target continues by providing the actual figures of the 'obese' population as:

from 8% for men and 12% for women in 1986/87 to no more than 6% and 8% respectively.

Of course these percentages still represent a great many people, all of whom are 'at risk' in relation to a variety of somatic problems, but will the diets, slimming pills and exercises work and help in weight reduction, and will the slimmer, more healthy individual be able to maintain that loss? And, if so few—relatively speaking—within the population are overweight and remain overweight, then who is buying all of the diet aids? Perhaps if the dieter knew a little more about the body mechanisms involved, the individual would be in a more powerful position with regard to selection of 'regimes' and 'maintenance programmes' on offer. What does the evidence tell us?

INTAKE, UTILIZATION AND OUTPUT

Food taken into the body is converted, via processes of chemical, mechanical and bacterial breakdown in the gastrointestinal tract, into substances suitable for absorption by the stomach and large intestine (10%) but mainly by the small intestine (90%). Glucose is derived from carbohydrates, amino acids from proteins ingested, and monoglycerides and fatty acids from fat intake, and in this form may be absorbed for utilization.

Material not required by the body for immediate use is converted to fat or to the insoluble glucose polymer, glycogen, and stored for future use. Glucose is the major energy source for all tissues, and, when necessary, the liver will convert the stored fat and amino acids into glucose for use.

Dieter's tip no. 1
All food taken in excess of body requirements will be stored.

Dieter's tip no. 2
All food means all food. Whether of a protein, fat or carbohydrate nature, excess will be stored.

Dieter's tip no. 3
When energy requirements exceed circulating glucose availability, stored material will be brought into play to provide added fuel, thus depleting stores.

With the exception of the cells of the nervous system, insulin, manufactured by the beta cells of the pancreas, is necessary to facilitate cellular uptake of glucose from the circulating blood. It reduces blood sugar levels not only in this manner, but also by accelerating conversion of glucose into storable glycogen and stimulating conversion of glucose and any other excess nutrients into fatty acids. Insulin also increases the build-up of proteins by cells.

HUNGER AND SATIATION

Despite the measures taken by any organism, no matter how simple or complex, to store available excesses of nutrients ingested, those stores require continual replenishment when normal activities are undertaken on a daily basis. Some animals, of course, overeat at the commencement of winter, storing as much fat as possible for both warmth and nutrition during hibernation. However, in order to survive that period of food abstinence, the animal must lower its metabolic rate and become inactive, merely ticking over in a state of suspended animation, until the spring, warmer climes and fresh vegetation appears to enable it to 'live' again. The fully awake, but store-depleted animal must now overeat until it reaches a weight at which it can match its energy requirements and yet still have a little 'put aside' for emergencies. This, as will be demonstrated below, is of great significance to the human 'dieter', but the fact is that the instinct for self-preservation in any organism initiates food-seeking behaviour, the feelings and sensations associated with which, we call 'hunger'.

The total mechanism for 'stock control and reordering of supplies' is less than completely understood but there would appear to be sufficient facts available to give an outline of the processes involved. Jean Mayer (1955), an American nutritionist, asserted that the body monitors glucose levels in the blood, via detectors called glucostats, specialized neurons which, it was proposed, fired at a higher rate when glucose levels were reduced, thus setting up the hunger drive and food-seeking behaviours. There is, indeed, monitoring of glucose levels in the lateral hypothalamus and also in the liver, which assesses nutrient absorption via the portal vein, sending information back to 'control' by way of the vagus nerve. However, experimentation in animals whereby the vagus nerve was severed (Tardoff, Hoffenbeck & Novin 1982) demonstrated no effect on eating behaviour, indicating that hunger and glucose level fluctuation appeared only obscurely connected. Further studies demonstrated that glucose levels within the blood fluctuate very little, despite the amount, nature or timing of food intake, and again the assumption must be that efficient conversion and storage of superfluous nutrients facilitates immediate reconversion and use when levels begin to signal a drop.

This is, of course, the point to reintroduce the example of the hibernating animal and his feeding patterns, pre- and postsleep, for it has been found that an experimental animal, deliberately starved and exhibiting signs of weight loss, will, when given the opportunity to feed freely, overeat until it regains the fat it has lost. Conversely, the animal who has been force fed until obese will, when in control of its own eating, undereat until the excess fat has been lost. There is a maintenance of total body fat at a reasonably constant level in adult animals and intake of food is regulated in relation to this. Somewhere within the brain there must be a representation of the amount of body fat necessary to individuals and their patterns of activity, in just the same way that the brain is aware of joint and muscle position.

Role of the hypothalamus

Dieter's tip no. 4
Your brain 'knows' how fat you are supposed to be. No matter your weight loss on the diet, when you 'free-feed', you will adjust upwards to your normal body weight.

Two areas of the brain appear to be of significance here, for damage to the lateral hypothalamus of a rat results in a refusal to eat or drink. If not fed artificially, the rat dies, but where intravenous feeding is undertaken for several weeks, the rat begins to recover its appetite, initially for wet food

but not for drink, and later for both food and drink. When feeding freely, the rat's weight is found to stabilize at a lower 'new' norm. Even in situations where the rat has been starved prior to the lesioning, when eating freely it will stabilize at a point of starved level (i.e. it will overeat for a time) but below that of its original weight. Lateral hypothalamic damage provokes a reduction and stabilization at a level below the previous norm (Mitchell & Keesey 1974).

Conversely, where tissue of the ventromedial region of the hypothalamus is destroyed, the rat will initially overeat for a period of up to 3 months, but then reduce its intake by an amount sufficient to maintain the new obese 'normal' weight. Should the new 'obese' rat find that food is restricted, its body weight is found to reduce to its original level and then be maintained. However, when allowed to feed freely, the obese level is achieved and again maintained (Hoebel & Teitelbaum 1966). It would appear, therefore, that both the lateral and ventromedial regions of the hypothalamus play a part in the set point for body weight, balancing each other to create the 'norm' to be expected and striven to be maintained, and indeed when precisely the same degree of damage is inflicted on both areas simultaneously, the animal exhibits no change in feeding behaviours, maintaining weight at its original, pre-operative level (Keesey & Powley 1975).

However, omitted from the above is the fact that, in damaging these specific areas of the hypothalamus, nerve fibres in the area may also suffer damage and therefore may influence observations. Indeed, Friedman & Stricker (1976), point out that damage to the nigrostriatal bundle, nerve fibres associated with the initiation not only of feeding but also other behaviours, inflicted at a point outside of the hypothalamus creates a variety of activation problems in the animal, including the refusal to eat and drink seen in the early stages of lateral hypothalamic lesioning. Similarly, branches of the parasympathetic nervous system pass through the area of the ventromedial hypothalamus, and, as these are seen to increase the rate at which nutrients are stored by the body at the expense of immediately available fuel, damage to these fibres will produce an animal constantly in need of circulating nutrients and therefore perpetually eating. The rat, therefore, behaves in the manner associated with that of a ventral medial hypothalamic-lesioned animal.

There is, however, no doubt of the new weight level achieved by hypothalamic-damaged rats and it is possible that the specific regions of the hypothalamus and the named nerve pathways are synergistic, working together to achieve a balanced body weight, suitable to the animal's function on a long term basis.

Other factors?

In addition to the long term overview of a set point for optimum survival potential, a more immediately acting mechanism is necessary to facilitate adjustment of eating patterns and the rate of metabolism to meet those long term goals for weight. The mechanism by which this appears to be achieved is via a circulating chemical substance, rather than by innervation, as demonstrated in the 'mouse experiments' conducted by Coleman & Hummel (1969). They surgically joined two mice, one obese and one normally lean, so that the animals shared a cardiovascular and extracellular fluid circulation, but had separate nervous systems. Therefore when the lean mouse began to undereat, just as if obese, this could not have been due to the influence of the obese mouse's nervous system, it had to have been achieved via a circulating messenger.

Insulin has been suggested as the regulator of body weight and therefore food intake and yet the cells of the nervous system utilize glucose directly and do not require insulin to achieve this uptake and indeed passage of insulin across the blood–brain barrier is achieved only with difficulty. Yet insulin is present within cerebrospinal fluid and there are receptor sites for this hormone within the brain, particularly in the olfactory lobe and hypothalamus. Indeed, microelectrodes implanted in the hypothalami of animals elicit a decrease in neural activity within the region after glucose is given by injection and an increase in activity in the same area following administration of insulin, thereby demonstrating adequate and diminished levels of circulating glucose respectively (Stricker

et al 1977). Further evidence to support insulin as an integral part of the initiation and termination of feeding behaviours is supplied by both Davis & Brief (1981) in their rat studies, and Woods et al (1979) in their experiments on baboons. Continuous infusion of insulin into the cerebrospinal fluid, or persistent application directly on to the neurons of the ventral region of the hypothalamus, induces firing of the cells and heralds a reduction in eating behaviours and therefore weight loss. As a passing thought, this could account for the demonstration of insatiable appetite and yet continuing weight loss associated with the onset of diabetes mellitus. If insulin is deficient or absent, neuronal firing within the ventral area of the hypothalamus will not occur and feeding behaviour will continue.

Of course if you had to wait for depleted stores to be replenished before ceasing food intake, you would be eating for quite some time at each stretch, for it takes 4 to 5 hours or more for complete gastric emptying, approximately the same period of time to journey through the small intestine, where most nutrients are absorbed, and then storage activities must be undertaken. Most of the day would be spent in breakfasting! Instead, the reality is that you eat until you have 'had enough' or are 'full' and then push your plate away. How is it that you know that you have eaten sufficient to keep the brain happy and the stores replete? The ventromedial aspect of the hypothalamus requires absorption to have taken place before it can make adjustments based on the blood sugar level and the amount of insulin circulating and although valuable as a mechanism, insulin is not secreted until glucose and fats enter the duodenum, which may again take some time, depending upon the nature of the food taken.

Janowitz & Grossman (1949) looked to the upper portion of the tract—the mouth and throat—in their efforts to locate satiety sensors and severed the oesophagus of a dog from the stomach in an effort to assess the effects of food entering the mouth upon feeding patterns. The researchers found that, whilst the animal ate a larger than usual meal prior to ceasing activities, it soon recommenced eating. The assertion that satiation sensors exist within this area was therefore proven, for the animal did desist from feeding activities, but the more rapid than usual return to eating indicates the short term nature of their effect. When redirecting attention to the stomach, it is obvious that satiety sensors are present within the area, for feeding via gastronomy satisfies hunger, and reduces food-seeking behaviours. Certainly stretch receptors in the stomach wall become activated when an animal risks injury by overfilling its stomach—the 'I just can't eat another bite' syndrome—and there is cessation of feeding. However, it would appear that the major satiation mechanism is mediated via the digestive hormones secreted by the gastrointestinal system during food digestion. There are a number of such hormones and the exact ones secreted depend upon the nature of the meal taken. The intestinal mucosa secretes, for example, cholecystokinin (CCK) directly into the blood supply in response to protein- and fat-based foods entering the duodenum. Amongst other effects, CCK stimulates the pancreas to secrete its enzyme-rich secretion, provokes contraction of the gall bladder and therefore release of bile, and slows the rate by which gastric emptying occurs. There are other such hormones—secretin, vasoactive intestinal polypeptide (VIP), gastric inhibitory peptide (GIP) and somatostatin—all of which circulate in response to specific foodstuffs within the gastrointestinal system and all of which appear to have a dual role. In their response to particular foods within the system, they achieve a tailoring of the appropriate digestive processes to match need. However, they also appear to interact with the nervous system to regulate intake. GIP, for example, is known to stimulate insulin production in response to glucose and fat entering the duodenum, and insulin is shown to influence feeding patterns. Injections of CCK have similarly been demonstrated as inhibiting eating (MacLean 1977). Hungry rats when transfused with the blood of well-fed peers demonstrate reduced feeding activities (West et al 1982) thus indicating that these circulating satiety factors pass directly to the brain to influence the point at which eating should be terminated.

The link between the neurotransmitter *noradrenaline* is acknowledged but vague. It is known, however, that preparations such as amphetamines release stored noradrenaline from axon terminals or inhibit its reuptake, and amphetamines can inhibit eating, hence their historical use as a diet aid. Passing through the lateral hypothalamus are several neural tracks that carry the transmitter and therefore it is present within the relevant locale. Noradrenaline, and the similarly structured adrenaline, do play a substantial role in the sympathetic activity, mediated via the hypothalamus, during stress. A reduced rate of digestive action and increased blood sugar level in the body's preparation for 'fight or flight' are demonstrable and hence connections between feeding, behaviours, the hypothalamus and the neurotransmitter appear strengthened.

One other point worthy of mention is that *endorphins* appear to increase the amount of food consumed during a meal. Endorphins are neuropeptides, the 'endogenous opiates', and are associated with suppression of pain, linked to memory and learning, regulation of body temperature, and sexual activity. There are connections, too, with the mental health problems diagnosed as 'schizophrenia' and 'depression'. Increased level of endorphins within the pituitary glands of genetically obese rats and mice suggest that there may be a relationship with feeding behaviours.

Metabolic rates

Metabolic rate influences intentional or naturally occurring diet reduction. The metabolic rate indicates the speed at which the synthesis and decomposition activities occur within the body, that is, the result of anabolic and catabolic reactions. An increase in the rate will elicit more rapid decomposition activities and foodstuffs broken down too quickly for the body to get the chance to do any storing activities. Unless the individual increases food intake, the inability to replenish utilized stores will result in weight reduction. A lowered metabolic rate will engender the converse, for food will be broken down more slowly and often incompletely and then stored. The individual gains weight easily. The sad truth for the dieter must be in the automatic response of the body to slow down metabolic activities when insufficient food is taken in to meet the brain's perceived needs. It is a protective mechanism designed to reduce energy expenditure and maintain store levels at the highest point possible for as long as is possible. The individual feels tired and energy-less, often complaining of feeling cold, as 'savings' are automatically made by the brain in whatever area possible, so that demands are reduced as far as possible in order to conserve those supplies. By this mechanism weight loss is reduced and it therefore falls to the higher cognitive powers of the human to initiate activities that will provoke a rise in metabolism, thus 'forcing' the brain to relinquish its hold on body stores, and facilitating weight loss acceleration.

Dieter's tip No. 5

Dieting, without a simultaneous increase in physical activity, may elicit disappointing weight loss. A combination of diet and exercise will be more likely to show results.

It would seem then that long term regulation of food intake is controlled by the brain's representation of the fat stores of the body. Insulin would appear to provide indication of the current status of stores and hence signal the need for intake of food and therefore eating behaviours. Cessation of eating would appear to be the responsibility of the digestive hormones, or gut peptides, in conjunction with the hypothalamus. So where is the dieter in all of this? At the moment things do not look too optimistic in relation to intentional weight reduction. But if an individual wishes to maintain a body weight conducive to looking good, when the cerebral 'fat controller' deems differently, is it physiologically feasible?

PSYCHOSOCIAL INFLUENCES

Sometimes the wolf children would get there first and whether it was meat for the table or a dead animal or bird that they had found—they were particularly fond of rotten meat—they did not care to be obstructed … it was a constant worry after witnessing their summary dealings with mice and cockroaches, that they would soon kill something larger.
MacLean 1977

Amala and Kamala had been raised by wolves in their den until 'rescued' by the Reverend Singh, in 1920, and taken to his orphanage at Midnapore. At that time, aged approximately 6 and 3 years respectively, their diet, method of locomotion, communication strategies and sleep–wake cycle reflected their socialization by the she-wolf as her cubs. The Singhs tried hard to 'civilize' the children into a more acceptable lifestyle, but the older one survived only a year and Kamala only 9 years. The doctor in attendance believed their deaths to be due in part to the attempt to change their dietary intake radically by suppressing the availability of the accustomed raw meat diet and imposing cooked mixed food for which their gastrointestinal tract was unprepared. This resulted in the generally weakened physical state and, in addition, gut irritability. Dysentery, fever and worm infestation further compounded the already lowered resistance and the exposure to human infections, for which sustenance by the she-wolf had given no immunity, found the children unprepared and unfit for human life and contact. Both children died of renal failure and even Kamala, an 'adolescent' 12-year-old by the time of her demise, demonstrated a very limited degree of 'civilized' behaviour as the result of her 9 years of human contact and 'assistance'.

We would probably find both our sensibilities and stomachs offended by the thought of killing dinner before eating it, or of being served with cockroach or mouse—raw or cooked—for this has not been a part of the socialization processes to which we have been exposed. Diet is one of the 'norms' of a culture, reflecting both traditional influences and the modifications concomitant in the changes of that society. In years past, an individual and family were reliant on what they themselves could produce, excess being exchanged or sold for other goods or services necessary. Today, few survive on the commodities that they home grow or rear and foodstuffs are mass produced on a large, more efficient scale and sold to the rest of the population.

Socialization in regard to eating may be deemed as relatively unimportant and yet it provides the rules governing the individual's dietary and social behaviour. At a party, an individual will eat whether hungry or not, because everyone else is eating and food is an integral part of every major milestone in life—christenings, weddings and funerals being examples. Meals may be the only times that a family comes together because of the different daily occupations and as such may be considered as priority by the family, or at least, the adult members—the rule makers—of that family. It represents the continuing nurturing responsibilities of the adults towards their offspring and is governed by rules and hence provides socialization opportunities. Exclusion from the meal table or from a meal is a punishment used by adults to express disapproval of behaviour—'You don't deserve to join us, please eat in the kitchen' and 'No supper for you, go to your room', being typical admonishments. Similarly it is used as a weapon by the child, knowing that it will evoke parental concern and therefore increased, comforting-style attention. It provides a consolation when things go wrong or the child is hurt—a grazed knee evokes the offer of a 'sweetie' to take away the pain and coming second in a competition or race deserves a chocolate bar on the way home. Sugary, sweet things are seen as a reward and the principle may be instilled early. Sweetness is something special and desired, reflected in the offering of chocolates to say 'I'm sorry' or 'I love you', the Christmas tree chocolate novelties and the Easter eggs. Food, and especially sweet food, may be seen to represent much more to the individual than mere sustenance.

The importance of all of the above to the dieter is that, whilst the human and every other animal is born with a prescribed number of fat cells, genetics only prescribes the *minimum* number of fat cells and, though this minimum number cannot be lost, they can be increased in number by overeating in both childhood and adult years. As the overweight child frequently becomes an overweight adult (West et al 1982), both genetics and upbringing may play significant roles within weight control. Knittle & Hirsch (1968) demonstrated that rats with twice the normal number of fat cells are double the body weight of their control group peers and Faust (1984) found that by removing half of the normal size rat's fat cells they developed to only half the sized of their siblings. Obeser people similarly show larger fat cells than their normal weight counterparts, and Faust et al (1978) suggest that it is the *volume* of these cells that provides the brain with its regulatory system. The assertion is that when fat cell volume decreases, the brain initiates food-seeking behaviours to restore the depleted volume to the set points discussed earlier.

The enzyme *lipoprotein lipase* is also of significance to the dieter for there is an increased level of this substance in the obese individual and animal alike. It is responsible for both the removal of fat from circulation and its storage in the adipocytes (fat cells), and when the obese restrict their food intake, the lipoprotein lipase level elevates further. It would appear that this higher level indicates continuing fat storage as a priority even where intake is restricted and may account for the periods of plateau experienced by dieters when they lose no further weight, or no weight at all, for often prolonged periods of time. It would certainly appear to be an integral part of the body's regulation of body fat and therefore weight control.

Upbringing and socialization processes may be seen therefore to influence eating behaviours and weight control. An association between food—especially sweet sticky food—and comfort, ease and contentment, and the curer of all ills, pains and disappointments, is a coping mechanism of dubious value and potential detriment to the individual.

People, whether obese, normally or underweighted, appear to fall naturally into two groups, those who show restraint in eating and those who do not. Studies (Herman & Polivy 1980, Ruderman 1986) consistently show the eating behaviours of the restrained eater are more similar to those of obese people than to the unrestrained eater. Restrained eaters consume more than their non-dieting counterparts, indicating their deprivation subsequently results in overeating, despite their original weight levels having been regained (Coscina & Dixon 1983). This would account for the common phenomenon of dieters who initially successfully lose weight only to exceed their original level when restraints are relaxed. Similarly it may be responsible for the binge eating associated with anorexia nervosa, though of course weight increase is not seen because of induced vomiting and purging behaviours.

Obese people often demonstrate different attitudes and psychological responses to food, which may reflect the elevated lipoprotein lipase level and resultant chronic hunger associated with this enzyme. Similarities have been drawn (Schachter 1971) between behaviours of obese individuals and those of the ventromedially hypothalamic damaged rat and yet no evidence of similar damage in these individuals has been demonstrated. However, overweight people are visibly more susceptible to food cues, such as the sight, aroma, texture and colour of foods, than their normally weighted peers and tend to be more selective in their choice of food and drink. They will drink less of a nondescript tasting milk shake and more of a flavourful one than the normally weighted person, for example. Despite their interest in food, Schachter (1971) found overweight people less likely to make an effort to gain available food. In studies where obese and normal-weight individuals were left alone in a room with a bowl of nuts—still in their shells—and a nutcracker, only 1 of 20 obese people used the nutcracker and ate a few of the nuts, in comparison to 10 of 20 normal weight subjects.

In our opinion, all of the above bodes poorly for the Government's weight-reducing target for the adult population. No matter how often an individual achieves a weight reduction, the brain will evoke its animalistic instincts and redress the balance, and indeed exceed the norm to ensure survival of the organism. The only way it would seem to us to achieve a reduction in obese adults is to educate parents into the necessity for sensible eating patterns in their children from birth and to inculcate the values of exercise for everyone.

PROBLEMS ASSOCIATED WITH EATING

There are a number of situations in which the individual is *unable* to control the intake of food and which may, therefore, produce a dependence upon others to ensure effective nutritional status. The most obvious of these is that of the young infant and the child and the previous identification of the reliance on parents' and carers' knowledge of how much food, how often provided and of what nature and balance is of value here. Education of nutritional needs and the advantages of exercise to the growing child are, however, not the only areas of importance for consideration here, as good food—low fat, high protein, low salt and sugar, and high in residue—is often more expensive than the 'stomach fillers' and therefore economics is a vital factor. The homeless, the unemployed, the one-parent families and the retired elderly people on no or low incomes to meet everyday needs at, what must be considered by anyone, a very basic level have little control over their diet.

We should also consider those at risk because of an actual physical limitation of movement, for example, the unconscious individual and those in whom the level of conscious awareness fluctuates, whether precipitated by injury, infection, metabolic disorder or tumour formation. Again these people are dependent for a varying period of time on the attention and support of others, as are those who, whilst conscious and aware, may not elicit a current appreciation of the need to eat. *Overactive individuals* excessively preoccupied with their own thoughts and with responding to even the most minor environmental stimuli, have no interest in such mundane matters as eating, and therefore show a drastic reduction in food intake and weight loss. The individual who, conversely, is experiencing the *psychomotor retardation* associated with *severely lowered mood*, or *apathy*, may again evince a disinterest in food, and diminished appetite, perhaps due to the overwhelming preoccupation with sad, distressing or negative ideation. Such depressed mood may indicate *organic impairment* or be a sequel to *psychoactive substance use*, in addition to representing the major problem in a *bipolar* or *depressive disorder*, or as seen in bereavement. Significant weight loss may be a feature of *dementia*, both Alzheimer and multi-infarct types. *Poor memory* may precipitate lack of awareness as to whether one has eaten or not, of the normal environmental cues that would suggest it is time for a meal, of the need to shop or prepare food for eating. Food that is prepared for, and presented to, the memory or intellectually impoverished individual may be hoarded, or used to feed the cat, rather than to fulfil nutritional needs, thus demonstrating poverty of judgement in addition to that of awareness and insight.

Within mental health care, individuals may be seen to refuse food and for a variety of reasons. 'Psychotic' individuals whose delusions include *persecutory beliefs* and fears related to being killed by some agency, may suspect all food and drink preparations as being poisoned or drugged and hence refuse them. Conversely they may believe that some vital part of their digestive system is missing, has been invaded or taken over by an alien being or animal, as with somatically orientated themes. Remember George's catatonia and ruptured duodenal ulcer (p 61–62)?

George would not be the only example from our repertoire of anecdotes in which investigation revealed a somatic problem in a body area which had been included in an individual's bizarre somatic delusions. It may at times represent the only way in which clients can communicate their physical sensations when the rest of their world is bizarre or unintelligible. Rats, mice and various insects 'gnawing' have all been indicated as causing problems and investigation has, on occasions, revealed tumours, ulcers and strictures within the gastrointestinal system. A thorough medical examination plus appropriate investigative procedures will exclude such problems. Similarly some

CASE STUDY

When George was well on the road to recovery and therefore resident once again in familiar territory, he responded to any query after his health and all-round attention by repeating the words 'rats, gnawing rats'! One or two members of staff recalled that a day or so prior to his illness, George had given out the odd mutter about rats!

individuals will demonstrate *negativism*, refusing to accede to any request, whether in relation to food and eating, or any other behaviour. The individual may display an apparently motiveless resistance to any activity or perform the complete opposite of what is requested.

Some individuals may feel profound *guilt* in regard to a real or imagined act or omission in the past and consequently exteriorize thoughts and behaviours relating to their perceived current unworthiness to accept food, comfort or care. Others fear they are in reduced circumstances and, believing themselves needing to pay for services offered, will refuse food, drink and any other attention. Both are relatively common features demonstrated by the elderly who, accustomed and proud of their independence from 'national assistance' over many years, return to such long-ago-held views when intellectual and memory impairments intercede and cause bewilderment. There is often little memory of the National Health Service (NHS), free at the point of demand, and if there is such an awareness, the individual may not recognize the environment as one of a hospital or other care facility. Of course, non-uniformed staff provide no clues to assist individuals who therefore may believe themselves in a hotel, restaurant or paying facility. It is not unusual for any organically impaired individual to refuse to eat for those reasons.

Eating disorders

Anorexia nervosa provides a further example of food refusal or severe curtailment. Predominantly a problem of girls aged 12–18 years of age, the theories put forward to account for the obsessive preoccupation with food and the pursuit of 'thinness' are numerous and inconclusive. Leibowitz (1983) suggests various brain structure/function abnormalities, for example, a noradrenaline-producing neuronal problem, to account for the behaviour of some anorexics, but there is little direct evidence to support this, and most clinicians believe it is a problem of a psychosocial nature. The Western image of the successful woman—the small breasts and narrow hips—as epitomized in adverts, films and the like is pressure to which all young women are exposed and therefore if it should be a strong influence on the anorexic, there must be some predisposition inherent in the youngster to achieve this influence. Crisp (1983) believes a fear of growing up, of achieving an independent identity and of adult responsibilities is translated into a fear of getting fat and yet other researchers suggest that eating may represent the only control over life and living that the youngster feels he or she may exert. Several studies have found high incidences of psychosocial problems within the families of anorexics, for example, psychoactive substance abuse, depression and psychosomatic disorders. Others point to the disordered body image perception as a key factor within development, though studies reveal that many women, particularly pregnant ones, demonstrate an overestimation of their own body size. Whatever the cause, the preoccupation with food and thinness is evident and may reach the point where 40% plus of body weight is lost. It therefore presents a life-threatening situation in need of efficient and effective management.

In some situations intake is seen to be ineffective for a variety of reasons. In anorexia nervosa, for example, binges may be a feature, where vast amounts of food, and often thousands of calories, are ingested within a short period. The individual then induces vomiting, or utilizes laxatives and diuretics, to prevent the absorption of those calories. This purge–binge behaviour is referred to as *bulimia*.

No aversion to food is seen in *pica*, where there is persistent ingestion of non-nutritious substances and these may range through materials such as plaster and paint, string and cloth, sand and pebbles, grass and leaves, insects and animal droppings. It is a problem associated with very young children, 1 to 2 years of age, and most often remits in early childhood. On occasions the problem persists into adolescence and very rarely into adult life. It is frequently associated with those experiencing problems of learning disability and 'schizophrenia', but may also be seen in a 'mild' form within pregnant women.

The eating–bingeing–purging behaviours associated with anorexia nervosa and bulimia combined with deliberate ingestion of large amounts of laxative preparations ensures no absorption of nutri-

ents that have been eaten. Of course, the anorexic is not the only candidate for inappropriate use of laxatives, which, in essence, achieve their purpose by irritating the intestinal mucosa. Many individuals, whether labelled 'sick' or 'well', are obsessed with their evacuatory processes, demonstrating that laxatives may be another substance which is abused.

An increase in *metabolic rate* may obviously result in more frequent defaecation and perhaps diarrhoea and therefore the individual, for example, experiencing the effects of hyperthyroidism, may complain of the problem. Similarly *irritable bowel syndrome*, considered psychogenic in origin, reveals no organic disease in the intestine or elsewhere in the body, the individual often being described as 'nervous, sensitive and anxious'. *Generalized anxiety*, or a specific emotional conflict, generates increased peristalsis as an integral part of parasympathetic arousal, and therefore any situation in which the flight–fight mechanism is operational over a protracted period of time may see diarrhoea as a problem requiring attention.

The psychosocial sequelae of *diabetes mellitus* may be ignored and yet the individual has to monitor diet and physical health obsessively, administer insulin or other medication as prescribed and take full responsibility for judgement of the need to increase/decrease dosage in response to unusual daily events. This requires high levels of adjustment and readjustment in relation to daily activities initially and may, quite reasonably, become the focus of intense preoccupation. Overwhelming parental concern and anxiety may filter through to the young child and hence disturbances may ensue. Overprotective parental behaviour may smother a child, or food may be excessively valuable in parental manipulation. Wilful self-neglect may be a part of adolescent rebellion and sexual dysfunction—approximately half of diabetic men may experience impotence (Davis 1978) and up to 35% of diabetic women may be inorgasmic (Ellenberg 1977, Kolodny 1971) for example—may contribute to relationship difficulties. Fear of the somatic sequelae of diabetes may result in *hypochondriasis* and episodes of hypoglycaemia and acidosis may damage brain tissue, both in those with early onset, that is before the age of 5 years (Ack, Miller & Weil 1961) and in adults (Ives 1963) where cerebral atherosclerosis may be the predisposing problem. The diabetic may find a good mental health nurse a boon in adjusting to the changes and potential obstacles and problems that may be an inevitable feature of living with insulin deficiency.

Obesity

Obesity indicates that calorie intake exceeds requirements and, rather than 'appearing overnight', tends to creep up on individuals. Whilst inherited fat cell numbers has to be a factor, obesity is either acquired via socialization processes or occurs as a direct result of changes in lifestyle that are not accompanied by a concomitant reduction in food intake. It is only occasionally that obesity is seen as a direct result of somatic health problems and where there is indication of physiological causation, it is symptoms other than the weight increase that provide the indicator of a problem. *Cushing's syndrome (adrenocortical hyperfunction)*, rare but more common in women, presents as a decreased glucose tolerance, hyperglycaemia, muscle wasting (due to excessive protein catabolism) and weakness. The excessive production of cortisol similarly provides an abnormal distribution of fat and atrophy of lymphoid tissue, and hence the individual presents with obesity of the head, neck and trunk (the classical symptom of *buffalo's hump*) on thin, wasted limbs. The oedematous, round bloated face—*moon-shaped face*—is again a classical sign.

Similarly *hypothyroidism* may be diagnosed on presenting problems, exclusive of increasing body weight. In congenital or childhood development, the limp, coarse-featured, thick-tongued appearance is unmistakable. The child looks 'puffy' and bloated, is pale, dry and cool skinned, and has problems in feeding and growth and development generally. Pulse is slow and temperature is subnormal, indicative of the reduced metabolic rate inherent in thyroid hormone deficiency. In adults, onset may be confused with depression or early organic impairment, but again, skin is dry, thickened and cold and the face is puffy with an enlarged tongue and lips. The individual feels weak, slow and lethargic, and there is a psychomotor retardation. Appetite is poor, despite the weight gain, and amenorrhoea is often a feature in women. Untreated, arteriosclerotic changes, cardiac insufficiency and coma may ensue and prompt treatment is therefore vital. One tip may be found within the hair distribution of the affected individual, as growth is reduced, head hair often becoming dry, coarse and sparse and eyebrows often disappearing or much reduced in quanity.

Lesions associated with the hypothalamus and its eating/appetite-related structures, may create problems associated with obesity and therefore will present with client problems associated with that specific lesion.

Research indicates, however, that overweight individuals tend to eat more when anxious, whilst normal weight individuals eat more in low anxiety situations (McKenna 1972) and other studies have demonstrated that this increased consumption occurs in relation to any emotionally arousing situation encountered by the overweight person (White 1977). Theories have been put forward to explain this increased eating both in anxiety-provoking situations and during emotional arousal in general. The scenario of food providing comfort during childhood, previously discussed, is important here and, where used as a panacea of all ills, it may be that differentiation between hunger and other feelings has never been attained. It follows, therefore, that obesity or significant weight increase may be a feature of *depressed* and *anxious individuals*.

SUMMARY

People eat to survive and therefore evolution has built in a system whereby a period of deprivation is automatically followed by overeating, thus maintaining optimum potential for species' survival. The social functions of food and eating have been introduced by the 'civilizing effect' of the advanced cortex of the human and with this 'advancement' complications may be incurred in respect of a purely biological function. Dieting individuals have to relearn the habits of a lifetime to find continuing satisfaction with their shape and weight, introducing and maintaining new routines and schedules, until habitual in nature. In regard, however, to the targets within The health of the nation (DOH 1992), we would sincerely suggest that resources be applied towards parents and parents in waiting, and to the young generation who are likely to be the frustrated dieters of the future. Good habits learned early are the foundation for healthy lifetime eating.

SLEEP

INTRODUCTION

Blessings on him that invented sleep! It covers a man, thoughts and all, like a cloak; it is meat for the hungry, drink for the thirsty, heat for the cold, and cold for the hot. It is the currency with which everything may be purchased, and the balance that sets even King and shepherd, simpleton and sage.
Andrews 1987

The words above are those of Miguel de Cervantes (1547–1616) and serve to illustrate the extent to which the sixteenth-century novelist, playwright and poet, creator of Don Quixote, was impressed by this simple, biological function. Of course, not everyone is quite so enamoured all of the time with sleep for, as with so many bodily functions, it may be taken for granted until it causes a problem. Whether it is an inappropriate 'nap', an inability to stay awake and alert at a point well past the normal bedtime, or sleep evading an individual, most people experience a difficulty on occasions. We will review the current knowledge relating to sleep, the manner in which it is mediated and the normal parameters associated with the event, prior to exploring difficulties that may be experienced.

TO SLEEP...

Sleep is an active physiological process, and not merely a failure of arousal. The most obvious of the human's circadian rhythms discussed earlier, it may be described as:

♦ a recurrent healthy state
♦ a normal, periodic, physiological depression of function
♦ a period of relative inertia and reduced environmental responsiveness
♦ a circumstance where overt responses are absent, and covert responses diminished
♦ a state clearly different from that of coma and stupor.

Were you to think about the overt signs of the onset of sleep, you may reflect upon the fact that an individual closes his eyes, that the normal breathing pattern changes, with respirations reducing the total flow of air breathed, and that the heart rate slows. Observations may also conclude that urinary output reduces sharply during the sleeping hours and that a stimulus of sufficient intensity—the ringing of the alarm clock or the sound of breaking glass—will provoke arousal.

However, more detailed reflection will elicit that you have far more knowledge than this about sleep and sleeping. For example, you will be aware that sleep is *species specific*, each animal having its own pattern and time for sleeping and assuming a position conducive to the activity. Some sleep in the day, others at night; some lie down whilst others remain standing and a glance at a wildlife programme—or around the house and garden—will confirm this specificity of the sleep pattern. Observations of the pet, caged bird will, for example, elicit that it sleeps standing up at night and yet the owl likes to roam in search of food at night, and tends not to be active during daylight. The family dog may go through the routine of pawing and scratching at the carpet, circling several times and then settling himself off to sleep, whereas anyone with knowledge of bats will know that these are also night-time activists which hang upside down, wrapped in their wings to sleep through the day. The members of the monkey and ape genre lie on their bellies along the branch of a tree and human beings, all things being equal, take themselves off to a special room in the late evening hours, lie down and cover themselves.

Sleeping positions

Every individual exhibits a routine which prepares them physically and emotionally for relaxation and sleep, and deviation from that routine may provoke a feeling of unease or discomfort. On nights when the individual is excessively tired some bits of the routine may safely be omitted without detrimental effects, indeed the whole set of activities may go to the wall, without even a notice!

Besides this routine, there are other comforts that may be necessary to attain the desired goal. Position in bed, for example, may be central to going off to sleep. The right arrangement of pillows and blankets or duvet evokes that feeling of familiarity and hence safety and relaxation. Many people find great difficulty in sleeping in a 'strange' bed and room—they cannot quite get comfortable. Body position assumed in preparation for sleep is similarly an individual preference—are you a 'diagonal' sleeper, corner-to-corner, a runner in mid-stride sort of sleeper, a hanger-on-to-the-edge of the mattress sleeper, or do you assume a fetal position? There is one position that each person feels comfortable in and it may not necessarily be any of the four identified above. If forced to move into a different position, for example, because of a plaster cast applied to a limb or an ache or pain, individuals may find that sleep eludes them, because they just 'can't get comfortable'.

A partner's sleeping habits may be significant. If you have spent many years occupying a bed alone, it may take a considerable degree of adjustment to accommodate a second person in the same bed, particularly if it is discovered that this individual is a teeth grinder and a snorer who likes to sleep diagonally across the bed, wrapped in the entire duvet! As an interesting and passing thought, animals seem to curl up when sleeping, perhaps to reduce exposure to predators of their soft unprotected underbellies. Do humans curl up for similar, evolutionary reasons? Similarly the positioning of animals' bodies against something flat, maybe even another animal, where possible, has been noted and could this be to prevent any enemy attacking them from behind, so to speak, and out

of eyeline? Many people prefer to sleep facing the bedroom door, rather than away from it. Is this, too, an evolutionary 'throwback'?

How much sleep?

It is known, for example, that the number of hours of sleep needed varies, not only with age but between individuals of comparable age and lifestyle. The newborn baby sleeps for most of the day, waking only for sustenance and comfort measures. As the days go by, the infant sleeps less so that, by 6 months of age, approximately 13 hours each day is spent in sleep, in two short 'naps' and a longer sleep at night. As a toddler, the two naps reduce to one and so on until in adulthood, the average period spent in sleep is about $7\frac{1}{2}$ hours. Again, however, the adult 'norm' must take account of those who seem to function best on less—as little as 3 hours a night for some—and those for whom 8 hours or more is a must. It is a very individual need. As people age, there is evidence to suggest that there is a tendency to sleep less at night and to awaken earlier in the morning, often before 5.00 a.m. (McGhie & Russell 1962). This may be of significance when looking towards problems associated with sleep. Most of us will have an acquaintance who is a 'night owl' who becomes active at night and also a 'morning lark'—the individual who is actually awake and fully alert and functioning before the first verse of the dawn chorus (Webb 1975). The particular rhythm in operation is as individual as a fingerprint.

You may also have experienced more or less successful attempts to change the sleeping time or pattern away from the norm. Night duty will require you to be awake and fully alert throughout the night-time hours, when you would normally be tucked up and asleep. You will therefore need to sleep during the hours when the vast majority of people are awake, moving about and generally making a noise. Night duty patterns rarely provide you with sufficient time to adjust to the change required, internal rotation often demonstrating three or four nights on and then the rest of the week off, or vice versa. Worse still for adjustment are split nights off duty—the sort of two on, two off, two on, one off pattern—requiring adjustment to differing cycles several times a week. Of course many nurses working predominantly on nights do accommodate well, having grown accustomed to the alterations required in order to function well in both situations. Humans also have the ability to accelerate and retard the sleep period while travelling across different time zones and the hour on/hour off game that is played with British Summer Time. Whilst more or less 'jet lagged' by both, people do adjust where necessary within a few days.

What happens during sleep?

You need to be relaxed at bedtime to succumb to sleep and once you lie back in that darkened room and close your eyes, the passage from wakefulness into sleep is actually an instantaneous one. William Dement (1976) demonstrated this fact exceptionally well in experiments in which recumbent and sleep-ready people, whose eyes had been taped open, were asked to respond by pressing a button each time a light was flashed. The light was flashed every second or two, and the 'guinea pigs'

showed no slowing of reaction, just an abrupt cessation of activity, indicating that, even with eyes taped open, they were fast asleep. The eyeballs deviate upwards, pupils constrict, but will respond slowly to light and a number of changed patterns of activity commence. The activity of the brain, demonstrable via EEG recordings, elicits a recurring ultradian rhythm of differing patterns of electrical impulses (Fig. 4.3).

The awake but relaxed brain shows activity at 8–12 vibrations per second (referred to as Hz or Hertz) at the rear of the head, and is described as *alpha rhythm*. This is transformed into the low voltage disorganized *theta activity* as drowsiness ensues, interpreted by some researchers as a sort of random neuronal firing—a running down—prior to passage to *stage three*, characterizing light sleep. Within stage three, the activity moves predominantly to the front of the head. *Sleep spindles*, sudden bursts of impulses that last for less than 1 second at a time but are synchronized at between 12 and 16 Hz, intersperse and interrupt low voltage slow activity. A series of *vertex sharp waves* and *K complexes* heralds the onset of *delta wave* activity and deep sleep. Activity is at 0.5–2

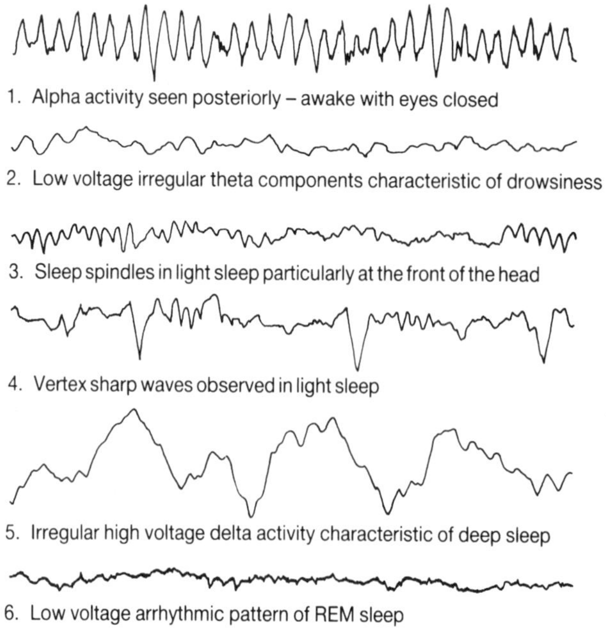

1. Alpha activity seen posteriorly – awake with eyes closed

2. Low voltage irregular theta components characteristic of drowsiness

3. Sleep spindles in light sleep particularly at the front of the head

4. Vertex sharp waves observed in light sleep

5. Irregular high voltage delta activity characteristic of deep sleep

6. Low voltage arrhythmic pattern of REM sleep

Fig. 4.3 The ECG in sleep.

Hz and sleepers are harder to awaken at this point, although something familiar—their name being called, for example—will cause arousal. This is the stage of *orthodox* or *non-rapid eye movement sleep*, to be followed by a sudden descent into *rapid eye movement* or *REM sleep*. Here the EEG resembles that of an awake and alert individual, hence the term *paradoxical sleep* is often applied. It shows a faster, low amplitude activity that is punctuated by bursts of phasic events during which eye muscles show rapid movement, hence the term rapid eye movement sleep. The term 'paradoxical' is appropriate for, despite the brain's apparently alert activity, muscle tone in general across the body shows a marked decrease and therefore complete relaxation of skeletal muscle, almost to the point of paralysis. The exact pattern of REM sleep varies from individual to individual and with age. The newborn infant spends approximately half of the sleeping time in REM sleep, and by the age of 5 years this has reduced to about a quarter or a fifth of total sleep. It then remains fairly constant through life at about 18% until old age. It is of interest to find that the premature baby spends about 75% of sleep time in REM, as will become obvious during the later discussion on dreams and dreaming, for it is during this REM period that dreaming occurs.

REM sleep

The adult who spends $7\frac{1}{2}$ hours asleep each night will experience between $1\frac{1}{2}$ and 2 hours of REM sleep. The first period is relatively short, lasting only 10 minutes or so, and occurs approximately 50–90 minutes after falling asleep. As the night wears on, REM periods become longer, interrupted only by return to stage two. The length of the deeper stages of sleep, characterized by the delta waves, tends to reduce throughout the night and therefore the indvidual's sleep becomes lighter after the first few hours. Strenous physical activity increases the period of time spent in delta (slow) wave sleep and yet does not affect REM time. It has also been noted that REM sleep is increased in hospital patients who demonstrate psychosocial problems and also by women in the premenstrual phase of the monthly cycle, which may be a time characterized by mild psychosocial symptomatology, such as depression, anxiety and irritability (Hartmann 1984).

During REM sleep, the rapid eye movements occur 40–60 times per minute and respiration and heart rate become rapid and irregular, in comparison to the almost absent eye movements and slow, regular breathing and heartbeat of non-REM sleep. There appear to be two distinct stages in REM sleep: one which is termed the *tonic phase* in which muscle tone is reduced and yet where, in men, an erection of the penis and, in women, increased vaginal blood flow is seen; the other is the *phasic period*, demonstrating the changes in heart and respiratory—and therefore blood pressure—rates mentioned plus an increase in cerebral blood flow, occasional myoclonic jerks and the conjugate eye movements. It has been suggested that REM sleep facilitates neural growth in the young (Roffwarg, Muzio & Dement 1968), which would account for the higher proportion of REM sleep in children than in adults. The finding that protein synthesis rate is at its highest level during REM sleep would also support this hypothesis.

Physiological responses

There are other important features known in regard to sleep; for example, *cell division* is seen at various phases throughout the night but maximally during slow wave sleep. Similarly *growth hormone* concentrations are seen to rise with the onset of deep sleep, and where sleep is delayed so is the rise in growth hormone, thus indicating that its release is related to sleep *per se* rather than a 24-hour clock timing. This is helpful where investigating a possible deficiency of growth hormone for a sample of blood taken an hour after the onset of sleep would provide an indication of the capacity of the hormone. In adults, the *plasma prolactin concentration* is seen to rise about 90 minutes after the onset of sleep, and then shows a series of increasingly large secretory bursts, to reach a peak between the hours of 5.00 a.m. and 7.00 a.m. A rapid fall follows and the daytime low is seen to be achieved by about 10.00 a.m. Again it is sleep related in onset, for if sleep is delayed then rises in prolactin levels are also delayed. However, it is not seen to be related to any one sleepwave pattern. The circadian rhythm of adrenocorticotrophic hormone (ACTH) and cortisol shows a series of secretory episodes that cluster between 3.00 a.m. and 9.00 a.m., and yet little is produced between 11.00 p.m. and 3.00 a.m. This boost so late in the sleep period is obviously designed to prepare the individual for the energy expenditure needed upon rising. It is interesting that abnormalities in the 24-hour concentrations of plasma cortisol have been noted in those who have severe depressed mood, with return to normal levels noted following 'treatment'. In prepubertal children, LH levels are low and show no rise during sleep. However, at puberty there is an increasingly strong episodic release of LH during sleep and this is seen with a corresponding increase in testosterone levels. By the time sexual maturity is attained, daytime waking and night-time sleeping patterns of the hormone's release are the same. The release of *renin* from the kidney is seen to be abruptly halted at the initiation of rapid eye movement and levels of vasopressin, the antidiuretic hormone, are also rhythmic in function, thereby reducing fluid loss during the night-time hours by limiting urinary output at a period of reduced intake.

We have mentioned the increased protein synthesis associated with REM sleep, and must also identify, therefore, that the body's energy and fat stores are replenished during sleep.

MEDIATORS OF SLEEP

The *reticular formation*, or *reticular activating system* (RAS), is composed of the structures which facilitate sleep and wakeful states. The *mesencephalic portion*, comprising of areas of grey matter in the pons and midbrain, when stimulated, prompts impulses to spread upwards to the thalamus and onwards to generally stimulate the cerebral cortex, thus creating *wakefulness* and *consciousness*. The *thalamic portion* of the reticular activating system, which is made up of grey matter in the thalamus, appears to have a slightly different role, for stimulation of specific parts of the thalamus activates particular areas of the cerebral cortex and thus provokes *arousal* from sleep. Arousal requires sensory input, which stimulates the reticular activating system, and this input may be in the form of proprioceptive stimuli, pain or physical discomfort, bright light and loud noises. The cortex is then activated. Conversely, however, the cerebral cortex may be the originator of impulses that activate the arousal process, via somatosensory, motor or limbic system signals, and this reciprocal energizing effect is evident throughout the conscious part of the day, through a multicircuit feedback loop. A similar arrangement is seen to be operating between the reticular activating system and the spinal cord, with impulses passing down through the cord to the skeletal muscles. The latter generate proprioceptive stimuli, which pass back via the cord and serve not only to sustain the activity of the reticular activating system, but also that of the cerebral cortex.

When it comes to sleep, several areas have been of interest to researchers. The *nucleus locus coeruleus* is a group of neurons which contain *noradrenaline*, and the *dorsal raphe nucleus* comprises of *serotonin*-enriched neurons. Both lie within the pons and recordings of the 'behaviour' of single cells within both areas demonstrate their maximum activity to occur during wakefulness. There is a progressive slowing of activity during the initial stages of slow wave sleep and a major depression of that activity prior to the end of the slow wave sleep phase. During REM sleep these cells are silent. Other pontine cells show a dramatic rise in activity prior to the EEG shift from slow wave to REM sleep patterns, indicating a responsibility in the transition from one stage to the other. It is clear, however, that this increase in activity is seen to be of a level 50–100 times that seen during wakefulness. These three groups of cells are thought to be connected to each other by various pathways and innervation, and it would appear that their activity is antagonistic. As activity increases in the REM-associated cells, a concomitant reduction in those related to consciousness and slow wave sleep is seen. Other substances produced within the area, for example, dopamine and acetylcholine, are known to be of importance within the wake–sleep cycle, though their exact role is obscure as yet. It is also possible that other pontine neurons are influential and have yet to be found. However, what does appear certain is that:

1. fatigue + withdrawal of afferent impulses → reduction in the alerting system → deactivation of cerebral cortex → sleep

   and

2. sleep + afferent impulses → stimulus to alerting system → activation of cerebral cortex → consciousness.

Early in the twentieth century, the French physiologist Henri Pieron (1913) demonstrated that the transfusion of cerebrospinal fluid from a sleepy dog to an alert one provoked the latter to fall asleep. In the 1970s, John Pappenheimer (1976) and his colleagues succeeded in isolating seven millionths of a gram of a substance—Factor S— from 3000 litres of human urine, which they believed to be a sleep-producing substance. It was discovered to be a tiny, five-amino-acid peptide and since this time, studies from as far afield as Japan, Mexico and Romania have elicited substances which appear to be produced by the brain and which appear to trigger different stages of sleep (Krueger & Karnovsky 1982). One such study demonstrated that a mere 600 molecules of the peptide *arginine vasotocin* induces sleep in a normal and alert cat. Sleep remains, to a large part, a continuing mystery.

Role of the pineal gland

We cannot ignore the role of the *pineal gland* in the cycles, including that of sleep, of animals, for, whilst no one can yet be sure, it may be that human physiological rhythms may be similarly influenced. The pineal gland converts the transmitter *serotonin* into the hormone *melatonin* and pours it directly into the bloodstream. Melatonin appears to have several functions in relation to both time and light, for example, it appears to cause a lightening in the colour of skin in certain lizards during the darkness hours and when injected into sparrows, they fall asleep. This conversion of serotonin to melatonin is achieved via the action of two enzymes produced within the pineal gland. One—*N-acetyltransferase*—determines the quantity of melatonin circulating and hence regulates cycles, for example, related to temperature changes and the sleep–wake cycle. It is a fact that, in many species of both nocturnal and diurnally active animals, the levels of N-acetyltransferase are always highest at night. This level may be 10 times that recorded in daylight hours and, for example, provokes chickens to roost and lowers their temperature. The mechanism by which melatonin levels are adjusted to match the normal variations of hours of light and darkness seen within the seasonal clock, is seen to be mediated via the pineal gland's sensitivity to light. Binkley's (1979) experiments with chicks kept in constant darkness elicited the normal N-acetyltransferase rhythm to continue. Those kept in constant lightness demonstrated a reduction in the levels of N-acetyltransferase circulating, whilst those exposed to alternating 12-hour periods of light and dark and which were then suddenly exposed to bright light during a dark spell, evinced a rapid drop in enzyme activity. It would appear therefore that the gland is sensitive to light, but it would also appear that there are certain times of the day when this sensitivity disappears and the rhythm is unalterable by environmental manipulation. The major influencing point appears to be related to light during dark periods and it may be, therefore, that the varying time of the early morning light is the resetter of the biological clock. Light reaching the pineal gland reduces the activity of N-acetyltransferase, thereby reducing the amount of melatonin produced and circulated. The chick's body temperature begins to rise and its daily activities ensue. Different species sense these light alterations in differing ways. The rat, for example, has a branch of the optic nerve, unnecessary for vision, which conducts light inputs to the pineal gland, whilst birds monitor the light levels directly through the bony skull in addition to the eyes. In the rat, the sympathetic nerves release noradrenaline which activates the pineal gland and hence the enzyme, and yet, in chickens, the same noradrenaline release inhibits pineal gland activity (Binkley 1979).

The human pineal gland, a small reddish-grey structure on the dorsal surface of the midbrain, which is attached to the roof of the third ventricle in the midline, also contains serotonin, melatonin and other active amines. However, its function is rather unclear, other than having an implication in the sexual development of the child at puberty. It does seem that there may be some similarities between the human function and that of the animals previously discussed. Humans, for example, may be seen to demonstrate a similar body temperature cycle to the chicken. An approximate 1 to 1.5°C difference is seen on the 24-hour cycle, with the lowest point between 2.00 a.m. and 5.00 a.m., and a peak in the afternoon. Body temperature is seen to influence the length of human sleep for those individuals on time-free schedules, and where no clock or environmental cues are provided to indicate bedtime is approaching. An individual retiring when his body temperature is at its lowest point sleeps for only 8 hours. In contrast, retiring when the body temperature is peaking results in a sleep period of up to 14 hours. Most individuals have no perception of this temperature change and yet when still awake in the early hours of the morning notice how cold and chilled they have become. Similarly an extra long sleep is attributed to being extra tired, overfull with late-night dining habits or consumption of an extra glass of an alcoholic beverage, when it may simply be due to falling asleep when the body temperature is high.

Sleep–wake cycles

Many studies, such as that of Michel Siffre (1963) a French cave explorer, have been conducted into the effects of living for a prolonged period of time without environmental cues to assist the body clock in timing of activities. Siffre, for example, lived in a carefully prepared cave, where no light could enter, for 6 months in Texas, USA. He ate and slept at will, wearing electrodes on his scalp to monitor his sleep cycles and passing specimens of urine up to the surface for analysis. When desirous of sleep, Siffre would contact the surface and artificial light sources would be extinguished. Each sleep–wake cycle constituted 'a day' and the

length of Siffre's days were seen to extend gradually, to the point that Siffre's believed 151-day stay was in reality 179 days long. You may recall that the hostage, Jackie Mann, similarly miscalculated the number of days of his confinement because of reduction/absence of environmental cues. Mann 'lost' only a very few days, but Siffre 'lost' a whole month.

It was noted with Siffre that, whilst his days lengthened to approximately 33 hours, his temperature cycle remained in a 24.8-hour cycle so that, at times, he experienced both the temperature peak and trough within his 'daytime' activity and indeed on his twelfth day experienced two highs and two lows during one 'day'. It's not at all surprising that at the end of his cave sojourn he was confused:

> Sullenly, mechanically, I stumble through my battery of tests. Just as I finish my laps on the hated bicycle, the telephone rings. Gerard tells me that it is August 10th, a stormy day, and the experiment has concluded; I am confused; I believe it to be mid-July. Then, as the truth sinks in, comes a flood of relief.

David Lafferty, however, who spent 127 days in a cave (Moore-Ede, Sulzman & Fuller 1982), found that, whilst initially his cycles were erratic, they did readjust. Some 'days' were 19 hours long—10 hours awake and 9 hours asleep—and others were 53 hours long—18 hours awake and 35 hours asleep—but eventually, towards the end of his investigation, he settled to a 25-hour day.

In support of the role of melatonin in the human sleep–wake cycle, Arendt et al (1987) at the University of Surrey, conducted experiments with potentially 'jet-lagged' individuals. You may have personal experience of the fatigue, insomnia and disorientation which may spoil the first few days of a holiday abroad, and it is a fact that individuals suffer less of a problem when travelling in a westerly rather than easterly direction. The 23–25-hour inbuilt clock is actually extending the hours of its day during this westward travel and this would appear easier to accommodate than the daylength reduction inherent in travelling eastward. After a long flight, the day–night cycle of home remains 'locked into' the system and it is the attempts to override the norm by assuming a new holiday clock that creates the symptoms of jet-leg. Arendt et al believed it to be the cyclical release of melatonin which maintains the inbuilt clock and therefore administered melatonin to jet-lagged volunteers during the evening when normally they would be sleepy. Far fewer of the volunteers complained of the ill effects of jet-lag than the control group who had been given a placebo.

A more gentle movement of the biological clock has been seen to be of value in shift work situations. A shift system comprising 1 week of night shifts each day, followed by a week of evening-shift working requires individuals to constantly turn back their clock by 8 hours each week and provokes insomnia, digestive problems, fatigue and irritability. Laboratory studies elicit the fact that animals exposed to such a rotating schedule have shorter lifespans and an increased level of heart disease, so it is an important factor in health. Czeisler et al (1981) utilized the natural preferences of the body for a forward adjustment rather than a backward-orientated one, and also suggested that shifts should rotate on a 3-weekly rather than a 1-weekly basis to facilitate an adjustment to the adjustment in 'time zone'. The workforce were happy and healthier and productivity rose by 22%. The workers found that a slight adjustment to their sleeping time, by going to bed a little later each week, made the transition even easier, in effect by gradually moving the inner clock forwards.

Perchance to dream?

It is not possible to leave the subject of sleep without a mention of dreams, and you may recall that REM sleep is the phase of the sleep cycle generally associated with the phenomenon. The studies of Aserinsky & Kleitman (1953) elicited the REM patterning of sleep and Dement & Kleitman's (1975) further investigations demonstrated that arousal immediately after the conjugate eye movements was more likely to evoke the report of a vivid dream, than arousal at any other part of the cycle. When Dement deprived individuals of REM sleep, by awaking them prior to its onset, subjects would show the signs of a sleepless night the fol-

lowing day and yet when woken the same number of times during other stages of sleep, a lesser degree of impairment was seen to follow. REM-deprived subjects similarly spent an increased amount of time in REM sleep the following night, as if to make up for the loss. Studies since the 1950s have pointed out that dreaming also occurs in slow wave sleep, for the subject awakened after only one hour of sleep and prior to the onset of the first REM period, often reports a dream. However, the more vivid and memorable dreams do appear to take place within the REM phase.

Of course it is a long time since Freud's Interpretation of Dreams (Freud 1954) and, though we would recommend it as reading of interest, a great deal of scientific knowledge has been accrued since then. It is of some amusement to think of dreams being symbolic, acceptable representations of the wicked, pleasure-seeking 'id', and yet many still adhere to the theory. Stranger still, in this regard, is the knowledge that the newborn baby spends half its sleeping time in REM cycle and that the dog, cat and rat indulge in REM sleep and therefore presumably some variety of dreaming. Dogs definitely dream during REM sleep, with paws twitching and little yelping noises! Without the human's higher cortex and therefore 'conscience', do they need to disguise their basic impulses, especially when one considers how little control they exhibit over instinctual behaviour when awake!

Crick & Mitchison (1983) suggested that, without the ability to dream, the cortex would be 'filled up' with out of date, uncorrected and superfluous information and that the organism would therefore require a very large cortex to continually absorb new information. Indeed, this appears to be supported by studies of the Australian spiny ant-eater (a marsupial) and the dolphin, both of which have an extraordinarily large cortex and neither of which demonstrates REM sleep ability. Crick believes the large cortex necessary because of the inability to unlearn material or revamp old learning in the light of further experience.

Sleep deprivation for three or more nights has been seen to produce both visual and auditory hallucinations, in addition to misperceptions. There are consistent reports of solid objects 'trembling', faces appearing from thin air and walls covered in insects and other items. Auditory hallucinations in the form of voices, talking about the subject, are similarly a regular complaint. Sounds familiar? It could be the clinical picture associated with a diagnosis of 'schizophrenia' and yet depressed mood has been successfully elevated via intentional sleep deprivation (Wehr et al 1979). The suggestion that dreaming is the brain's mechanism for removing old and incorporating new learning seems a sensible one when one views the mixed-up nature of many dreams. Events or information of the day appear often to be linked up with yesterday's activities and memories of many years ago, during sleep, in an apparently logicless sequence and certainly cause either amusement or bewilderment on the part of the subject. The new learning being incorporated, or replacing old memories, would appear a safe bet. However, the current state of physiological knowledge has many gaps with regard to sleep.

The evolutionary protective mechanism of sleep as the basis for all subsequent sleep-related activities also seems a realistic purport. Remaining tucked away from marauding predators during the night-time hours of darkness, when visual acuity has to be less effective, is an eminently sensible idea. The fact, too, that a period of inactivity and sensory deprivation is necessary to stock up on depleted food stores, provide a period of rest, recuperation, growth and repair of organs and to amend stored memories in the light of continuing inputs, would support the value of a prolonged and regular reduced awareness and response. Sleep is a necessary part therefore of the optimum potential for survival of any organism and thence should be viewed as valuable in its own right.

PROBLEMS OF SLEEP

Many of the everyday problems associated with sleep may be attributed to the adoption of a lifestyle which is not conducive—and may, indeed, be preclusive—to regular, restful sleep patterns. Children may never acquire the sleep hygiene measures necessary to ensure a lifetime of efficient

sleeping, and sleep may be viewed as a waste of a third of the valuable waking time.

Sometimes people are less than helpful to their body rhythms, because of their attitudes to sleep, as one of something to do when there is nothing better on offer and not really of sufficient value to warrant specific attention. Whilst most people will not be happy to go past lunchtime without eating, and would certainly be really put out if their monthly/weekly income was unavailable on the correct day, the importance of *regular sleep hours* is often overlooked. Of course, there are many distractions to divert the individual's attention away from bedtime. Late and all-night television broadcasting, with all the best films screened during the bedtime hours, seems far more enthralling a proposition than bed at 10.30 p.m., especially if there is no deadline for getting up in the morning, as with the unemployed person, the afternoon shift worker or the college student. Entertainment, and leisure services in general, are encroaching more and more on the hours traditionally viewed as those for sleep, with midnight cinema shows, late night restaurant and sports facilities all extending their opening hours to provide services for the more demanding population needs. There is more leisure time available and, in relative terms, the vast majority of the population have money to spend in excess of that needed for pure survival needs. Time and money are only two of three criteria necessary to enable the individual to go out and play; one needs the energy to spare in such activities and again, in comparison with our ancestors, today's generation expends far less physical exertion in their jobs and in general leads a far more sedentary lifestyle. *Daily exercise* promotes an increased blood circulation, raises the metabolic rate and assists in ridding the body of its toxins, as well as assisting in respiratory function and healthy bone and muscle maintenance. Steady daily exercise helps to promote sleep. No one would suggest a return to the days of 16–18 hours of hard graft, but the newfound freedom from such major time constraints and commitments must be used to the human advantage and not detriment. Regular sleeping hours and daily exercise are two important sleep enhancers.

A third important factor again relates to the

same general theme, for the individual needs to put aside *sufficient time* for sleep. There appears little point in spending a mere 3 or 4 hours in sleeping when the individual's biological activities undertaken during the period are programmed to personal requirements and require 6 or 8 hours each night to complete. How can a person expect to feel refreshed and alert with so much unfinished business still to be attended to, which can only build up like an intray of unanswered mail? The duration of sleep which provokes this 'alert and refreshed' state is the amount needed to be set aside nightly to maintain health and well-being.

The environment is yet another area of importance when promoting sleep hygiene measures, for it used to be the case that a bedroom was solely, or almost solely, used for sleeping, but this is often no longer the case. Children often utilize a bedroom as a play area and hence it is filled to the brim with bright, attractive and stimulating material. It is an area associated now with socialization, friends being invited into the room and it being used as an entertaining area, rather than of peace, quiet and rest. For some, this valuable personal space may become inextricably linked with feelings of discomfort, isolation, punishment or physical and/or emotional pain. The child continually excluded from adult or family interactions and 'sent to his room' is more likely to resent the facility and associate it with negative, tumultuous emotions rather than the placid, peaceful, contented feelings which need to be engendered within a sleeping area. The physically and/or sexually abused child may feel fear and terror in regard to the environment where the injuries have been perpetrated. Such feelings are not conductive to restful sleep.

Of course, it is not only the child who may experience an environment unconductive to sleep. The student who lives in a hall of residence, with just one room available for all activities, may find similarly new and different associations being acquired in regard to what should be, in essence, sleeping quarters. Whilst communal cooking, eating and lounge facilities may be provided, the 'bed-sit' may become the centre for studying, socializing and sleeping. Adults who have access to a lounge in which to watch television may still insist on watching it in bed and hence again dilute the association with a sleeping area. The bedroom needs to be as free from distractions as possible and engender feelings of tranquillity, comfort and safety. Decor, too, needs to be restful rather than stimulating.

The individual gets used to the general sounds within the external environment too, and again changes may cause disturbances to sleep:

> Mother's home is situated on the outskirts of a busy little town, whilst I live in the heart of the country and recently, when I'd got an overnight trip away, she came to 'dog-sit'. On my return, I was astounded to hear that she 'hadn't slept a wink all night for the noise'. The 'resident' owl, the cows and other farm animals in the locale had kept her awake when the passing—and often quite heavy—traffic outside her own home never disturbs her!

Whilst the problems identified above may provoke consistently *ineffective and inefficient sleeping routines*, the term *sleep disorders* is reserved for sleep problems of more than 1 month's duration, rather than transient sleeplessness or other disturbance associated with a short-lived psychosocial stressor or poor sleep habits. Sleep disturbance may be the initiator of other biopsychosocial problems or may be a sequela of mental health or somatic health difficulties, and therefore may represent a frequent complaint of the client or his significant others in many and varied care situations. Nurses will often wonder whether such problems represent a primary or secondary health deviation and it is therefore essential to ask the questions appropriate to elicit as much information as is possible, in order that relevant assistance may be provided.

THE DYSSOMNIAS

Dyssomnia is the generic term applied to problems associated with the *amount, quality* or *timing* of sleep. The group includes *insomnia*, where the duration or quality of sleep is insufficient for normal and expected levels of daytime functioning, *hypersomnias*, where despite an adequate night's sleep, the individual complains of excessive day-time drowsiness, and *sleep–wake schedule disorders*, where the individual's pattern of sleeping and waking is seen to be out of synchronization with what is considered to be the norm of the environment. A second generic group of problems, the *parasomnias*, are associated with the occurrence of abnormal events, either during sleep itself or in the twilight stage between sleep and wakefulness. These include problems related to dreaming, that is *nightmares and terrors*, and those relating to *sleep walking (somnambulism)*. Whilst all occur as a primary problem in the absence of any biopsychosocial health deviation, many may be seen as a secondary exteriorization to some other problem of health.

Insomnia may be diagnosed in response to client—or family—complaints related to:

1. a difficulty in initiating sleep
2. difficulty in maintaining sleep

or

3. non-restorative, though normal duration, sleep.

McGhie & Russell (1962) described insomnia as being reported with increasing frequency in older age groups, from less than 10% in the 15–24-year age group, to around 18% in the 45–54-year band and approximately 40% of 65+ year olds. They also note that 'symptoms' change with advancing age, as those in the younger group tend to complain of non-restorative sleep, whilst the older age groups complain of initiation–maintenance problems. Women appear to experience problems at twice the rate of their age-matched male peers—14% as opposed to 6% (Kripke & Gillin 1985). The frequency of insomnia in men, whilst consistently lower than in women, shows a sudden increase in the 65–74-year-old age group, and this may be related to the changes in general routines and exercise levels brought about by retirement. Researchers have discovered that individuals tend to overestimate the amount of sleep lost. One such study (Carskadon, Mitler & Dement 1974) found that less than half of a group, who complained of protracted and severe sleep loss, were actually awake for 30 minutes during the night, and it has

been suggested this overestimation may be due to one of two factors. It may be, for example, that, because there is no memory of having slept, the 'insomniac' remembers only the wakeful period, or that perhaps restless or light sleep may be interpreted as wakefulness and hence a miscalculation occurs.

In *primary insomnia*, sleep often becomes a major preoccupation with the individual anxious for the entire waking hours in relation to the difficulties experienced. The person tries hard to fall asleep, but this merely increases the prevailing tension and therefore sleep continues to be evasive. Often subjects report being able to sleep when not trying, for example, they may fall asleep easily in front of the television or in the cinema. Similarly, the individual may describe an improvement in the problem when sleeping in an unfamiliar environment. Often the individual reports a lifelong sleep difficulty, although others may be able to pinpoint some event or psychosocial stressor in adult life which coincided with the onset of sleep disturbance. On occasions primary insomnia may be a complication of an insomnia which occurs as an integral part of a mental health or organic health problem. The client may 'get into the habit' of sleep disturbance during this time so that even when there is a resolution to the original problem, the sleep disorder remains.

Insomnia and mental disorders

Insomnia related to another, non-organic, mental health problem is frequently encountered, for many individuals experiencing lowered or elevated mood, or anxiety, will describe such disturbances. Where the diagnosis, for example, is one of *dysthymia*, a lowered mood, not associated with hallucinatory experiences or delusional ideation, there may be difficulties expressed with regard to initiation of sleep, but once asleep, the individual may be undisturbed for the rest of the night. In contrast, the individual experiencing a *major depressive episode*, with its concomitant absence of insight into reality, may initiate sleep relatively easily but exteriorize wakening in the early hours of the morning. 'Dysthymic' clients experience their lowest mood 'trough' of the day late in the evening just prior to bedtime, whilst individuals diagnosed as suffering a 'major' depressed mood awaken at their lowest mood point. Both may be of significance when nursing a client who has expressed or may be considering suicidal thoughts, for it is when mood is at its lowest point that such thoughts may find expression in enactment, and whilst close observation of this client is a priority 24 hours of the day, intense scrutiny during the quiet hours, when the client is expected to be asleep, and yet may not be, is of prime importance. You should be aware, however, that it is not only clients with a label of 'depression' who may experience a profound lowering of mood as an integral or concomitant feature of their total mental health problems and therefore any individual exteriorizing such mood deviation—for no matter how fleeting a period—may suffer severe sleep disturbance (and also ideas of self-harm).

Preoccupation with mental activities and imagery quite naturally will provoke unease, restlessness, agitation and perhaps motor acceleration and therefore any individual experiencing such problems is likely to find sleeping problematical. Clients exteriorizing elevated mood—as in diagnoses such as *cyclothymia* and *bipolar mood disorder* of a *mixed or manic nature*—may exhibit no inclination or desire to sleep, being unable to relax the body and quieten the mind for a sufficient period to allow sleep to encroach. Anxiety or fear for one's own health or safety and well-being may provoke a similar high level of mental alertness and a concomitant bodily tension and therefore preclude sleep initiation. This would encompass a wide number of individuals within care provision and not only those traditionally associated with anxiety. Individuals, for example, who demonstrate obsessive ideation and compulsive, ritualistic behaviours may be too tense to sleep easily, whilst people who are utterly convinced of the fact that someone is either intent on killing or 'interfering' with them or their mind or body during sleep may be understandably unwilling to drop their guard to allow sleep. Young people experiencing anorexia nervosa and its associated problems may appear to have no sleep disturbance at all, for they seem to initiate sleep with no trouble and may still be fast off when approached next morning to get up,

and yet the total sleep duration is often considerably reduced. How? The individual is frequently awake during the very early hours of the morning and may, within that wakeful period, exercise vigorously with no carer to observe the phenomenon. Bingeing and purging activities may similarly be quietly performed without other people's awareness.

Insomnia and organic disorders

It would be unreasonable, too, to assume that problems associated with somatic health during the day would miraculously disappear just because it is time for bed, and it is, therefore, a relatively common event to see *insomnia* that is *related to a known organic factor*. For example, the pain, stiffness or general discomfort associated with a broken bone, arthritic joints or the rigidity of Parkinson's disease may, indeed, be perceived as increasing at night, during the protracted period of enforced immobility and when environmental distractors and comforters are reduced in both quality and quantity. Some individuals may experience horror at the thought of lying down in bed, and people experiencing the effects of a left-sided heart failure are amongst this number. The difficulty in breathing (*dyspnoea*) that they experience is significantly exacerbated when lying flat (*orthopnoea*) owing to pulmonary oedema, which 'clogs up' the alveoli and reduces the oxygen-filling capability of lung tissue. The individual may awaken suddenly during the night, often understandably panicked by inability to breathe easily—*paroxysmal nocturnal dyspnoea*. *Asthma* may also awaken the individual at night and cause early morning wheezing and dyspnoea, and, in fact, some paroxysmal disorders may be seen to begin with the REM sleep phases of the sleep cycle, for example, *duodenal ulcer pain* and *migraine*, causing disturbance in the early hours. Angina and cardiac arrhythmias occur more frequently in REM sleep, too, as do deaths from myocardial infarction. Whilst it is not clear during which phase of sleep infarcts occur, they usually happen between 5.00 a.m. and 6.00 a.m., when REM sleep predominates. Some people may experience *seizures* on a regular basis during sleep and the characteristic electroencephalographic 'epileptic discharges' may be seen to be activated in either REM or slow wave sleep, depending on the type of disorder. You are probably only too well aware of the disturbed sleep associated with a persistent cough in a short duration respiratory tract infection, but such a problem may be a long term feature in a variety of respiratory problems and may be the result of both intrinsic stimuli (neoplasia, inflammation, foreign bodies and scar tissue formation are examples) and extrinsic stimuli (pleurisy, oesophageal growths, mediastinal lymphadenopathy) in addition to a psychogenic or attention-seeking origin. Sleep disturbance may serve to weaken the individual further and this type of intermittent night-time wakening may be a common feature in a variety of somatic health problems. The *pruritus* of jaundice and the *nocturia* (voiding during the night hours) associated with impaired renal function provide two such instances.

Within mental health care provision, individuals experiencing organic *impairment* may likewise exteriorize sleep problems. *Delirium* may be seen to provoke problems of both the insomnia-type and disturbances in the sleep–wake cycle later elucidated. The individual may be hypervigilant or hypersomnolent, and vivid dreams and nightmares may be seen to blend imperceptibly for the client into hallucinatory experiences during waking. There may be crying, moaning, muttering and calls for help during the night hours, thus disturbing the sleep of others within the environment. Delirium may be an integral feature experienced during a variety of somatic as well as mental health orientated problems—systemic infections, metabolic disorders, renal and hepatic disease and head injury to name but a few—and colleagues within all specialties of care should be aware of such sleep problems.

Psychoactive substance use and abuse is a frequent cause of delirium within the sphere of psychosocial health care and therefore this insomnia–hypersomnia pattern may be problematical. Withdrawal from substance use may elicit similar symptomatology and those experiencing the effects of a psychoactive-substance-related organic mood disorder may have difficulty initiat-ing sleep. However, it is not only the 'illicit' drugs that may provoke a sleeping problem, for steroids, bronchodilators and central adrenergic blocking agents given 'therapeutically' over prolonged periods may engender an insomnia disorder.

Insomnia, whether primary or secondary in nature, is bound to result in excessive daytime fatigue, impaired daytime functioning and general irritability. Some may experience disturbances in mood, in memory and concentration and attention spans, and social and occupational functioning may become seriously disrupted if problems are protracted.

Hypersomnia

Hypersomnia on the other hand may engender disruption from day one, for, despite night-time sleep of an adequate amount, there are complaints of either excessive daytime sleepiness, sleep attacks or a prolonged transition from sleep to wakefulness, often referred to as *sleep drunkenness* (Roth, Nevsimalova & Rechtschaffen 1972). That hypersomnia may be associated with other, *non-organic, mental health problems* has already been mentioned in passing. It may be a feature of *depressed mood*, in *bipolar disorders*, and in some other mood disorders, such as *major depression* or *dysthymia*. Similarly, hypersomnia may be a feature in the sleep of those diagnosed as 'schizophrenic' and where 'somatoform disorders' exist, but in the majority of instances the individual asserts that this excessive sleepiness is the result of non-restorative sleep. We have also made previous mention of hypersomnia in relation to a *known organic factor*, as in delirium and illicit and prescribed drugs, and other abused substance use/withdrawal.

Hypersomnolence may be a *secondary* phenomenon to a wide number of cerebral problems (trauma, tumour, vascular accident, inflammation and infection), in endocrinological dysfunction, for example hypothyroidism, and in respiratory, renal and hepatic failure (Guilleminault et al 1983). They may also be secondary to primary sleep disorders of which the subject is totally unaware. *Sleep apnoea syndrome*, for example, may result in daytime sleepiness because of persistent, short duration periods of respiratory cessation throughout the night. An individual may stop breathing in this way for one of two reasons; there may be a hyposensitivity of the respiratory centre to carbon dioxide or an upper airway obstruction to respiration, although mixed aetiology has been demonstrated. The commonest causes of obstruction would appear to be tonsillar hypertrophy, obesity or a sleep-induced hypotonia of the pharyngeal muscles, although deformity of the mandible has also been indicated as a predisposing factor (Lugaresi et al 1973).

The 'Pickwickian syndrome', named by Burwell et al (1956) after the fat boy in Dickens' novel, is, as the name suggests, seen in grossly overweight children. Some experience only mild headaches in addition to the sleep apnoea, but daytime somnolence does, of course, result in poor school performance. Other children may exhibit *cyanosis, right-sided heart failure* and *polycythaemia* (an increase in the number of erythrocytes and therefore an increase in the concentration of haemoglobin) in addition to the night-time periodic respiration and daytime sleepiness. There continues to be a dispute in regard to the specific aetiology of the problem (Passouant, Cadilhac & Baldy-Moulinier 1967, Schwartz, Seguy & Escande 1967).

Whatever the cause, each episode of apnoea may last from 10 to 80 seconds or more, and there may be anywhere in the region of 30 to several hundred such episodes each night. Individuals must partially or fully arouse in order to breathe, although they are oblivious to the fact. There is a period of loud snoring and snorting, followed by a resumption in respiration. Gross movement of the extremities, sleep walking and enuresis (involuntary voiding of urine) may all be exhibited. If awakened at night, the individual may demonstrate automatic behaviour, amnesia, temporal disorientation, poor judgement and hypnagogic hallucinations. Daytime performance may be interspersed within microsleeps, or a generalized excessive sleepiness. Complaints may be made regarding decreased sexual drive and potency, personality changes and headaches and on examination hypertension and sinus tachycardia may be evident. Whilst it has been asserted that up to

10% of the population suffer from this syndrome, 'normal' sleepers may experience occasional apnoeic episodes too.

Primary hypersomnias may occur in short or long periods and, amongst the former, '*sleep drunkenness*' is by far the most common example. Subjects complain of not being able to wake up 'properly' for some considerable period after actually getting out of bed, which may extend to up to 4 hours. This half-awake/half-asleep period is accompanied by confusion, disorientation, retarded and uncoordinated motor activity and a desire to go back to bed. Subjects will sleep, if left undisturbed, for up to 20 hours with no spontaneous waking and yet still experience daytime somnolence. Night-time sleep is rapidly initiated, often within seconds of putting the head on the pillow, and is extremely deep. Headaches, depressed mood and personality changes have frequently been reported, and occurrence is seen to be slightly higher in men. Whilst it may be seen to follow a period of sleep deprivation, in Roth and his colleagues' detailed study (Roth, Nevsimalova & Rechtschaffen 1972), one-third of presenting individuals had a family history of such problems and most people demonstrated a lifelong tendency towards sleep drunkenness symptomatology. It presented as a relatively common experience within this particular study of hypersomnia sufferers, with an approximate incidence of 30% of problems seen.

Kleine–Levin syndrome

In contrast Kleine (1925) and Levin (1936) described a much rarer type of hypersomnia which now bears their names. This syndrome is characterized by periods when the appetite is excessive (*bulimia*) and the individual will eat ravenously, and often anything in sight, yet if food is not available, neither complains of hunger nor demands food. The eating behaviour is compulsive, greedy and wolfish in nature and this is followed by a period of profound sleepiness, where the individual will sleep day and night, rousing only to eat, drink or perform evacuatory functions. During this period the individual is as easily awoken as any normal sleeper, but is irritable, bad tempered and may be physically aggressive. When awake, too, the individual demonstrates marked cognitive impairment—confusion, disorientation, muddled and depersonalized thinking and speech and memory disturbances—and perceptions may be littered with vivid imagery which the individual finds difficult to differentiate from dreams. Auditory hallucinations and delusional ideation may also be exteriorized. Emotional and motor agitation and unrest are also a feature, with fidgety movements and generalized unease. Abnormal—for the individual—levels of sexual behaviour have been reported (Critchley 1962, Garland, Sumner & Fourman 1965) with frequent masturbation and hypersexuality.

The Kleine–Levin syndrome is seen to affect adolescent boys predominantly, though atypical cases have been documented where onset has been seen in an adolescent girl (Duffy & Davison 1968), in women (Gilbert 1964) and in middle age (Gallinek 1954). An 'attack' may last for days or weeks, but typically are infrequent, the average being two per year though as many as 12 have been described. The onset is usually spontaneous, although it may be seen that a period of stress or flu-like condition may precede its onset. Indeed, whilst death during an attack is rare, a post-mortem examination of one fatality indicated the possibility of a viral aetiology (Carpenter, Yassa & Ochs 1982) though this has not been confirmed. In between attacks, the individual reverts to 'normal' characteristics and behavioural patterns, although mental health problems may exist for a short time before and after the episode. Onset and cessation of an attack may be gradual or abrupt in nature, and the individual may have only partial, or a complete lack of, awareness of the episode. The episodic problems of bingeing and somnolence appear to reduce in both frequency and duration with time, and ultimately cease completely (Gallinek 1954).

Diencephalic abnormality has been suggested to account for the eating–sleeping behaviours of the syndrome, but no abnormalities within biochemistry, electroencephalography or physiology have been elicited during attacks. The problem for the client, and the professional must be in the syndrome's rarity and the apparently 'psychotic'

symptomatology which may predominate within the clinical picture, for as Critchley (1962) and others observe (Robinson & McQuillan 1951), the client may present with distinct schizophrenia-like symptomatology. The need for a comprehensive and accurate analysis of actual problems experienced by the individual, regardless of the symptomatology to be expected in a specific diagnosis applied, and the willingness to consider alternative explanations for behaviours exhibited, is therefore a necessary characteristic for all carers within mental health service provision.

Narcolepsy

Probably first described by Westphal (1877) but named by Gelineau (1880), narcolepsy is, by contrast, much easier to recognize. Individuals experience an irresistible desire to sleep during the daytime, and awake easily enough from such naps, feeling refreshed and alert, experiencing no more episodes for several hours. The nap usually lasts for a period of 10–15 minutes and if such individuals are prevented from napping, or awakened during the sleep, they may be extremely irritable. Naps most frequently occur at junctures of the day when events or activities are more conducive to drowsiness, for example, after meals and where environmental stimuli are reduced or monotonous, but some individuals experience the problem when talking, eating, dancing—even when making love—and attacks may lead to life-threatening situations if they occur during periods of driving, swimming or operating machinery.

In 75% of individuals presenting, there is evidence of other, additional features. *Cataplexy*, a sudden loss of emotional tone, appears to be evident in 70% of narcolepsy sufferers, and tends to occur following an emotion-provoking event, for example, after laughter or tears are evoked. Where all muscle groups are involved, the individual will fall to the floor, unable to move or speak, and possibly sustaining injury. Often the individual will remain standing, however, and reaction is appropriate to a limited muscular involvement, as the individual may drop something he was previously holding, or elicit a jaw- or head-dropping movement. Such attacks rarely extend beyond a minute's duration and the individual is always alert and fully aware of what is happening. Cataplectic attacks rarely occur more than once a day, and subjects may learn to avoid precipitating situations. Cataplexy has been described within one family, where 11 children were affected and attacks were laughter induced (Gelardi & Brown 1967). The researchers believed it to be transmitted via an autosomal dominant gene and described only three of the children as evincing any—even if dubious—signs of narcolepsy, though *sleep paralysis* was occasionally demonstrated. Whilst rare, such an account is of value when attempting to discover the aetiology of such problems.

Sleep paralysis, mentioned above, is again a relatively common accompaniment to narcolepsy, with an estimated 30% of narcoleptic individuals exhibiting the problem. There is a sudden inability to move either just before sleeping or immediately upon waking, which may occur in relation to both nocturnal and diurnal sleep periods. Abrupt in onset, there is a *flaccid paralysis* which is usually seen to encompass all muscles, although on occasions the individual may find some degree of eye movement possible. Duration does not usually exceed one minute, though one case has been reported where the paralysis exceeded an hour, and the experience may be dispelled by touch or by calling the individual's name. In a similar manner to cataplectic attacks, some rare instances of sleep paralysis occurring without narcolepsy have been described (Bowling & Richards 1961) which affected 10 people from two families.

Hypnagogic hallucinations are reported by a slightly smaller percentage of narcolepsy sufferers than is sleep paralysis, and are commonly experienced via the auditory modality, though visual, tactile and multimodal perceptual disorders are also seen. They predominantly arise as the individual passes into sleep, but on occasions may occur during the transition from sleep to wakefulness, when they are referred to as *hypnopompic hallucinations*. You may have experienced similar bedtime experiences and both hypnagogic and hypnopompic hallucinations are 'normal' phenomena. The difference between the 'normal' and the 'narcoleptic' is that in the former, the perceptual experiences are often of a word or a brief image that has little emotional meaning to the individual, whilst the latter experiences vivid, intense and complex visions, often bizarre and sometimes unpleasant in content. They may be difficult to distinguish from a dream, because of these characteristics and are always accompanied by strong emotional reactions, and, whilst the subject may respond to his experience whilst it operates, there is the recognition, once awake, of the true nature of the hallucinatory experience (Zarcone 1973).

Narcolepsy has its onset predominantly in the 10–20-year-old age group and it is rare to see a new subject of the 40-year-old-plus age group. Again it appears more common in boys and there is, in one-third of subjects, a family history evident. As has been identified, narcoleptic attacks as a sole problem presenting is less frequently seen— only 30% of instances, but to see all potentially associated features, that is cataplectic attacks, sleep paralysis and hypnagogic hallucinations, is much more rare at only 10% of all subjects with narcolepsy. The disturbed nocturnal sleep associated with narcolepsy demonstrates rapid initiation of sleep but subsequent restlessness and frequent wakeful periods. Many individuals, some 60% of those subject to both narcolepsy and cataplexy, experience vivid dreams, of an unpleasant and often terrifying nature, whilst where narcolepsy is a sole feature, the incidence is approximately 20% (Gelardi & Brown 1967). Daytime sleep is not, however, associated with dreaming.

Whilst no such disturbance has been demonstrated in those experiencing narcolepsy alone, those individuals who exhibit one or more of the other accompanying features of sleep paralysis, hypnagogic hallucinations or cataplectic attacks, show REM sleep occurring out of the normal sequence during nocturnal sleep, with REM occurring immediately or very quickly after the onset of sleep, and also during the daytime 'catnaps'. The features of hallucinations and sleep paralysis both occur during this early REM phase, as do cataplectic attacks. In addition, or perhaps because of, this out-of-synchronization of the REM phase, the other stages of nocturnal sleep are disturbed accounting for the restlessness and frequent awakenings. It has been suggested

(Rechtschaffen et al 1963), in the light of these EEG findings, that narcolepsy assumes a midpoint on a continuum that extends from hypersomnia at one extreme and narcolepsy plus cataplexy at the other.

You will recall the emphasis we laid on the basic circadian rhythms, of which sleep is one example, and of the importance of environmental cues in the individual's awareness of when it is time to eat and sleep. Problems related to the *sleep–wake cycle* are seen to occur because of a mismatch between environmental norms and the individual's circadian rhythm, and again you may recall the 'jet-lag' and 'shift work' examples previously offered within the introductory discussion on sleep and its norms.

Sleep–wake schedules may be seen to be *advanced* or *delayed* in relation to the societal norms. Where an advance is seen, the individual is really desirous of sleep early in the evening, perhaps as early as 6.00 or 7.00 p.m. and is awake around 2.00 or 3.00 a.m., happy and alert. In delayed schedules, the reverse is seen with the individual actually wanting to sleep at around 3.00 or 4.00 a.m. and, if allowed, will sleep until perhaps 10.00 or 11.00 a.m., therefore finding great difficulty if needing to be at work or seeing the children to school at 8.30 a.m. An advanced sleep pattern is often a feature of older people and hence the nurse must be aware of this as a normal routine for an individual rather than merely assuming that it is indicative of depressed mood, especially when one recalls that the need for sleep appears to reduce as age advances. The delayed sleep pattern is more likely to be a problem for the younger age group individuals and particularly those who have no rigid occupational or social commitments.

A third variation of the problem may be seen when there is no real 24-hour routine to life, and the individual is able to nap at will throughout the day, thus disrupting the circadian cycle of one major period of inactivity per day. The elderly and the bedridden individual may form part of this group of subjects, as may those individuals who fit their sleep into the voids created between work and socialization activities, thus demonstrating a *disorganized sleep–wake schedule.*

A *frequently changing pattern* of sleep–wake cycles may be seen to occur, yet again, as a result of lifestyle, in those jet-setters and shift workers, for example, who continually interfere with the normal routines of the body. You may recall that changes in 'time zone' require a period of adaptation to synchronize internal rhythms and environmental needs, and often an individual may try to mix the old and the new requirements, thus creating problems. The shift worker on night duty for a 3-week period organized thus by his employer in order to ease the transition from one time zone functioning level to another, may attempt at the weekends when off duty to revert to a pattern of daytime wakefulness and night-time sleeping, thereby throwing the cycle's stability yet again. Having previously referred to the health problems associated with frequently changing schedules, it may be recognized as a detrimental practice.

For many of the individuals who experience sleep–wake schedule problems, the answers lie in their own hands in the need to assume a daily routine conducive to environmental norms and circadian cycles, for in a preponderance of instances daytime naps and night-time revelling interfere with normal sleep requirements. For shift workers and jet-setters, the answer is predominantly in maintenance of new 'time zones' until another change is on the horizon and then a gradual adjustment towards the new requirements, to prevent a total derangement of the cycle and an easier transition phase. Gradual sleep-time advance or retard may be of a similar value to those individuals experiencing an innate cyclical problem, and may be a far more advantageous option than medication-induced conventional sleep patterns or being tired for large parts of the morning.

Within mental health care, problems of the sleep–wake schedule may be associated with a variety of situations in which there is a lack of awareness of environmental reality or an inability to recognize, or accede to, the demands of the body for sleep and rest. Clients experiencing problems associated with organic deterioration and hallucinatory experiences and delusional ideation are therefore prime candidates, and may need intensive night hour assistance and support.

THE PARASOMNIAS

The parasomnias, the second category associated with problems of sleep experienced, are characterized by 'abnormal' events that occur either during sleep or in the transition from wakefulness to sleep. Whilst disturbing the quality or quantity of sleep attained, as, in the dyssomnia group, individuals' complaints are not related either to that disturbance or sleep loss as such—the individuals concerned or their partners or families, centre concerns upon the event(s) experienced, and thus a differentiation is immediately possible and necessary. Are clients having problems in initiating or maintaining sleep, or are they experiencing some 'happening' within the night-time sleep period which engenders fear to sleep or which wakens them and precludes a return to rest?

Who has not had the experience of a bad dream and awoken in the darkness, heart thumping and momentarily panicked that fantasy may indeed be reality, only to find that the bed and surroundings are safe and familiar, and breathe a sigh of relief? On the majority of occasions, having assured the security of the environment and of self within it, the individual will settle back to sleep, and it is only on rare occasions that the sleeper will remain disturbed and awake for the rest of the night. The REM phase of sleep is that commonly associated with dreaming and certainly this is the period when the vivid, bizarre and seemingly illogical visual images, which are labelled by individuals as 'dreams', occur. The individual 'running' or 'seeing' in his dream is actually experiencing the brain activity associated with these activities, and if it was not for the fact that his brain and skeletal muscles were 'disconnected' at this point via the loss of muscle tone, the individual would be running or seeing in actuality at that moment. In contrast, the dreams occurring in non-REM sleep are far less visual in nature, more logical and related to events occurring in waking life and are not as emotionally intense as REM dreams. Muscle tone is relaxed but 'connected' and available for use if necessary, as slow wave sleep predominates. The distinction is important when considering the potential events of sleep.

Dream anxiety, or *nightmare, disorder* occurs during periods of REM sleep, which whilst occurring throughout sleep on a cyclical basis, occurs in longer phases as the night wears on, the longest period occurring prior to waking. Nightmares may then occur at any of these REM phases but become more frequent at the end of the night, when the period is more abundant. The observer will, of course, note very little physical indication of the sleeper's turmoil because of the lack of muscle tone and therefore no large movements are possible although, as the individual arouses from sleep, movement is regained.

Nightmare content may be recalled in detail on waking, and typically relates to a threat to the individual's biopsychosocial integrity—to physical survival, to personal security, whether of a social or material nature, or to self-esteem. The nightmare theme may be a recurring one, is ultra-detailed, vivid and appears, to the sleeper, to be of a prolonged duration, and is often able to be recalled in the morning as efficiently as immediately upon waking after the experience. The nightmare content is extremely distressing and frightening and the individual, whilst gaining a rapid grasp of the reality of the situation, is often loath, or has great difficulty, in regaining sleep.

The years associated with childhood and the teens are most frequently those of the onset of the problem, and children tend to 'grow out' of the disorder. Where beginning in adults, it does tend to be rather more persistent and often continues for years. Nightmares are reported to occur as frequently as four or more times a week and therefore may provoke considerable disruption of the sleep pattern, regardless of the degree of fear or anxiety associated with the potential for the event. Many sufferers (about 60%) will describe the onset as related to some major life stressor that has occurred and indeed the frequency of nightmares is seen to increase at times of stress. In some instances, a change in the sleeping environment may engender a significant reduction in episodes experienced, as may physical fatigue.

Nightmares may be an integral problem, though not the primary problem, for many individuals seeking mental health assistance. Children, for example, who are experiencing a separation from a loved one, may describe nightmares comprising of people or monsters trying to hurt them, or people they love. Typically, too, they are afraid of the dark and unhappy to sleep alone, frequently finding protection and security by crawling into the bed of a sibling, parent or other significant adult. The child is little different to the adult, who may respond to estrangement, feelings of alienation or distrust, in a similar fashion.

Individuals experiencing the problems associated with organic cerebral impairment may find that their nightmares merge with hallucinatory events and may signify just one aspect of a disturbed sleep pattern that may also include insomnia and daytime hypersomnolence. Certain drugs have nightmares as a potential side-effect, for example, beta-blocking agents and thioridazine, and withdrawal from REM-suppressing substances, for instance, alcohol or tricyclic preparations, will generally create a 'rebound' or compensatory increase in REM sleep and thus increase the likelihood of vivid dreams and nightmares.

In contrast, *sleep terror disorder* occurs during the slow wave, stage three and four delta rhythm activity and tends to occur during the first third of nocturnal sleep. Otherwise termed *parvor nocturnus*, individuals frequently sit up in bed with a scream (remember, there is full muscle tone in non-REM sleep), eyes open, pupils dilated and breathing rapidly. The picture is one of pure terror, the skin is pale, there is cold and profuse sweat, the hairs on the arms stand erect (*piloerection*) and the pulse is accelerated. Their facial expression tells it all. At that moment they are totally unaware of the presence of any other person and are unresponsive to any attempt of comfort. The episode lasts for a period of up to 10 minutes, and when it subsides, individuals may recount a very fragmented nightmare scene and recall feeling the terror associated with it. They will, however, settle back to sleep and have no recall in the morning of the incident.

Where onset is in children, it appears to stand alone as a problem, with no apparent other psychosocial symptomatology. On occasions onset, which tends towards the 4–12-year-old age group, may be seen to follow a febrile illness, and the frequency of episodes may be variable, occurring on consecutive nights or with several days or weeks

in between. Again the child tends to 'grow out' of the problem during adolescence. However, the adult does not tend to be so lucky, for where onset is in the 20–40-year-old age group—and it rarely occurs later than this—the course is often a chronic and persistent one, and is often associated with general feelings of anxiety towards life and living. Yet again, sleep terrors tend to occur more frequently in boys/men than their female peers and there would appear to be a higher incidence in first degree biological relatives than within the remainder of the population. Cerebral pathology should always be excluded at the outset, via an efficient and comprehensive neurological examination to ensure no underlying pathology is provoking the problem.

Sleep walking (*somnambulism*) may damage health; many, including Scott (1981), have described children within care who have fractured limbs as a result of their nightly wanderings. Sleep walking, too, occurs within slow wave sleep and may actually be initiated by lifting a child to his feet during this phase of the cycle, demonstrating the fact, amply, that the child is not responding to a dream. Again, more common in children, and boys rather than girls, it makes only a rare appearance in adulthood. Usually the activity witnessed is a gentle-paced aimless meandering, although, on occasions, running, jumping or searching behaviours may be seen. Sometimes the pattern of behaviour is very stereotyped and repetitive, totally purposeless in nature. The child will often reply to questions posed monosyllabically and some children will perform simple commands whilst experiencing this state. The episode may last half an hour or more, with the child then returning to bed and if awaken, contrary to popular belief, the child will display confusion and disorientation, but will gradually return to full awareness and have no recall of the incident. The problem tends to disappear as the child ages and matures into adolescence. There would appear again to be an increased familial prevalence of the problem, and an association with both *sleep-talking* (*somniloquy*) and *bed-wetting behaviour* (*nocturnal enuresis*).

Where sleep walking is seen during adulthood, both onset (usually around the time of puberty) and episodes (about four or five a year) are associated with psychosocially traumatic events. These include separation from a parent, for a variety of reasons, the birth of a sibling or school change and the investigations of Sours, Frumkin & Indermill (1963) highlighted disturbed and difficult family situations and interactions as a common feature within the group they studied. Similarly, the majority of subjects had displayed antisocial behaviours—'theft, delinquency and acting out'—and demonstrated high levels of anxiety and depressed mood. Some of the group (9 of the 14) were diagnosed as 'schizophrenic' or of a 'schizoid personality', whilst others were considered to demonstrate symptomatology consistent with 'hysterical conversion disorders'.

Very seldomly, sleep walking may be associated with an organic focus, for example, temporal lobe epilepsy, but, in general, it appears to be due to a partial arousal out of slow wave sleep due to an abnormality—perhaps a lack of mature development—of the sleep-associated mechanisms.

Sleep talking (*somniloquy*) is the production of speech, or other meaningful sounds, during sleep, of which the subject is totally unaware. Again more common in boys and seen within the slow wave phase of sleep, it is often associated with sleep-walking children. *Bruxism* (*teeth grinding*) tends to occur in stages one and two of sleep and may lead to erosion and wearing down of the teeth. Aetiology and incidence is relatively vague.

Whilst not a 'sleep disorder', as such, *nocturnal enuresis* is an abnormal event that may punctuate sleep and hence warrants a fleeting mention. A behavioural problem, believed to occur in 10% of 7-year-old and 3% of 12-year-old boys, it may occur during any sleep stage but is more common in slow wave sleep. It is less common in girls (3% and 2% for the respective age groups).

Micturition (the passage of urine) is heralded by a burst of EEG activity within stage four or one and two, though when it does occur during REM sleep, the child may recall a dream in which he or she was urinating. However, in the majority of instances, the child awakes with no memory either of the dream or of voiding. Sufferers do outgrow the problem, with only 1% of 18-year-old young men still experiencing a problem, and almost a non-existent incidence in young women of this age group.

The problem does tend to show a familial link, and developmental delay in bladder musculature and physiology that results in a low bladder threshold, and therefore involuntary voiding, may predispose the difficulty. Lax, inconsistent and delayed toilet training and psychosocial stress, for example sibling rivalry in response to a new baby, may also precipitate such involuntary voiding. Whilst not usually seen in relation to a coexisting mental health problem, more psychosocial problems are seen to exist within these children than in the general population.

Conclusions

Sleep is fascinating, and although an activity that everyone participates in, there are still many gaps in knowledge relating to the subject. Problems of sleep may indicate a significant biopsychosocial health status deviation or merely poor habits and a lack of understanding in relation to the great value of regular efficient sleeping within daily functioning. We assert the importance of a comprehensive, objective assessment of the individual's health needs and problems to ensure effective assistance is provided. The role of education, in regard to all aspects of sleeping patterns and routines, is important in the promotion of optimum psychosocial and somatic health.

SUMMARY

We have explored only some of the themes associated with the personal motivation resulting in exhibited behaviour and space precludes a more detailed and extensive analysis of both this area and that of social motivation. It is our hope that there is sufficient here to provoke both observation and reflection and to encourage you to look for similarities, as well as differences (or modifications) in behaviours exhibited by human beings and animals alike. To achieve the real degree of civilization desired rather than the superficial veneer so far attained requires more individual and societal attention, reflection and debate.

DISCUSSION QUESTIONS

1. We have been limited in space and able to explore only moving, eating and sleeping as specific behaviours affected by the experience of mental health problems. Sexual behaviour is another area worthy of detailed investigation, however, that is commonly seen to be affected by emotional and cognitive difficulties.

   How do our sexual identity and behaviour develop? What are the influences that impact upon that development and later exteriorization of a sexual identity? What exactly is 'normal' sexual behaviour and where does acceptable behaviour end and inappropriacy begin? How is sexual behaviour affected by the experience of mental health difficulties?

2. We are aware that some behaviours carried to excess are unhealthy. Smoking, drinking too much alcohol, unprotected sex and speeding on urban roads are examples of the type of thing we mean, and that you may be able to relate to. Why do some people do these things? Until we know, we can't generate effective health promotion strategies to reduce the incidence of these behaviours.

   Discuss the issues and motivation/ideation with your peers. Attempt to generate strategies that may help to alter behaviours. Try these strategies out on others within the learning environment. Assess their effects on stated behaviours.

3. Examine the ways in which 'normal', everyday behaviours have been perceived to be affected by a client experiencing mental health problems. The client's permission must be sought and gained and feedback should be in writing where appropriate, but always to the supervising nurse.

FURTHER READING

Abraham S, Llewellyn-Jones D 1987 Eating disorders: the facts. Oxford University Press, Oxford

Allen Hobson J 1989 Sleep. Scientific American Library, New York

Borbely A 1986 Secrets of sleep. Penguin, London

Brain W R 1985 Brain's diseases of the nervous system. Oxford University Press, Oxford

Brunner L S, Suddarth D S 1986 The Lippincott manual of medical surgical nursing. Harper & Row, London

Duker M, Slade R 1988 Anorexia nervosa and bulimia: how to help. Open University Press, Milton Keynes

Hinchliffe S, Montague S 1988 Physiology for nursing practice. Baillière Tindall, London

Hinwood B 1993 A textbook of science for the health professions, 2nd edn. Chapman & Hall, London

Lishman W A 1978 Organic psychiatry: the psychological consequences of cerebral disorder. Blackwell Scientific, Oxford

Roth I (ed) 1990 Introduction to psychology, vols 1 and 2. Laurence Erlbaum Associates in conjunction with the Open University, Milton Keynes

REFERENCES

Ack M, Miller I, Weil W B 1961 Intelligence of children with diabetes mellitus. Paediatrics 28:764–770

Andrews R 1987 Routledge dictionary of quotations. Routledge & Kegan Paul, London

Appleby L, Forshaw D 1990 Postgraduate psychiatry: clinical and scientific foundations. Heinemann Medical, Oxford

Arendt J, Aldous M, English J, Marks V, Arendt J H 1987 Some effects of jet lag and their alleviation by melatonin. Ergonomics 30(9):1379–1393

Aserinsky E, Kleitman N 1953 Regularly occurring periods of eye motility and concurrent phenomena during sleep. Science 118:273–274

Bearn A G 1972 Wilson's disease. In: Stanbury J B, Wyngaarden J B, Fredrickson D S (eds) The metabolic basis of inherited disease. McGraw-Hill, New York

Beck E, Daniel P M, Alpers M, Gajdusek D C, Gibbs C J 1966 Experimental 'Kuru' in chimpanzees. A pathological report. Lancet 2:1056–1059

Beck E, Daniel P M, Gajdusek D C, Gibbs D J 1969a Similarities and differences in the pattern of the pathological changes in scrapie, Kuru, experimental Kuru and subacute presenile polioencephalopathy. In: Whitty C W M, Hughes J T, MacCallum F O (eds) Virus diseases and the nervous system. Blackwell Scientific, Oxford, pp 558–569

Beck E, Daniel P M, Matthews, W B et al 1969b Creuzfeldt–Jakob disease: the neuropathology of a transmission experiment. Brain 92:699–716

Binkley S 1979 A timekeeping enzyme in the pineal gland. Scientific American 240:66–71

Bowling G, Richards N G 1961 Diagnosis and treatment of the narcolepsy syndrome. Cleveland Clinic Quarterly 28:38–45

Burwell C S, Robin E D, Whaley R D, Bickelmann A G 1956 Extreme obesity associated with alveolar hypoventilation—a Pickwickian syndrome. American Journal of Medicine 21:811–818

Campbell R J 1989 Psychiatric dictionary. Oxford University Press, Oxford

Carpenter S, Yassa R, Ochs R 1982 A pathologic basis for Kleine–Levin syndrome. Archives of Neurology 39:25

Carskadon M A, Mitler M M, Dement W C 1974 A comparison of insomniacs and normals: total sleep time and sleep latency. Sleep Research 3:130

Coleman D L, Hummel K P 1969 Effects of parabiosis of normal with genetically diabetic mice. American Journal of Physiology 217:1298–1304

Coscina D V, Dixon L M 1983 Body weight regulation in anorexia nervosa: insights from an animal model. In: Darby P L, Garfinkel P E, Garner D M, Coscina D V (eds) Anorexia nervosa: recent developments. Allen R Liss, New York

Crick F, Mitchison G 1983 The function of dream sleep. Nature 304:111–114

Crisp A H 1983 Treatment of anorexia nervosa. What can be the role of psychopharmacological agents? In: Pirke K M, Ploog D (eds) The psychobiology of anorexia nervosa. Springer, New York

Critchley M 1962 Periodic hypersomnia and megaphagia in adolescent males. Brain 85:627

Crowley W F Jr, Beitins I Z, Vale W et al 1980 The biologic activity of a potent analogue of gonadotrophin releasing hormone in normal and hypogonadotropic men. New England Journal of Medicine 302:1052–1057

Czeisler C, Richardson G S, Coleman R M et al 1981 Chronotherapy: resetting the arcadian clocks of patients with delayed sleep phase insomnia. Sleep 4:1–21

Davis H 1978 Sexual dysfunction in diabetes. Medical Aspect of Human Sexuality 12:48

Davis J D, Brief D J 1981 Chronic intraventricular insulin infusions reduce food intake and body weight in rats. Social Neuroscience Abstract 7:655

Dement W C 1976 Some must watch while some must sleep. W H Freeman, New York

Dement W C, Kleitman N 1975 The relation of eye movements during sleep to dream activity: an objective method for the study of dreaming. Journal of Experimental Psychology 53:89–97

Denko J D, Kaelbling R 1962 The psychiatric aspects of hypoparathyroidism. Acta Psychiatrica Scandinavica 164(suppl.):1–70

DOH (Department of Health) 1992 The health of the nation. HMSO, London

Duffy J P, Davison K 1968 A female case of Kleine–Levin syndrome. British Journal of Psychiatry 114:77

Ellenberg M 1977 Sex and the female diabetic. Medical Aspect of Human Sexuality 11:30

Faust I M 1984 Role of the fat cell in energy balance physiology. In: Stunkard A T, Stellar E (eds) Eating and its disorders. Raven Press, New York

Faust I M, Johnson P R, Stern J S, Hirsch J 1978 Diet induced adipocyte increase in adult rats: a new model of obesity. American Journal of Physiology 235:E279–E286

Fourman P, Rawnsley K, David R H, Jones K H, Morgan D B 1967 Effect of calcium on mental symptoms in partial parathyroid insufficiency. Lancet 2:914–915

Freud S 1954 The interpretation of dreams, translated by Strachey J. George Allen & Unwin, London

Friedman M I, Stricker E M 1976 The physiological psychology of hunger: a physiological perspective. Psychological Review 83:401–431

Gallinek A 1954 Syndrome of episodes of hypersomnia, bulimia and abnormal mental states. Journal of the American Medical Association 154:1081–1083

Garland H, Sumner D, Fourman P 1965 The Kleine–Levin syndrome. Some further observations. Neurology 15:1161

Gelardi J A M, Brown J W 1967 Hereditary cataplexy. Journal of Neurology, Neurosurgery & Psychiatry 30:455–457

Gelineau Dr 1880 De la narcolepsie. In: Brain W R 1985 Brain's diseases of the nervous system. Oxford University Press, Oxford

Gilbert G J 1964 Periodic hypersomnia and bulimia: the Kleine–Levin syndrome. Neurology 14:844–850

Guilleminault C, Faull K F, Miles L, Van den Hoed J 1983 Post-traumatic excessive daytime sleepiness: a review of 20 patients. Neurology 33:1584

Harlow J M 1848 Passage of an iron rod through the head. Boston Medical and Surgical Journal 39:389–393

Hartmann E 1984 The nightmare. Basic Books, New York

Herman C P, Polivy J 1980 Restrained eating. In: Stunkard A J (ed) Obesity. W B Saunders, Phildelphia

Hinchliff S, Montague S 1988 Physiology for nursing practice. Baillière Tindall, London

Hoebel B G, Teitelbaum P 1966 Effects of forcefeeding and starvation on food intake and body weight on a rat with ventromedial hypothalamic lesions. Journal of Comparative and Physiological Psychology 61:189–193

Huxley J 1958 Evolution. Allen & Unwin, London

Ives E R 1963 Mental aberrations in diabetic patients. Bulletin of the Los Angeles Neurological Society 28:279–285

Janowitz H D, Grossman M I 1949 Some facts affecting the food intake of normal dogs and dogs with oesophagostomy and gastric fistula. American Journal of Physiology 159:143–148

Keesey R E, Powley T K 1975 Hypothalamic regulation of body weight. American Scientist 63:558–565

Kleine W 1925 Periodische Schlafsucht. Monatsschriftfur und Neurologie 57:285–320

Knittle J L, Hirsch J 1968 Effect of early nutrition on the development of rat epididymal fat pads: cellularity and metabolism. Journal of Clinical Investigation 47:2091

Knobil E, Neill J, Ewings L A, Greenwald G (eds) 1988 The physiology of reproduction. Raven Press, New York

Koenig H 1968 Dementia associated with the benign form of multiple sclerosis. Transactions of the American Neurological Association 93:227–231

Kolodny R 1971 Sexual function in diabetic females. Diabetes 20:557

Kripke D F, Gillin J C 1985 Sleep disorders. In: Klerman G L, Weissman M M, Applebaum P S, Roth L N (eds) Psychiatry vol 3. Lippincott, New York

Krueger J M P Jr, Karnovsky M L 1982 The composition of sleep promoting factor isolated from human urine. Journal of Biological Chemistry 257:1664–1669

Lavie P, Kripke D F G 1975 Ultradian rhythms! The 90 minute clock inside us. Psychology Today 8:54–65

Leibowitz S F 1983 Noradrenergic function in the medial hypothalamus: potential relation to anorexia nervosa and bulimia. In: Pirke K M, Ploog D (eds) The psychobiology of anorexia nervosa. Springer, New York

Levin M 1936 Periodic somnolence and morbid hunger: a new syndrome. Brain 59:494

Lugaresi E, Coccaena G, Ontavani M, Brignanv F 1973 Effects of tracheostomy in two cases of hypersomnia with periodic breathing. Journal of Neurology, Neurosurgery and Psychiatry 36:15–26

Mayer J 1955 Regulation of energy uptake and the body weight! The glucostatic theory and the lipostatic hypotheses. Annals of the New York Academy of Sciences 63:15–42

MacLean C 1977 The wolf children. Allen Lane, London

McGhie A, Russell S M 1962 The subjective assessment of normal sleep patterns. Journal of Mental Science 108:456

McKenna R J 1972 Some effects of anxiety level and food crises on the eating behaviour of obese and normal subjects. Journal of Personality and Social Psychology 22:311–319

Mitchell J S, Keesey R E 1974 The effects of lateral hypothalamic lesions and castration upon the body weight of male rats. Behavioural Biology 11:69–82

Moore-Ede M C, Sulzman F Z, Fuller C A 1982 The clocks that time us. Harvard University Press, Massachusetts

Pappenheimer J R 1976 The sleep factor. Scientific American 235:24–29

Passouant P, Cadilhac J, Baldy-Moulinier M 1967 Physiopathologie des hypersomnies. Revue Neurologique 116:585–629

Pieron H 1913 Le probleme physiologique du sommeil. Masson, Paris

Rechtschaffen A R, Wolpert E A, Dement W C, Mitchell S A, Fisher C 1963 Nocturnal sleep of narcoleptics. Electroencephalography and Clinical Neurophysiology 15:599–609

Robinson J T, McQuillan J 1951 Schizophrenic reaction associated with the Kleine–Levin syndrome. Journal of the Royal Army Medical Corps 96:377–381

Robinson K C, Kallberg M H, Crowley M F 1954 Idiopathic hypoparathyroidism presenting as dementia. British Medical Journal 21:1203–1206

Roffwarg H P, Muzio J M, Dement W C 1968 Ontogenetic development of the human sleep–dream cycle. In: Webb W B (ed) Sleep—an experimental approach. Macmillan, New York

Roth B, Nevsimalova S, Rechtschaffen A 1972 Hypersomnia with sleep drunkenness. Archives of General Psychiatry 26:456–462

Ruderman A J 1986 Dietary restraint: a theoretical and empirical review. Psychological Bulletin 99:247–262

Schachter S 1971 Emotion, obesity and crime. Academic Press, New York

Scheinberg I H, Sternlieb I, Richman I 1968 Psychiatric manifestations in patients with Wilson's disease. In: Bergsma D (ed) Wilson's disease. Birth Defects Original Article Series 4, no. 2. The National Foundation

Schwartz B A, Seguy M, Escande J P 1967 Correlations EEG, respiratoires, oculaires et myographiques dans le 'syndrome Pickwickien' et autre affections paraissant apparantees: proposition d'une hypothese. Revue Neurologique 117:145–152

Scott D F 1981 What is sleep? World Medicine, June 27 1981, 57–58

Siffre M 1963 Hors du temps. Julliard, Paris

Sours J A, Frumkin P, Indermill R R 1963 Somnambulism: its clinical significance and dynamic meaning in late adolescence and adulthood. Archives of General Psychiatry 9:400–413

Stricker E M, Rowland N, Saller C F, Friedman M I 1977 Homeostasis during hypoglycaemia: central control of adrenal secretion and peripheral control of feeding. Science 196:79–81

Surridge D 1969 An investigation into some psychiatric aspects of multiple sclerosis. British Journal of Psychiatry 115:749–764

Tardoff M G, Hoffenbeck J, Novin D 1982 Hepatic vagotomy (partial hepatic denervation) does not alter ingestive responses to metabolic changes. Physiology and Behaviour 28:417–424

Walker S 1969 The psychiatric presentation of Wilson's disease (hepatolenticular degeneration) with an aetiologic explanation. Behavioural Neuropsychiatry 1:38–43

Webb W B 1975 Sleep: the gentle tyrant. Prentice-Hall, New Jersey

Wehr T A, Wirz-Justice A, Goodwin F K, Duncan W, Gillin J C 1979 Phase advance of the sleep–wake cycle as an antidepressant. Science 206:710–713

West D B, Williams R H, Braget D J, Woods S C 1982 Bombesin reduces food intake of normal and hypothalamically obese rats and lowers body weight when given chronically. Peptides 3:61–67

Westphal K F 1877 Eigen Hiü mluche mit Eimshaffen. Verbundene Aufälle. Arch Psychnevenkrar. British Medical Journal 7:631–635

White C 1977 Unpublished Ph.D. dissertation. Catholic University, Washington DC

Woods S C, Lotter E C, McKay L D, Porte D 1979 Chronic intracerebroventricular infusion reduces food intake and body weight in baboons. Nature (London) 282:503–505

Zarcone V 1973 Narcolepsy. New England Journal of Medicine 288:1156–1166

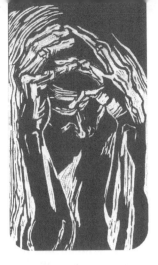

Chapter Five

Cognition

F Clifford Johnson   Lynne D Smith

 AIMS

- ◆ To review and consolidate previous learning in relation to cognition
- ◆ To explore the characteristics associated with:
  - (a) perception
  - (b) attention
  - (c) thinking
  - (d) memory
  - (e) language in health
- ◆ To determine problems which may be experienced in relation to the above abilities and which may indicate deviation from health status

KEY ISSUES

Definitions

Explanations

Relevant biopsychosocial development

Relevant theoretical perspectives

Illusions and hallucinations

Problems of attention

Problems of the form, content and nature of thinking

Memory distortions and difficulties

Language and speech problems

INTRODUCTION

Imagine:

a young woman, sitting on a bench, in the park, waiting for a friend. During the first few minutes, she is busy compiling a mental list of all the information she wants to share with her friend, but then she begins to shiver and notices how cold it has become.[a] Looking around her, she notes that the wind has strengthened and is whipping the dry, scrunchy-sounding, orange-gold leaves around the paths and between the shrubs. They congregate around her feet, the base of the bench and in the closed doorway of the cricket pavilion behind her. The trees are beginning to sway, and the windows behind her are rattling. The wooden verandah begins to creak and moan and the wind starts to howl. It's getting dark too, and shadows are forming around the foliage in the vicinity of the bench.[b] Whilst not afraid, the young woman is not feeling particularly comfortable either, as she snuggles deeper into her coat, reflecting that this was a less than ideal location to meet.[c] Looking about, the place is desolate, although she can hear traffic on the nearby road. She looks at her watch—it's five past four—her friend will be here any minute. Even as she's thinking it, she hears the iron gate, at the park entrance nearby, clang shut, and looks expectantly in that direction. Even in the dim light and shadows, she knows the figure is not that of her friend, and settles back on the bench.[d] A few moments later, a stranger passes her seat, just as the metal gate resounds again. This time the young woman, sure of the identity of the silhouetted figure, leaves the bench and hurries forward to meet her friend. They leave the park.

Some days later, the two friends are discussing a future meeting and on this occasion decide that the coffee shop should be the venue to meet.[e]

The scenario utilized hopefully reminds us of the operations inherent within cognition, that is, the vehicles via which an individual gains knowledge and understanding of both external reality and physiological status, thereby preparing for management of the situation presenting.

An analysis of the scenario identifies five distinct processes which culminate in cognition, namely:

(a) Perception, *that is, the organization and interpretation of stimuli received into meaningful knowledge.*
Longman's Dictionary of Psychology and Psychiatry 1984

Within the scenario, the young woman has not been sitting with her eyes closed, whilst compiling her agenda for the forthcoming meeting, but even so was able to focus her concentration upon it during the period of time that the environment matched her expectations or remained relatively unchanged. However, when a change in stimulus occurred—she began to feel cold—she becomes specifically aware of her environment and begins to *perceive* her surroundings rather than mechanically *observe* them.

(b) Attention, *represents conscious awareness, sensory clarity and central nervous system readiness to respond to stimuli received. It is a focusing on specific aspects of the environment and is a selective process, influenced by a variety of factors.*
Campbell 1989

The fictitious woman on the bench moves her centre of concentration to her environment, to facilitate assessment of the situation, by absorbing cues and clues available to her. She now clearly *attends* to the aspects of her surroundings that may influence subsequent activities.

(c) Thinking, *where images and ideas, representing objects and events experienced, are manipulated, using previous knowledge and general understanding of the situation to arrive at strategies by which changes in status may be managed.*
Campbell 1989

The young woman has done this, for she has identified the unsuitability of the environment for her purpose. Indeed her thoughts generate further focusing upon her immediate situation as she searches for more data to assist in activity planning. She is not only exposed to the elements within the present circumstances but notes the potential hazards to continued well-being in relation to the relative isolation and loneliness of the location. Therefore, she seeks information with regard to the proximity of people—the road and gate of the park—and an estimation of when company, in the form of her friend, may be expected.

> (d) Memory, *the ability to register, retain, recognize and recall past experiences for utilization at a subsequent time.*
> Campbell 1989

She has employed memory, in conjunction with thinking activities to come to conclusions about her current situation, but, in addition, possesses sufficient details within her store of knowledge, in regard to the size, shape and general appearance of her friend, to know that the indistinct figure at the gate is not the person expected. The results of this experience—the perceptions, thoughts and feelings—will be stored too, for future use and consideration.

> (e) Language *is the mode by which thought and activity is made available to conscious awareness. It is the basic vehicle utilized to structure experiences and, other than for those few aspects of conscious thought when mental images are utilized or objects are rotated in space, is therefore depended upon to achieve conscious awareness. It may be vocal or utilize other methods but in essence is the manner in which communication between parties also occurs.*
> Longman's Dictionary of Psychology and Psychiatry 1984

The young woman awaiting her friend utilized language to assess mentally her circumstances and to label the stranger as too fat/thin/short/tall to be her companion, to be wearing the 'wrong' sort of clothes or walk differently from her friend. In addition she manages her disquietude in regard to the environment by making alternative arrangements for the next meeting. She may not verbalize the 'why' but she utilizes language to inform, or negotiate, the where.

Cognition is the result of perception, attention, thinking, memory and language. The individual experiencing mental health problems may exteriorize a variety of divergencies from expected characteristics and it may therefore be valuable to explore briefly the basis for each process and the parameters and characteristics associated with it, prior to analysis of specific problems that may be evinced and the strategies that may be employed to manage/ameliorate their existence.

PERCEPTION

WHAT IS PERCEIVED AND HOW

We defined the process of perception as that encompassing the organization and interpretation of stimuli received, into meaningful knowledge. Such stimuli are recorded via a variety of sources, and, whilst we may automatically refer, at this point, to those senses that monitor the external environment, that is, the visual, auditory, tactile, olfactory and gustatory senses (Table 5.1), there are others to be considered.

The maculae and cristae, for example, are sense organs positioned within the semicircular ducts of the ear. These monitor the position of the head relative to the ground—*static equilibrium* or *gravity*—and sudden movements of the head, such as rotation, deceleration and acceleration—*dynamic equilibrium*—respectively. Impulses pass, via the vestibulocochlear (VIII) nerve, to the vestibular nuclei of the medulla, the cerebellum, thalamus and somatosensory cortex of the brain. Fibres from the vestibular nuclei transmit information to the nerves that control eye movements (III, IV, VI) and to the accessory (XI) nerve nucleus which helps control the head and neck. Other fibres from the lateral vestibular nucleus, forming the vestibulospinal tract, transmit impulses to skeletal muscles, regulating the response of body tone to head movement. Pathways between the vestibular nuclei, cerebellum and cerebrum enable the cerebellum, which is continuously receiving sensory updates, to exercise a key role within the maintenance of balance (Tortora & Anagnostakos 1984).

Table 5.1	Sensation and the pathway to interpretation					
Sensation	Receptor	Quality	Sensing system	Primary relay level	Secondary relay level	Tertiary relay level
Vision	Rods Cones	Brightness Colour Size Motion Contrast	Retina	Retina	Lateral geniculate Superior colliculus Hypothalamus	Primary visual cortex Secondary visual cortex
Hearing	Hair cells	Pitch Tone	Cochlea	Cochlear nuclei	Lemniscal, collicular and medial geniculate nuclei	Primary auditory cortex
Touch	Ruffini corpuscles	Pressure	Skin and internal organs	Spinal cord or brainstem	Thalamus	Somatosensory cortex
	Merkel discs Pacinian corpuscles	Temperature Vibration				
Smell	Olfactory receptor	Floral Fruity Musky Pungent	Olfactory nerves	Olfactory bulb	Piriform cortex	Limbic system Hypothalamus
Taste	Taste buds at tip of tongue Taste buds at edge and base of tongue	Sweet Salt Bitter Sour	Tongue	Medulla	Thalamus	Somatosensory cortex

There is, too, the *kinaesthetic sense*, which provides the individual with an awareness of the activities of muscles, tendons and joints, which muscles are contracted and the degree of tension resultant within tendons. It is via this sense that individuals are able to judge the movements and positions of limbs when they walk without the use of their eyes, or in the darkness, by recognizing the location and rate of movement of one part, in relation to the other parts, of the body. There are joint kinaesthetic (or proprioceptive) receptors located within the capsule, and around ligaments in the area of the joint, providing feedback on the changing degree of angularity of the joint. Muscle spindles, comprising sensory neurons, are positioned within most skeletal muscles, and provide information in relation to the degree of stretch within muscles. Tendon organs provide similar information relating to tendon tension, from their situation at the junction of muscle and tendon. All three types of proprioceptor pass impulses for conscious utilization, via ascending tracts in the spinal cord, to the thalamus and cerebral cortex, whilst those resulting in reflex action pass, via spinocerebellar tracts, to the cerebellum (Tortora & Anagnostakos 1984).

The above provides just two examples of sources of data, other than the five senses often considered to comprise perception. There are others—for example, baroreceptors monitor blood pressure, thermoreceptors respond to temperature changes and chemoreceptors measure levels of oxygen, carbon dioxide and hydrogen ions within arterial blood (Hinchliff & Montague 1988). In addition, the endocrine system assists by maintenance of blood chemical levels within activities designed to ensure internal optimum balance, or *homeostasis*. Perception involves the use of information from various origins, and is rarely dependent upon just one source of stimuli reception. It is considered, therefore, to be resultant from *cross-modal transfer*, utilizing and integrating a combination of material from several sources. Indeed, the young woman within the scenario provided utilized data from visual, auditory and tactile senses to gain an understanding of her environment.

Despite the source of data employed, perception is dependent upon a stimulus being received by a specialized receptor. The stimulus is, at this point, converted from its original, physical, form (e.g. light, heat or sound) into action potentials, or nerve impulses, which are a representation of the event in the form of an electrical message. In this form, the information is despatched to an initial receiving unit, which, again, is sensitive to that specific form of sensation. This unit monitors the frequency of the impulses and the total number of receptors transmitting the information, indicating the extent of the object/event perceived. An example may be advantageous, and that of the stimuli emanating from an orange may be suitable. The colour, size, shape, fragrance and the distance from the orange's position, would all be noted in a primary receiving unit and passed to a secondary processing centre, where further judgements about the stimuli are made. The next step in the chain is transfer to an integrating centre, where sensations available from other sources (e.g. in the case of the orange, olfactory and visual receptors) and information from past experiences is added to the original data, via links with other similar centres. Thus cross-modal transfer is facilitated. Neural connections with motor areas of the brain provide for motor activity as a potential response to stimulus awareness (Hinchliff & Montague 1988).

The qualities of a stimulus (e.g. the pitch, loudness and location of a sound) are processed in parallel, via the specialist receptors, and conducted to the appropriate area of the brain—in the instance of sound, to the primary auditory cortex (Kandel & Schwartz 1981). Associated cells, within the immediate area of the primary centre, receive impulses from the area and will respond to certain aspects to produce an overall stimulus. A useful

analogy may be that of an orchestra—each individual member playing an instrument contributes to the composite sound produced, and yet on its own is only capable of eliciting a tiny fraction of the proposed end result. It is only when these parallel processes are combined that the perception of the complete stimulus is achieved. Once the entire details of any specific stimulus have been 'learned', it only requires the detection of a small number of these details in the future to enable recognition to take place.

MAKING SENSE OF PERCEPTIONS

In the same way as the qualities or specific aspects of a stimulus may be perceived, so a complex experience, or percept, may be broken down into its two or more distinctive elements. You will no doubt be aware of the research of Gestalt psychologists (Kohler 1952) in relation to the perceptual organization of these elements of the stimulus, namely that:

1. Where two or more distinct elements comprise a stimulus, a proportion of the stimulus is perceived as 'figure' and the rest as 'ground'. There are many visual examples of this—a girl (the figure) seated by a tree (background), a house (figure) within a landscape (background), a train (figure) standing at a platform of the railway station (background)—but also auditory ones, too, for example, the voice of the soloist against the background of the chorus, the sound of the river or a bird's song against the rest of the outdoor noise, or one voice amongst many others at a party.
2. There is a tendency to organize into ordered relationships, generated by the pattern of stimuli.

Similarity

There is a tendency to perceive three alternating groups of a two row/line pattern, even though the letters are consistently spaced apart (Fig. 5.1). Individuals incline towards uniting similarities within the percept.

aaaabbbbaaaabbbb

aaaabbbbaaaabbbb

Fig. 5.1 Similarity.

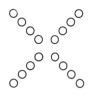

Fig. 5.2 Continuity.

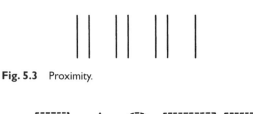

Fig. 5.3 Proximity.

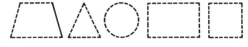

Fig. 5.4 Closure.

Continuity

Individuals perceive dots as straight lines rather than unconnected items and, in addition, 'see' two continuing lines rather than four short ones (Fig. 5.2). The overall perception is one of a letter 'x', a meaningful symbol, rather than a pattern of dots. There appears a natural opposition to breaking a continuous line, shape or design.

Proximity

Individuals tend to 'see' three pairs of lines, plus one extra on the right-hand side of the figure (Fig. 5.3). It could be interpreted as seven lines, or one plus three pairs of lines—the 'one' being the first line on the left. However, the likelihood is that the perception is of three pairs plus one line.

Closure

Although incomplete, individuals tend to perceive complete geometrical shapes, in what appears to be a strong inclination to 'close' incomplete stimuli (Fig. 5.4).

In addition, individuals perceive the elements within their environment as remaining relatively stable despite changing conditions or altering the position from which they are viewed, for example, the individual recognizes a pillar box, despite its cylindrical shape being distorted by bushes or a snow drift that is obscuring most of it. It is recognized when viewed from above and appears as a circular, one-dimensional structure, and also from

a two-dimensional sketch. Similarly it is 'known' to be red in colour, even when viewed in the darkness of late evening, and of an approximately constant size, the individual never having to lie face down on the ground to slip a letter into the box's opening!

Context

Individuals experience an element of a percept within a frame of reference provided by the context or setting in which it occurs. The perception of the size of an element is one aspect of this contextual setting. An example may assist here and, hence, a return to the example of the red pillar box may be valuable. When viewed from a distance the pillar box *appears* smaller than it actually is, and becomes progressively larger, the nearer an individual moves towards it. The individual recognizes the effect of distance on the apparent size of a structure, and does not consider for one moment that the real size of the object is actually changing. Similarly when both a building and the pillar box are viewed from a distance and appear to be of a similar size, the observer automatically accommodates the impression by inferring the house to be positioned at some considerable distance beyond the pillar box. The observer 'knows' that houses are much larger than pillar boxes and relates size to contextual setting.

Colour

Individuals are aware of the 'true' colour of a variety of objects and items within everyday life and will perceive that colour regardless of the wavelength of the light reaching the eye. Therefore, no matter the distance at which a tree is observed, the leaves are perceived as green, and, despite the dimness of an environment, an orange is 'seen' as orange in colour.

Location constancy

In regard to elements of a percept which do not generally move, despite the observer moving and the retinal image changing, objects are 'seen' to remain in the same place. Sometimes, indeed, individuals fail to recognize a familiar face or object because its contextual/location constancy changes. Bank managers may be familiar and easily recognizable figures in the location of their usual environment (the office, the desk and its contents, filing cabinets, etc.), dressed in a suit. However, meet them on the beach hundreds of miles from home, wearing cut-off jeans, tee-shirt, sporting a rude slogan or a three-day growth of beard and we may 'know they are familiar but can't place them'.

Shape constancy

The individual is aware of the 'real' shape of an article and perceives it to be that shape, no matter the angle from which it is viewed and despite the fact that a substantial portion may be occluded from view. Searching for a comb, should we see the last 'tooth' of it projecting from underneath a book, we will recognize just that one tiny aspect as the whole comb, and stop searching.

PROBLEMS OF RECOGNITION

Physiologically speaking, the systems involved in perception must be intact. The appropriately sensitive receptors must be available to monitor stimuli available within the environment and sensory pathways are required to transmit data to the responsible primary and association areas of the cortex for interpretation. However, despite fully functioning physiological processes, on occasions individuals fail to *recognize* the stimuli perceived.

Agnosia is a term utilized to describe an inability to recognize an object despite intact sensation, and may take numerous forms. All are characterized by a lack of awareness and feeling of familiarity when encountering people, places, events or objects that have been encountered before and often 'known' on a daily basis. *Tactile agnosia*, or *astereognosis*, follows lesions in the dominant parietal cortex, especially the posterior aspects of the area and demonstrates a lack of ability to perceive, and identify, an object by touching and manipulating it alone. Whilst no defects are found within the sensory tract, a problem is identifiable within the processes of higher level correlation of proprioceptive sensation. *Finger agnosia* is an inability to interpret which finger has been touched by an examiner, and is commonly seen in childhood schizophrenia and also in children experiencing minimal brain dysfunction. *Anosognosia* is a denial of disability, particularly a part of the body evidencing disease or paralysis and *autotopagnosia* (or *somatotopagnosia*) is an inability to identify or orientate the body or the relationship of its individual parts.

Neuropsychologists working in Marseilles described the problems of a 19-year-old male patient who suffered the effects of bilateral temporal lobe lesions (Sirigu, Duhamel & Poncet 1991). Intellectually, linguistically and perceptually, he experienced no significant impairment and yet his ability to recognize visually a wide variety of objects was quite profoundly deficient. The individual knew how to manipulate the objects and yet was unable to define either their function or the context in which they were utilized. The problems experienced by Paulette V., who had suffered a cerebrovascular accident some years previous, were described by Sergent & Poncet (1990). Since the stroke, Paulette had been unable to recognize faces as familiar or known to her (*prosopagnosia*) although able to match pictures of faces, even utilizing differing views of the same faces. Paulette was unable to recognize a slide showing the face of Dr Poncet, even though he sat next to the screen, and yet she could describe the facial features and approximate age of the doctor's face upon the screen. They concluded that there was a disturbance in the interaction between pertinent memories and facial representations, thus the latter remained meaningless.

The above are merely a few of the problems associated with *recognition* of objects via perceptual experiences when the sensory system remains intact. Physiological deficits are often readily identifiable—visual and auditory impairment are relatively easy to elicit during an efficient neurological examination, as is paresis or paralysis. However, when the client describes his world as colourless and perceived as shades of grey, it may be useful to discuss the matter with him further. Whilst rare, there is a problem associated with total colour blindness, termed *achromatopsia* (Zeki 1991), where congenital absence of retinal cone cells, injury, inflammation or exposure to lead, or other toxic substances, render the individual unable to distinguish colour. Similarly, lesions outside of the striate cortex have been shown to cause cerebral akinetopsia—visual motion blindness—and again whilst rare, these do occur. The two examples provided are obscure but hopefully serve to emphasize that it is unwise to accept clients' complaints, no matter how vague or 'florid', as automatic indicators of mental health status. Neurological disorders and dysfunctions may provoke seemingly bizarre symptomatology and present as deviation in mental health.

PROBLEMS OF PERCEPTION

We are aware that, at times, perceptions may mislead or confuse the individual with ambiguities, via illusions. An illusion may be described as a 'distorted perception or memory; a misinterpretation of sensory stimuli' (Campbell 1989) and you may have seen examples of such illusions before (Figs 5.5–5.10). We may also have seen instances of 'reversible figures' in the past, where two differing images may be perceived but not simultaneously (Figs 5.11–5.13). However, illusions are not merely the result of either the artist's or psychologist's contrivance of an interesting possibility. They occur both within health, and disturbances of somatic and psychosocial equilibrium in a variety of situations and circumstances.

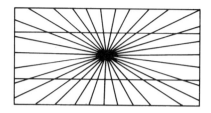

Fig. 5.5 Are the horizontal lines parallel, or bent?

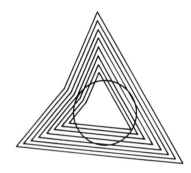

Fig. 5.6 Is the circle perfect?

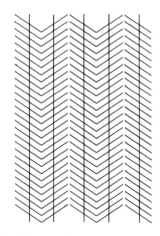

Fig. 5.7 Zoller's illusion of direction.

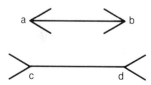

Fig. 5.8 The Mueller–Lyer illusion of length.

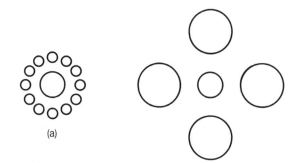

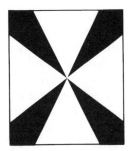

Fig. 5.9 Which of the central circles is larger?

Fig. 5.12 The Köhler cross: a black or a white cross?

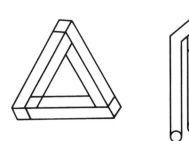

Fig. 5.10 Are these objects possible?

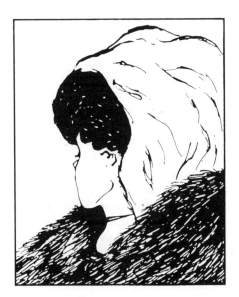

Fig. 5.13 The Beauty or the Hag (after Boring 1930).

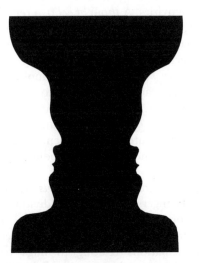

Fig. 5.11 Rubin's vase: face profiles, or a vase?

Pareidolic images are one example of *sensory deception* which we may have experienced. A pareidolic image is a vivid perception of visual images in response to an indistinct stimulus. The image and the percept coexist, and the image is usually recognized as 'unreal'. The commonly quoted example is that of objects, faces or scenes 'seen' within the flames of a coal fire. The individual sees the coal, the flames and the image—fantasy within reality.

An *eidetic* image is vivid and usually visual although it may be auditory in nature. It closely resembles actual perception and is very detailed in composition. It occurs mainly in children—10% show a strong inclination and some 50% demonstrate a tendency (Leask, Haber & Haber 1969)—

and may extend beyond adolescence in those who display an artistic ability or photographic memory. It may be referred to as primary mental image and the individual is able to scan a visual display even after the display has been removed. The image, whilst at times interfering with consequent stimuli, may be recalled with photographic accuracy long after the event or experience. Gardner & Roylance (1982) believe that the increasing ability of adolescents and adults to classify and relabel items weakens this figurative preciseness of memory and hence explains virtual absence from the older person's repertoire.

Pareidolic and eidetic images are examples of an illusion, that is, the *misinterpretation* of existing *stimuli*, and a relatively 'normal' phenomenon. A similar form of eidetic imagery may be seen to occur in individuals with somatic disorder, for example, tetany (calcium deficiency due to hypoparathyroidism) and Basedow's disease (hyperparathyroidism causing demineralization of bone) (Professional guide to diseases 1989). Systemic infections, particularly in the immature or ageing brain, metabolic disorders, such as hypoxia, hypercarbia, hypoglycaemia, thiamine deficiencies, and postoperative states may also elicit the experience of imagery. Individuals regaining consciousness following head injury, or seizures, may similarly demonstrate illusions (Green 1982), and within mental health care, those experiencing withdrawal from alcohol and those experiencing hallucinogen-induced organic problems provide examples of the exteriorization of illusions (Appleby & Forshaw 1990).

Lyttle (1986) utilizes an example to facilitate differentiation between an illusion and a hallucination:

The alcoholic in delirium tremens (alcohol withdrawal delirium) may be startled by the pattern on the wallpaper as it resembles snakes to his fevered eye (illusion)—the snakes may then proceed to slide down the wall and climb up the counterpane (hallucination).

Hallucinations represent another example of sensory deception and may be defined as 'a false perception occurring in the absence of an external sensory stimulus' (Lyttle 1986). They occur simultaneously alongside 'real' perceptions of the environment, and may be described as *elementary* or *complex* in nature. Elementary, or simple, hallucinations may take the form of a discrete noise, for example, as in a buzzing, banging or shuffling sound, whilst complex hallucinations may be a combination of sounds heard, as in voices or music. They are classified according to the sensory mode via which they are perceived.

Visual hallucinations may be clearly defined people, objects or animals, geometrical patterns, symbols or flashes of light. *Lilliputian (microptic) hallucinations* are those visual images that are seen as much reduced in size, for example, little people. They appear as a feature in typhoid, cholera and scarlet fever, temporal or temporosphenoidal tumour presence and are reported by some individuals experiencing petit mal epilepsy. Intoxication via alcohol, chloral, ether and trichlorethylene may also provoke Lilliputian hallucinations.

Auditory hallucinations may be of noises, but are commonly experienced as voices. They may be friendly or intimidating, clear or unintelligible, recognized as belonging to someone known or considered to be that of a stranger. Both *second* and *third person* auditory hallucinations are reported, and the latter often involve voices keeping a 'running commentary' on the individual's actions, or arguing or discussing the individual and his activities. A *thought echo*, a repetition of a thought, is frequently considered as an auditory hallucination because the individual reports 'hearing' the echo.

Gustatory hallucinations are unpleasant tastes which often lead the individual to believe that his food is poisoned, and may occur in conjunction with *olfactory hallucinations*, again often of an unpleasant nature, and frequently perceived as being of poisonous gases, introduced to kill the individual.

Tactile (or haptic) hallucinations are often experienced as fingers touching the individual's skin, of sexually orientated sensations, pain or extremes of temperature. The term *formication* describes tactile hallucinations relating to bugs or vermin crawling in or under the skin, often associated with the experience of cocaine delusional disorders.

Kinaesthetic hallucinations are false sensations related to body movement, and one of the most common problems seen relates to a phantom limb. The individual feels that a lost limb is really present, finding great difficulty in correlating the absent limb and perceptions of body image. It is a 'healthy' response, that is, an expected one, and in time, as the amputee adjusts to reorganized body image, will disappear. Sometimes, however, individuals retain an 'extended phantom'—of the same length as the missing limb—for years, whilst others experience a 'retracted phantom' (a shortened missing limb) or a 'telescoped phantom', where toes are felt to be protruding from the stump.

Other hallucinations may be experienced, for example, *reflex hallucinations* occur when a stimulus in one sensory mode provokes an hallucination via a different sensing system. Such a reflex may relate to, for example, experiencing an auditory sensation in response to a tactile stimulus.

Functional hallucinations are experienced in conjunction with a real background stimulus, for instance, hearing water and perceiving voices in responses to the sound. *Extracampine hallucinations* occur when the individual experiences stimuli that are located out of range of the sensory field. The individual 'hearing' another person talking in Moscow, from his position in London, without either the aid of a telephone or other 'eavesdropping' type of device, provides an example of this type of sensory deception.

Dissociative hallucinations, commonly elicited in individuals experiencing bereavement or grief, are feelings associated with the presence, or closeness of someone or something, to the degree where they can *almost* see, hear and feel the 'intruder'. Sometimes the term refers to bimodal hallucinations, where the image 'seen', 'speaks'. *Autoscopic hallucinations* may be dissociative in nature and relate to seeing self, that is, 'standing' outside of the body and watching one's own activities from a distance. Again these are commonly experienced by individuals following bereavement. *Pseudohallucinations* is the term utilized to describe those images that occur in the mind of the individual rather than within the external environment, or to

those sensations and experiences which are perceived as unreal and yet where there is no ability to exert voluntary control over the image.

Mention has been made elsewhere (Chapter 4) of the 'normality' of hypnogogic and hypnopompic hallucinations—those visual or auditory perceptions occurring when falling asleep and waking up—and of those associated with febrile conditions, exhaustion and fatigue, and oxygen lack.

Indeed hallucinations may be induced experimentally by electrical stimulation of the temporal lobe, amygdala and hippocampus, plus other areas of the brain. They may occur as a feature of the aura of epileptic seizures, when they may be of the visual, olfactory or gustatory mode. Irritation of the vestibular apparatus of the ear may provoke false sensory perceptions, mainly visual and tactile in nature. Multiplication and diminution of the image, loss of colour and sometimes of half of the image, are evoked when the subject is subjected to a passive rotating movement. Similar *vestibular hallucinations* may be seen with those false perceptions experienced within alcohol-related mental health problems and in psychosis, vestibular hallucinations may be portrayed in sensations of the body's lightness or heaviness. In severe hypothyroidism (myxoedema) and a small proportion of individuals experiencing vitamin B_{12} deficiency they are vivid. Individuals suffering from neoplasia or injury to the temporal lobe also exteriorized the hallucinatory experience. Within the sphere of psychosocial health, many individuals experience such a problem—those who are severely depressed in mood, often those who demonstrate psychomotor acceleration, as in 'hypomania', the 'schizophrenic' and the individual utilizing psychoactive substances or experiencing the sequelae of their use.

Illusions and hallucinations are sensory deceptions but, in addition, some individuals may show problems associated with *sensory distortion*. The intensity of perceptions may be heightened by alterations in physiological thresholds—for example, the individual utilizing lysergic acid diethylamide (LSD) may perceive vivid and intense colours. Similarly emotional status may affect perception, for the individual experiencing depressed mood may encounter a colourless, grey or drab world, whilst the hyperactive and overoptimistic person may perceive a bright, exaggerated and florid environment. *Dysmegalopsia* may be experienced as the spatial form of objects alters. An example would be *microspia* where objects are perceived to be smaller than they actually are and which may be a feature of temporal lobe epilepsy and psychoactive substance utilization. Distortion of the size perception accuracy—part of the 'physical appearance' construct—is seen within the diagnostic category of anorexia nervosa, where individuals perceive themselves 'fat' despite actual emaciation. *Depersonalization* and *derealization* are sensory distortions, occurring where anxiety, depressed mood, schizophrenia, or temporal lobe epilepsy are featured, as well as in 'normal folk'. Depersonalization is the term utilized to describe the individual's feelings of lost personal identity, of being 'different', changed or strange and unreal. Derealization relates to similar feelings about one's environment, and the two may frequently be seen to coexist.

CONCLUSIONS

We have provided examples of sensory deception and distortion and, not by any means, an exhaustive list. Whilst providing an overview of the problems of perception that may be encountered by the nurse because of an individual client's experience, we have also attempted to reinforce the fact that such problems are not solely encountered within mental health-related care. The nurse in the adult, somatic-care-orientated ward, the nurse within child care services and carers within facilities for those experiencing learning disability, may all witness such problems. There is therefore a requirement for all care workers to be able to recognize perceptual problems and employ strategies and interventions to manage the presenting situation.

ATTENTION

Our definition of attention was that attention represents conscious awareness, sensory clarity and

central nervous system readiness to respond to stimuli received (Campbell 1989). We also stated that attention is influenced by a variety of factors and that it is selective in nature.

Returning to the scenario at the beginning of the chapter, the young woman's initial concentration was focused upon compiling the mental agenda of discussion topics for her meeting and that it was only when she *perceived* a change in her bodily status that she deliberately and consciously 'tuned in' to her surroundings and situation. People are constantly assailed with stimuli from competing sources and any sensory system that attempted to process every minute fragment of information available would quickly be overwhelmed with data and yet impotent to construct anything meaningful or valuable to the individual. Imagine . . .

just one instance from the past when, above a cacophony of noise, a voice has emanated forth. 'Be quiet, I can't hear myself think!' . . . and then, observe and register the composition of the room/environment in which you are currently seated. Look at the walls and decoration, the floor and its covering, the windows and the curtains. Take in the furniture detail—are there chairs, what type, how many and what colours? What about a table—is there one, what shape and size is it and what is it composed of? Is there a television, music centre or a video player? Are there books, pictures, photographs and ornaments—how many and what are the detailed features of each? How is the room heated and illuminated and who is sitting there within the environment other than you?

It is a myriad of different shapes, colours, sizes, textures and materials and the light and shade of the room is not static but ever subtly changing. Now imagine that every aspect of the room is communicating its detail to you simultaneously and continuously—a little like a speaking clock telephone service—repeating its vital statistics, current status, temperature, state of repair—and every particle of dust that settles upon it! A constant recorded message emanating from each element of the room, registering every fractional change in image would rapidly overwhelm you. There would be no time to register or record details provided and no opportunity to concentrate on one piece of furniture or other environmental feature, because of the equally demanding competition from the rest of the room. Chaos!

Attention is therefore of necessity a selective process. Physiologically speaking, some sensory receptor cells respond intensely to a novel stimulus, but as the stimulus continues, the response fades. This process is termed *adaptation*, and the speed and degree of adaptation occurring are seen to vary both in relation to the sensory modality involved and the prevailing circumstances or conditions. In this way, changes in environment or the status of self are incorporated into existing knowledge, to maintain the individuals' mental constructs—their current perception of the world or environment. Without adaptation, the imagery utilized to introduce this section would be the reality.

THEORIES OF SELECTION

Having decided that individuals are selective in their attention to the environment, how is this limited attention achieved? Broadbent (1958), utilizing *dichotic listening* tasks (i.e. sending one message to a person's left ear and a different one to his right ear simultaneously), found that the individuals participating made fewer errors when repeating messages back from 'one ear at a time' rather than trying to combine data from both ears and repeat material as it was presented (Fig. 5.14).

Broadbent found that people tested tended to repeat information back in this way which led him to theorize that individuals were only able to attend to one channel—in the above example, one ear—at a time, and that, furthermore, individuals found it difficult to change from one sensory channel to another at a rate of more than twice a second. His model suggests that information to the unattended ear is predominantly lost, though some elements may be held in the short-term memory store for a reduced period of time. Broadbent's *single channel model* asserts that it is the physical characteristics of the input (e.g. the

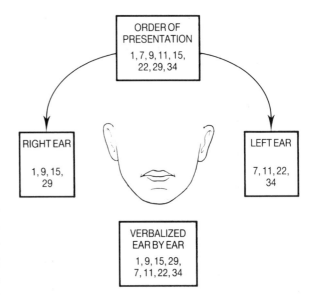

Fig. 5.14 Dichotic listening I (from Broadbent 1958).

source of the impulse, its strength and the number of times it is repeated) rather than the meaning of it that engenders attention and that understanding of the input occurs at a later stage after the filtering process. The model is limited, for it provides no explanation for those occasions when individuals are attending to one aspect of their environment but are distracted by, perhaps, overhearing a familiar name, or voice. Broadbent's theory would suggest that, if attention is not being paid to the channel, material incoming via that channel is all but lost, and yet we know that such distractions are frequently experienced.

Gray & Wedderburn (1960) found, utilizing similar experiments of dichotic listening, that material could be combined from both ears and sorted to make sense, in a category by category response by participants, thus reducing the validity of the Broadbent model (Fig. 5.15).

Speech shadowing, utilized by Treisman (1964) required the participant to repeat aloud material simultaneously being played into one ear, whilst an unconnected message was being played in the non-attending ear. Treisman found that individuals could shadow the attending ear's material, but could also follow the information accurately when, unexpectedly within the duration of the

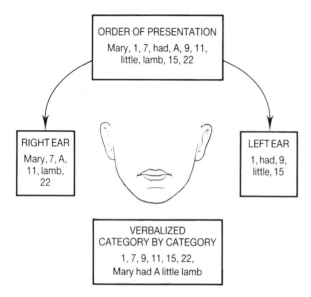

Fig. 5.15 Dichotic listening II (from Gray & Wedderburn 1960).

experiment, the inputs to both ears were changed over. The non-attending ear became the attending ear often without the participant even noticing the change in channel. In addition, she discovered that bilingual participants were aware that the passage of French language being played into the non-attending ear was a direct translation of the passage of English prose being played into the attending ear. Treisman & Gelade's *attenuation model* (1980), whilst agreeing with that of Broadbent with regard to the physical qualities of a stimulus being the attention-grabbing factor, asserts that the material inputting from non-attended channels is attenuated, or modified rather than lost. We would liken the process to turning down the television volume prior to answering a phone call—the background noise is still there but reduced. This model suggests, too, that both attended and relevant unattended (attenuated) stimuli pass through a second filtering system to ascertain their value for attention. Treisman & Gelade stated that a *threshold value* was required to be reached by stimuli in order that they pass through the second filter for attention, and that all attended stimuli would automatically reach this threshold. In addition, they suggested that some stimuli within the environ-

ment, for example, an individual's own name or those of other significant individuals, and words such as 'help' and 'fire', or screams, may have a permanently low threshold to facilitate passage through the filter. Temporary low thresholds, they asserted, were awarded to environmental features or other stimuli which had a relevancy of the moment.

The attenuation model, whilst more effective than Broadbent's single channel model, does not explain how information is processed to provide understanding. Deutsch & Deutsch (1963) tried a different analysis. The *late selection model* proposed that information is not selected until its meaning has been evaluated, and that filtering therefore occurs only after data have been recognized and their relevance or worth have been determined. Within this hypothesis, *all* inputs are screened at a high level and items selected as important are passed upwards for conscious attention. Research has provided some support for the late selection model via conditioning experiments, and those utilizing shadowing of ambiguous sentences. However, Dawson & Schell (1982) found that conditioned responses were only evident when the word stimulus was fed into the left ear of the subject, and Wexler (1988) found that such a conditioned response depended not only upon which ear was used but also on the personality of the subject.

The late selection model would appear to be an extreme hypothesis, occupying the furthest end of a continuum that begins with Broadbent. From processing only attended material to processing *all* data appears too much of a quantum leap. Atkinson et al (1987) propose a simplified theory, which draws upon elements of many and which they term a '*contemporary theory*'. The theory postulates that conscious perception and recognition of a stimulus may only occur when the *recognition* threshold of a specific neuron is reached and is dependent upon three factors. *Stimulus input* of a sufficient intensity and of an appropriate sensitivity will activate the specific neuron towards the recognition threshold, whilst an *attentional set* adds an internal input to the neuron relating the current context or relevancy, and the individual's motives and expectations. This added attentional set results in partial activation or inhibition of the neuron, with *selective attention* achieved via active neurons suppressing the activity of others. Reciprocal inhibition is suggested as the process by which less active neurons are suppressed and most active neurons are boosted towards the recognition threshold. The theory continues that the processing of stimuli is parallel to a point but that where attention is required, serial processing must take over to accommodate the fact that attention is limited to a small number of items at a time.

There is certainly little doubt regarding the features and characteristics of stimuli that attract attention and these may be viewed daily in the work of advertisers. A loud noise attracts where a soft one would not and repeated loud noises will attract attention even more effectively. Bright colours, changes in, or flashes of, colour have been utilized in neon-lighting adverts to good effect, but any novel or incongruous feature will do the trick and you may find it is a valuable exercise to spend a few moments analysing the features of adverts that draw attention to a product.

'Attention set' is certainly of importance too, for, just as the dieting individual may constantly, and almost to the exclusion of all else, perceive food-related stimuli, and the person who is attempting to give up smoking may be able to smell cigarette smoke within a half a mile radius, so current interests and basic needs will influence attention. Similarly an activity already in progress may significantly influence attention. The athlete awaiting the starting pistol hears no background noise for example, and, similarly, the individual engrossed in a good book will attend to little else within the environment.

SUSTAINED ATTENTION

Sometimes, in situations where prolonged duration vigilance tasks are needed to be performed, attention suffers. Mackworth (1950) studied *sustained vigilance* in response to problems encountered within military operations during World War II, where the operator's task was beyond his control and his responsibilities centred around watching a radar screen for activity (particularly enemy activity), and lapse in concentration or attention could prove dangerous for a large number of individuals. Mackworth's findings in relation to performances similar in nature to those undertaken by military personnel elicited a rapid reduction in attention within the first 30-minute phase of the test, as accuracy of reporting stimuli dropped to 85%. Within the second and third 30-minute periods of testing, the decline noted was more gradual—74 and 70% accuracy in reporting respectively. Mackworth elicited the results of decline in arousal by stimuli presented and therefore reduced attention levels. Oswald (1960) demonstrated that prolonged exposure to repetitive and monotonous stimuli evoked electroencephalogram (EEG) patterns characteristic of sleep in subjects. Indeed, prior to sleep, subjects experienced short lapses of consciousness, of which they were totally unaware. Wilkinson (1963) compared subjects' performance under 'normal' circumstances with that produced following sleep deprivation and with that exteriorized during exposure to noise. Within both of the 'abnormal' situations, performance was seen to decline and yet when combined (i.e. the subject was both sleep deprived and attempting to perform in a noisy environment), levels of performance were representative of those evoked under 'normal' circumstances. It may be logical to assume that poor performance following sleep deprivation may be the result of underarousal, and that witnessed during exposure to high levels of noise, the result of overarousal. The two combined may therefore cancel each other out to facilitate 'normal' performance supporting a theory of an inverted 'U'-shaped performance curve (Fig. 5.16).

There are, according to this theory, optimum levels of arousal—not too little and not too much stimulation—required to evoke optimum levels of performance. Certainly Wilkinson's work would support such a theory, and therefore manipulation of the environment may be a realistic method of increasing attention thereby improving performance. You may have noted that prolonged periods of study are ineffective—attention wanders and no matter how frequently the passage has

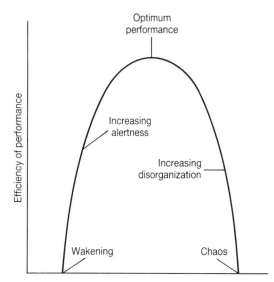

Fig. 5.16 Levels of alertness.

been read, it still is not absorbed or understood. A change of activity—not more of the same, by reading a different passage—will restore attention at this point. For example, stopping reading after each couple of pages and jotting down notes of points required to be remembered or taking a complete break for 5 minutes and *doing* something different within the period, rather than dwelling on one's tardiness over a cup of coffee, will relieve the monotony of presenting stimuli.

PROBLEMS OF ATTENTION

Everyone is at times inattentive. The woman on the bench in the park exhibited inattentiveness whilst preoccupied with making her mental list of subjects to be discussed with her friend, and most individuals will be able to identify with this phenomenon. Short mental activities such as this are an integral part of daily function, and for those periods of time attention is turned inwards. In a similar fashion, most individuals have experienced a situation where too many issues are prevailing and consequently they cannot attend to one because of interference from another or others. These are problems encountered fairly frequently and most people learn to manage such situations

more or less effectively. Temporary lapses in outward attention may, of course, be detrimental to health, should they occur, for example, whilst crossing a busy road or driving in heavy traffic. Many everyday activities may be performed almost by an 'automatic pilot', facilitating thinking about other things rather than the activity itself. Driving is one area where perhaps individuals do not always attend to the degree necessary to perform safely.

Problems associated with inattention are more common than you may think. In childhood, for example, attention deficits may be seen in combination with impulsiveness and hyperactivity, and this creates varying levels of difficulty within all settings. Some impairment in social and school functioning is always evident and follow-up studies show that in approximately one-third of such children, problems persist in later life. Attention deficit may be seen in children, without the added hyperactivity, but little is known about this, and more investigation is required.

An inability to attend or concentrate is a common problem experienced by those individuals experiencing maladaptive reactions to identifiable psychosocial stressors, termed adjustment disorders. These are evidenced within 3 months of the onset of stressor(s) and may take many forms, but will remit soon after the stressor ceases or when adaptation is achieved. Similarly inattention is a feature associated with depressed mood or hyperactivity in adults with anxiety, and those individuals experiencing the effects of psychoactive substance use. Poor attention levels may be responsible for complaints regarding 'poor memory', and differentiation of the actual difficulties experienced must therefore be employed.

The withdrawal from, and inattentiveness to, the environment described within discussions relating to schizophrenia were once thought, too, to be due to an excessive preoccupation with mental imagery and one's own thoughts and feelings. However, studies have demonstrated that, at least within the early stages of the experience, there is an inability to attend selectively to the environment and that therefore withdrawal is used as a defence against the bombardment of senses by the multitude of stimuli which compete for attention. The continuous distraction by the environment precludes adequate or effective general performance, by inability to exclude any aspect of surroundings. It may be that complete withdrawal may be the only alternative to the chaos of attempting to interact with the environment.

To be able to attend, of course, one has to be conscious and this area of function is the responsibility of the mesencephalic portions of the *reticular activating system* (RAS). When asleep, for example, inputs via sensory receptors stimulate the RAS into *general consciousness*, then pass upwards to the *thalamus*, causing the widespread cortical activity, termed *arousal* (Tortora & Anagnostakos 1984). The RAS acts as 'the brain's chief watchguard', monitoring stimuli and forwarding only essential material to the conscious mind. Consciousness may be altered by various factors, from meditation to medication, and from somatic disorder to mental health problems. Hence problems associated with attention again may be encountered within all fields of health care, not solely that related to psychosocial service provision.

THINKING

The following definition of 'thinking' was used in the introduction to the chapter:

> the process by which images and ideas, representing objects and events experienced, are manipulated, using previous knowledge and general understanding of the situation to arrive at strategies by which changes in status may be managed.
> Campbell 1989

Thinking is something 'automatic' in nature, something that individuals take for granted. It represents a process that is continuous, from the time of awakening until the moment of drifting back off to sleep, and yet it is an area which most individuals never dream to analyse in relation to self. However, thinking is an area that has attracted the attention of philosophers, scientists and physicians for hundreds of years.

SOME THOUGHTS ON THINKING

Aristotle addressed the subject of thinking from his general philosophical framework and generated three primary laws to explain the *continuity* of thought and to elucidate the principles of memory.

1. Ideas are combined or *associated* because they are *similar* in some way, for example, bread and rolls have a similar *taste and function* within the eating process. Similarity of *location* provides another relevant association, therefore shoes and socks, table and chair, and garden and flowers are ideas that are associated.

2. The second law of association relates to the *contrast* between concepts, and therefore the association between up and down, in and out, black and white, and yes and no, are explainable.

3. The principle of *contiguity* suggests an association via concepts which have a relationship in *time or space*. Therefore an association exists between schools and learning, churches and worship, pens and writing, beds and sleeping and the like.

Aristotle and the early *philosophical association-ists* (Warren 1921) maintained that any specific concept may be accounted for by one of the primary laws, but that, in addition, one concept may generate several associations (Fig. 5.17).

Later associationists attempted to trace the construction of complex ideas, though it was generally accepted by all that the process involved a combination of all elements involved in some way. James Mill maintained that any idea, no matter how complex, was composed of discrete elements, each of which maintained its own identity, and which amalgamated with others to form a group. This view later gave way to the understanding that a complex idea involved a fusion of the properties of each individual element, and that such fusion evoked characteristics of properties in the whole which were not evident in the separate elements. This understanding was eventually accepted by the associationists and the view generally held became that related to the coalescence

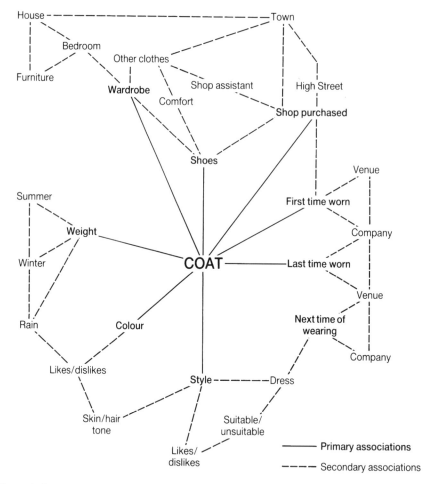

Fig. 5.17 Potential associations.

of elements to form a different, whole and complex idea.

Attempts were also made to account for the *specific selection* of associations by providing a series of secondary laws. It was asserted that concepts *most frequently* associated in the past were likely to remain so in the future—for example, school would continue to be associated with learning rather than a one-off visit to the seaside, which occurred at the age of 5 years. Where two associations had been made with almost equal frequency in the past, say school and learning and school and friends, it was believed that the *most recent* association would take precedence, and that where a conflict occurred between the frequency or recency of an association, the one evoking the

most vivid or *emotionally significant* association would predominate.

Herbart theorized regarding the manner by which conscious experience was *organized*, thus providing another set of principles for the combination of ideas and thoughts. He suggested that some concepts attract each other, that is, are *congruent*, whilst others repel or inhibit each other and are termed *incongruent*. Herbart believed that congruent material combined to make up the *apperceptive mass*—the existing body of knowledge and experience—which became the centre for the organization of conscious experience. Incongruent material, which is irrelevant or which does not 'fit' into the overall scheme, Herbart believed to be either rejected, and excluded from conscious experience, or 'made to fit in', according to its importance to the individual (Warren 1921).

Wundt (cited in Watson 1963) became known as the 'father of psychology' in respect of his activities, which separated the work of philosophers from that of 'scientists', who wished to conduct a more objective study of the mind. Wundt declared that the scientific methodology available was not applicable to the study of higher mental processes, such as thinking. However, observations of social phenomena, for example, language, and studies of reaction time, particularly those related to the focusing aspects of consciousness, provided Wundt with insight into the complexity of the subject, and, in addition, some objective information concerning thought. He asserted that thought and association were two different entities, and that thinking followed some logical sequence whilst association did not. He believed that associations did not, of necessity, make sense, for example, the individual who, when buying a book, gets soaking wet in a sudden downpour of rain, may associate the two events and yet there is no logical connection between them. The situation of needing the book for a specific purpose and the event of purchasing it, provide a logical consideration and, therefore, a logical connection. According to Wundt, cognitive connections are made upon logical considerations, relevancy and appropriacy.

Titchener (1909) also a structuralist like Wundt, arrived at his conclusions regarding thought and thinking via studies of the process of attention. For Titchener, the conscious content of an individual's mind comprised various elements, or ingredients, and that any one element could be explained or described through the patterning of the others present. Much like a kaleidoscope may produce various images from a set number of different coloured pieces of glass, by adjustment of the pattern into which they fall, so any one element of conscious content depended upon the configuration of the others. Titchener believed that cognitive activities, such as thinking and attention, were composed of *images*, somewhat similar to those of sensation, in that they possessed characteristics such as quality, intensity, clarity and duration, and yet dissimilar, in regard to their 'transparency'. By this, he was referring to the images' characteristics of being less objective, appearing less realistic and being more easily destroyed than those of sensation. By equating thought with variations in the conscious content, he provided facility for the particular meaning of an image to be determined, not only by the appearance of the salient stimulus at a specific time, but also by the conscious content of the mind within the prevailing circumstances.

Titchener's European colleagues, however, objected to such a peremptory dismissal of the area of cognitive function, and with reference to this discussion of thought, whilst agreeing that images could occur within thinking processes, asserted that *imageless thought* was the typical component comprising the processes of thinking.

William James (1890) considered the processes of thinking, reasoning and believing were biological in essence and resultant from the elaboration of sensory processes within the central nervous system. He believed these processes to be dynamic in nature and that, therefore, any attempt to break down the overall processes into subunits of 'ideas' or 'images' was both pedantic and artificial, engendering a rigidity where, in his view, the essence was of fluidity and flexibility. He believed thinking to be the vehicle by which biological needs were met by the individual, facilitating adjustment to the environment, goal-directed behaviours to achieve basic needs, and the anticipation of difficulties, and generation of solutions to problems encountered on the way. According to James, it is an irrational process, directed by biological need. He did not differentiate between the roles of thinking and memory within this process. He believed both to be dependent upon two separate and differing sequences. The first of these he referred to as *sagacity* or *insight*, and described this as a creative ability, combining the capacity for perspective with the ability to select the relevant features of the problem from the accompanying minutiae. Thus a 'sagaciously structured' problem is one that has been clearly identified with regard to its detailed nature, and which has been examined from a variety of points of view. Having achieved this sequence, the second one begins operation, with an arousal of previously learned associations and the application of these to the decision, or choice of solution, to arrive at a reasonable course of action within the circumstances.

Whilst not differentiating between thinking and remembering, James did distinguish between thoughts and beliefs. The latter he asserted to be more closely related to emotion than to thought and reasoning, because of their *coercive* nature. He considered that beliefs determined an individual's psychological reality, by exerting pressure upon the person to perceive the world in accordance with those beliefs. Beliefs were, he asserted, established on the basis of biological need or instinct and their continued existence served only to gratify that need. Hence beliefs were irrefutable.

Tolman (1932) developed his theory relating to *cognitive maps* from his work with rats. He had observed that rats *learned* about a maze during his experiments, rather than merely utilizing a series of responses to deal with it. He discovered that, given the opportunity, the rats would select the shortest pathway between two points even if they had no previous experience of that specific path and were on unfamiliar territory. He believed that the rats had constructed a 'map' which represented the salient features of the maze and the spatial relationships involved. In addition, Tolman considered the rats not only to be aware of the relationships among stimuli, but also to have generated expectancies about their meanings and a readiness to respond in appropriate ways. It was as if the rats had 'visualized' the journey from A to B and the activities necessary to complete the journey successfully and in the shortest period of time.

Tolman asserted that human beings create cognitive maps, too, and in their instance, such maps are not solely related to locations. People exhibit 'maps and expectancies' relating to what self and others should, or would do within a number of different situations, and he concluded that individuals possess a symbolic representation of all biopsychosocial aspects of their environment, plus their potential reactions to them. These anticipations, maps and the ability to mentally 'try out' scenarios presenting held no meaning in themselves, for he asserted that they were derived from, and relevant to, whatever purpose was influencing behaviour.

It was Tolman's belief that consciousness (*awareness*) and thinking occurred only within situations where behaviour could not be automatically evoked, for example, in novel situations where anticipations and predictions could not be inferred with any certainty. The absence of knowledge was not considered to be the cause of consciousness or thinking, but merely provided an *opportunity* for their utilization. Where new relationships emerge from productive thought, engendering new anticipations and novel responses, he coined the term *inventive ideation*, to indicate an especially creative process. In general, however, Tolman believed that once the novelty had diminished within a situation, conscious awareness and thinking were also reduced, allowing automatic processes and habitual responses to assume responsibility for continuation of activities at the earliest appropriate opportunity.

To understand the beliefs of Sigmund Freud (1922) and psychoanalytical theory in relation to thought and thinking, a brief review of his considerations of consciousness and personality is required. You may recall that Freud characterized *conscious activity* as that encompassing an awareness of events occurring both within the individual and his external environment. In addition, however, he believed that there were other occurrences of which the individual was unaware, situated within the *unconscious*, and again material which, whilst the individual had no current awareness of it, could be recalled into consciousness at will, within the *preconscious*.

With regard to personality, Freud delineated three regions—the *id, ego* and *superego*. The id he described as a composition of primitive and unsocialized biological urges and drives, guided by the *pleasure principle*, and maximizing the pleasure of the moment, uncaring of eventual consequences. The ego assumed the role of mediator between the id and the real world, seeking realistic outlets for id impulses whilst simultaneously keeping within expectations of the environment and avoiding painful experiences of injury, rejection and punishment on behalf of the id. The guiding feature of the ego was referred to as the *reality principle*. The superego provided the region of the personality that included the person's moral values and ethics—the conscience—which often influences behaviour without the individual's awareness, via social learning taking place prior to the child's ability to understand or verbalize such material. The superego basically interacts with reality and the external world and is, therefore, like the ego, necessarily conscious in nature.

To recap, Freud believed the mind to be influenced by animal drives (id), moderated by the demands imposed by reality (ego) and censored by moral values (superego). Of necessity, the individual is aware (conscious) of the demands of the ego (reality) and of some of the material of the superego (moral values and ethics). However, the individual is totally oblivious (unconscious) of the true nature of his animal urges, because awareness would create distress. Awareness constituted only the salient stimuli, impulses and memories necessary to performance, with the preconscious providing a reservoir for the additional resources necessary.

Freud maintained that the infant, at the mercy of, and solely influenced by, the pleasure principle (the id), can neither perceive nor think, but reacts both impulsively, and automatically, to maximize satisfaction of biological urges and drives. Gradually, however, the child becomes aware of the need to adjust behaviour to the reality of the situation, because of the pain that may result from its disregard. To avoid such pain—rejection, punishment and injury—the individual evokes thoughtful behaviour, to analyse and respond appropriately to the demands of reality. Thoughtful behaviour represents a more mature stage of development and signals the influence of the ego. Freud asserted that once an individual exhibited sufficient maturity to maintain a realistic orientation, he was able to revert to the drives of pleasure principle only when the ego was rendered inactive—in sleep, fantasies, neurotic and psychotic symptomatology.

Freud believed thought to be a symbolic representation, rather than an entity in itself, and that these symbols, words and images are representative of objects, events and feelings and are mostly learned. The child is unable to think until such learning has taken place. In addition he believed thought to be symbolic in another way, being an expression of unconscious material, and therefore a mechanism via which primitive, repressed urges may be satisfied. This type of symbolism, he determined, was often a product of cultural and racial heritage and found expression within fantasy, day dreaming and aimless mental wanderings. His interpretation of dream symbolism is an extension of this element of the theoretical perspective. According to Freud, then, thought is a learned symbolism, relating to feelings, events and objects, which originates with the reality principle and which assists the ego to moderate the relationship between the id and the external reality.

We have identified just some of the many perspectives that have been applied to thought and thinking. There are many others, including those of Adler, Harry Stack Sullivan, Lewin, Hebb, Piaget and others, plus those attributed to Gestalt, phenomenological and cybernetic schools of study (Neel 1969). Limitations of space alone preclude their outline within this section, though we would suggest their perusal to be valuable in relation to any detailed study of the area. In providing broad examples of 'thoughts about thinking', we have attempted to provide insight into the widely differing perspectives held and promulgated by philosophers and psychologists. However thinking arises and whatever influences are applied to the process, individuals do think, and in some recognizable ways.

TYPES OF THINKING

McKellar (1957) differentiated between two different types of thinking processes. The first—*autistic thinking*—related to that mental activity which is more or less subjective and removed from reality. It represents the narcissistic, egocentric material that daydreams and fantasies are made of and the type of thinking experienced within dream states. The second category identified by McKellar is that of *realistic* or *imaginative thinking* and in this he is referring to a more logical, rational, goal-directed thinking, in which words and symbols, representing objects and events, are manipulated mentally rather than in reality. Realistic thinking is the process inherent within problem solving and scientific thinking, and any goal-directed activity requiring the ability to *reason*. McKellar believed realistic thinking to be influenced by learning and experience.

Experimental psychology has been, for the most part, concerned with realistic thinking, and yet there is evidence—if one looks for it—of autistic trends in the everyday thinking of adults, who would, no doubt, consider themselves objective and logical beings. Autistic thinking is, for example, a prerequisite for spiritual beliefs. 'In sure and certain hope' is reliant upon faith, not logical, objective evidence and yet millions of people worldwide believe in a God, of some specific name, of an after-life and of this existence being a preparation for another, better one. People either have faith or they do not. Individuals who are superstitious are similarly a little less than logical for, whilst there was frequently a sensible basis for a superstition in the past, circumstances change and actions or beliefs are now no longer relevant. Whether one believes that the 'third light' from a match is unlucky, a broken mirror brings 7 years' bad luck or walking under a ladder bodes badly, there is no longer a logic to underpin the beliefs held. Prejudices and stereotypes are irrational, as are the 'miracle' cures that promise to ameliorate everything from obesity to shyness. Anyone utilizing a sweeping generalization in a statement or accepting a 'quick fix' to solve a personality problem has got to believe in magic!

We believe that any relaxation of attention or redirection of thoughts from goal-orientated activities is an opportunity for autistic-orientated thought. Indeed mental health nurses encourage it—'For the next few moments I want you to close your eyes and relax. Imagine yourself walking along a beach ...'. Everyone has fantasies and daydreams. Many people 'relive' a particular incident within their minds, where they engender a more effective self—'I should have said that ... if only I'd have thought about saying ...'. On any continuum of thought where the autistic type provides one extreme and realistic thought the other, the vast majority of people will be seen to move

somewhere between the two extremes at various times of the day.

Realistic thinking is goal orientated and logical, being subject to the influence of learning and experience. You may find it valuable to undertake a small analysis of the day's events in regard to the number and type of activities that required a deliberate effort of thought. A day at home may include, for example:

> Switched off alarm clock ... got up, washed and dressed ... listened/watched news ... made and ate breakfast ... jobs around the house ... an hour in the garden ... shopping ... more food ... reading ... listened to music/TV ... got showered and changed ... out with friends ... home ... bed ... slept.

Who has such a simple, selfish and wonderful day? You, will, no doubt, have to include activities related to a partner, children and relatives. Walking the dogs, cleaning the car and arguing with a salesperson in a shop may also figure, but of your list, how many of the day's activities were 'routine' and undertaken with habitual action or reaction, and how many really required thinking about? Whilst constantly thinking, many of your daily activities *will* be undertaken on automatic pilot and those that require 'thinking about' *are* those in which an obstacle of some nature prevents goal achievement. They are those situations that require the individual to utilize the reasoning process to effect a removal of the impediment and facilitate goal success. If the individual applied logic to the situation, the answer to a new problem is to be found externally, within the nature of the problem and internally, via the stored memories of previous learning experience. Inhibition of the irrelevancies of a situation facilitates organization of the information available in a way that will lead to solution. That would be logical and rational. The question to ask, of course, is do individuals do this within the reasoning process?

Unless prevented from acting freely, the individual will randomly apply various responses when faced with a novel problem to achieve a solution. One has only to think of completing a jigsaw to see our meaning. The individual will try to fit a piece of the jigsaw into a specific place even though the colour shading is inaccurate, the shape is wrong and the part picture upon the piece is totally out of tune with the area. The individual will even turn the piece of puzzle around to try to fit it in, perhaps two or three times before deciding it is the wrong piece. People are most likely to attempt a solution via trial and error when faced with unfamiliar tasks which can be physically manipulated. Many people prefer to utilize trial and error thinking—even Edison tried hundreds of substances, one by one, rather than reasoning through the qualities necessary in a substance to render it an effective filament for his incandescent light bulbs. His response to critics of his trial and error methods was, 'Now I know hundreds of things that won't work!'

In some situations trial and error thinking may be the most practical solution. Ruger (1910) set up experiments with people who had to solve a wire puzzle. He found that an analysis of the solution *followed after* the solution was reached and not before, and that understanding was achieved in two distinct stages. First subjects would analyse which bit of the puzzle they had successfully manipulated and then retrace the movements utilized to attain that success. After several attempts, subjects would finally experience an abrupt understanding and perform speedily and successfully from this point onwards. 'The penny dropping' and suddenly 'seeing the light' are phrases used to describe *insight*.

We are certain that there is no need to recount the classic tale of Archimedes, his bath and running naked down the streets of Syracuse, but the anecdote reinforces the abruptness of the understanding associated with insight. The mental restructuring of the situation that is required to attain insight may occur *prior* to solving the problem and will result in a reduced period of time taken to achieve the desired outcomes. The Gestalt school of psychology—particularly Wolfgang Kohler (1925)—was responsible for extensive investigation in this area.

Harlow (1949), in his experiments with monkeys found that, after several exposures to tests where the animals were required to 'select the odd one out', the monkeys seemed to understand the concept of 'oddness' and became very adept at choosing the correct—that is the odd—object from the group offered. He argued that the monkeys were not simply learning to respond to a specific stimulus, because they would select the appropriate object in one test, where its selection in a previous test had proved incorrect, and hence the monkeys had failed on that occasion to gain a record. Harlow argued that the monkeys had developed a 'learning set', a state of mental preparedness to solve this particular type of problem.

Luchins (1959) asserted that humans develop such a readiness, too, and that, with sufficient experience, in any one particular method of problem-solving activity, individuals would tend to choose that method, above easier and quicker ways of solving the problem. He discovered that such *mental sets* may be both a hindrance and a help, for though they may assist an individual to find a solution quickly in some situations, they may also prevent alternative possibilities being looked for and used. Glucksberg (1962) found that the use of mental sets precluded an ability to think of using objects outside their normal function—something he termed *functional fixedness*—and that, because of this, solutions to some problems were unavailable to the individual. The Gestalt psychologists believed that, partly because of this tendency to adopt mental sets and partly due to the nature of thinking itself, individuals could be reluctant to accept new modes of activity and alternative ways of problem solving.

LOGICAL REASONING

'Logic' is the branch of philosophy that is concerned with analysis of *inferences* and *arguments* (Salmon 1973). An 'inference' is the formation of a conclusion based upon available evidence, whilst an 'argument' is that conclusion plus the evidence. Such evidence used to support this conclusion may involve one or more theoretical statements, called *premises*, and the strategies of logic facilitate an analysis of the reasoning involved from premises to conclusion.

Pierce (in Steiner 1978) asserted that the major stages of inquiry comprise of three kinds of reasoning: *deduction*, *induction* and *reproduction*.

Deduction is reasoning that commences with the 'general' and proceeds to the 'particular', as specific conclusions are drawn from more general premises or principles. An example may assist:

1. If A were true, then B would be true.
2. A is true.
3. B must be true.

Some arguments are *deductively valid*—that is, it is impossible for the argument (conclusion) to be false if the premises (the statements that build the conclusion) are true (Skyrms 1986):

◆ To be a registered nurse, you must pass the appropriate examinations.
◆ Jayne works as a registered nurse.
◆ Therefore, Jayne passed the examinations.

This sort of argument may be evaluated in two ways: the first requires an analysis as to whether the conclusion follows logically from the premises; the second requires an assessment of the truth—or otherwise—of the statements used. Deductive arguments may comprise of all true statements, as with the above example, or they may contain one or more incorrect or false statements. When the latter applies, the argument is referred to as *deductively invalid*, for example:

◆ All hawthorn berries are red.
◆ This berry is red.
◆ Therefore this is a hawthorn berry.

The conclusion reached is not supported by the evidence of the premises. The information provided within the premises is neither implicit nor explicit enough to arrive at such a conclusion. Now if *only* hawthorn berries are red, that would be a different matter.

Inductive reasoning describes the exact opposite process to the above, for a generalization is arrived at from a number of specific observed instances. It is less well developed than deductive reasoning (Pospesel 1974) and is based on the assumption that what is true of randomly selected members of a group or classification, is true for all members of the group:

◆ Susan's husband drank too much and always became violent.

◆ Margaret, Josie, Pam and Ann were also married to men who drank to excess and then became violent.
◆ All married men are alcoholic, wife-beaters.

The conclusion reached is generalized well beyond the small number of instances observed, to the whole group or class of 'married men'. Similar assumptions may be seen to be applied by pollsters in election campaigns:

◆ 56% of the survey stated that they will vote for Party A.
◆ Therefore 56% of the population will vote for Party A.

Excluding for the purposes of this analysis, the fact that some of those surveyed in the poll (a) may have deliberately lied, (b) may change their mind before actually voting, (c) may not actually make it to the polling station, (d) may spoil their ballot paper by placing a tick rather than a cross against the candidate's name, or (e) may not be entitled to vote, this conclusion is based on limited evidence and therefore can clearly be erroneous. The population sample may, for example, have been only 25 people, 14 of whom may have been approached as they came out of Party A's election headquarters! The survey may have been limited in any number of ways—the age group selected, sex, occupational group, area of domicile, etc.— and hence the conclusion would be disputable. However, the valid–invalid assessment utilized in relation to deductive arguments is not applied to those of inductive arguments. An inductive argument is viewed in terms of the *probability* of the premises leading to a given conclusion, therefore degrees of high, medium and low probability may be applied to any inductive argument. An appropriately sized, representative sample used in the survey, or several such surveys used in combination to achieve a premise, may be awarded a higher level of probability than the one provided as an example.

The third type of reasoning identified by Pierce (in Steiner 1978) was that of retroduction, which he viewed as the first stage in the analysis of a 'surprising phenomenon', to generate a potential explanation. Once an explanation of some description was available, he believed deductive reasoning could be employed to develop it and that, finally, inductive reasoning could be used to assess the degree of probability of the hypothesis in practice. Retroductive reasoning does not seek to establish a 'truth', but merely to originate ideas about a phenomenon, which may then be evaluated. It is therefore of value in areas where little is known about a subject and innovation is required to advance current knowledge and understanding. An idea or conjecture related to a new area of study or observation may be devised from previous knowledge in a different field, for example, explaining brain activity and function via the workings of a telephone switchboard, as an analogy. In relation to human activities of an everyday nature:

◆ In situation 'A', behaviour 'X' was successful.
◆ Situation 'B', whilst relating to a different problem, has some similarities.
◆ Perhaps the principles of behaviour 'X' could be modified to produce behaviour 'Y' and achieve the goals desired.

Applying Pierce's theory the individual may then deduce the conclusions of the activity—'if I do "this", then "that" will follow' and later use inductive reasoning to analyse the probability of the conclusion actually being the outcome—'but, if I do "this", then "that" may not necessarily follow; the result may actually be … or …'—and, therefore, the potential value of any specific activity undertaken.

The question begs: 'Do human beings use logical reasoning?' Hudson (1966), in an extensive study of school children, analysed the cognitive patterns that characterized those who selected 'arts' or 'science' subjects. He discovered two distinctly varying *cognitive styles*, which he termed *convergent* and *divergent* thinking. Convergent thinkers tended to choose science subjects, and exhibited an extremely logical and linear-focused style of reasoning. Those considered as divergent thinkers exhibited more intuitive and impulsive thinking, would utilize a range of potential options in problem-solving activities than their convergent peers, and tended towards the art-type subjects at school. Discrete convergent and diver-

gent thinkers each represented approximately 30% of the population tested, whilst the remaining 40% of the sample tended to mix the characteristics of the two, emphasizing different styles in different situations. Hudson's study found support in that conducted by Pask & Scott (1972) and therefore it may be that some individuals are more 'logical' in cognitive styles than others.

Those then, who may be more logical in their reasoning—how logical are they? Wason & Johnson-Laird (1970) discovered that, despite two statements being 'logically equivalent', individuals take longer to process a negative statement than a positive one, for example:

◆ *Statement 1*—If the carpet is blue, the curtains will be red.
◆ *Statement 2*—If the carpet is not green, the curtains will not be yellow.

Individuals took more time and found it more difficult to process the information presented in a negative form, as in Statement 2, than in a positive form, as in Statement 1. In addition, Wason & Johnson-Laird asserted that humans utilize a less than formal logic, for they utilize their broader knowledge to analyse what is *likely* or *probable* to occur within problem-solving activities, rather than what is *definite* or *certain* in the situation, as logic would dictate. Rips (1986) demonstrated that people tend to use 'shortcuts'—*heuristics*—by applying previous experiences and learning to a situation or problem requiring a solution. Such previous experience facilitates ease of application of the problem-solving strategy—it is already in the individual's repertoire—and may be successful in its outcome. Johnson-Laird (1983) suggested that, rather than reasoning a problem through, individuals showed evidence of applying a concrete example to the situation presenting, so that instead of mentally manipulating concepts or language, images representing the problem are utilized. The image content, he believed, of the concrete representation would be selected by the nature and content of the problem to be addressed. Again the evidence suggests people to be less logical than philosophers would have us believe.

Tversky & Kahnemann (1973) demonstrated that, in tests to ascertain how individuals arrive at a judgement regarding probability and the degree to which something is likely, people frequently ignore—or at least fail to take into account—evidence available to assist in determining probability. Despite the fact, for instance, that subjects were presented with a neutral character description which related to one or other of a group of 70 lawyers or 30 engineers, the subjects assessed the probability of the description being that of an engineer as '50–50'!

Individuals are not necessarily logical in reasoning and problem-solving activities and, whilst this may be viewed in some quarters, particularly by philosophers and purists, as detrimental to functioning, it would appear to others to be far more sophisticated and of a higher cognitive order than logic. Human reasoning encompasses more than mere logic, for it uses previous knowledge of past experiences and learning, of social context and meanings, and personal choices to come to a conclusion. The human being does far more than 'compute' information to arrive at an answer to a problem—people 'think' about problems.

PROBLEMS OF THOUGHT AND THINKING

Minor 'aberrations' of thought content and thinking patterns are relatively common within the mentally healthy individual and you may not only be able to identify with some of the examples provided here, but also be able to proffer one or two of your own. Discussions within preceding pages of this section identified the frequently illogical basis for thoughts and beliefs, for example, the shades of autistic thinking evident within superstition and religious, or spiritual, beliefs. It is relatively easy to recognize elements of *magical thinking* within the above examples, that belief or certainty that, somehow, specific thoughts, words or actions may precipitate or prevent a particular outcome, thus thwarting the laws of cause and effect. Children commonly exteriorize such thinking patterns in activities like refusing to step on the cracks in the paving of a street and it represents an integral part of development and growing

up. Adults, too, may rely on charms and rituals to provide a sense of security, safety or continued well-being. People talk about 'tempting fate', believing that to think about or verbalize the possibility of an event or occurrence, may be sufficient to provoke its happening. Others speak of lucky charms or significant items—footballers may believe their skill increased by wearing a specific pair of boots, golfers have favoured putters that they are unable to hole a ball without and gamblers may have 'lucky dice', with which they 'just can't lose'.

Frequently such talismen and amulets provide the wearer with a sense of increased confidence, optimism and self-esteem, thus facilitating enhanced performance. The individual feels good and therefore functions well—the self-fulfilling prophecy. Such a reliance on an external object, however, detracts from the individual's ability to recognize and value the power, skill and personality characteristics which essentially generate the successful, or otherwise, outcome and which are built in and readily accessible to the person. You may recall the Walt Disney film of 'Dumbo the Elephant'. Dumbo was able to fly, he believed, because of the influence and power of a magic feather. He was confident until he dropped the feather and then panicked, believing himself incapable without it. His mouse-friend and mentor convinced him otherwise just in time to prevent Dumbo's sad demise from a great height. You may wonder why we recount this tale, but it would seem very clear to us that a token may initially be a boon in promoting confidence in one's own abilities, but the sooner the individual realizes that this is exactly what it is and that he or she alone is in control of 'fate' and the hand that is dealt, the more effective the efforts made towards reaching optimum development will be.

Many people experience a transitory *blocking of thought* processes, where a train of speech is interrupted before a thought or idea has been completed. Often it happens to the individual who is uncomfortable or anxious within a situation, in an interview, at the end of a driving test or in the middle of a soliloquy or speech of some kind. You have no doubt—at least once in a lifetime—experienced that dreaded pause, when you find it impossible to recall what you were saying or meant to say, and therefore are unable to continue. That dreaded 'drying up' of the actor, on stage and in mid-flow, which requires one, or several, prompts from off-stage, happens to everyone at some time and is provoked by some feeling of 'threat' to one's own psychosocial integrity and well-being. Such an elevated level of anxiety is inhibitory to performance and the individual whose confidence levels are sufficiently poised to facilitate the view of 'what is the worst case scenario, resultant from my failing to achieve the desired outcome?' is one who will perform more effectively, for there is the realization that life will not come to an end because of a 'negative' event. There will be a great deal of learning achieved, just by the experience, and hence there is a potential value to the individual which may far exceed that of actually achieving the desired ends. There will be another opportunity and all is not lost.

Many have experienced differences in the speed of their thought processes, as they accelerate or retard. An increased *pressure of thought*, as ideas move more rapidly through the mind, may be more noticeable in two distinctly different situations. The first occurs when the individual is overjoyed or excitedly anticipating some event. The individual finds great difficulty in concentrating or attending as the thoughts that preoccupy flit through the mind, one often leading to another via association. Similar patterns of acceleration may be experienced in those who feel anxious or overwhelmed, as thoughts flow in rapid succession regarding things that have to be done. Conversely, when a person is severely fatigued or stressed, thought processes may *retard*, and a great effort of will may be necessary to accomplish reasoning activities. Those who are sad and distressed, or somatically discomforted, may find their thought processes slow and stultified, heavy, cumbersome and difficult to achieve. Boredom and insufficient stimulation may evoke retardation of thought in a similar way.

We mentioned elsewhere the relative normality of *obsessional thoughts*, those persistent, recurrent and intrusive ideas that many people experience. You may recall individuals who are compulsive 'picture straighteners', 'precise folders' of paper or linen, 'centre-ists', who need one article to be positioned symmetrically on top of another or other precise activities. To resist the desire to respond to the thoughts that generate such activities may create discomfort and unease, though the recognition exists that the action is meaningless and futile. These small obsessional thoughts provide the individual with feelings of 'same-ness' and stability, and hence security, plus feelings of control over the environment, which again promotes ease and confidence.

Thought aberration, particularly *delusional ideation*, may accompany a number of primarily somatic health problems. A delusion may be defined as a false belief, which cannot be shared by others of the same culture, or social standing, and which cannot be altered by logical argument or contrary experiences. The central nervous system of 75% of individuals suffering from systemic lupus erythematosus—a multisystem disease—is characterized by inflammation and biochemical and structural changes in collagen fibres of connective tissues throughout the body, and delusions, accompanied by problems of perception, may be a feature requiring attention for some. Similarly, individuals experiencing the cerebral infective process, termed encephalitis, may present within mental health facilities because of bizarre thoughts and odd behavioural changes. Cerebral neoplasia and perceptual disturbances (temporal) may present with delusions, the individual experiencing the effects of an overactive thyroid may complain of thought acceleration and the person whose thyroid is underproductive, may demonstrate slow, sluggish, dull thinking or conversely delusional thoughts. Vitamin B_{12} deficiency may provoke significant thought disorder in approximately 10% of individuals concerned, whilst drug preparations, for example, steroids and cardiac glycosides, may also affect the quality and speed of thought processes. Preoccupation of thoughts with distressing facts and fears may, of course, be a problem for anyone experiencing somatic ill health, its treatment or sequelae.

Within mental health care, problems of thought and thinking may, for ease of description, be subdivided into those relating to:

1. thought content
2. form of thought
3. thought possession
4. stream of thought
5. judgement and decision making.

We have referred previously, within this section, to the delusional ideation that may be associated with somatic ill health, and, in particular, neurological disease and dysfunction. At that juncture, meaning was given to the term 'delusion'—that is, a false belief, which cannot be shared by others of the same culture, or social standing, and which cannot be altered by logical argument or contrary experiences. One may assume, then, that all false beliefs may be delusional and indicative, therefore, of deviation in psychosocial or somatic health. However, that assumption would be erroneous, for many individuals may demonstrate *overvalued ideas*, which whilst indicative of eccentricity, may not be considered as evidence of a deviation in mental health status. An overvalued idea assumes an integral and important role in the individual's life because of its associated emotions and personal significance. These, too, are immune to rational argument, but differ from delusions in that they become comprehensible in the light of the individual's previous experience or in relation to the beliefs of his family or his subculture. Commonly quoted examples of the phenomenon include a belief that the world is flat; that a daily purgative is essential to health and that modern-day wet summertimes are due to space exploration.

Delusions represent problems of *thought content*, and, as such, are associated with those who lack insight or contact with reality, that is the individual ascribed the label of '*psychotic*'. A delusion may be referred to as *primary*, or *autochthonous*, in nature, when it arises fully formed and without any identifiable precursors. There may be no apparent relationship with the subject's prevailing mood (though on occasions and in reprospect, mood may be considered aberrant) or with any recent event. The subject *suddenly knows* that he or she is God, that the two hemispheres of his brain have been transposed or that he or she has a personal and profound mission in the world. Jaspers (1963) suggests that this *sudden delusion idea* provides one example of a *primary delusional experience*, and that this, plus the second example of a *delusional perception*, may both arise from a *delusional mood*. He described a delusional perception as that event which occurs when a full delusional meaning is ascribed to a normal, innocuous perception that is totally unrelated—for example, running water evoking the subject's belief that he or she is God. Subjects believe that their environment has dramatically and inexplicably changed; it is usually unpleasant and self-referential. They are convinced—or at least strongly suspect—that mundane events are of tremendous significance, but they remain perplexed and apprehensive, as they attempt to make sense of their environment. Grandiosed or paranoid ideas (see later discussion) may be entertained and quickly discarded, and the problem resolution is seen either in the form of recovery or development of a stable delusional system. Delusional mood may be diagnosed retrospectively, following the emergence of a sudden delusional idea or perception. Sometimes, however, the term is used loosely by practitioners, who may attribute little diagnostic importance or specificity to its presence.

Individuals may present with the problem of a persistent delusion and very few other, associated problems. Behaviour does not appear 'odd' or bizarre, and, whilst on occasions, the delusion may be accompanied by perceptual problems—notably visual or auditory hallucinations—these are neither distressing nor prominent for the individual and his or her daily performance. When present in this, almost isolated form, the label of *delusional disorder* may be assigned to differentiate between this and more complex problem experience. You may observe that an individual's delusions tend to follow one or more distinct themes of content. *Somatic type* delusions may be exteriorized by a belief that certain parts of the body are malfunctioning, harbouring a parasite or emitting a foul smell. Subjects may believe that insects inhabit their skin or have burrowed beneath it, causing an infestation, or perhaps that organs, or body parts, have become distorted in size, shape or appearance. All available evidence refutes the individual's beliefs, but he or she will frequently present to somatically orientated health care facilities with his apparent problems.

Jealousy may similarly assume a delusional theme, with the subject certain that his or her partner is unfaithful and yet there being no just cause for this belief. The subject may prevent the partner from leaving the house alone, may initiate a surveillance upon the individual's every move and collect 'evidence'—in the form of creased clothing or use of a new perfume—to support this belief. The subject may actually confront the partner with the supposed infidelity, as, indeed, he or she may accuse a 'lover' of these activities, and violence may ensue.

The belief that one possesses a great, and, hitherto, unrecognized skill, talent or knowledge, for which there is no apparent basis or evidence, is characteristic of the *grandiose type* of delusion. Beliefs that one has a special relationship with a well-known personality—a film star, politician, footballer and so on—whilst less common, similarly occur and where this is exhibited, the well-known personality is often accused of being an imposter, and not the 'real' individual at all. Where grandiose delusions have a religious content, subjects may assume elevated, if not leading, positions within cult movements.

In *erotomanic-type* delusions, individuals believe themselves romantically and spiritually united with someone—often a public figure, sometimes a complete and utter stranger—whom they will avidly pursue, whether by telephone, letter, via sending gifts and cards, or by following the individual in daily life or through the person's publicity. The 'erotic' connotation of the descriptor would suggest a sexual desire as the basis of the fantasy relationship, but this may not be so, the beliefs and desires being 'pure and unsullied', idealistic and loving rather than lusting in nature. Sometimes, people experiencing this delusional theme may come to the notice of the police because of the harassment, stalking or attempts to 'rescue' their loved one from some imagined threatening individual or situation. Often, however, the subject maintains a secrecy around their beliefs and desires and is unwilling to discuss or share them with anyone, even their closest relatives or peers.

The *persecutory theme* is one of the most commonly encountered, and may be simple or complex, and single, or multiple and intertwined, delusional ideas. Most revolve around an injustice of some sort—the individual is being cheated, mistreated, excluded from events or being drugged or poisoned—and the subject feels 'hard-done-by', often angry and sometimes is overtly violent towards the believed perpetrators of his problem. On occasions, the subject may persistently attempt to gain legal redress for the imagined injustices—*querulous paranoia*—and initiate proceedings via the courts, repeatedly and determinedly using all channels and avenues available to him.

The above themes—somatic, jealous, grandiose, erotomanic and persecutory—may be viewed as embellishments, expansions and explanations of a primary delusional idea or perception and hence may be referred to as *secondary delusions*. They may feature in association with other characteristic problems within a variety of discrete diagnostic 'psychotic' categories utilized by medical colleagues including schizophrenia, bipolar affective disorders, psychoactive substance use and misuse, and organically precipitated problems.

*Delusions of control—passivity—*may be seen when the individuals believe that their thoughts, feelings, actions or will are being determined, influenced or controlled by an external or alien power. When related to movement, it may be referred to as *motor passivity* or *made acts*, to sensation as *somatic passivity* or *made sensations*, and to emotions as *emotional passivity* or *made emotions*. Individuals believe themselves to be the passive recipient of some external influence and in essence, have an experience that simultaneously acquires a delusional interpretation or explanation. Passivity phenomena are characteristic of the multiple problems categorized as 'schizophrenia'.

Delusions of reference are characterized by the subject's belief that events, objects, overheard conversation and similar mundane occurrences not in reality relating to the individual, have great personal significance, are self-referential, and may have been deliberately arranged to influence or affect him or her personally. Any event may be misconstrued by the individual and ascribed as an important indicator of his or her beliefs regarding the situation. The specific manner in which a pint of beer is pulled, the method used to fold a table cloth, or the particular direction in which a shopper fills his trolley may all be highly significant to the individual experiencing this problem. *Ideas of reference* is the term applied to a similar phenomenon but of lesser intensity and therefore not reaching delusional proportions. These may be exteriorized by the mentally healthy individual as well as many individuals experiencing a deviation in mental health status.

Problems associated with the *form of thought*, or *formal thought disorders*, are those that relate to the *process* of thinking and the consequent expression of those thoughts. They include the difficulties associated with conceptual or abstract thinking, particularly experienced by those individuals diagnosed as suffering from schizophrenia and organic impairment, and, whilst several authorities have described the various problems associated with form of thought, differing terminology has been utilized in describing those problems.

Bleuler (1950), for example, identified a distinct lack of connection between the individual's ideas, and termed this *loosening of association*. As a result of this loosening, Bleuler believed that the subject's use of concepts becomes imprecise and fluctuates, and he identified three Freud-orientated factors which he believed contributed to the problem. The first he termed *condensation*, describing the merger of two or more associated ideas to form a false concept; the second he related as *displacement*, where a correct idea was replaced by an incorrect, but associated one; the third he named *misuse of symbols*, and this described the concreteness of interpretation of a symbol, rather than its abstract, more 'symbolic' meaning.

Cameron (1938) similarly noted this lack of connection of ideas, and termed it *asyndesis*, and, in addition, the imprecise, idiomatic and shifting conceptual expression, which he labelled as *metonyms*. He described the subject's confusion by other themes when attempting to consider one subject, and called this *interpretation of thoughts*, and the lack of organized thinking, the inability to set parameters to a topic or to differentiate between central themes and peripheral, unimportant, details as *overinclusivity*.

Schneider (1959) considered that healthy thinking exhibited characteristics of *constancy, organization* and *continuity* and that, in 'formal thought disorder', these were disrupted to produce *transitory, drivelling*—the mixing of the elements of a complex thought—and *desultory* thoughts. He similarly identified problems of *fusion, omission, derailment* and *substitution* as occurring. He regarded fusion as the enmeshing and weaving together of separate thoughts in a confusing manner; omission refers to the exclusion of major parts of a thought; derailment is the term used to describe the individual's penchant of moving from one train of thought to another, without logical connection; substitution was the term used to describe the replacement of one thought by another, unconnected, one.

Certainly the term '*knight's move thinking*', which illustrates the peculiar 'angled' thought pattern demonstrated by the individual experiencing the multiplicity of problems categorized as schizophrenia (as illustrated by the 'L' shaped movement of the knight piece on a chess board) would approximate to both Schneider's terms of derailment and substitution. In addition, problems of overinclusivity and concrete thinking are commonly encountered within the individual's exteriorization of his mechanism or form of thinking. Further discussion on problems associated with derailment, incoherence and poverty of content are undertaken within the final section of this chapter and relate more easily to language.

Problems associated with *thought possession* are relatively easy and quickly related. In 'normal, healthy' individuals, their thoughts are their own, and remain inside their head unless they choose to verbalize and hence share them with others. Whilst they may be persuaded, or manipulated, to think in a particular way, individuals are in ultimate control of that thinking, which occurs in response or reaction to their environment and experiences. Individuals may demonstrate problems within aspects of the above, for, as an example, they may believe their thoughts to be foreign or alien to themselves and that they have been placed there by others—*thought insertion*. Similarly, individuals may experience, what they believe to be, a sudden removal of thoughts by an outside individual, agency or authority—*thought withdrawal*—or that one's own thoughts are available to others, that they are being *broadcasted* and that others speak with those thoughts.

The above are commonly verbalized by individuals who are diagnosed as 'schizophrenic' and, whilst not delusions but experiences, may acquire embellishment and stability via additional delusional ideation.

Problems related to the *stream of thought* are, again, frequently exteriorized. We have already mentioned *thought blocking* as a common experience accompanying anxiety but for some individuals there is a sudden cessation of the train of thought, which leaves a vacant expanse within the cognitive function without evidence of anxiety. Subjects find that when their thoughts resume, they follow a totally unrelated train and will continue in that new vein unperturbed. Anxious individuals will frantically search their mind for the lost thread and desperately try to remember what they were thinking or verbalizing, but this is not so with the person whose mental health status is significantly altered. *Perseveration* is similarly indicative of a major mental health disruption, as a thought—it may also be a word or phrase—is repeated persistently, long after it has become irrelevant. Both thought blocking and perseveration may be exhibited by the individual categorized as schizophrenic, and thought perseveration may also be a problem for the individual experiencing temporal lobe epilepsy.

The speed of the stream of thought may similarly create difficulties for both the individual and others. We previously mentioned the minimal levels of acceleration and retardation which the mentally healthy individual may experience on occasions. However, the degree of the problems that may be experienced by the individual may be prolonged, extensive and create severe disruption to life and living. *Retardation of thought* is a common problem for those who are intensely depressed, and may form part of an overall psychomotor retardation, with poor concentration, attention, memory and motor activity reduction. *Pressure of thought* describes an increased speed of flow of thoughts and ideas through the individual's mind, whilst *flight of ideas* relates to a more accelerated thought pattern, in which ideas are linked or associated and continue to flow without respite. Both pressure of thought and flight of ideas are associated with the generalized psychomotor acceleration and increased rate of activities and functions indicative of elevated mood problems. They are, therefore, a problem in situations where mood and affect are aberrant—that is in those using psychoactive substances, for example, hallucinogens, phencyclidine, or similar preparations, those experiencing organic impairment and deterioration, of various aetiological factors, and those experiencing a primary mood disturbance, often categorized as 'affective' or 'bipolar disorder', of elevated or mixed mood.

Circumstantiality may also serve to slow down or retard thought processes and this occurs when trivial details are persistently included within thinking processes. The individual then has so many items to consider within any reflective period or decision-making process that a conclusion is well nigh impossible to achieve. The normal speed of thought may similarly be reduced if other, recurring, and intrusive thoughts persistently interrupt thinking. We have previously mentioned obsessions, that is, those repetitive thoughts—or perhaps actions—which one feels compelled to resist and yet is unable to do so successfully. When excessive, the individual may experience a life that is organized around such obsessional thoughts and their overt responses—compulsive, ritualistic activities. However, there are many examples of recurring, intrusive thoughts—perhaps relating to hopelessness, suicide, or a preoccupation with having been assigned the wrong gender role by society. Individuals may find themselves returning time and time again, and often unwillingly or without deliberate intention to a recurring often distressing theme, thus inhibiting thought processes related to daily living.

Judgement may be impaired within the cognitive functioning of those whose mental health is giving rise to concern. The ability to collate all available information, to weigh it, piece by piece and then make decisions in the light of projected value, anticipated outcomes and rationale within overall goals, may be disturbed within any state of intoxication, for example, and therefore there may be a problem in excessive utilization of alcohol, cannabis, opioids, inhalants and other psychoactive substances. Similarly, because of elevated mood and accelerated thought processes, individuals experiencing hyperactive functioning, those diagnosed as 'mood disorders—manic/mixed', and those whose cognitive abilities are deteriorating due to organic impairment from a variety of causes, may exhibit such uncertain judgement. Certainly any individual who demonstrates impulsive, antisocial or extremely dependent behaviour will exteriorize problems associated with judgement and decision making, as will anyone who, for whatever reason, finds attention and concentration limited or easily disrupted.

Problems of thought and thinking may create significant disruption in the individual's life and total functioning and represent a considerable challenge to carers.

MEMORY

INTRODUCTION

Memory is the diary we all carry around with us.
Oscar Wilde 1969

This observation, made by Miss Letitia Prism to her student, Cecily, in Oscar Wilde's comedy of manners The importance of being earnest, could not be more succinct or accurate, and hence provides an effective analogy for use here.

The diary that many individuals rely on, and carry around in a handbag or pocket, has two distinct functions. It provides a record, and hence a reminder, of what an individual has spent time doing, when and where. In addition, however, it enables the individual to plan, predict and anticipate the future thereby assisting in the organization of current and continuing activities.

Memory is very similar in action, for where the diary is a written record of previous events and occurrences accessible via visual scanning, the memory provides a store of past learning, related to the experiences of life and living, that is able to

be accessed in various formats, in a variety of different ways, for use in current activities. The value of memory is not appreciated by the individual until it does not provide the service that has come to be expected. Most people have 'forgotten' something, somewhere, sometime—that is, have failed to recall a name, an important date, the time of a meeting, and the like. Many have experienced 'losing' a piece of information—a word, perhaps, which elicits the exact meaning wished to be conveyed—and having to enter into a long drawn out explanation of material, associated with the 'lost' item, to compensate. Behaviours learned in the past are often automatically evoked by the adult who, if required to explain how an action is to be achieved, may now be unable to 'remember' exactly what processes are performed and in which order they are carried out. The experienced driver trying to teach a novice is a prime example of this, driving having become so integral to the behaviour evoked by opening a car door and sitting in the driver's seat, that the individual no longer has to think about the series of activities or manoeuvres required. When one considers the traumas often associated with learning a complex set of interrelated movements for the first time, such as is involved in driving, it has to be a relief to realize that such activities do become an integral aspect of functioning. If one had to learn to dress and tie shoe laces every morning, no one would ever get out of the house! It is irritating enough to forget one item of vocabulary in a day, but imagine being unable to recall something done only a few minutes ago—not just once, but as a common regular occurrence of everyday life.

SURGICAL SEQUELAE—A CASE HISTORY

In 1953, a young man was referred to a hospital in Hartford. Connecticut, USA, for advice and assistance from the neurosurgeon, William Scoville. The young man, known to the world as HM, was, at that time, 27 years old and had, from the age of 16, suffered severe epileptic seizures, with terrible frequency. Neurological examination depicted the temporal lobe as the focus of the fits and both hemispheres appeared equally affected. Medication had failed to effect any relief and therefore surgical intervention, in a manner never previously attempted, was deemed appropriate. The surgeon removed parts of both temporal lobes, including the hippocampus and amygdala. Miraculously the seizures ceased, and the team were, of course, delighted, until, within a few hours of surgery, it became obvious that HM was experiencing difficulties in a different area of function. He was unable to recognize care staff, or even find his way back to his room in the hospital. It was soon discovered that HM was unable to remember any new fact or experience.

HM had good recall for the early part of his life and for those elements learned during that time, so, for example, his linguistic abilities, and psychomotor skills of walking, dressing and eating remained intact. His level of intellect was unimpaired and, using standard intelligence tests, his IQ was, in fact, a little higher following surgery than preoperatively. However, HM lived entirely in the present, being able to recall objects, people or experiences only whilst they remained in his short term memory. Brenda Milner, of the Neurological Institute of Montreal, who had known the individual for over 25 years, presented as a stranger every time they met. She reported (Milner 1972) that 10 months after the operation, HM and his family moved to a new house not far away from their previous residence. A year later, HM was still unable to provide his new address to questioners and proved unable to go home alone, for he continually returned to his old address. Milner described his ability to repeat the same jigsaw puzzles, day after day, without showing any evidence of the practice effect, and to read repeatedly the same magazines without any evidence of familiarity with, or recognition of, their contents. An individual who chatted with HM and then left the room for a few minutes, returned as a stranger, for HM had no recollection of either the individual or the previous discussions held.

HM and his family moved to Boston in the late 1970s, and were supported by Massachusetts General Hospital. Material and events stored within his memory up to a period of 3 years before the operation were available to him. That stored within the year or two preceding surgery had suffered some impairment and he could remember little since surgery. As a result of the unforeseen sequelae, the procedure was never performed again, for whilst the well-meaning surgeon achieved his objectives in preventing further epileptic seizures, it was at a devastating cost to the individual and his family.

HM, sadly, became one of the best-known amnesiacs in the world, but from his experience, much was able to be deduced:

1. The hippocampus and the medial part of the temporal lobe play a role in the processes inherent in memory consolidation—that is, the physical and psychological changes that occur as the brain organizes material that may become part of permanent memory.

2. The part played by these structures appears to be related to making memories, rather than their storage (his memory for up to 3 years preoperation was intact) or recall.

3. Memory may continue to be consolidated for some considerable time after learning has taken place.

ACCIDENTAL EVIDENCE—A SECOND CASE STUDY

NA presents another saddening lesson in the search for the biological basis of memory, this time via injury (Squire 1984). He was on army service in the Azores, in 1960, when during some friendly horseplay in the barracks with a room mate, a fencing foil penetrated his brain, via his left nostril. His recollections after the accident are that he really had no control over immediate activities or himself—'I really became someone outside of my body … I didn't really care too much about it because I didn't think it was me'. NA recalls the details of the actual accident with clarity. He did not experience pain, but a sensation of 'shock' felt by his brain. He tried to remove the foil but found it to be stuck hard, so he persuaded his companion to try. The foil was withdrawn with relative ease, again with only a sensation of a shock felt by his brain. After a few seconds, a thick clear substance began to run from his nose, which would not stop flowing.

NA did eventually collapse after the accident but not for some minutes and not until after he had walked down some stairs. He spent months in hospital, often seeming to watch events that were happening to him from outside of himself, sometimes feeling that these things might be happening to him and on other occasions certain that they were. For much of this period he was unsure of who these events were happening to.

After the accident, NA went to live with his mother, and, about a year following the accident, suddenly was able to pull the fragments of his identity together, to become a 'whole person', and yet remained amnesic. Computerized axial tomography (CAT scan) enabled Squire to identify the area damaged by the fencing foil. The area of damage proved to be that of the dorsal medial nucleus of the thalamus, that area of the limbic system that lies quite close to the hippocampus and amygdala. The damage was on the left-hand side of the brain structures, an element of importance when identifying the exact nature of memory loss experienced.

According to Squire, the fact that pre-1960 memory was intact whilst post-1960 memory demonstrated impairment, would indicate a 'difficulty in laying down new memories', that is, a disruption of the learning process itself rather than the retrieval process. This assertion is strongly contested by other scientists who believe the memory store to be the area damaged. Squire connects all three phases—learning, storage and recall—but asserts that the storage of memory probably functions in the larger, overlying areas of the brain, within the cortex. The thalamus, he believes, is part of the system that establishes and forms memories and that elaborates them over time.

The damage to NA's brain was on the left-hand side of the organ, where it is known that centres concerned with speech and language are situated. NA's visual memory was existing, as Squire demonstrated via a test utilizing cards with black and white line drawings upon them. All of the drawings were of everyday objects, and half an hour after being shown them, NA could recall that he had been shown the cards and that one was of a fork. He was unable to recall the reason for being shown the cards, but could at least remember being shown them. A second test, comprising of written words on cards, was followed 30 minutes later by Squire's posing a question as to whether NA remembered *either* of the tests. NA recalled the cards with drawings upon them, but had no recollection of the word-card test.

The inference would seem to be that there is a system for learning verbal material and a separate one for learning visual material.

DRINKING TO FORGET

Amnesia is also seen to occur in Korsakoff's syndrome, a result of vitamin B (thiamine) deficiency which is progressive in nature and a relatively common sequel to chronic alcohol misuse. Treatment, if the problem is discovered early enough, is with extensive doses of the deficient vitamin.

The problems associated with memory in Korsakoff's syndrome are not only related to forming new memories, but in addition, to predamage events. There are problems associated with thinking and problem solving, shown in tests requiring differing strategies to be utilized, to solve a puzzle. For example, a test may be conducted with a number of cards, each of which depicts a different geometrical shape. Given no information, subjects will pick up cards, one at a time, until they are told that one in particular is 'the right card'—for example, the circle-card. In subsequent tests individuals select that same card and are told that they are correct on each occasion. When on the next trial, the experimenter changes the solution to a different card, say a card depicting a square, subjects choose the circle-card and are told they are incorrect. Instead of trying a different geometrical design, individuals experiencing the Korsakoff-related amnesia will continue to select the circle-bearing card and will do so despite being told on each occasion that this is the 'wrong card'. They will persevere with the strategy long after it has proved inadequate or incorrect in the problem-solving experience. 'Normal' subjects—and indeed HM and NA—would try different cards until they selected the right card.

Proactive inhibition is the term used to describe the interference of old learning on new learning related to the same topic. For example, when learning successive groups of words all belonging to one category—say the names of birds—the content of earlier lists learned interferes with those learned later. The phenomenon disappears when later word groups to be learned relate to a different category, for example, types of dogs. The individual experiencing amnesia associated with Korsakoff's syndrome, demonstrates no improvement when categories are changed, continuing to display proactive inhibition.

The damage of Korsakoff's syndrome includes the same thalamic nucleus that NA damaged in his fencing accident, but, in addition, there is neuronal loss in both the cerebral cortex, particularly the frontal lobe, and in the cerebellum. The question to ask would seem to be 'Is the long term memory deficit of Korsakoff's syndrome due to cortical loss, or does cognitive dysfunction—problem solving and concept formation difficulties—prevent reconstruction of past memories?'

Studies by Moscovitch (1981) of individuals who do not demonstrate amnesia and yet who have sustained trauma to the frontal lobe reveal that such people have similar problem-solving difficulties as those experiencing Korsakoff's syndrome. The answer to the question becomes more obscure at this point, because further questions related to the different degrees of damage that have been sustained, and exactly where such damage lies, may be significant. Plus, of course, damage may have been incurred in those alcohol-related Korsakoff's syndrome sufferers through head traumas that have not been accounted for.

MEMORY AND LEARNING

To conclude the valuable information gained from the unfortunate experiences of HM and NA, an identification of the continuing abilities of such individuals to learn is available. Whilst cognizant of the fact the individual would not remember the new learning, Cohen & Squire (1981) taught a group of amnesic individuals the skill of mirror reading. It took 3 days for the individuals to become adept at the task—about the same time as 'normal' subjects—though of course, they could not remember ever having worked on the skill before, and none could later remember the words he or she had read. The group retained a high level of skill for the entire period of testing, some 3 months. Indeed, Cohen (1981) found HM capable of learning to solve puzzles and repeat the successful solution, though he had no recall of working on the puzzle in the past and appeared not to know what was expected of him.

Cohen & Squire suggested that problems such as those experienced by HM were not related to retrieval of memory as many had suggested, but indicated a failure to store as much information as others do, to facilitate problem solving (Cohen & Squire 1980). In the light of this, they advanced the theory that the brain handles and stores two kinds of information in different ways. *Procedural knowledge* is that related to how to do something, which probably developed early in the evolutionary period, and, at a later juncture, there will be an exploration of evidence which would support the existence of such a memory. However, in addition to procedural knowledge, they suggested the existence of an 'explicit, accessible record of individual previous experiences, a sense of familiarity about those experiences', which they termed *declarative knowledge*. It is this latter type of knowledge that they believe to be processed in the temporal region and parts of the thalamus, and which requires a remodelling and adjustment of neural circuitry in those areas, differing from that of procedural knowledge, in which only structures directly involved in the procedure being learned seem to be changed biochemically or biophysically.

It is of interest to note that, in relation to learning, the rates of forgetting shown by HM, NA and individuals experiencing Korsakoff's syndrome, show some differences. Where the primary injury site was the medial dorsal thalamic nucleus, as in the case of NA, and those with Korsakoff's syndrome, the individuals 'forgot' at a normal rate, as compared with that of a control group of 'normal' people. HM—and individuals receiving bilateral electroplexy by the way—demonstrated an abnormally rapid rate of forgetting. It would appear, therefore, that the hippocampus, amygdala and related structures are necessary in memory consolidation, that is, the transfer of declarative material to long term memory. The thalamus, on the other hand, may be necessary to perform the initial coding of certain kinds of declarative information and material.

In the introduction to the chapter, we asked you to imagine being unable to recall something done only a few minutes before, on a consistent, everyday basis. Perhaps the words of NA may assist:

> There are, I guess, many missing pieces but I don't remember that I miss them. I don't remember what it is I'm missing, so I don't pay much attention to it.

LEARNING AND THE BRAIN

A combination of the work of anatomists, psychologists and neuroscientists has, over the past century, provided a wealth of knowledge in relation to the effects of learning upon the brain.

The brain of a newborn baby is approximately a quarter of the size of that of the adult. At 6 months the brain has assumed almost half the size of that of the adult and at the age of 2 years, 75% of the final dimensions. The number, size, shape and function of neurons is decreed at conception via genetic inheritance and no new brain cells are created after birth. The increase in the size of the brain of the developing infant is accounted for in part by the increasing size of the neurons, their increasing number of connections via axon growth and dendrite branching, new glial cells and myelin sheath growth. However, the remainder of this growth would seem to be related to the interaction between the individual's genetic plan and the environment.

Animal experiments, in the main, have provided evidence that denial or reduction in sensory input will inhibit development. Woolsey & Wann (1976) found that each of a mouse's whiskers relays sensory data, via two synaptic relays, to a group of cells—a barrel—within the cerebral cortex. Removal of one row of whiskers shortly after birth shows a failure of the related cortical barrels to develop, with cells shrinking and losing their function. In addition, however, the barrels of

adjoining rows of whiskers will be larger than normal, showing a compensatory mechanism in operation, to make up for the deficit experienced. This compensation is termed *plasticity*. Hubel & Wiesel (1977) demonstrated similar results in a kitten. One of the kitten's eyes was covered shortly after birth and within a few months, the kitten was unable to see through that eye. The 'defect' was not in the eye or its structure, but due to a failure of the visual cortex to develop. Conversely, Rosenzweig (1984) showed that rats raised in an 'enriched environment' developed more extensive cerebral cortices than those 'deprived' and raised in isolation. A large cage, plenty of company, and objects to play with resulted in an improved learning ability within maze experiments. The 'pampered' rats could run faster and more reliably than their lonely rat counterparts, their learning in relation to the maze being swifter and more accurate. The cortical neurons evinced more spines in the enriched rats, these spines acting as extra receivers of impulses at synaptic relays (Globus et al 1973). The size of these synaptic contacts was seen to be 50% larger than those of the deprived rat (Mollgaard et al 1971) and far more frequent in number (Greenough, West & DeVoogd 1978).

The cortex of humans may be seen to be similarly affected. Freeman & Thibes (1973) found abnormal cortical development in the brains of adults who had an astigmatism at birth, which had gone untreated. An astigmatism is a refractive error, where horizontal and vertical curvatures of the cornea of the eye are uneven, producing differences in focusing of light rays. Whilst some may fall upon the retina, others may fall short and others may be carried beyond the retina, causing blurring of the image. Freeman & Thibes (1973) demonstrated a reduced cortical response from the area of the cortex related to the dimension that had always been blurred. Dennis (1960) demonstrated the effects of severe sensory deprivation in his study of infants in Iranian orphanages. Babies were handled, in essence, only once a day, for bathing, otherwise human contact was negligible. Feeding was achieved via bottles propped upon pillows and any physical attention required was performed in the cot, where babies lay all day. To prevent draughts, the cot sides were covered hence reducing potential stimuli even further. The study showed that many of these orphans were unable to sit up, unaided, at the age of 21 months, something usually achieved by 9 months, and that less than 15% could walk at 3 years of age, where most children are walking well before the age of 2 years. The normal stimulation of the brain was absent and therefore infants failed to develop and learn the skills associated with normal milestones. The cortex failed to develop.

Curtiss (1977), a psycholinguist, described the sad account of Genie, a 13-year-old girl who came to the attention of Californian welfare authorities in 1970. Genie's father was severely mentally ill and her mother almost blind. From the age of 20 months, Genie had been confined solely to one room, kept naked and tethered to a commode chair, by a harness designed by her father. Fed only baby food and milk throughout her short lifetime, the girl weighed 26.8 kilograms when discovered, and did not know how to chew food. She was unable to recognize words or speak—father had forbidden mother to talk to her throughout her incarceration—had no control over bowels and bladder, and was unable to straighten her arms or legs, having only experienced free movement of her hands and feet. Father committed suicide soon after the discovery of Genie, but mother asserted that Genie had been a normal, healthy baby. Father had apparently hated children, and had placed a previous baby, aged 2 months, in the garage because it cried. That baby died of pneumonia.

During the following 6 years, Genie was provided with a great deal of general and expert assistance. She made great advances in some areas—she learned to use tools, to draw and had some ability to orientate herself and find her way around, for example, in a supermarket. In simpler instances, Genie could relate cause and effect and yet her linguistic skills remained at a level similar to a 2 year-old child. In 1977, her IQ on non-verbal tests showed a low–normal score of 74 and EEG patterns indicated that Genie was utilizing the right hemisphere of her brain for both language and non-language functions. Normally the specialist skills relating to language would be sited in the left hemisphere.

Curtiss asserts that language acquisition provokes or facilitates the hemispheric specialization pattern that is normally seen and that failure to acquire language may engender cortical degeneration and atrophy of those areas relating to linguistic functions.

WHAT HAPPENS WHEN AN ORGANISM LEARNS?

Neuroscientists have investigated the simple learning that occurs in animals at an unconscious level—that is, that learning which occurs without the organism's awareness of a change in behaviour.

Habituation is said to occur when a stimulus, which initially provoked a response, is presented so frequently that the organism fails to respond to it any more. The organism becomes accustomed to the stimulus and its meaning to the environment and the organism's own survival, and simply ceases to react to its presence. Kandel & Schwartz (1982) studied a marine snail, *Aplysia californica*, and demonstrated that changes at a cellular level accompany habituation. *Aplysia* demonstrates a reflex action implicit in survival. It has a gill-withdrawal ability, which facilitates retraction of the gill and hence its protection in rough waters or when debris may cause damage. In quiet water, the gill is extended to allow the *Aplysia* to breathe. When conditions become adverse, retraction occurs, being controlled by one ganglion, containing six motor and 24 sensory neurons. Connections between the two are provided both directly, via excitatory synapses, and indirectly, via interneurons. Repeated stimulation in the laboratory, provoked initially a less vigorous withdrawal and after 10 stimulations, no withdrawal was elicited at all. Less neurotransmitter substance was released by sensory neurons across the synapse to motor neurons, which, because they were in receipt of a lower level of activation, performed less intensely. A short term habituation results because of decrease in excitation at the synapses of the existing neural pathway. The researchers discovered that after no further experimentation, the gill-withdrawal reflex returned to its usual vigorous activity within a few hours. This return is due to a change in the amount of transmitter substance released at the same synaptic junction. It is brought about by the release of another chemical transmitter substance, by other sensory fibres in response to stimulation of another part of the organism. This is termed *sensitization*, and reflects a second type of simple learning, in essence, a reversal of habituation. The animal learns to respond vigorously to a previously neutral stimulus.

The study has parallels in the behaviour of the newborn human infant who demonstrates a capability for habituation. A sensing device attached to the soother of a 4-hour-old baby detected a cessation of sucking at the onset of a tone, loud enough for the infant to hear. After a few seconds—presumably of listening to the tone—sucking was recommenced, and it was only when a tone different from the first was played that the infant stopped sucking again to listen. The first tone had been habituated (Bronshtein & Petrova 1967).

Pavlov's (1927) experiments with dogs and classical conditioning are well recorded and frequently cited. In Pavlov's experiments, a stimulus which naturally produces a particular reaction, is paired a number of times with another stimulus. The natural stimulus becomes representative of, and elicits the same reaction as, the primary stimulus. To achieve conditioning, the two stimuli must be presented close together.

Alkon (1983) had demonstrated neural changes occurring in response to conditioning in another genus of marine snail, *Hermissenda crassicornis*. This particular snail naturally feeds in well-lit water near the surface of the sea and therefore instinctively moves towards light. Like *Aplysia*, it dislikes turbulence, as it tends to injure the delicate appendages of the organism, and therefore, in response to rough water, will contract its foot, reducing the speed of its movement towards light. Alkon and his colleagues paired turbulence with a preceding light, conditioning the snails to associate light with the onset of turbulence. The snails slowed their rate of movement towards light, their feet contracting when they saw light, and this response was maintained for several weeks. The researchers found the response had been mediated on three different levels.

Anatomically speaking, light generates impulses in two types of photoreceptors in the snail's eyes, which are in turn transmitted to interneurons, motor neurons and muscles. Water turbulence is detected via hair-like structures in, what are the equivalent of, the snail's ears. Impulses are similarly transmitted along an interneuron–motor neuron–muscle pathway, but some axons have synapses with the light sensitive, receptor axons, allowing the two systems to interact.

Of the photoreceptor cells in the eye, one is excitatory and one inhibitory. When the latter is activated, impulses along the neural path, which drive muscle contractions allowing movement towards light, are inhibited. The hair cells usually maintain these inhibitory receptors in a state of rest and during turbulence, that resting state is increased. When turbulence ceases—after the light had flashed—the hair cells release their effect on the inhibitory photoreceptor, allowing it to become excited, impulses to pass, and dampening down of the movement towards light. Following conditioning, the light alone will cause these inhibitory photoreceptor cells to exert their role.

In addition to the above, Alkon noted *biophysical* changes in the cell membrane. To recap on the physiology, you may recall that:

A neuron at rest is polarized, the inside of the cell being negative in respect to the outside environment. The potassium concentration is higher inside the cell than outside it. The concentration of sodium is higher outside than inside the cell

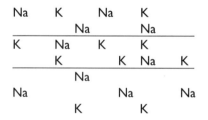

Owing to the effects of a chemical transmitter or in response to a sensory stimulus, channels in the cell membrane open, allowing sodium (and calcium) ions to flood in, causing depolarization. Similarly potassium channels open, allowing potassium to move from an area of high concentration to an area of low concentration, outside of the cell membrane. When

movement across the cell membrane is at an appropriate level, a wave of activity—the nerve impulse—is able to pass through the length of the axon. When activity ceases, the reverse process occurs, and the cell membrane returns to a state of rest.

Before conditioning, the photoreceptor cell receives inhibitory messages from the hair cell and thus the photoreceptor cell is kept at rest and negatively charged by allowing potassium ions to pass out. When the light flashes, the photoreceptor becomes excited, and sodium ions, followed closely by calcium ions, pass into the cell. At this precise moment, the turbulence commences, prompting the hair cell to increase its inhibitory action on the photoreceptor cell, and upon cessation of the turbulence, the hair cell relaxes its influence. The photoreceptor cell assumes a more positive charge as further calcium channels open, allowing an increase in the concentration of calcium within the cell cytoplasm. Potassium channels close, preventing further loss of these ions, and the cell is depolarized. Passage of the impulse then inhibits the snail's movement towards the light. This excited state may last for days and within this time a flash of light alone will cause continuing cessation of movement.

Alkon (1983) demonstrated that the behaviour exhibited could persist for weeks, with the photoreceptor cell maintaining its excitability and inhibiting the muscle action that would move the snail towards the light. Levels of calcium had been seen to be elevated within the photoreceptor cell during training but these reduced to normal levels once training had been discontinued, and yet the learned response persisted. It had been noted that these previously high levels of calcium had activated enzymes that combine proteins and phosphate molecules. This *phosphorylation* was thought to both change the character of the protein and the ion channel specificity, which may directly reduce the outflow of potassium from the cell, and thus maintain the excited state. It seems, too, that once activated, these phosphorylating enzymes continue to function despite the return of calcium levels to normal.

Simple learning in lower life organisms may be seen, therefore, to create changes in anatomical, biophysical and biochemical neural mechanisms, and remembering that human beings *evolved* to their current abilities, it is sensible to assume that such simple cellular learning has been preserved, even though the complex and complicated nervous system of vertebrates may have additional mechanisms and systems for memory storage.

Certainly Kandel & Schwartz (1982) point to the similarities between the signalling properties of the nerve cell of a snail, cat, monkey and human, stating that the kind of chemical substances used as transmitters and patterns of synaptic interactions closely resemble each other. They comment that 'one has reason from just the tradition of biology to feel that the basic processes like these are very likely to be similar in simple animals and complex ones'.

WHAT IS STORED AND WHERE?

Individuals who have sustained damage to the *cerebellum* report that they have lost the ability to move automatically and now have to consciously perform each step of a complex movement, for example, lifting a cup and actually stopping it at the right position before it 'hits' the mouth. McCormick et al (1982) believe that a wide number of classically conditioned, learned responses may be stored in the cerebellum. Experiments with rabbits indicated that a memory trace, associated with eyelid conditioning, developed in one particular area of the cerebellum called the deep cerebellar nuclei. Destruction of the region destroyed the memory trace and completely removed the conditioned response. With the area removed, the rabbit was unable to relearn the conditioned response, thus indicating the relative contribution of the cerebellum to the storage of memories of learned responses.

We have already mentioned the apparent role of the *hippocampus* in relation to memory, via the case study of HM's surgery and its sequelae. O'Keefe & Nadel (1978) in studies of the brains of rats, found some neurons within the hippocampus respond only when the animal is in a certain position within familiar territory. The rat may be moving about, and a specific cell be quiet until a particular location is reached, when the cell will fire vigorously. As the rat moves its position, the nerve cell activity ceases, only to refire when the rat returns to the precise position. O'Keefe & Nadel found that different cells scattered throughout the hippocampus fired in response to different regions of the rat's cage, thus prompting the researchers to suggest that the animals keep a mental map of their immediate environment 'in mind' in a sort of short term memory facility. They believe that in simpler animals, the hippocampus may store information relating to environments previously encountered, helping the animal to plan continuing exploration of that environment. It has been demonstrated that removal of the rat's hippocampus reduces the effectiveness of its ability to find its way around a maze, thus supporting the hypothesis.

Olton, Becker & Handelman (1980) found that, when foraging for food, 'normal' rats learned about their environment to the point where they would remember where they had already been and never retraced their steps to cover a path twice. However, when the hippocampus was removed the rat frequently retraced its path, apparently unable to remember where it had been before. It appears, therefore, that the hippocampus provides a short term memory related to current activity.

Thompson, Berger & Madden (1983) identified the role of the hippocampus in the conditioning of rabbits. With no hippocampus, conditioning was still possible, but with disruption of neuronal activity in the hippocampus, the rabbit was unable to learn a conditioned response. Thompson found that a slight delay between the presentation of conditioned and unconditioned stimuli provoked hippocampal neurons to commence firing activities as if the hippocampus was maintaining a state of readiness for the arrival of the unconditioned stimulus. Tasks of increasing complexity seemed to require increased neuronal activity within the hippocampus and evidence accumulated to demonstrate continuing firing long after stimulation has ceased. This *long term potentiation* appears to evoke neuronal structural changes and hence may be indicative of learning (Swanson, Teyler & Thompson 1982).

The *cortex* of the brain is the probable ultimate home of many memories but the actual way that these are spread out, or how this is achieved, is as yet unknown. It is possible that cerebral cortical cells have the ability to change the strength of their responses to incoming signals in a manner similar to that of the hippocampal cells, and that initial cortical activity is responsible for short term conscious memory. This may then be transferred to the hippocampus for processes aimed at conversion to long term storage and then returned to the cortex, where it results in permanent neuronal change, and long term storage.

The role of transmitter substances has been implicated within learning and memory, particularly noradrenaline secreted by the adrenal medulla, at times of arousal. Whilst unable to cross the blood–brain barrier, noradrenaline is seen to consolidate memory formation. McGough (1982) demonstrated that animals given a small amount of the substance following the use of pain as a punishment showed a greater propensity and better memory for correct behaviour.

Increased protein synthesis is seen in animals during learning, as demonstrated by Rose, Bateson & Horn (1973) in their work with chicks. The imprinting behaviour exhibited by chicks as they become attached to, and follow, the first moving object they see—usually the mother—was shown to be associated with an increased production of protein in the chick's brain, within 2 hours of exposure to the stimulus being imprinted. It is suggested that the extra available protein may be transferred to the synapse to facilitate a temporary increase in its effectiveness and hence may provide the basis for learning.

Whilst researchers continue to uncover elements of the memory-learning processes, a great deal remains to be clarified to facilitate a complete understanding of the subject area.

PROBLEMS OF MEMORY

Most people forget something at some time, and there is usually a simple reason for this. On occasions, the individual has not attended effectively to the exposed stimulus and does not, therefore, absorb the data available. This inattention may be due to a variety of factors—disinterest or boredom, a lack of perceived relevance of information to self, excessive preoccupation with other data, or activities, are examples—but whatever the causation, the result is the same, for an individual may not expect to recall material which has not yet been learned and retained.

At times, too, an individual attempts to recall information which was only in temporary storage, long after it has disappeared. The telephone number which one expects to use on a single occasion only, would not be available within memory the following day, for example. Whether because of decay (Brown 1964) or because new information disrupts or replaces previously stored data (Tulving & Madigan 1970), the original memory has disappeared and is unavailable for recall. We have already mentioned retroactive inhibition, the process whereby new learning interferes with and influences previously learned material, which has not had time to consolidate and be transferred into permanent storage sites. This knowledge may infer that theories of disruption or replacement may provide a more reasonable hypothesis for the loss of transiently stored material than those of decay.

The process of forgetting material from remote memory storage may be due to similar processes, but, in addition, may be a problem associated with an ineffective retrieval process. It is noted, for example, that, utilizing computerized information retrieval systems, the 'correct' word or command—that is, a word already within the system—is needed to access the desired information. The computer is not capable of substituting a similar meaning word for the one entered; the operator must utilize the appropriate terminology. It may be that formal retrieval processes are used within the human brain in relation to memory recall and that some part of this process is disrupted.

Freud, of course, would have asserted that forgetting is 'motivated', and the means by which unacceptable, unpleasant or threatening scenarios or data are removed from conscious awareness. His original work, later embellished and expanded by Anna Freud, asserted that the defence mechanism of *repression* was the primary vehicle via

which the elimination from consciousness was achieved and that under free association or hypnosis, recall was possible (Freud 1986). However, Eysenck & Wilson (1973) declared there to be little experimental evidence available to support Freud's hypothesis.

You may be aware, from personal experience, of other factors which may influence recall abilities, for example, excessive tiredness and fatigue, the general malaise associated with colds and influenza, and the 'saturated solution' scenario, where your mind is so full of the events of the day, that you are just not able to give of your best. Any situation which has a detrimental effect on attention and concentration may affect recall abilities. Stress and anxiety may have quite opposite effects in that individuals experiencing longstanding and cumulative stressors may be so overwhelmed that they forget a variety of aspects of life and living, and yet, given an 'acute' and threatening situation, they may be able to recall the tiniest and most obscure detail of the event.

The case studies of HM and NA demonstrate that cerebral trauma, whether accidentally or surgically induced, may create memory problems, and, even a relatively 'innocuous' bump to the head, may evoke an amnesia that may persist for minutes or hours. Frequently an individual does not recall the incident that precipitated damage or bodily injury, for example, there may be no recollection of a road traffic accident or the few minutes preceding or following it. However, sometimes there may be a persistent and recurring memory or 'dream sequence', where the precise nature of the incident—the actual movement of impact, say—is relived, time and time again, as in *post-traumatic stress disorder*. Certainly where an individual exhibits memory disturbances that are accompanied by sensorimotor symptomatology— paraesthesias and/or hemiparesis—evidence of recent injury to the side of the head opposite to that showing the sensorimotor impairment should be excluded.

Previous examples of memory problems associated with temporal lobe damage have been provided, but any irritable focus of the cerebrum may evoke a disturbance. Temporal lobe seizures, for example, may disrupt memory for a period of minutes or hours. Where verbal memories show disturbance, the focal area of irritation is found within the left hemisphere, whilst graphic and verbal amnesia is due to right hemispheric dysfunction. Cerebral tumours within the temporal lobe may precipitate early cognitive deficits, as may cerebral abscesses and a subdural haematoma, the latter being more common in alcohol-dependent individuals (approximately 50%; Lishman 1987) and the elderly, for obvious reasons of limitations or difficulties in mobility.

Cerebral hypoxia may similarly precipitate memory problems. Those associated with carbon monoxide poisoning, for example, may be accompanied by sensory disturbances—tingling and numbness—and be profound in nature. Vertebrobasilar circulatory disorders, whether caused by ischaemia, embolus, haemorrhage or infarct, may be abrupt in onset, last for some hours and then end as abruptly as they commenced. On occasions, there is a global loss of recent memory associated with feelings of bewilderment in an otherwise alert and responsible individual (transient global amnesia). For others, there is blurred, or double vision, vertigo, dizziness, nausea and vomiting, and ataxia. Remaining symptomatology subside to a vast extent as the episode is resolved, but amnesia remains.

Individuals, recovering from the effects of herpes simplex encephalitis, a viral disease affecting predominantly the medial temporal and orbital regions of the cortex, may demonstrate a residual amnesia associated with olfactory and gustatory hallucinations, and, similarly, those experiencing cerebral involvement due to syphilitic infection, may exteriorize problems associated with memory.

It has previously been noted that endocrine and metabolic problems may exteriorize as, or precipitate, deviations in mental health status and are significant, too, in relation to memory disturbances. Addison's disease (primary adrenal insufficiency), hypopituitarism, hypothyroidism, under- or oversecretion of parathyroid glands and hypoglycaemia may all encompass problems associated with memory.

Within mental health care, one may hear several terms utilized to describe the particular 'shade' of memory problem experienced by the individual. One such term may be *psychogenic amnesia*, where there is an abrupt inability to recall personal details and information and yet no organic reason is elicited to explain the phenomenon. One such type of psychogenic amnesia has been identified in the example relating to the inability to remember the details surrounding a road traffic accident and on occasions, this amnesia may extend to the period of 2 days or so following the trauma. This is termed a *localized* (or *circumscribed*) *amnesia* and is characterized by this inability to recall the events occurring within a 'circumscribed' period of time. *Selective amnesia* is less common and is the failure to recall some—but not all—of the events of a circumscribed period. Utilizing the previous example of the road traffic accident, victims may recall a passer-by assisting them from the car and, at some time within the episode, sitting at the side of the road, and yet nothing else of the event. *Generalized amnesia*, a total inability to recall any aspect of previous existence, and *continuous amnesia*, where amnesia extends from a specific event and includes present functioning, are more rarely seen. The psychogenic amnesias are associated with stress or an intolerable life event, for example in war situations and other life-threatening or psychosocially devastating experiences. It usually disappears abruptly, leaving the individual completely recovered.

Another, less common, absence of recall is again exhibited at times of great personal distress, and has been well documented in times of war and following natural disasters. *Psychogenic fugue* is the term used when individuals demonstrate a total lack of recall for their previous life, assume a new identity and move away from their home location, abruptly and unexpectedly. With the assumption of the new identity, individuals frequently assume a new personality, which often tends to be more extroverted, disinhibited and socially gregarious than that hitherto displayed. They appear well integrated and competent within socially complex situations, and are therefore accepted by others as 'legitimate' and as presented. On occasions, the fugue state is less well developed and is incomplete. There may be little more than abrupt, purposeful travel which is of brief duration. Although a new identity may be taken, it may be less well systematized and patchy in development. In these situations, social contact may not be so extensive and may be avoided by the individual. Again, on occasions, psychogenic fugue may be associated with acts of violence, either related to person or property. Such fugue states may last for hours, days or, occasionally, months. Recovery is usually abrupt and reoccurrences are rare; the problems which tend to be exteriorized are those related to the social implications of the abrupt disappearance and return, and because there is no recollection of events or experiences that took place during the fugue period. Differentiation needs to be made between such problems of a psychogenic nature, and those automatisms and fugues associated with typically temporal lobe epilepsy. Lishman (1987) makes the point that many experienced clinicians view all epileptic fugues as essentially psychogenic in nature, and asserts the inextricable link between organic and psychogenic factors. Despite this potential dispute between researchers regarding the aetiology of such experiences, the nurse's management of the individual, being tailor-made to the exteriorized and potential client needs, will differ due to the problems which may be concomitant in the experience of epilepsy *per se*.

Amnesia associated with herpes simplex encephalitis, head injury, hypoxia and cerebral circulatory disorders has previously been mentioned in relation to the somatic aetiology of memory problems. In mental health care, such *amnestic syndrome* is relatively rare, but when demonstrated tends to be by those people exhibiting a chronic use of alcohol and the consequent thiamine deficiency. Recent memory shows impairment via the individual's inability to learn new material, and that which has been learned is quickly forgotten—termed *anterograde amnesia*. As a result of this the individual so affected demonstrates disorientation related to time, ordering of events and frequently place and person.

Retrograde amnesia may cover a period of months or years prior to the onset of the problem and may be patchy and incomplete. *Remote memory* related to learning beyond the retrograde gap is relatively unimpaired and therefore speaking, writing, calculation and other early learned skills remain intact. Some individuals lack the awareness or insight to appreciate the impairment of memory, whilst others will acknowledge it, but be unperturbed by it. The gaps in memory may be filled by *confabulation*, that is the recounting of 'imaginary' events, but this tends to disappear with time. Individuals often demonstrate apathy, shallow affect and a distinct lack of initiative, though superficially they may appear gregarious and companionable. When related to alcohol utilization, individuals may be experiencing profound neurological deficits, for example, cerebellar ataxia, peripheral neuropathy and myopathy. Alcohol amnestic disorder is also referred to as *Korsakoff's syndrome*.

Memory impairment is commonly associated with any situation in which *delirium* is evident. Memory disturbance is related to recent events, and is associated with disorientation to time and place, though in relation to persons it is rare. Thinking is often disorganized and speech irrelevant, rambling and incoherent. Psychomotor activity may be severely aberrant, with restlessness and hyperactivity at one end of a continuum, and sluggishness and stupor at the other. Rapid fluctuations from one extreme to the other are common, and the individual may grope or strike out at non-existent objects. Misinterpretations, illusions and hallucinations are common, and frequently via the visual mode, although any sense may be involved. The sleep–wake cycle may be severely disturbed, with drowsiness, which may assume semicoma level, or hypervigilance and insomnia. Emotional disturbances may be exhibited, with lability, or a constant emotional tone displayed throughout. Physiologically, various autonomic symptoms—tachycardia, palpitations, elevated blood pressure, dilated pupils, etc.—are common. Psychoactive substance utilization may precipitate such problems, for example, it may be seen 24 hours after the use of amphetamines, cocaine, phencyclidine and similar-acting preparations. It is similarly evident during withdrawal from alcohol, sedative, hypnotic and anxiolytic preparations, and in the intoxication phase associated with opioid, sedative, anxiolytic and hypnotic substances.

Memory impairment associated with dementia is accompanied by problems of abstract thinking, impaired judgement and other higher cognitive deficits, plus changes within the personality characteristics demonstrated. The problems of memory may be moderate and predominantly relate to recent events, or be severe, showing marked anterograde and retrograde amnesia. Thinking difficulties, of an abstract nature, are exhibited via difficulty in managing novel tasks and processing new or complex information. Problems associated with judgement are particularly evident where frontal lobe damage is a feature of the cerebral deterioration. Inappropriate, rude and coarse speech and behaviour may be exteriorized, with impulsive, reckless or antisocial activities—for example, sexual overtures to strangers, shoplifting, incautious gambling or risky business ventures—often being a problem. *Aphasia, agnosia* and *apraxia*, the failure to name articles, recognize them and carry out motor activities respectively, may all create difficulties for both individuals and their carers. Personality characteristics may demonstrate a profound alteration or accentuation, with, for example, previously neat and tidy individuals becoming either slovenly and unkempt, or obsessively hyperattentive to the minutest detail of their appearance. Where some awareness of the extent of the deterioration is retained, fear or depression may be evident, and delusions, of a persecutory or jealous nature, may also be exteriorized. Dementia may be the unfortunate sequelae in a number of situations, for example, following:

1. vascular disease, when it is termed multi-infarct dementia
2. central nervous system infection—tertiary neurosyphilis, accquired immune deficiency syndrome (AIDS) related disorders, viral encephalitis, fungal and tuberculous meningitis and Creutzfeldt–Jakob disease (CJD)
3. cerebral trauma
4. toxic/metabolic disturbances—bromide intoxication, pernicious anaemia, folic acid deficiency, hypothyroidism, posthypoglycaemic and post-anoxic states
5. normal pressure hydrocephalus
6. neurological disorders—Pick's disease, Parkinson's disease, Huntington's disease, multiple sclerosis and cerebellar degeneration.

Absence of memory is not the only problem that may be experienced, for there may be *distortions of recall (paramnesias)* exhibited by some. We have previously mentioned confabulation, where past fictitious events are described in some detail to 'fill in' the gaps evident in memory. Berlyne (1972) supports the earlier distinction, provided by Bonhoeffer (1909) between two distinct types of confabulation. One is brief in content, may often be related to a real event which has become misplaced in time or context, and has to be provoked. This may be referred to as the *momentary type* of confabulation. The second type, the *fantastic type* or *delusional confabulation*, is rarer to encounter, but relates to impossibly, far-fetched accounts of events or experiences that could never have taken place, for example, the detailed memories of being born. Often the content is grandiosed in theme, and the 'memories' are sustained and elaborated, with no stimulus required for their exteriorization.

Retrospective falsifications are memories which are modified by the individual to be consistent with current thoughts, beliefs, experiences and mood. This may be exhibited by all individuals at one time or another—'Nothing ever goes right for me, I remember nothing but a catalogue of disasters and mistakes, just like this one'—it happens when the individual feels down and deflated. Where depressed mood is of a prolonged and severe nature however, such retrospective falsifications may be a common and persistent feature.

Retrospective delusion, on the other hand, is the term used to describe individuals' 'back-dating' of their delusional ideation, to a point within their life history which is well before the actual origination of the false belief. Individuals may claim, for example, that their recently acquired persecutory beliefs have been held for some years. *Delusional memories* are exhibited when a delusional interpretation is applied to a previous experience. Both problems may be exteriorized by individuals diagnosed as 'schizophrenic'.

Doppleganger or *reduplicative paramnesia* are terms used to describe the belief that an exact replica of an individual or place exists somewhere, and this is associated with problems in the non-dominant parietal lobe.

Similarly, *distortions of recognition* may occur and create potential problems for an individual. People may, during a totally novel experience, event or situation, feel that they have seen this exact situation before. They do not know where or when, and yet there is an illusion of familiarity and recognition which they cannot eradicate or account for. This is referred to as *déjà vu*, and happens to most people and one time or another. Quite the opposite experience is encountered in *jamais vu*, for in a familiar and previously met event, place or situation, the individual feels a distinct lack of recognition, and strangeness and unfamiliarity. Again, *jamais vu* may be experienced very occasionally by the individual who has no problems related to mental health status as such, but both phenomena are a more common feature for those subject to temporal lobe seizures, and within mental health care situations. There are other distortions of recognition, for example:

◆ *Déjà entendu*—the feeling that something has already been heard or perceived
◆ *Déjà eprouve*—that something has already been tried out or tested
◆ *Déjà fait*—that something has already been done, or has happened to the individual before
◆ *Déjà pense*—that 'an idea' has previously been thought
◆ *Déjà reconte*—that something has already been told or recounted
◆ *Déjà voulu*—that feelings of wanting or desiring something are the same now as they have been in the past; something has already been desired.

These feelings associated with false recollections are common occasional experiences within the general population, but may be far more frequently encountered within those requiring mental health care.

Positive or *negative misidentifications* may create problems for some. In the former, strangers are 'recognized' as friends or relatives and responded to as such. In the latter situation, friends and family members are not 'recognized' as in any way known or significant to the individual or his life, and are therefore treated as strangers. The *Capgras syndrome*, describes the individual's belief that either significant others, or himself, or both, have been replaced by identical doubles. It is also referred to as the *illusion of doubles*, and often follows changes in the quality of significant relationships. Negative feelings are directed towards someone previously loved, and it may be that the individual is unable to manage this dichotomy. The misidentification of the spouse having been replaced by an imposter may facilitate coping. It may be common in situations where persecutory ideation is a feature, or where mood is significantly depressed. The *Fregoli phenomenon* or *illusion*, named after an actor who was renowned for his ability to change his appearance, relates to the belief that a persecutor has assumed the guise of a variety of people who are encountered in everyday life. In the *Amphitryon illusion*, individuals believe their spouse alone to be a look-alike imposter, whilst in the *Soaias illusion*, friends, acquaintances and other relatives are considered to be such. All again relate to the persecutory type theme of thought problems.

Hypermnesia is the term used to describe an excessive retention of memories, which are recalled in very fine detail. You may have observed such abilities in show business personalities, who have made a career out of their enhanced abilities to remember. There is, for example, one individual able to remember 36 digits at a time and this he achieves by linking each number proffered with a consonant of the alphabet, which he then converts into words by adding vowels. The words provide an image within the individual's mind and hence enable him to recall the original numbers. Certainly there are references from a variety of sources to indicate that the eidetic imagery utilized in childhood (Gardner & Roylance 1982, Leask, Haber & Haber 1969) (refer to section related to perception) may continue to be employed by adults. Cicero (1927) relates the story of the poet, Simonides, who attended a banquet thrown in honour of Scopas, a nobleman, in order to provide part of the evening's 'cabaret'. After Simonides left the stage, the roof of the building collapsed, killing, and mutilating beyond all recognition, Scopas and many of his guests. Simonides' 'photographic memory' facilitated the task of the relatives claiming the correct body of their loved one, for he could remember, precisely, the position of each individual seated within the auditorium.

Similarly, Luria (1987), a Russian neuropsychologist, in his book The Mind of a Mnemonist, recalls his studies of a Russian reporter, who worked for a newspaper in Moscow, in the 1920s. This individual was able to reproduce the most detailed reports of events and situations without ever taking a written note. Luria observed that this individual's memory apparently had no limits for capacity or durability, the reporter being able to store the required information quickly—in minutes—and yet recall it days and weeks later. Luria actually tested the individual 30 years after their original work together and was astounded to discover that the newspaper man still retained, in perfect detail, that information first learned during their initial experiments together, all those years before.

In relation to those experiencing such a deviation in mental health status, there is a wonderful book, initially published in 1909, which recounts the experiences of Clifford Whittingham Beers during his encounters within American institutions and asylums at the turn of the twentieth century (Beers 1962). In it, he describes the thoughts, feelings and behaviours associated with his, initially, severely depressed mood and then his overoptimistic, grandiosed and hyperactive state. He similarly identifies the 'care' and 'attention' he received during that time. The following is a selected abstract from that work:

that one's memory may perform its function in the grip of Unreason itself is proved by the fact that my memory retains an impression, and an accurate one, of virtually everything that befell me, except when under the influence of an anaesthetic or in the unconscious hours of undisturbed sleep. Important events, trifling conversations, and more trifling thoughts of my own are now recalled with ease and accuracy: whereas prior to my illness ... mine was an ordinary memory when it was not noticeably poor.
Beers 1962

The recollections contained within the book would certainly appear to bear out the statement above, for the author goes on to elucidate the events fixed within his 'supersensitive memory'. The individual experiencing elevated mood and psychomotor acceleration frequently exhibits such a retentive memory for detailed events occurring to him, as may those individuals eliciting delusional ideation of a persecutory theme. Hypermnesia may be related to hypnosis, fever or cerebral trauma. In addition, it may be elicited during neurosurgical procedures, where the temporal lobe is stimulated, and where delirium is a feature.

We have continually mentioned *insight*, that is, individuals' awareness and understanding of the *status quo*, whether that relates to the specific nature of a puzzle or problem, the way forward within a situation, or their own biopsychosocial health and well-being in the current environment or circumstances. The problems experienced by those requiring mental health assistance may be seen to form a continuum on the scale of 'no problems recognized' to 'Help, I need assistance' (Fig. 5.18). At each stage of the continuum, the particular individual experiencing the problem will need specific assistance. This failure to be aware of the status of a situation may relate to any aspect of functioning, for it is just as likely that an individual will ignore or deny that a problem exists at work, within a current relationship or within somatic health status.

All require and will respond to the same principles of therapeutic intervention—time, assistance to ventilate problems, education and strategies designed to facilitate movement forwards. Warmth, emotional support and understanding are demonstrated in the approach utilized by the carer and are of importance regardless of the field of practice.

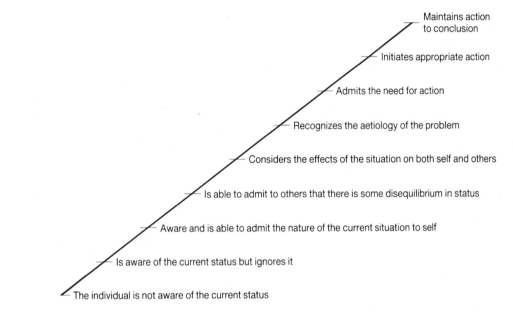

Fig. 5.18 Degrees of insight.

LANGUAGE

INTRODUCTION

The term language has previously been defined as:

the mode by which thought and activity is made available to conscious awareness. It is the basic vehicle utilized to structure experiences and, other than for those few aspects of conscious thought when mental images are utilized or objects are rotated in space, is therefore depended upon to achieve conscious awareness. It may be vocal or utilize other methods but in essence is the manner in which communication between parties also occurs.
Longman's Dictionary of Psychology and Psychiatry 1984

Language is yet another skill that the individual takes for granted, only perhaps valuing it appropriately when unable to find the words necessary to express current thoughts and feelings—one becomes speechless—or perhaps when someone demonstrates eloquence, fluidity and versatility in respect of his or her native, or another, tongue. Most of the time, little credit is given to the value

of language in the evolutionary process and yet Julian Huxley, the eminent biologist, has asserted that:

for their (our pre-human ape ancestors) transformation into man a series of steps were needed. Descent from the trees; erect posture; some enlargement of the brain; more carnivorous habits; the use and then the making of tools; further enlargement of the brain; the discovery of fire; true speech and language; elaboration of tools and rituals.
Huxley 1969

Wendt, again in the attempt to differentiate between animals and humans goes so far as to say:

certainly we modern men are chiefly distinguished from all other living animals by the development of speech and our ability to think in abstract terms— but where word symbolism and the formation of abstract concepts began in fossil hominids is of course something we cannot determine.
Wendt 1972

Language is a remarkable phenomenon. Directly as a result of it, the knowledge and wisdom accrued by humans over centuries, become accessible to the individual in the here and now situation. Individuals are then able, if they so desire, to learn via lessons of the past, to build on current knowledge and disseminate new information to others. By utilizing language, people are able to name, describe, explain and often predict the components of their worlds and experiences. Once a name, and characteristics or descriptors are applied to people, places, objects, situations and other environmental variations, information may then be filed away within the appropriate memory frameworks, to be recalled at a later date for use. What, then, does the term 'language' infer?

CHARACTERISTICS

Brown (1973) asserted that, before any system of communication could qualify as a language, three distinct criteria needed to be fulfilled. The first he termed *semanticity* and by this he meant that the symbolic representations utilized to convey meaning must denote the same thing to all users of that language. This is sensible, if you consider the point, for if our words are communicated with one meaning intended but, when received by you, are interpreted as something entirely different, the result may be that you may now believe that you have been instructed in the care of hardy annuals in the garden, rather than in the analysis of the problems associated with an individual's mental health! Secondly, Brown (1973) identified the need for communication to relate to past, present and future elements of life and living, and this he termed *displacement*. Again, this would appear eminently sensible when one considers the limitations imposed by verbalizing only about the present. There would be no 'had a nice day?'—it relates to the past—and no 'Where shall we go tomorrow?'—it's all in the future! Reflection would be nigh impossible, as would planning or anticipating, for there would be no appropriate, meaningful terminology to apply to such situations. *Productivity* was the term applied to the third criterion, and in this, Brown was referring to the need for communication to facilitate the combination of a limited number of symbols into an

unlimited number of varying uses. A simple example would be the way that, within the English language, it is possible to change a statement into a question by using the same words but altering the order or sequence of those words—'I shall get you a cup of coffee' easily becomes 'Shall I get you a cup of coffee?' The addition of the appropriate punctuation at the end of the sentence provides a visual clue to the intent of the words, whilst in verbalizing the sentence the individual's tone of voice would provide the added clue. However, without either, the offer of a cup of coffee would be inferred by the specific meaning of the words used.

Certainly the manner in which *concepts* are utilized within language would support Brown's criterion of productivity, for consider how many extra words would be needed within a vocabulary, for example, if every variation in an object's shape, size, colour, composition or location required it to be allocated a new name. Imagine the situation where only one, very specific shade, of red carpet was termed a carpet, and all of the other shades of red carpet were allocated individual names, as would be all shades of all other colours available. A 'carpet shop' would only be able to sell one particular shade of red carpet—if a vendor wanted to sell more than just examples of this one item, he or she would have to run a 'floor covering shop!' Now it would seem to us that this would be a very precise way of doing things, but remembering that colour is only one of the variations possible in carpet selection, the mind boggles when wandering in the direction of the number of words needed to describe each and every variation with an individual name! Think of the chaos of asking for a patterned, multicoloured carpet! Concepts, then, are a boon. They provide the individual with a mental impression of the properties commonly associated with an object, event, activity, etc. and therefore one word may encompass a significant number of variations on that one theme.

Rosch (1973, 1975) asserts that there are two distinct categories of concepts. The first she refers to as classical concepts, in which all characteristics are exhibited by every member of the group, for example:

◆ Bachelors have to be unmarried adult men.

◆ Wives have to be married, female and, in our legal system, 16 years old plus.

◆ Nephews and nieces have to be the offspring of the individual's sibling(s).

◆ Squares have to have four sides of equal length joined at 90° angles.

◆ Circles have to be plane figures, bounded by a single curved line, every point of which is equidistant from its centre.

Classical concepts are less commonly encountered than the second type, which she identified as *probabilistic concepts*. The term describes those situations in which members do not always share the same properties or characteristics, or where, perhaps, there is not one common feature shared by all members of the group. All birds, for example, do not fly, all chairs do not have arms, all books may not be for reading. Despite this, one is aware that there are sufficient features in common, for an individual member to be assigned to a particular group, and that a penguin is, for instance, 'probably' a bird. Rosch suggested that most everyday concepts are of this type.

Labov (1973) believed that individuals are significantly influenced in their conceptualization of objects by the context of their surroundings, and that because of this there was a necessary vagueness, or *fuzziness*, regarding the boundaries of many concepts. A useful example may be that of the chamber pot, which, as we are sure you will be aware, used to sit under most people's beds prior to the introduction of 'plumbed in' water closets within house structures. Nowadays, where observed at all, they tend to be adorned with a plant. The concept is fuzzy, for, under a bed, or at first glance, it would be recognized and viewed as something to urinate into, whilst in the middle of the dining-room table, it is hopefully otherwise defined. Similarly a cup may only be conceptualized as such when used to drink from. When positioned upon a dresser or display unit, with its saucer placed behind it, it is more likely to be viewed as an ornament, or considered a financial investment and irreplaceable.

Rosch (1975) asserted that, in addition to recognizing and accumulating knowledge regarding the properties of concepts, individuals have insight into their relationships with other concepts. Fruit, for example, is a division, or *subset*, of food, and other subsets may include vegetables, meat, grains and fish. She believed that the properties of concepts and their relationships to each other, formed a *hierarchy*, thus creating finer, more detailed delineation of the overall concept:

Mother: What would you like for lunch?
Son: I don't know—what have we got?
Mother: (opens fridge door) Well, a sandwich, something on toast, meat and veg?—give me some idea.
Son: I don't know—what is there?
Mother: Well, there's ham, corned beef—
Son: I don't feel like meat.
Mother: (in addition, now opens cupboard door) There's tuna or sardines—
Son: Haven't we got something else?
Mother: How about beans or spaghetti on toast?
Son: No thanks, I don't want toast.
Mother: What about bacon and egg or fish and chips?
Son: There's never anything to eat in this house! I'll have a cheese and tomato sandwich please.

Concepts have to be learned and analysis of the properties and relationships which link elements of the world are acquired over the years, but, in addition to concepts, other components of language have to be learned.

LINGUISTICS

It is highly probable that most individuals fail to recognize the complexities of language until, at some point following their initial mastery of their native language, they embark on trying to acquire a second one. It is at this point that the individual recalls a teacher, within the past, differentiating between nouns and verbs, or adjectives and pronouns, though these have, most likely, never *appeared* to influence one's speech since that period. It is often when one realizes the difference in the sounds of letters in the new language, compared with the old, or that verbs are conjugated to provide variation in tense and person that an individual is more likely to appreciate the task of the child as he masters his native language. For example, the child is required to learn the precise sounds each letter makes and that sometimes one letter may make more than one sound, depending upon its combination with other letters. There are more exceptions to learn, for example the differing sounds of pairs of letters—cough and about, please and lease, and chop and chaos—and that some words sound the same but are spelt differently and convey very different meanings—by and buy, sore and soar, sail and sale. The study of the specific sounds and how they function to indicate a change in meaning is termed *phonology* and Ladefoged (1975) defined the smallest sounds, which may be distinguished by their contrasts in words, as *phonemes*. The word apt, for instance, has three phonemes—a-p-t—whilst, by replacing the 't' with an 'e' to form the word 'ape' would only provide two phonemes, due to the long 'a' sound produced by the a–e combination. Of course, the child, unlike the majority of adult learners, absorbs and remembers the sounds of language long before those sounds are correlated with the appropriate symbolic letter. Children may have no problems learning and verbalizing their native language and yet encounter great difficulties in reading and writing, as may be seen later in this section, and, of course, children who are deaf, or reared in an environment of severe sensory deprivation, may never hear the sounds required to be amalgamated to form language.

Phonemes combine to create larger, more complex units of sound, termed *morphemes*, for example, the words 'turn' 'excite' and 'develop' are all morphemes. These cannot be reduced further and yet still have sensible meaning. They can, however, have other morphemes added to them. For instance turn + 'ed' = turned, or + 'ing' = turning, or + a single s = turns and this, in English, changes the *tense* of the verb, or in the case of 'turns' may convert the word to its *plural* form, as in 'We took turns on the swing'. Of course there are other ways in which added morphemes are utilized, for example to create *comparatives* and *absolutes*—

tall, taller, tallest and dark, darker and darkest—and other contrasts—excite, exciting, unexciting, and develop, developed and undeveloped.

Having said all of the above, one has most surely heard the errors of childhood language, such as 'mummy, is it time we goed now?' or 'Do it be for me?'. It, again, takes time to learn *syntax*—the rules that govern the ways in which words may legitimately be combined, to form meaningful sentences in a language. Similarly, the child requires to understand the actual meaning of words utilized, and many parents have, no doubt, experienced great embarrassment as a youngster repeats a word that has been overheard, perhaps in 'adult' conversation, and yet has no idea of the meaning or nature of the term. This knowledge of word meaning is referred to as *lexical knowledge*, whilst *semantics* is the term utilized to convey that necessary understanding of combined sounds, as words, phrases or sentences. Certainly if language is to be utilized to the full and employed in both verbal and written form, it is necessary to understand that the symbols selected to form an alphabet represent words with meanings.

It is possible, of course, to have a detailed linguisitic knowledge and yet fail to be understood, and a useful example may be provided by the situation where a non-English speaking tourist detains a passer-by to ask directions to the nearest lavatory. His speech is, probably, grammatically perfect and yet he is unable to share the meaning of his communication. It appears a very simplistic observation to make, but it is vital that speaker and listener share enough common ground or knowledge, and have enough relevant information, to understand what is conveyed by the language used. We make the point to remind you that professional groups utilize a language which may not be completely or correctly understood by those who are not a part of that group. Therefore, it is necessary to be willing and able to discard the terminology and jargon associated with the professional tongue, to facilitate communication appropriate to the experiences and norms of the listener. Language is utilized to achieve an aim relevant to a specific social context and in this sense is a very self-referential activity. Whether an individual is seeking or conveying information, persuading, influencing, negotiating, demanding or instructing, the use of language is *pragmatic*, for it achieves the individual's aims and purposes.

Language is, it would seem, a complex skill, with regard to the elements which need to be mastered. However, having looked previously at thinking, and acknowledged that the vast majority of thinking is achieved via language, it seems appropriate to examine the relationship between the two cognitive functions.

LANGUAGE AND THINKING

There are three main perspectives with regard to the relationship between language and thought:

1. Thinking is dependent upon language.
2. Language is dependent upon cognitive development.
3. The two functions develop separately and amalgamate early in childhood.

For many years, it was believed that all individuals think in similar ways, but in the second and third decade of the twentieth century, two individuals, working separately from each other, put forward theories in opposition to that commonly held view. An anthropologist and linguist, Edward Sapir (1949) and Benjamin Lee Whorf, an insurance company fire prevention officer and avid spare-time linguist, both asserted that people's languages confine and constrict methods of perception and thought, and hence, individuals in various parts of the world both perceive and think about their world in different ways. The *Sapir–Whorf*, or *linguistic relativity hypothesis*, proposes that the environment and way of life experienced within the different cultures of the world engender the development of a unique view of that world and its important features. This specificity evokes a vocabulary, concepts and grammar appropriate to the needs experienced and that, therefore, determines the parameters and nature of thinking. Thus, in learning the native language, children also learn the concomitant and implicit view of the world expressed via that language, for vocabulary is not available for, what are considered, culturally unimportant or irrele-

vant features. *Linguistic determinism* is, then, the hypothesis that language determines thinking. Whorf produced a great deal of evidence to support his beliefs, which included his work with the Hopi Indians, who, he pointed out, have no expressions or words relating to time—past, present and future—as European languages have, and who, often, have just one word to describe a whole performance:

> 'The light flashed', we say in English. Something has to be there to make the light flash; 'light' is the subject, 'flash' the predicate ... A Hopi Indian ... says Reh-pi—'flash'—one word for the whole performance, no subject, no predicate, no time element.
> Stuart Chase (in Carroll 1956)

The emphasis is placed on what actually happened—not the 'how, when, why, how or where' of it happening. These factors would appear unimportant to the Hopi and are therefore not delineated, thus, according to Whorf, altering the perception of the event and the thinking associated with it.

A second, commonly quoted, example used in support of the hypothesis relates the fact that the Eskimo people have more words to describe snow—27 in fact—than are available in English. There are specific names, for instance, for drifting snow, packed snow, fluffy snow and words for the snow suitable for igloo construction and for sledging on, indicating the importance of the feature within their way of life and not that of Europeans. Therefore, according to Whorf, each of the two cultures will adopt a unique view of their world, the parameters of which will be provided by language.

There has been evidence both to support and refute the Sapir–Whorf hypothesis in the years since its inception. As early as 1932, Carmichael, Hogan & Walter confirmed the fact that verbal labelling significantly *influences* perception and hence thinking. In their studies, two experimental groups were given the same neutral drawing. Each group, however, was given a different verbal label in association with the picture. When later requested to reproduce the previously viewed drawings, subjects were found to produce very different drawings, according to which verbal label had been offered.

Carroll & Casagrande (1958) studied the language of the Navaho Indians, and compared children of the same age, who spoke Navaho only, English only and both languages. The Navaho language places great emphasis on the form of objects, with separate verbs, for example, to describe the performance of handling an item, which is dependent upon the qualities of the object being manipulated. There is, therefore, a verb used in relation to handling long, flexible items, such as string, another for handling long rigid items, such as sticks, and yet another related to the handling of flat and flexible articles, such as pieces of cloth. American children, in contrast, learn object recognition first in relation to size, then colour and finally form or shape, so that some items will initially be recognized as big or little, then red or green and finally round or square. In their studies, Carroll & Casagrande discovered that children who spoke only Navaho were more aware of the form of an object than their English-only speaking peers, and were able to recognize items by their form. A surprising second comparison, however, between the English-only speaking children and the English–Navaho speaking group of youngsters, revealed the former to be more adept in recognition of the form of objects than the latter, and this Carroll & Casagrande accounted for by the experience gained by the English-only speaking children within preschool nursery education.

Slobin (1979) maintains that the Sapir–Whorf hypothesis is too strong an assertion, for whilst he agrees that language may *influence* thought, he refutes its action as a *determinant*. He identifies points of emphasis in other languages—French and German—which do not appear in English, for example, the familiar and polite terms used for the second person pronoun. In English, the term 'you' is consistently used, with no differentiation made between a personal or formal reference. This is not so in French, where 'tu' and 'vous' are used, or in German, where 'du' and 'sie' are delineated. Slobin remarks that in all forms of speech, the French and German speakers are required to incorporate an assessment of the social relation-

ships involved within communication, whilst English speakers are not so obliged. This does not mean, avers Slobin, that social relationships are not recognized, or that they are not considered within intercourse, it merely indicates that the English language does not emphasize the need to do so.

Berlim & Kay (1969) analysed the ways in which different languages label and differentiate colours and their variations in shade. Native speakers were presented with over 300 coloured squares and asked to name them in their own language. All languages had at least two terms for, what were described by the researchers as, *focal*, or *main colours*, whilst some languages identified as many as 11 words. The best example of a colour—the best example of red, yellow or green for instance—was identified as such regardless of the language used, but despite the lack of a specific word to name a shade of colour, shades were still recognized as being related to the appropriate focal colour. Heider (1972) similarly found that the Dani, of Indonesian New Guinea, had only terms to distinguish two main colour features. The word 'Mola' means light, and 'Mili' means dark, and yet native language speakers were able to perceive and recognize focal colours better than the non-focal examples. Language did not influence perception and thinking, but only items of sufficient relevance or significance to life had warranted a unique label. Perhaps language may influence thinking, but it certainly does not appear to determine it.

Piaget, of course, believed language depended on, and indicated the level of, cognitive development attained:

language and thought are linked in a genetic circle ... In the last analysis, both depend on intelligence itself, which antedates language and is independent of it. Piaget 1968

Whilst he would acknowledge the important role of language in extending the range of symbolic thinking, Piaget asserted that language represented only one element of such symbolic function, which, in addition, included the rudimentary forms of symbolic play and imagery. Development of intelligence, he proposes, begins at birth and predates the acquisition of language, and, therefore, Piaget believed that the initial thoughts of the child are expressed via images and activities, which he termed *autistic thought*. The child, he believed, was unable to understand the linguistic expression of a concept until competent to master the concept *per se*. Certainly, there is some everyday evidence to support that specific element of the theory:

> When are we going to the park, mummy?
>
> Tomorrow, dear.
>
> When's tomorrow, Mummy?
>
> It's the day after this day, dear.
>
> When's this day over, Mummy?
>
> When we've been to sleep tonight and then wake up in the morning, that will be tomorrow, dear.
>
> The child ponders.
>
> When are we going to the park, Mummy?

This child has no understanding of the concept of 'tomorrow', has no understanding of when he will be taken to the park, or when it will be his birthday or Christmas day, or can reference any other future element in time.

Piaget believed that babies develop impressions or outlines of their world via their experiences and that such outlines or schemas are embellished and new ones created as the world is explored. In the same way that children are able to understand that they can 'pretend' that four dining-room chairs appropriately positioned are their car, that is, they have learned the one is a symbolic representation of a 'real' object in their life, so they are able to understand that a word represents an object. Children's initial speech is, Piaget believes, merely an expression of their own thoughts—a sort of running commentary on their world and their activities within it—and that only at a later point in cognitive development, will the 'social aspects' of language be introduced, as they begin to incorporate the responses or interjections of a significant onlooker into account.

Again, direct observation would support Piaget's assertion of the egocentric and self-absorbed nature of early language displayed. One only has to watch children in a preschool setting to note that whilst within the group, the younger children are actually playing alone, and that, whilst talking, they are not actually communicating with the child next to them. However, Piaget did not pay any credence to the fact that exposure to language itself may assist the child to absorb and understand new concepts. Returning to the example of the 'tomorrow' concept, the child does learn via explanations and experience when 'tomorrow' will arrive, that is, the concept of time.

Vygotsky (1962), a Russian psychologist, believed that thought and language initially develop as separate entities, and whilst continuing in this fashion to a greater or lesser extent into adulthood, also combine to form a third and major component of the thinking–language processes. Like Piaget, Vygotsky believed that:

1. Children think before they speak.
2. They build up schemas related to their experiences of their world.
3. Early thinking is comprised of images, perceptions and actions.
4. Initially, speech is egocentric and basically a verbalization of thinking.
5. Symbols begin to double for 'reality'—the four chairs standing for a car—at around the age of 2 years.

Vygotsky referred to this early thinking as *prelinguistic thought*. However, he diverged from the theory put forward by Piaget in his assertions that language develops simultaneously throughout this period, as the child practises the sounds that will amalgamate to form speech. This he refers to as *preintellectual language*.

The crux of the matter for Vygotsky was the differentiation he made between *inner speech*, which reflected personal thoughts, and *external speech*, which represented social communications with others. He proposed that early speech is thoughtless speech and purely social in nature, for the child's ability to reason and think about his environment, and experiences, has no language available to describe it. However, about the age of 2 years the thoughtless speech and languageless thought processes begin to merge, with words used as representative symbols for thoughts. Vygotsky believed that only at this merging point within cognitive development could individual social development begin, as children explore their world and that of others with the aid of language. Similarly, children absorb the sociocultural norms that surround them, as thinking and language create two interlinking circles, and activity in one area generates a concomitant response in the other. Vygotsky believed that the egocentric speech of early childhood, rather than disappearing in the light of social speech, actually continues, but in the child's head. He found that both children and adults, when faced with a difficult or complex task, would verbalize their egocentric speech via thinking aloud. Certainly, individuals are aware of the continuation of languageless thought into adulthood, because of their ability to manipulate images, not just words, within their minds.

The theories of Sapir–Whorf, Piaget and Vygotsky seek to explain the relationship between thinking and language, and certainly you may consider elements of each to be feasible even if you cannot accept one perspective in its entirety. The next, seemingly logical, point requiring analysis would appear to be related to the methods via which children master their native language.

ACQUISITION

Jakobson (1968) studying the language of babies and young children, concentrated his attention on the sounds and sound patterns (phonology) that were used regularly and appeared to be employed by the child with distinctive meaning.

It may be a valuable exercise, at this point, for you to analyse the parts of the mouth and the way the tongue is utilized in making the sounds symbolized by the alphabet. Is there, for example, a significant difference in the way in which the sounds of vowels and consonants are produced, and are all consonants formed by the same movement?

Jakobson believed that the child initially differen-

tiates between vowels and consonants in very broad terms, though these broad terms do not immediately include an ability to distinguish between the sounds within either group. Each group is then further embellished, for example, by a distinction between consonants produced nasally and non-nasally, and later between those that are produced in various sites of the mouth, to build up an extensive 'menu' of available sounds. He uses embryological development as a simile for the process, with an initially undifferentiated group of sounds, repeatedly subdividing until the sound system is fully differentiated. The original work by Jakobson was published in 1941, and, since this time, elements have been questioned by others researching the field. One example of dissonance is seen in relation to his proposals that the order of acquisition of contrasts was consistent for all children and all languages, for Menn (1985) amongst others, has refuted the actuality of such proposals. Jakobson was, however, a pioneer in the field, for previous studies in phonology had concentrated on the number and specific sounds available in a child's vocabulary at different ages.

Stampe (1969) asserted that the child's phonological development is determined by ease of articulation, and is best described in terms of simplifying functions that affect whole groups of phonemes, rather than single sounds. He maintains, for instance, that whilst able to perceive the difference between the 'k' or 'g' sounds (velar stops) and the 't' or 'd' sounds (alveolar stops), the latter are easier to articulate and therefore 'cup' is pronounced 'tup' and 'girl' becomes 'dirl'. One sound replaces another. Similarly one sound may be seen to influence the pronunciation of a second sound in the same word, for example 'kekkle' and 'goggie' for 'kettle' and 'doggie', despite the child's ability to make the sound of 't' and 'd' as in 'tap' or 'bed'. Others have shared Stampe's belief in the child's ability to differentiate between sounds, though the factors involved in the order of acquisition of speech sounds continue to be disputed. Dodd (1987) would assert that visual as well as auditory cues are utilized by the child to learn the required sound system for language development.

Early studies of grammar and its development in the child, concentrated on the quantity of material learned—the number of words used, how many different types of words are employed and how much of speech conformed to adult grammatical rules. Studies during this time, for example, by Gesell (1950) merely established the fact that the length of speech and the amount of that speech which complies with grammatical rules, increases with age. However, Brown (1973) asserted that, even in the earliest stages of speech production, there is order and regularity within that speech, both in the type of words used and the way in which they are combined. This regularity could not be accounted for in grammatical terms alone, and Bloom (1970) asserted that meaning, too, was a vital element requiring consideration alongside grammar. Semantics, the meanings of words used, is discussed below, but one aspect of grammar is certain and that is, it is not produced by imitating adult speech alone. Rarely can it be considered that a child will hear an adult state 'I no go', 'I not want', 'I goed', 'I feeled it', or similar errors of speech, and yet these are terms used at a particular point in language development by all children. Children definitely learn rules, rather than merely imitating adults, for they recognize that, for example, adding an '–ed' to a verb will—in some situations—change present tense to past tense—for example, I wanted, I wished. The child applies the rule consistently across all verbs only later absorbing the exceptions observed. The grammatical complexity of children's speech is seen to increase with their general maturity (Crystal 1984), and a full set of sentence types is in use by the age of 5 years (Wells 1985).

We have previously mentioned Bloom (1970) and his emphasis on meaning within early word combinations used by children. He asserted that the meaning of words uttered could be construed by the context in which they occurred, and used the example of 'mummy sock' to prove his point. When the child is offering mummy one of her own stockings, the child's meaning is inferred as 'there, mummy, this is one of your stockings', that is 'mummy's sock'. However, where the child is sitting barefoot, with a sock in his hand, his speech may be translated into, 'mummy please put my sock on'. Children consistently string more words together, adding common linking words (the, on,

at) and those of relationships (my, your) until grammatical sentences are produced. First words produced are proper nouns—mummy and daddy—progressing to common nouns where differentiations have to be absorbed—dogs and cats (small), horse and cow (big)—and where full meaning of the noun is rarely understood despite the term being used. It is common to hear one term misused by an overgeneralization, where, for example, all animals are dogs, which is termed *overextension*. Similarly, misuse of a word may occur as the child overspecifies, with only, for example, the family pet, or a particular breed of dog, labelled as an instance of the word. This is referred to an *underextension*.

The linguist, Noam Chomsky (1959) believed that the capacity for human language is an innate element, as are the internal 'rules' that enable the individual to decide whether sentences both convey the meaning intended and are grammatically appropriate. Chomsky asserts that people do not use the same 'stock' sentences time and time again, but are constantly creating new ones. If an individual were only able to repeat sentences previously heard, speech and language would be severely limited, but he maintains that *because* humans are born with the rules of grammar, they are capable of inventing and understanding sentences never previously heard. Chomsky stated:

> *One can only conclude that children do not build grammars primarily from the evidence they hear, but according to an inner design—a genetic program.*
> Chomsky 1980

He compares the development of grammar to the growth of the child's physical organs, with the environment providing both activation of the system and its support, in exactly the same way as oxygen and nutrients facilitate the growth of an embryonic heart. The fact that children learn a culturally specific language which reflects their native environment and therefore varies greatly between cultural groups does not deflect Chomsky (1986) from his proposals. He asserts that the inner rules relate to a *universal grammar*, which provides an automatic knowledge of the general form any language should take. Hyams (1986) raises objections to such a hypothesis on the grounds that all languages do not conform to the same grammatical rules, citing the norm of saying 'went' in Italian, whereas, in English, a subject is grammatically necessary, as in 'she went'. Chomsky replies to such criticisms by proposing that environmental influences will modify such parameters as are necessary to meet cultural aberrations.

Chomsky is a prolific writer and his work is very valuable in any detailed study of linguistics. However, his theories suggest that individuals produce perfectly grammatical sentences, which frequently they do not. A point of some interest, though, is the work of Werker & Tees (1985) who discovered that babies lose their initial potential to recognize all possible sounds in languages as they begin to assimilate a single dialect. Eight-month-old babies, immaterial of their nationality, immediately detect and react to changes in sounds which adults fail to recognize. By the time the child reaches 12 months, this ability to recognize such subtle shifts in sound is lost if exposure to them is not undertaken on a regular basis.

FACTORS IMPLICIT IN DEVELOPMENT OF LANGUAGE

You may recall the lack of verbal recognition and memory associated with Genie, the 13-year-old girl discovered after being confined to a small room under conditions of extreme physical restraint and sensory deprivation from the age of 20 months by her parents (Curtiss 1977). You may recall, too, that Genie had failed to acquire language skills despite intensive expert assistance. The cerebral hemisphere specialization that one would expect to occur had failed to develop and Genie's language-related cerebral structures had degenerated. Similarly in this area of memory and learning, we recalled the work of Dennis (1960) with children in Iranian orphanages and their slowness to develop, due to sensory deprivation. All spheres of growth were severely retarded and the children failed to reach any of the expected milestones of the early years.

It would be a relief to believe that these were isolated instances, but, unfortunately, this is not the case. There are many historical examples of children deliberately isolated in attempts to analyse the nature and development of language. The Egyptian pharaoh, Psammetichos, the Holy Roman Emperor, Frederik II and King James IV of Scotland are all alleged to have used such experiments (Curtiss 1981) and within the twentieth century, alone, there were a number of instances of children isolated from human contact and interaction besides Genie:

Anna, a 5-year-old girl, found tied to a chair in a store room of the family farm, where she had been since babyhood. Removed to a children's home and later to an institution for the elderly infirm, Anna was cachexic and frail physically, and expressionless and apathetic. She was thought to be deaf and probably blind. Once removed to a foster home and one to one attention, however, Anna began to acquire both cognitive and motor skills. Anna was, for some reason, transferred to a private home for 'retarded' children and after 2 years there, was reported to be uttering single words and attempting conversation. She died, aged approximately 10 years old, of jaundice.

Isabelle, a 6 year old, was kept isolated because of her illegitimacy. She and her mother, who was both deaf and mute, were housed in a darkened room, away from the remainder of the family, who had rejected them. After their escape, the child was admitted to a children's hospital for orthopaedic surgery and physiotherapy, necessary due to rickets and abnormal bone development. In hospital she was withdrawn and mute, showing extreme hostility to strangers, especially men. Her acquisition of language was quite remarkable, however, for within 2 months she was singing nursery rhymes, could read and write within a year, and after 18 months possessed a vocabulary of some 2000 words and could create stories.
Davis 1967

Space precludes more examples than proffered above, but many more are documented—the Koluchova twins (1976), Mary and Louise (Skuse 1984), Alice and Beth (Douglas & Sutton 1978) and Adam (Thompson 1986) are just a few. Similarly there are recorded examples of children being raised from babies, as 'Wolf children',

Victor, the 'Wild boy of Aveyron' (Itard 1801) and Amala and Kamala of Midnapore (Singh & Zingg 1942), who experienced isolation from humans, but adopted the animal parent's language and way of life. Other studies, too, of institutional care and its effects on the development of children, for example, Skeels' (1966) comparison between a group of children raised in an unstimulating orphanage and a second group who had been transferred from the home to an institution for 'retarded adults' at about 20 months of age, and Dennis' study of a poor foundling home in Beirut, Lebanon (Dennis 1973), all direct attention to the importance of environmental stimulation in language development.

Bruner (1983) and others have stressed the importance of a stimulating environment in the prelinguistic period on the acquisition of speech. Certainly psychosocial deprivation at this point has been shown to impair preverbal vocalization and babble (Provence & Lipton 1962) and Dennis (1941) discovered that, whilst babies still expressed preverbal sounds within situations of minimal verbal interaction, they did not progress to use any sound that corresponded with a 'real' word during the 61 weeks of his study.

Piaget (1967), of course, would assert that the lack of opportunity to play in such isolated and deprived circumstances would inhibit a child's progression to the level of cognitive function necessary for thought, and hence language, to develop. His belief in symbolic function, including mental imagery and symbolic play, as the precursor and facilitator of an appropriate level of sensorimotor behaviour to engender the representational skills necessary for thought and language, firmly places language in the primary role of personal communication strategy first, and social interaction strategy second in importance. Yet others (Gopnik & Meltzoff 1985, Tomasello & Farrar 1984) have asserted that the earliest words used usually relate to social relationships and are uttered in social contexts.

Certainly malnutrition was a common factor experienced by the isolated children referred to above, but many studies have indicated that this alone fails to produce permanent mental impairment. In conjunction with social and intellectual deprivation, cognitive development is depressed. In many of the case histories provided which relate to 'wild' children, whilst linguistic abilities were poor on discovery, progress was rapid after rescue and the implementation of strategies to enhance psychosocial development, for example, play school attendance and speech therapy. Many of the children actually reached age-appropriate lanaguage skills within a few years of rescue, with little difference in acquisition between those removed at an earlier or relatively later age. Lenneberg (1967) suggested that to proceed normally, language must be acquired during the first 12 years of life and the story of 13-year-old Genie, who never achieved more than the single word speech associated with a toddler, may be used as evidence to support his proposals for this critical learning period.

Common sense would indicate that the child must be able to hear efficiently in order to identify and discriminate between the speech sounds of a lanaguage. Therefore any loss or distortion of auditory stimuli within the early years of language development may significantly impair its acquisition. The visually impaired child, too, may be disadvantaged during the preverbal period of speech development. In normally sighted children, partners in an interaction will utilize the direction of the children's gaze as indicative of their focus of attention, and also their visually directed gestures, such as pointing to objects that stimulate them, to choose topics of interaction. These are absent or greatly reduced in the visually impaired infant and therefore cues to assist the partner are missing, engendering difficulties in understanding the child's desires or intentions. Rowland (1983) found that, in such situations, whilst affective states could be communicated successfully to an adult, sightless babies vocalized less than, and in different patterns to, sighted babies. Rowland suggests that listening becomes so important in the baby's assessment of the environment that perhaps his lack of vocalization is to prevent 'clutter' of the auditory cues. It must be difficult to relate the word 'tree' to something that is noiseless and out of reach, and to try to associate 'dog' with certain tactile, olfactory and auditory cues, and yet generate the concepts relevant. Structural abnormalities of the speech apparatus, such as cleft palate and lip, do not necessarily preclude normal speech production, for in most instances surgical repair is instigated before the child starts to talk. Articulatory abnormalities are higher for these children than the normal population; often the child exhibits a more nasal quality in verbalizing consonants. Some conductive hearing loss may also result from the impaired functioning of the Eustachian tube (auditory tube), with a concomitant phonological developmental difficulty. Motor speech impairments (*dysarthria*) result from problems within the central or peripheral nervous system. Children experiencing such problems as cerebral palsy may exhibit an ability to talk but verbalizations are often slow and distorted. In extreme situations, the child may be unable to speak at all, termed *anarthria*.

The examples provided above serve hopefully to remind us that language acquisition and speech production are complex biopsychosocial skills, involving processes which, as yet, are incompletely understood.

PROBLEMS ENCOUNTERED WITHIN MENTAL HEALTH CARE

Throughout we have attempted to emphasize the fact that problems encountered within mental health care are also encountered in other spheres of care delivery and those associated with language are no exception.

The cerebral hemispheres function asymmetrically, with one hemisphere, termed *dominant*, determining language, and the favoured, or *preferred*, hand, foot and eye use. People talk of being left or right handed, referring to the side of the body most favoured, and the vast majority of the population—90%—are right handed with the left hemisphere dominant. The remaining individuals, though left handed, may have a right hemisphere dominant (30%) or a left (70%). Various tests for dominance are available, for example, an EEG demonstrates greater alpha wave suppression in the dominant hemisphere during verbal thought.

Language is mediated via different areas of the cortex of the dominant hemisphere, although they are interconnected. Any problem occurring within any of these areas, or along the interconnecting network of fibres associated with them, may affect the ability to speak, write or understand language.

Broca's area is associated with the mechanisms by which words are selected, articulated and constructed to form sentences. Damage in this area (frontal cortex) may produce *primary motor dysphasia*, otherwise termed cortical motor, expressive or Broca's dysphasia, and whilst comprehension remains relatively unaffected, speech is slow, sparse and hesitant. Its rhythm and intonation are disturbed and the individual experiences great difficulty in word finding, with 'wrong' words being utilized and often being incorrectly pronounced. Individuals often recognize errors made and in attempting to correct them, become irritated and annoyed. They may compensate by miming words 'lost' or using gestures, but when offered the correct word, can recognize and select it. Sentences are abbreviated with words omitted, but are meaningful. Problems of writing reflect those of speech.

Wernicke's area, spanning the temporal and parietal cortex, posterior to the medial end of the Sylvian fissure, is associated with comprehension of language, both spoken and written, therefore lesions here reflect those functions. *Primary sensory dysphasia*, otherwise termed receptive or Wernickes dysphasia, demonstrates a defective appreciation of the meaning of words and grammatical constructions. The individual is less able to respond to instructions and has difficulty in repeating back phrases provided. The cortical system for analysing incoming speech is affected, and therefore speech is affected, with words used incorrectly, *neologisms* (new words, distortions or combinations of existing words) and errors of grammar and syntactical construction. Speech is fluent and easy, unlike Broca's dysphasia, with rhythm and inflexion preserved and no articulatory defects, though it may be pressurized. Individuals are unaware of linguistic errors, and are unable to recognize a 'correct' word when offered. They seem unable to discard words already used and speech is often *contaminated* by previously used words. Both these individuals and those experiencing Broca's dysphasia demonstrate *perseveration*, that is, repetition of a word or phrase long after its relevance is past. Whilst the individual may be able to read a single word aloud with no problems, reading of longer sentences is jumbled and contaminated, with no comprehension and therefore an inability to carry out written instructions.

A lesion in the dominant temporal lobe, which is adjacent to the primary receptive area for hearing, is rare but, when occurring, produces an agnosia for spoken words which are interpreted as sounds, but not words. The individual hears because pathways in the non-dominant hemisphere are intact, but information related to speech cannot reach the receiving centre in the dominant hemisphere. Speech and writing are fluent and without error, and the term used for the problem is *subcortical auditory dysphasia* or pure word deafness. Similarly, lesions of the left visual cortex and the splenium of the corpus callosum evoke pure word blindness, or *subcortical visual aphasia*. Visual input is possible to the right hemisphere only and therefore access to the language systems of the left hemisphere is not available. The individual speaks normally and can understand the spoken word. Difficulties relate to comprehension of visually perceived language, that is, written words. Pure word dumbness, or *subcortical motor aphasia*, creates a picture of individuals able to comprehend both spoken and written language, and who are able to express themselves in writing, thus indicating that their inner speech is unaffected. Their problem relates to articulating speech, which may be complete or achieved with great difficulty (dysarthria). Where speech is achieved, it is slurred, and individuals cannot repeat words heard, or read alone, neither can they verbalize at will. *Agraphia*—an inability to write—may be seen to occur in any general dysphasia, or as a problem associated with movement difficulties termed *apraxias*. However, a pure motor agraphia is thought to be associated with an interruption of the pathway from the left angular gyrus to the hand area of the left motor cortex. Speech is unimpaired, as is understanding of written and spoken words. Spontaneous writing or that related to dic-

tated material is disturbed, though individuals may be able to copy written words provided for them.

Nominal dysphasia (amnesic or anomic aphasia) is the term describing difficulty in evoking names at will. Individuals may be able to describe the object, its use and even recognize the name if offered to them, but its name eludes them. Speech is fluent, but at times word-finding pauses may be demonstrated, or individuals may have to go 'all around the houses' to make their point—*circumlocution*. Sometimes, individuals exhibit difficulty in comprehension or execution of oral or written commands, demonstrating that internal speech is affected. Nominal aphasia is associated with both diffuse cerebral dysfunction but also with lesions of the dominant temporoparietal region.

There are other disturbances of language, for example, lesions that disrupt links between Broca's and Wernicke's areas—*conduction dysphasia*—and where it is thought that the links between these areas remain intact and yet the area is isolated from other parts of the cortex—*syndromes of isolated speech area*. However, sufficient examples have been provided here to provoke consideration of somatic aetiology for disturbances of speech exhibited by an individual rather than an automatic assumption that they are indicative of a primary deviation in mental health status.

Neologisms have previously been mentioned in relation to primary sensory dysphasia. New words are created, standard words may be given a new and highly idiosyncratic meaning or more than one word may be combined. Within mental health care, the use of such new words is indicative of a lack of contact with reality and is therefore observed in individuals who are subject to a 'psychosis'. It is always necessary to incorporate an assessment of the individual's cultural and educational experiences prior to labelling an aberration of speech, a neologism, for errors of speech, and meaning may, on occasions, be an integral, though incorrect, part of 'normal' speech.

Circumlocution has also been mentioned, as indirect speech which is delayed in reaching the point, because of difficulty in word finding. *Circumstantiality* is a similar meandering of speech but on this occasion is due to the inclusion of unnecessary and tedious details, and parenthetical remarks. The latter are meaningful and connected clauses, related to the point of the speech, which the speaker never loses sight of. Circumstantiality is a feature frequently encountered within the mentally well, but may be a feature of those categorized as 'obsessive–compulsive personality disorders' and schizophrenia. You may recall within the section on thinking, that *loosening of associations* was mentioned. Circumstantiality demonstrates connections between areas of speech whereas in the individual experiencing loosening of associations, the original point is lost, and thoughts and speech wander off in a new and unrelated direction. *Tangentiality*—statements either totally unrelated to each other, or only obliquely so, are juxtapositioned—may be the verbal evidence to support loosening of association, and is demonstrated where the individual exteriorizes the complex problems labelled as schizophrenia.

Perseveration, mentioned in relation to both primary sensory and motor dysphasias, may also be evidence of mental health difficulties. The persistent repetition of currently irrelevant words is associated with organically evoked mental health problems and also others which demonstrate a lack of contact with reality. *Echolalia*, however, is the term used to describe the constant repetition, or echoing, of words or phrases of others. The intonation of the individual's voice during this persistent repetition may be mocking or staccato, or conversely the individual may 'mumble'. This may be exhibited by those experiencing pervasive developmental disorders, such as autism, and again by those demonstrating the mental health related sequelae of organic impairment, and 'schizophrenia'. Words selected for use in speech may be seen at times to depend on their sound rather than their meaning. *Rhyming* and *punning* (the construction of poor quality jokes) are features associated with *clanging* or *clang association*, evident in those experiencing psychomotor acceleration problems and where contact with reality is disturbed. *Word salad* may be the term used to described the jumbled, incomprehensible speech exhibited by some 'psychotic' individuals, particularly those experiencing the

multiplicity of problems labelled together as 'schizophrenia'. Similarly *'talking past the point'* may be demonstrated by this individual, who provides an answer to a question posed which, whilst related to the topic itself, is inappropriate and incorrect.

Slurred speech, previously mentioned in relation to subcortical motor dysphasia, is associated with intoxication due to various psychoactive substances when seen within mental health care. Alcohol, opioids and inhalants may all evoke the problem. *Incoherence* is differentiated easily and quickly from slurring, for, whilst there is a lack of logical, or meaningful connections, between words or phrases, changes in subject matter and the inclusion of irrelevances, words emitted are not dragged or drawn out in articulation. Speech may be *pressurized*, reflecting the speed of thoughts experienced by the overactive individual, or may demonstrate the *interruptions* of flow associated with blocking of thoughts and ideas. Similarly, *mutism* or *elective mutism* may be features indicating a mental health problem. The severely depressed individual may initially show a slowing of the stream of speech which may dry up completely, but such silence may be the result of hallucinatory experiences, or delusional ideation, or extreme difficulty in thinking. Elective mutism, demonstrated by children, is a persistent refusal to talk though gestures and odd monosyllabic responses may be evoked. This is often situationally specific, occurring in a discrete social setting. Only rarely is total mutism seen, but the excessively shy, withdrawn or isolated child, or conversely the controlling, negativistic child, may exhibit the problem. On occasions, there may be delayed language development or articulatory problems, but in the main, such children will have normal language skills.

There are a myriad of problems associated with language and speech production, but a selection has been included to encourage further observation and reflection on the linguistic functions and abilities demonstrated by people within care. An efficient neurological examination may preclude an incorrect diagnosis of somatic problems which may require neuromedical or surgical intervention but the nurse's observations may be the prerequisite and provoking factor that results in more detailed investigation.

SUMMARY

This has, of necessity, been a brief exploration of the cognitive functions specifically and commonly affected by mental health problems and, with the preceding chapters relating to affect and behaviour, is far from all encompassing. Some workers have spent a lifetime studying one tiny aspect of cognitive function and refinements to our current knowledge are taking shape daily.

In layman's terms, a 'thought', or indeed a 'memory' is difficult to make concrete. We can describe the content of each but to try to describe the actuality of a thought is beyond most of us. We can state how it 'materialized' from out of the blue, or came as a protracted effort through a tortuous pathway, but when it comes to specific characteristics, it is a bit like an elephant: we'll recognize its presence if we need to.

Perceptions are often unnoticed and received at an unconscious level. We talk about 'gut feelings' but so many of these are perceptions that, whilst we were unaware of their significance at the time, somehow seem to permeate into consciousness and prod us into action.

Concentration and attention are faculties that we only notice by their intensity or absence. There seems no real midway, merely excesses. The intense attention to some stimuli, which means you are unaware of everything else in your surroundings, including time passing, is contrasted by the need to reread this paragraph for the fifth time because your attention wandered.

We know that we learn and try to create optimum learning conditions when necessary, but we all know, too, that the words of a favourite song are learned effortlessly, whilst the names and order of the cranial nerves need swotting. When that song is rereleased 20 years later and you can sing along, much to the embarrassment of your loving offspring, you'll probably be unable to remember the names of the cranial nerves, though you may recall the rude mnemonic you used at the time to help them stick.

These head-bound functions are the products of electrochemical activities in the body, just the same as so many other functions, and just as likely to develop malfunction. Exclusion of underlying pathology is so important, before looking for the combination of affective, behavioural and cognitive difficulties suggestive of mental disorder, and we have emphasized the need for nurses to expand their knowledge to increase awareness of the similarities and differences between the two. This is all neurology, just a difference in the focus of concentration and attention, that is all.

Finally, the incidence of mental disorder within the population as a whole has been explored, using available statistics. In recognition of the reasons why these official statistics are less than the whole story in regard to mental illness, it must

DISCUSSION QUESTIONS

1. Language is the medium via which we describe our world, both internal and external. It is the method used to express our joys and frustrations, our successes and failures, our hopes and fears. Similarly, it is the medium required to describe our symptoms, hurts and horrors.
   How may we assist someone with limited hearing or linguistic difficulties to express themselves in regard to their health problems?
2. What cognitive functions are required to demonstrate a sense of humour? Where does it come from and how does it develop? Does it change with age and with culture? Discuss this within a group setting and develop your own theories to test. Test the theory.
3. Telepathy is just one of many skills that some claim to have, whilst the vast majority of the population can only sit back and wonder. The power of the mind is said to be of sufficient strength to move objects, find water, minerals and lost people and items. What is the evidence for these powers? Select a specific area of interest and explore it. Are you more, or less, convinced after your studies?

be concluded that those clients who do seek the help of a professional or self-help group are the tip of what may be an iceberg of enormous proportions.

Remembering all that has been stated in the above, the next step in the logical progression through the study of mental disorder is to explore those functions of affect, behaviour and cognition and the problems associated with each, which may indicate mental disorder.

FURTHER READING

Brain W R 1985 Brain's diseases of the nervous system. Oxford University Press, Oxford

Bruce V, Green P 1988 Visual perception, physiology, psychology and ecology. Lawrence Erlbaum, London

Brunner L S, Suddarth D S 1986 The Lippincott manual of medical surgical nursing. Harper & Row, London

Gellatly A (ed) 1986 The skilful mind. Open University Press, Milton Keynes

Hinchliff S, Montague S 1988 Physiology for nursing practice. Baillière Tindall, London

Hinwood B 1993 A textbook of science for the health professions, 2nd edn. Chapman & Hall, London

Lishman W A 1978 Organic psychiatry: the psychological consequences of cerebral disorder. Blackwell Scientific, Oxford

Loftus G R, Loftus E F 1976 Human memory: the processing of information. Lawrence Erlbaum, Hillsdale, NJ

Roth I (ed) 1990 Introduction to psychology, vols 1 and 2. Lawrence Erlbaum in conjunction with the Open University, Milton Keynes

Thouless R H 1974 Straight and crooked thinking. Pan, London

REFERENCES

Alkon D L 1983 Learning in a marine snail. Scientific American 249:70–84

Appleby L, Forshaw D M 1990 Postgraduate psychiatry: clinical and scientific foundations. Heinemann Medical, Oxford

Atkinson R L, Atkinson R C, Smith E E, Hilgard E R 1987 Introduction to psychology, 9th edn. Harcourt Brace Jovanovich, Florida

Beers C W 1962 A mind that found itself. Doubleday, New York

Berlim B, Kay P 1969 Basic colour terms: their universality and evolution. University of California Press, Los Angeles

Berlyne N 1972 Confabulation. British Journal of Psychiatry 120:285–292

Bleuler A (transl Zinkin J) 1950 Dementia praecox or the group of schizophrenics. International University Press, New York

Bloom L 1970 Language development: form and function in emerging grammars. MIT Press, Cambridge, MA

Bonhoeffer K (transl Marshall H) 1909 Exogenous psychoses. Zentralblatt fur Nervenheilkunde 32:499–505. In: Hirsch S R, Shephard M (eds) 1974 Themes and variations in European psychiatry. John Wright, Bristol

Boring EC 1930 A new ambiguous figure. American Journal of Psychology 42:444–445

Broadbent D 1958 Perception and communication. Pergamon, Oxford

Bronshtein A I, Petrova E P 1967 The auditory analyser in young infants. In: Brackbill Y, Thompson G (eds) Behaviour in infancy and early childhood. Free Press, New York

Brown J 1964 Short term memory. British Medical Bulletin 20:8–11

Brown R 1973 A first language: the early stages. Harvard University Press, Cambridge, MA

Bruner J 1983 Child's talk: learning to use language. Norton, New York

Cameron N 1938 Reasoning, regression and communication in schizophrenics. Psychological Monographs 50(1)

Campbell R J 1989 Psychiatric dictionary, 5th edn. Oxford University Press, Oxford

Carmichael L, Hogan H P, Walter A A 1932 An experimental study of the effect of language on the reproduction of visually perceived forms. Journal of Experimental Psychology 15:73–86

Carroll J B (ed) 1956 Language, thought and reality:

selected writings of Benjamin Lee Whorf. MIT Press & Wiley, Cambridge, MA

Carroll J B, Casagrande J B 1958 The function of language classifications in behaviour. In: Maccoby E et al (eds) Readings in social psychology, 3rd edn. Holt, New York

Chomsky N 1959 Review of Skinner 1957. Language 35:26–58

Chomsky N 1980 Rules and representations. Columbia University Press, New York

Chomsky N 1986 Knowledge of language: it's nature, origin and use. Praeger, New York

Cicero M T 1927 Tusculan disputations, text and English translation. Harvard University Press, Loeb Classical Library, Cambridge, MA

Cohen N J 1981 Neuropsychological evidence for a distinction between procedural and declarative knowledge in human memory and amnesia. Ph.D thesis, University of California

Cohen N J, Squire L R 1980 Preserved learning and retention of pattern analysing skill in amnesia: dissociation of knowing how and knowing that. Science 210:207–209

Cohen N J, Squire L R 1981 Retrograde amnesia and remote memory impairment. Neuropsychologia 19:337–356

Crystal D 1984 Who cares about English usage? Penguin, Harmondsworth

Curtiss S 1977 Genie: a psycholinguistic study of a modern-day 'wild child'. Academic Press, New York

Curtiss S 1981 Feral children. In: Wortis J (ed) Mental retardation and developmental disabilities, Vol. xii. Bruner/Mazel, New York

Davis K 1967 Final note on a case of extreme isolation. American Journal of Sociology 45:554–565

Dawson M E, Schell A M 1982 Electrodermal responses to attended and unattended significant stimuli during dichotic listening. Journal of Experimental Psychology: Human Perception and Performance 8:82–86

Dennis W 1941 Infant development under conditions of restricted practice and of minimal social stimulation. Genetics of Psychology Monographs 23:143–189

Dennis W 1960 Causes of retardation among institutional children: Iran. Journal of Genetic Psychology 96:46–60

Dennis W 1973 Children of the creche. Appleton-Century-Crofts, Englewood Cliffs, NJ

Deutsch J A, Deutsch D 1963 Attention: some theoretical considerations. Psychological Review 70:80–90

Dodd B 1987 The acquisition of lip-reading skills by normally hearing children. In: Dodd B, Campbell R (eds) Hearing by eye: the psychology of lipreading. Erlbaum, London

Douglas J E, Sutton A 1978 The development of speech and mental processes in a pair of twins: a case study. Journal of Child Psychology and Psychiatry 19:49–56

Eysenck H J, Wilson G D 1973 The experimental study of Freudian theories. Methuen, London

Freeman R D, Thibes L N 1973 Electrophysiological evidence that abnormal early visual experience can modify the human brain. Science 180:876–878

Freud S 1922 Introductory lectures on psychoanalysis, 10th impression. George Allen & Unwin, London

Freud S 1986 The essentials of psychoanalysis. Pelican, London

Gardner H, Roylance P J 1982 Developmental psychology: an introduction. Little Brown, Boston

Gesell A 1950 The first five years of life. Methuen, London

Globus A, Rosenzweig M R, Bennett E, Diamond M C 1973 Effects of differential experience on dendritic spin counts in rat cerebral cortex. Journal of Comparative Physiology and Psychology 82:175–181

Glucksberg S 1962 The influence of strength of drive on functional fixedness and perceptual recognition. Journal of Experimental Psychology 63:36–41

Goldenson R M, Barrows H S 1984 Longman's dictionary of psychology and psychiatry. Longman, New York

Gopnik A, Meltzoff A N 1985 From people, to plans, to objects. Journal of Pragmatics 9:495–512

Gray J A, Wedderburn A A I 1960 Grouping strategies with simultaneous stimuli. Quarterly Journal of Experimental Psychology 12:180–184

Green B 1982 Intensive care for neurological trauma and disease. Academic Press, Orlando

Greenough W T, West R W, DeVoogd T J 1978 Subsynaptic plate perforations: changes with age and experience in the rat. Science 202:1096–1098

Harlow H F 1949 The formation of learning sets. Psychological Review 56:51–65

Heider G R 1972 Universals in colour meaning and memory. Experimental Psychology 93:10–20

Herbart J F 1891 Textbook of psychology. Appleton, New York

Hinchliff S M, Montague S E 1988 Physiology for nursing practice. Baillière Tindall, London

Hubel D H, Wiesel T N 1977 Brain mechanisms of vision. Scientific American 241:150–162

Hudson L 1966 Contrary imaginations: a psychological study of English school boys. Metheun, London

Huxley J 1969 Evolution. McDonald, London

Hyams N M 1986 Language acquisition and the theory of parameters D. Reider, Dordrecht

Itard J 1801 In: Maison L (ed) 1972 The wild boy of Aveyron. NLB, London

Jakobson R 1968 Child language, aphasia and phonological universals. Janua Lingaurum, Series Minor, 72. Mouton, The Hague

James W 1890 The principles of psychology. Holt, Rinehart, Winston, New York

Jaspers K 1963 Translation by Hoenig J, Hamilton M General psychopathology. Manchester University Press, Manchester

Johnson-Laird P N 1983 Mental models: toward a cognitive science of language, inference, and consciousness. Harvard University Press, Cambridge, MA

Kandel E R, Schwartz J H 1981 Principles of neural science. Elsevier, North Holland, New York

Kandel E R, Schwartz J H 1982 Molecular biology of learning: modulation of transmitter release. Science 218:433–442

Kohler W 1925 The mentality of apes. Harcourt Brace, New York

Kohler W 1952 Gestalt psychology. Vision Press, London

Koluchova J 1976 The further development of twins after severe and prolonged deprivation: a second report. Journal of Child Psychology and Psychiatry 17:181–188

Labov W 1973 The boundaries of words and their meanings. In: Bailey C J N, Shuy R W (eds) New ways of analysing variations in English. Georgetown University Press, Washington, DC

Ladefoged P 1975 A course in phonetics. Harcourt Brace Jovanovich, New York

Leask J, Haber R N, Haber R B 1969 Eidetic imagery in children. Psychonomic Monograph Supplements 3:25–48

Lenneberg E H 1967 The biological foundations of language. Wiley, New York

Lishman W A 1987 Organic psychiatry: the psychological consequences of cerebral disorder. Blackwell, Oxford

Longman's dictionary of psychology and psychiatry 1984 Longman, London

Luchins A F 1959 Primary–recency in impression formation. In: Hovland C I (ed) The order of presentation in persuasion. Yale University Press, New Haven

Luria A 1987 The mind of a mnemonist: a little book about a big memory. Harvard, Cambridge, MA

Lyttle J 1986 Mental disorder: its care and treatment. Baillière Tindall, London

Mackworth N H 1950 Researches in the measurement of human performance. MRC Special Report Series 268. HMSO, London

McCormick D A, Clark G A, Lavord D G, Thompson R F 1982 Initial localisation of the memory trace for a basic form of learning. Proceedings of the National Academy of Sciences USA 79:2731–2735

McGough J J 1982 Memory consolidation. Lawrence Erlbaum, Hillsdale NJ

McKellar P 1957 Imagination and thinking. Cohen & West, London

Menn L 1985 Phonological development: learning sounds and sound patterns. In: Berko Gleason J (ed) The development of language. Merrill, Columbus, OH

Mill J 1906 A system of logic. Longmans, London

Milner B 1972 Disorders of learning and memory after temporal lobe lesions in man. Clinical Neurosurgery 19:421–446

Mollgaard K, Diamond M C, Bennett E K, Rosenweig M R, Lindner B 1971 Quantitative synaptic changes with differential experience in rat brain. International Journal of Neuroscience 2:113–128

Moscovitch M 1981 Multiple dissociations in the amnesic syndrome. In: Cermak L S (ed) Human memory and amnesia. Lawrence Erlbaum, Hillsdale, NJ

Neel A F 1969 Theories of psychology. University of London Press, London

O'Keefe J, Nadel L 1978 The hippocampus as a cognitive map. Oxford University Press, Oxford

Olton D S, Becker J T, Handelman G R 1980 Hippocampal function: working memory or cognitive mapping. Physiological Psychology 8:239–246

Oswald I 1960 Falling asleep open-eyed during intense rhythmic stimulation. British Medical Journal 1:1450

Pask G, Scott B C E 1972 Learning strategies and individual competence. International Journal of Man–Machine Studies 4(3):217–253

Pavlov I P 1927 Conditioned reflexes. Oxford University Press, Oxford

Piaget J 1967 Play, dreams and limitation in childhood. International University Press, New York

Piaget J 1968 Language and thought from the genetic point of view. In: Piaget J (ed) Six psychological studies. University of London Press, London

Pospesel H 1974 Propositional logic. Prentice-Hall, Englewood Cliffs, NJ

Professional guide to diseases 1989. Springhouse Corporation

Provence S, Lipton R C 1962 Infants in institutions: a comparison of their development with family reared infants during the first year of life. International University Press, New York

Rips L J 1986 Deduction. In: Sternberg R J, Smith E E (eds) The psychology of human thought. Cambridge University Press, Cambridge

Rosch E 1973 On the internal structures of perceptual and semantic categories. In: Moore T E (ed) Cognitive development and the acquisition of language. Academic Press, New York

Rosch E 1975 Cognitive representations of semantic categories. Journal of Experimental Psychology 104(3):192–233

Rose S P R, Bateson P P G, Horn G 1973 Experience and plasticity in the nervous system. Science 181:506–514

Rosenzweig M R 1984 Experience, memory and the brain. American Psychologist 49:150–162

Rowland C 1983 Patterns of interaction between three blind infants and their mothers. In: Mills A E (ed) Language acquisition in the blind child: normal and deficient. Croom Helm, London

Ruger H A 1910 The psychology of efficiency. Archives of Psychology 19:15

Salmon W C 1973 Logic. Prentice-Hall, Englewood Cliffs, NJ

Sapir E 1949 Language, culture and personality: selected essays. University of California Press, Berkeley, CA

Schneider K 1959 Clinical psychopathology. Grune, New York

Sergent J, Poncet M 1990 From covert to overt recognition of faces in a prosopagnosic patient. Brain 113:989–1004

Singh J A L, Zingg R M 1942 Wolf children and feral man. Harper Bros, New York

Sirigu A, Duhamel J R, Poncet M 1991 The role of sensorimotor experience in object recognition. A case of multimodal agnosia. Brain 114(6):2555–2573

Skeels H M 1966 Adult status of children with contrasting early life experiences: a follow up study. Monographs of the Society for Research in Child Development 31:3

Skuse D 1984 Extreme deprivation in early childhood 1. Diverse outcomes for three siblings from an extraordinary family. Journal of Child Psychology and Psychiatry 25:523–541

Skyrms B 1986 Choice and chance: an introduction to inductive logic. Dickenson, Belmont, CA

Slobin D 1979 Psycholinguistics, 2nd edn. Foresman, Glenview, IL

Squire L R 1984 Memory and the brain. In: Friedman S et al (eds) Brain, cognition and education. Academic Press, New York

Stampe D 1969 The acquisition of phonemic representation. Proceedings of the Vth Regional Meeting of the Chicago Linguistic Society 433–444

Steiner E 1978 Logical and conceptual analytic techniques for educational research. University Press, Washington, DC

Swanson L E, Teyler T J, Thompson R F (eds) 1982 Hippocampal long-term potentiation: mechanisms and implications for memory. Neurosciences Research Program Bulletin 20(5). MIT Press, Cambridge, MA

Thompson A M 1986 Adam—a severely deprived Colombian orphan: a case report. Journal of Child Psychology and Psychiatry 27:689–695

Thompson R F, Berger T, Madden J 1983 Cellular processes of learning and memory in the mammalian CNS. Annual Review of Neuroscience 6:447–491

Titchener E B 1909 Lectures on experimental psychology of the thought processes. MacMillan, New York

Tolman E B 1932 Purposive behaviour in animals and men. Appleton Century, New York

Tomasello M, Farrar M 1984 Cognitive bases of lexical development: object permanence and relational words. Journal of Child Language 11:477–495

Tortora G J, Anagnostakos N P 1984 Principles of anatomy and physiology. Harper & Row, New York

Treisman A 1964 Verbal cues, language and meaning in selective attention. American Journal of Psychology 77:206–219

Treisman A, Gelade G 1980 A feature-integration theory of attention. Cognitive Psychology 12:97–136

Tulving E, Madigan S A 1970 Memory and verbal memory. In: Mussen P H, Rosenzweig M R (eds) Annual Review of Psychology 21:437–484

Tversky A, Kahnemann D 1973 On the psychology of prediction. Psychological Review 80:237–251

Vygotsky L S 1962 Thought and language. MIT Press, Cambridge, MA

Warren H C 1921 A history of the association: psychology. Scribners, New York

Wason P C, Johnson-Laird P N 1970 A conflict between selecting and evaluating information in an inferential task. British Journal of Psychology 61:509–515

Watson R I 1963 The great psychologists: from Aristotle to Freud. Lippincott, Philadelphia

Wells G 1985 Language development in the preschool years. Cambridge University Press, Cambridge

Wendt H 1972 From ape to Adam. Thames & Hudson, London

Werker J F, Tees R C 1985 Cross-language speech perception: evidence for perceptual reorganization during the first year of life. Infant Behaviour and Development 7:49–63

Wexler B E 1988 Dichotic presentation as a method for single hemisphere stimulation studies. In: Hugdahl K (ed) Handbook of dichotic listening: theory, methods and research. Wiley, Chichester

Wilde O 1969 The importance of being earnest. In: Complete Plays. Methuen, London

Wilkinson R T 1963 Interaction of noise with knowledge of results and sleep deprivation. Journal of Experimental Psychology 66:332–337

Woolsey T A, Wann J R 1976 Areal changes in mouse cortical barrels following vibrissal damage at different postnatal ages. Journal of Comparative Neurology 170:53–66

Zeki S 1991 Cerebral akinetopsia (visual motion blindness), a review. Brain 114(2):811–824

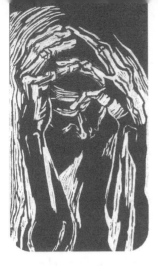

Chapter Six

Mental health problems

Lynne D Smith

AIMS

- ◆ To outline commonly encountered diagnostic categories, with their variations within the A, B, C format explored in the previous chapters

KEY ISSUES

DSM-IV classification system

Disorders of mood

Anxiety

Problems of somatic health

Schizophrenia

Dementia

Psychoactive substance misuse

INTRODUCTION

In Chapter 2, it was asserted that problems associated with mental health do not stand alone, but are seen to generate or coexist with other problems relating to mental health status. We do not, for example, experience a low mood and no other problems. Low mood may be considered the prime problem, but it is seen to affect behaviour and cognitive function in a manner that significantly interferes with the ability to function on a daily basis.

It may be recalled that we used the jigsaw to indicate the enmeshing nature of mental health status (Fig. 6.1) and that it was asserted that:

a problem of + a problem of + a problem of
affect   behaviour   cognition
= diagnosis of mental disorder

This is therefore the format used in the brief outline of some of the commonly encountered diagnostic categories, with their variations.

Chapter 1 introduced the International classification of diseases (10th edition, ICD-10 1992) as a set of criteria upon which to assess problems experienced. This chapter will introduce a second classification system, that of the Diagnostic and statistical manual of mental disorders (4th edition, 1995) to provide insight into an alternative set of criteria, well used within the UK. Abbreviated to DSM-IV, this set of criteria views mental disorders as comprising very specific symptomatology. Any variations within the symptomatology experienced by the client are viewed and treated as a separate, coexisting problem. Whereas ICD-10 would describe 'moderate depression with somatic symptoms', DSM-IV would describe the same client as experiencing a 'major depressive episode' plus 'an undifferentiated somatoform disorder'. The two systems do not mix easily and therefore health care professionals need to clarify which operates in their care area.

MOOD DISORDERS

Depressive episodes

Problems associated with lowered mood are required, in DSM-IV, to have been present for 2 weeks before a diagnosis of *major depressive episode* (Fig. 6.2) is awarded. Similarly, such feelings are required to be evident for most of the day and on nearly every day during this 2-week period, and represent an obvious departure from previous status. Coexisting alongside this lowered mood, there is a loss of joy in life, a reduction in pleasure related to all activities and a loss of self-interest. Self-perception is often related to inadequacy of function and worthlessness, and this may achieve delusional proportions, whilst guilt may be evident as a result of these feelings or past activities or events.

Anxiety and fear—for one's own health, for the well-being of others and for the future in general—may be present and irritability and loss of control may be demonstrated.

Facial expression reflects sadness, eye contact may be lost and there is often tearfulness, or evidence of recent and prolonged crying. Movement levels may demonstrate retardation or, conversely, agitation, as the individual paces, wrings the hands, pulls or rubs skin, clothing, hair and other objects in the vicinity. Appetite is often poor,

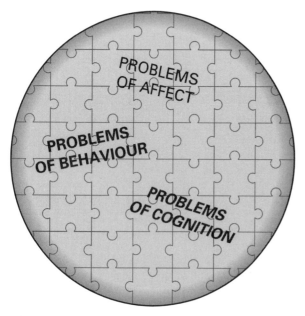

Fig. 6.1 Aggregation of problems to provide a diagnosis.

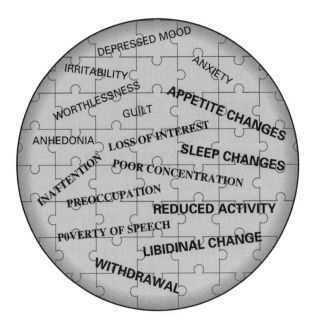

Fig. 6.2 A major depressive episode.

resulting in lowered energy levels, constant fatigue and weight loss, though on occasions 'comfort' eating may be seen. The fatigue is compounded by sleep problems, with failing to sleep (initial insomnia), waking during sleep (middle insomnia) and early morning wakening (terminal insomnia) all common complaints. Again, on occasions, sleep may be seen to be excessive (hypersomnia), with frequent daytime naps or longer periods of night-time sleep described.

Cognitively, the individual frequently experiences a difficulty in thinking, inattention and problems related to concentration. Thinking is slow and preoccupied, often with somatic health or dying, with the belief expressed that all would be 'better off' if the individual were dead. Speech is slow and monotone, and often considerably reduced in amount, at times to the point of mutism. Commonly, where delusional ideation and hallucinatory experiences occur, there is a reflection of the sad, negative mood within the content expressed (mood congruence); more rarely is there incongruence.

Variations on the theme of depressed mood are commonly diagnosed. Episodes, for example, may be single or recurrent, or may be elicited in con-junction with episodes of intense psychomotor activity and elevated mood as a *bipolar disorder*. It may be experienced at all stages of life. In children, it is associated with agitation, rather than retardation, and an emphasis on complaints surrounding somatic health are commonly made. Hallucinations are usually auditory in nature and mood congruent. Adolescents often demonstrate overtly antisocial behaviour, examples being negativism, aggression, withdrawal and psychoactive substance use. The 'leanings' of the normal adolescent are greatly exaggerated and often completely out of character. Exteriorization of problems associated with depression in the elderly population may be confused with those of organic impairment and hence precise diagnostic techniques are required to elicit the true picture.

Major life changes, which may evoke feelings of inadequacy and stress, may precede depressed mood. Loss of a loved one, by death, divorce or separation, or some other important element of life, for example, a job or property, may precipitate difficulties, as may chronic, physical ill health. Leaving school, changing workplace, childbirth and retirement may all evoke stress and therefore problems of this type.

Manic episodes

A *manic episode* (Fig. 6.3), conversely, demonstrates problems for the individual that are almost at the opposite end of the continuum, for mood is persistently and inappropriately elevated, with an infectiously euphoric face being presented to the world. The overoptimistic and expansive approach to life engendered prompts pleasure-seeking activities and disinhibited behaviour, which, if thwarted, may provoke responses ranging from irritation to anger.

There is a pronounced increase in motor activity, which is goal directed and yet which demonstrates no appreciation of the implications of repercussions of actions. Such individuals exhibit well-intentioned—though none the less irritating—and continual meddling and interference in whatever interaction or event takes their fleeting attention or interest. Sleep pattern is disturbed, with an apparent reduced need for prolonged

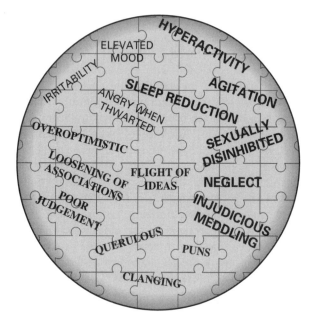

Fig. 6.3 A manic episode.

periods of rest. Two or three hours will furnish the individual with limitless energy and unrestrained activity. Social convention and inhibitions are thrown to the wind, as individuals follow their immediate desire, and therefore tactless, offensive and often sexually frank behaviour ensues. The individual finds no time for the basic activities of eating and self-care, being far too preoccupied with the environmental and thought-provoked stimulation of the surroundings. Work activities and social relationships inevitably suffer.

Individuals exhibit grandiosity, in the form of grossly inflated beliefs concerning their own characteristics, abilities and experiences, and present, therefore, as self-opinionated and arrogant. Flight of ideas reflects in pressurized, loud and rapid speech, which often becomes incoherent and unintelligible. As thoughts race, individuals display distractability and frequent shifts in attention towards external stimuli. In turn, speech shows evidence of word selection via sound rather than by meaning, in rhymes, clang association and silly puns.

Manic episodes may similarly be precipitated by psychological stressors, but may also be seen following treatment for depressed mood, that is,

antidepressant medication and electroplexy, and mood disorders are a frequently observable feature of psychoactive substance use.

ANXIETY

The diagnostic category of *generalized anxiety disorder* (Fig. 6.4) is reserved for those individuals who experience excessive or unrealistic anxiety or apprehension, relating to two or more activities or circumstances, on more days than not during a 6-month period. Depressed or irritable mood may feature due to the individual's perceived sense of inadequacy to meet current needs to perform.

Somatic experiences reflect the hyperarousal of sympathetic innervation of the autonomic nervous system and are therefore seen in all spheres of function. Muscle tension gives rise to shaky, aching muscles and general feelings of fatigue. Shortness of breath, difficulty in breathing and rapid, shallow breathing may feature, and lightheadedness, dizziness and palpitations are all common symptoms. Cold and clammy or alternatively flushed skin are characteristic, and gastrointestinal problems, such as dysphagia, nausea, diarrhoea

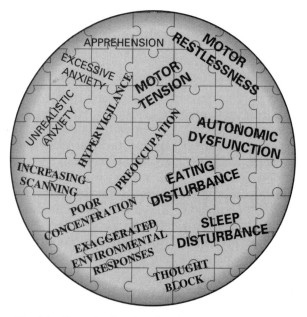

Fig. 6.4 Generalized anxiety disorder.

and 'butterflies', often serve to reduce the desire for food. An increased desire to micturate is also a common complaint, and sleep is disturbed, with difficulties in going off to sleep, or remaining asleep, creating added feelings of fatigue.

There is a preoccupation with areas of concern, and therefore inattention and poor concentration may be complaints. Thought blocks may be elicited and words 'lost' within explanatory dialogue. The individual's perceptual functions are on a state of high alert, and hypervigilance and hyper-attentiveness to environmental nuances are both observable, via exaggerated responses to minor changes in the surroundings.

Separation anxiety disorder

Anxiety is a common element of many diagnoses. In children and young adults, for example, *separation anxiety disorder* may be seen following detachment from a loved one. Such youngsters demonstrate a need for familiar surroundings, clinging behaviour and often somatic symptomatology such as nausea, vomiting, diarrhoea and headaches. In older children, dizziness, palpitations and fainting may occur. Fears of harm befalling the loved one and of never being reunited are commonly expressed, and young children may be afraid to sleep alone, as bad dreams and nightmares create further anxiety.

Avoidant disorder

Avoidant disorder of childhood and adolescence may similarly be diagnosed where social anxiety is a problem. Such children are withdrawn, shy and embarrassed in unfamiliar company and yet sociable and happy with those known to them. The problem is rarely seen in isolation and often accompanies a generalized anxiety disorder, or an *overanxious disorder*, where problems associated with a preoccupation and concern with past or future events is seen. Children worry about their competence in a variety of situations and the perceptions of others regarding their performance are a major concern. The somatic problems associated with autonomic arousal are frequently observed.

Fears

Panic attacks, or relatively short lasting and discrete periods of intense fear and terror, may occur without any obvious precipitating event or as an integral feature of other anxiety-provoking situations. *Phobias* represent a persistent and focused fear of a specific situation, event or object, which evoke the autonomic anxiety response. There is a recognition of the unreasonable nature of the fear, but continued avoidance of the stimulus, wherever feasible. Intense anxiety is elicited if exposure occurs, and an integral aspect of the phobia is often related to the possibility of humiliating oneself during such an exposure. Where the stimulus is a commonly encountered one within everyday life and living experiences, work and social routines and relationships may be significantly impaired.

Post-traumatic stress disorder may follow the experience of a situation encompassing characteristics of terror, intense fear, helplessness and fear of death. Traumas beyond the comprehension and believed physical endurance of many, for example, rape, combat, earthquakes and torture, may engender a recurrent reliving of the trauma, an avoidance of stimuli associated with it or an emotional detachment from the world. Recurrent nightmares may further disturb already difficult sleeping patterns. Irritability, loss of control and aggression may be problems, as may be generalized and exaggerated responses to environmental cues. Withdrawal, diminished interest, poor attention and concentration spans may all be experienced.

Obsessive–compulsive disorder

Obsessive–compulsive disorder is the term reserved to describe the problem compilation associated with obtrusive, repetitive thoughts and the physical manoeuvres instigated to eradicate, neutralize or prevent that thought content from occurring. The obsessive thoughts are recognized as belonging to, and being generated by, the self and initially behaviours may be resisted as senseless or unreasonable activities. Anxiety and tension created by resistance may be seen to be released only by the performance of stereotyped, ritualistic movements, which commonly include handwashing, touching, checking and counting procedures. The problems may be seen to begin in childhood, adolescence or early adult years.

PROBLEMS ASSOCIATED WITH SOMATIC HEALTH

Hypochondriasis

Hypochondriasis (Fig. 6.5) is the category used to describe an amalgamation of problems engendered by an unwarranted fear or belief that one has a physical disease, although there is no actual evidence found upon medical evaluation to support such a belief. The fear may be accompanied by frustration and anger in the response to doctors, who are unable to support the individual's fears with a concrete somatic diagnosis, and depression is also common, both as a response to this medical failure and also to the persistent sensations and perceptions experienced.

Clients may, because of their beliefs, present themselves as 'delicate' or 'fragile' in health and indulge in doctor-shopping activities, trailing from one expert to another in the hope that one of them will recognize what all of the others have failed to diagnose. Several body systems may be involved within the focus of attention at any one time, or, conversely, the perceived signs and symptoms may be transferred from one system to another. Social and occupational functioning may be affected to a greater or lesser degree, dependent upon the intensity of the beliefs and the nature of the symptoms expressed.

Whilst the belief regarding the somatic disorder may be intense, it is not of delusional proportions, in that the client may consider medical suggestions of exaggeration of the symptoms as a possibility, and indeed that such symptoms do not exist at all. Uncertainty, whilst possibly elicited, does not, however, reassure the client that there is no abnormality or illness present. The person shows a preoccupation, therefore, with the functions or perceived sensations related to the part of the body under focus.

Malingering and non-compliance

There are many variations on the theme of somatically orientated problems, ranging from *malingering*, where there is an intentional production or excessive exaggeration of health problems, which is motivated by external incentives, such as avoiding work, legal prosecution or obtaining drugs, to *non-compliance with medical treatment*, due to denial of a real illness, contrary religious beliefs and value judgements made to the relative value of treatment. Whilst neither can be attributed to mental illness, as such, they may usefully be seen to form the parameters of somatic health related problems.

Body dysmorphic disorder

Body dysmorphic disorder is exhibited as an excessive preoccupation with an imagined or real, but slight, body defect, in an individual who appears 'normal'. The focus of this preoccupation may be related to imaginary wrinkles, spots or lumps, or to the size, shape or symmetry of features. Repeated medical advice may be sought to

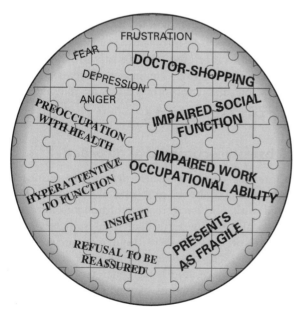

Fig. 6.5 Hypochondriasis.

correct the perceived flaws, and ideation may assume delusional proportions, as a separate *delusional disorder—somatic subtype*.

Conversion disorder

Conversion disorder is the term used to describe problems associated with a loss of function or an alteration in some aspect of bodily function that, whilst suggestive of underlying somatic pathology, is put forward as a physiological expression of a psychological desire or conflict. It has been suggested that exteriorization of the problem in a physical form fulfils two different motives or needs for the client. The first relates to the achievement of a 'primary gain', by preventing the need for a conscious awareness of the psychological conflict. An individual, for example, may witness a traumatic event and, rather than admitting or acknowledging the trauma, unconsciously 'develop' a blindness, or the person who fears hurting a loved one, following an intense argument, may 'develop' a paralysis of an arm. The symptom may also supply, therefore, an 'insurance policy' against the occurrence of the feared activity and offer a potential solution to the continuance of such a psychological conflict.

Similarly, a 'secondary gain' may be achieved via the provision of a legitimate reason for avoidance or prevention of a traumatic event or situation. A wife, about to leave her husband and the marital home, would be less inclined to do so were he to develop a paralysis from the waist down. Soldiers would be looked upon more kindly were they to develop a paralysis of a hand and therefore be unable to fire their weapon, than were they to voice their anxieties about killing others.

There are, of course, the often quoted examples of 'glove' and 'stocking' paralyses—that is, a loss of function over a discrete, symmetrical area, which, physiologically, is impossible to experience. 'Convenient' development of any symptomatology must always be thoroughly investigated to ensure that there is no physiological or somatic cause operating, but the feature *la belle indifférence*, where there is an apparent lack of concern regarding the physical symptomatology present, may be significant to the diagnosis.

Individuals who exhibit recurrent, multiple somatic health complaints over a period of several years that, upon medical investigation, are not apparently caused by physiological abnormality or disease processes, may be considered as experiencing *somatization disorder*. Descriptions of symptomatology may be vague or delivered in a dramatic or exaggerated manner, and medical assistance may have frequently been sought over a period of many years. Problems may be considered to reflect neurological dysfunction, such as paralyses, paraesthesias and blindness, or cardiovascular manifestations, such as chest pain and dizziness, or gastrointestinal pathology, for example, pain or disordered bowel function. Dysmenorrhoea, or sexual dysfunction or disinterest, is also relatively common. Anxiety or depressed mood may often be elicited by a skilled practitioner, and life or relationship problems exposed.

Complaints solely related to the experience of pain that, again, are unable to be accounted for by medical findings, may acquire the diagnosis of *somatoform pain disorder*. The presence within individuals or their environment of some conflict-evoking stimulus may be readily demonstrated, or, conversely, such pain may be seen to facilitate avoidance of an unpleasant or intolerable activity or situation. Often the symptoms develop immediately after some traumatic event or experience, which individuals refuse to admit may have a bearing on their ill health.

SCHIZOPHRENIA

The problems that are seen to combine within the diagnostic criteria of *schizophrenia* (Fig. 6.6) need to have been in evidence for a minimum period of 6 months in order to fulfil the diagnostic criteria. This may include symptomatology that is put forward as indicative of three phases associated with the development of the overall picture of full presentation, namely the *prodromal*, *acute* and *residual* phases. The first and last phases are essentially the same and in reality this demarcation of separate developmental stages may be observable only in hindsight. In essence, the three

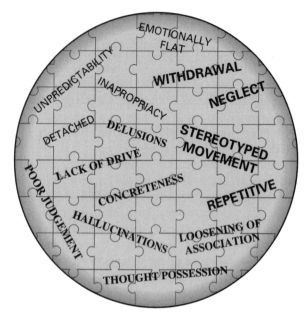

Fig. 6.6 Schizophrenia.

phases represent an increasing–plateauing–decreasing severity of problems experienced.

Prodromal and residual phases

Within the prodromal and residual phases, those significant to the individual may describe features which indicate a clear deterioration from previous levels of performance and functioning, and which suggest an apparent change in personality characteristics. Affect may be blunted, shallow and inappropriate to events. Behaviour is often described as 'odd' or 'bizarre', with evidence of hoarding or collecting activities, particularly related to rubbish or unassociated, unconnected items, which may assume great importance in the individual's life. There is frequently a complaint that such individuals are talking to themself in public, that they have isolated themself from previous seemingly satisfactory relationships and interactions, and that there is a deterioration of previous roles and functions. Self-neglect is obvious in all spheres of personal and social care, and the individual demonstrates a reduction in drive, interest and energy. Speech may be poor in quantity and content, often eliciting vagueness, circumstantiality and overelaboration. Odd beliefs may be indicated within speech content, which are not reflective of the prevailing culture, and misperceptions and illusions may be frequent. A minimum of two of the above problems must be present to warrant diagnosis as prodromal/residual symptoms of schizophrenia.

Acute phase

The acute, active phase is very precisely defined within three sets of criteria. One of these three sets of criteria must have been in evidence for a minimum period of 1 week before diagnosis of the acute phase of schizophrenia is made—that is, the individual either:

1. must demonstrate at least two of the following:
   (a) flat or inappropriate affect
   (b) catatonic behaviour
   (c) delusions
   (d) loosening of associations
   (e) hallucinations, which must be experienced several times a day, for a week, or several times a week for several weeks
2. express bizarre delusions, for example, relating to thought possession, or control of behaviour by outside agencies

or

3. demonstrate prominent hallucinations, commonly auditory in nature and often related to one or more voice, commentating upon the individual's behaviour or actions.

Types of schizophrenia

Self-care, relationships and occupational spheres of activity demonstrate considerable deterioration over previous or anticipated levels of performance. DSM-IV identifies four 'types' of schizophrenia, which, whilst conceded to be less than stable over time, and variable with regard to treatment implications and prognosis, are based upon the predominant symptoms evident upon clinical examination.

Catatonic

The *catatonic type* is indicated by gross disturbances in behaviour and cognition. Stupor may be
evident, whereby the individual elicits a decreased
level of reactivity to the environment and its
stimuli, and which is often associated with mute-
ness and a drastic reduction in motor activity,
sometimes to the point of total immobility.
Conversely, catatonic excitement may be evident,
or there may be a rapid transition from one
extreme to the other, from stupor to purposeless,
excited motor activity. Neither seems to be provoked by environmental stimuli. An apparently
motiveless resistance to the desires or instructions
may be exhibited, termed negativism, and a rigidity of stance may similarly be observed. Catatonic
posturing, where individuals voluntarily assume
obviously uncomfortable and bizarre positions,
which they may maintain for prolonged periods of
time, may also be a feature.

Disorganized

The *disorganized type* is characterized by grossly
inappropriate affect, bizarre behaviours, which
may include grimaces, mannerisms and stereotyped patterns of movement, and severe loosening
of associations and incoherence. Delusions and
hallucinations may be less persistent and more
fleeting and fragmentary than are experienced by
other individuals.

Paranoid

The problems usually linked with schizophrenia—
flat and inappropriate affect, disorganized behaviour and loosening of associations—are not
evident within the *paranoid type*. Delusions,
which are more systematized and may be related
to one or more themes, and related auditory hallucinations are the essential features here, with
anger, argumentativeness and aggression all possible. Anxiety may be unfocused where demonstrated, and behaviour may appear to be precise, and
consciously thought out, particularly where interactions with others are concerned. An obvious
lack of warmth and a stilted, formal manner is
characteristic of such interactions.

Undifferentiated

Where the individual fails to meet the criteria of
the above three categories, the term *undifferentiated type* may be used, and in situations where
there is no evidence of a prodromal stage, or
where similar symptomatology appears following
events of an intensely stressful nature, the term
brief reactive psychosis may be made. Affect may
be intense and rapid shifts may be observed.
Behaviour may be catatonic or disorganized in
nature, and cognition may show features such as
loosening of associations, delusions, hallucinatory
experiences and incoherence. Symptomatology is
seen to resolve within a month.

Schizophreniform and schizoaffective disorder

Schizophreniform disorder is said to demonstrate
identical symptomatology to schizophrenia, but
the duration of problems does not exceed
6 months, with a full return to levels of premorbid
functioning evident after that time. Similarly,
where there is a mixture of symptomatology associated with both mood disorder and schizophrenia, the term *schizoaffective disorder* may be
applied.

Induced psychotic disorder

On occasions, significant others involved in a relationship with the individual experiencing a 'psychotic disorder' may similarly exteriorize and
share the delusional ideation exhibited by the
client. In a sort of 'contagion', there has very often
been a close relationship shared, which has been
'undiluted' because of reduced social contact with
others outside of the situation. Symptomatology
disappears from the 'well person' when the two
individuals are separated. The diagnostic category
used to describe this type of episode in the well
person is *induced psychotic disorder*.

DEMENTIA

Whilst acknowledging the fact that the term
'dementia' (Fig. 6.7) may be used by many to infer

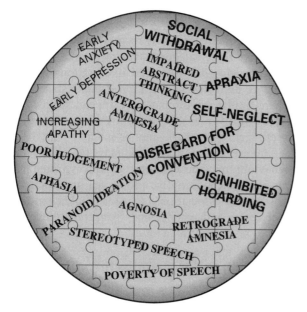

Fig. 6.7 Dementia.

a progressive and unremitting course and eventual severe cognitive impairment as the prognosis, DSM-IV clearly describes the term in relation to the clear presenting clinical picture rather than its outcome. Definitive statements indicate the potential degree of reversibility as dependent upon aetiology and early recognition and treatment.

The individual may present as anxious or depressed within the early stages of deterioration, often as a response to the awareness and appreciation of the deficits arising in previously efficient functioning. This may result in withdrawal from social interaction, excessive organization of activities and overelaboration of details relating to events experienced, in an attempt to conceal memory problems and cognitive/intellectual difficulties. Psychosocial stressors impact severely upon the already struggling individual, with further deterioration as its result. Paranoid ideation may engender anger and its verbal and motor consequences. Diagnosis is made only when intellectual impairment is of sufficient degree to provoke repercussions within occupational and social functioning spheres.

Primary problems relate to the impairment of short and long term memory functions, and the implicit difficulties of vast gaps in personal and common knowledge. Difficulties are evinced within abstract thinking, with the individual unable to identify similarities or differences in objects or situations, and impairment in the ability to define words and concepts. Judgement is therefore unreliable. There may be a failure to recognize everyday objects, despite intact sensory pathways, or agnosia, and similarly an inability to perform motor activities despite intact understanding and motor function, or apraxia. Constructional activities, for example, reproducing three-dimensional figures, may also create difficulties for the individual. Family and friends frequently observe an accentuation or alteration in previous personality characteristics.

Primary degenerative dementia

Where neurological disease, for example, cerebral tumours, infections and metabolic dysfunctions, and trauma via head injury, have been excluded, problems that develop insidiously and show a progressively deteriorating course may be diagnosed as a *primary degenerative dementia of the Alzheimer type*. Evidence to support such a diagnosis may be commonly observable after the age of 50 years, when it is termed *presenile*, or after 65 years of age, when it is defined as *senile* in nature. On occasions, delirium, delusions or depression may be significant individual and predominating symptoms, hence the term dementia is applied to the overall diagnosis.

Multi-infarct dementia

Dementia-related problems may be seen within an overall pattern of abrupt onset, patchy degrees of deterioration in intellectual function and a stepwise, rather than gradual, progression and course. *Multi-infarct dementia* is due to cerebral and systemic vascular disease, which results in small, but multiple, areas of cerebral tissue softening and death, hence the pattern of deterioration seen. Neurological signs are evident, often with a concomitant deterioration in physical function. Dysarthria, dysphagia and a characteristic small-stepped gait may be observed. Physical examination reveals problems associated with circulation, for example, hypertension or heart disease. As with Alzheimer-type problems, significant delirium, delusions and depression may feature, and therefore the main category is amended to indicate this. Lability of mood, with sham tears alternating with laughter, is a commonly encountered problem.

PSYCHOACTIVE SUBSTANCE DEPENDENCE

DSM-IV identifies 11 groups of substances that may be used by people to achieve a change in mood or behaviour on a non-medical basis:

1. alcohol
2. amphetamines, and other similarly acting sympathomimetics
3. caffeine
4. cannabis
5. cocaine
6. hallucinogens
7. inhalants
8. nicotine
9. opioids
10. phencyclidine (PCP), and other similarly acting arylcyclohexylamines
11. sedatives, hypnotics and anxiolytics.

Despite the specific substance used, dependence elicits some common features (Fig. 6.8), as well as some individual differences, and symptomatology must be evident for a period of 1 month to meet the criteria awarded within this system of classification.

Whilst mood problems may be evident, particularly in relation to depression, anxiety, irritability, anger and lability, it is often unclear as to the degree to which this is induced by the substance used or was pre-existing, and, in some instances, a precipitating factor in initial use. A large and increasing amount of time is spent in activities relating to procurement, use and recovery from use, which may provoke withdrawal from social situations and normal role performance. Indeed, there may be occasions where, during daily activities and occupational pursuits, the individual is

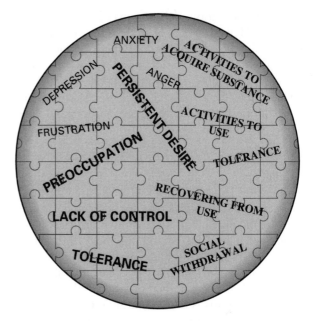

Fig. 6.8 Psychoactive substance abuse.

observed to be intoxicated. Though cognizant of the problem and its detrimental effects on biopsychosocial functioning, individuals are unable to control their intake of the substance and are in fact aware of developing a tolerance for it, requiring increasing amounts to achieve the same desired effect.

Some substances induce characteristic symptoms of withdrawal from use. These may relate to mood, in the form of depression, anxiety and irritability, psychomotor agitation, sleep disturbances and fatigue, as with, for example, amphetamines and cocaine. In withdrawal from alcohol, sedative, hypnotic and anxiolytic substances, problems experienced may include autonomic nervous system hyperactivity. Each substance, barring cannabis, hallucinogens and PCP, which are not identified as evoking withdrawal symptoms, produces a characteristic pattern of features associated with abrupt cessation of use.

Delirium

Delirium may be a sequel associated with the use of cocaine, amphetamines, PCP and similarly acting preparations. Rapidly developing, and often of only brief duration, delirium may be heralded by emotional disturbances of anxiety, fear, irritability, depression, anger, euphoria or apathy, which may be consistent in exteriorization or which may fluctuate rapidly and unpredictably, as lability. There may be a reduced level of consciousness, psychomotor retardation or acceleration, and possibly sleep disturbances of insomnia or excessive daytime sleeping. The individual experiences a reduced ability to maintain or shift attention, with a concomitant reduction in reactivity to the environment. Thinking may show disorganization, irrelevancy and wandering, as indicated by the nature of speech, and there is often disorientation to time, place and person. Memory difficulties and perceptual disturbances may similarly be present, and, as delirium may occur in relation to a wide and varied number of health-related problems, diagnosis is dependent upon the history of use of an evoking substance within the preceding 24-hour period.

Organic delusional disorder

Organic delusional disorder may be a feature of amphetamine, PCP (and similar, related substances), cannabis, cocaine and hallucinogenic preparations. The former, for example, may evoke a highly organized paranoid state, with ingrained persecutory delusions, as may cannabis and cocaine. Hallucinations, whilst exteriorized, are a less prominent symptom. Where hallucinations are equally or more prominent, a diagnosis of *hallucinosis* may be added to, or substituted for that of delusional disorder, as may be seen related to alcohol ingestion.

Perception disorder

On occasions, a *posthallucinogenic perception disorder* may be seen, where there is a reliving of one or more of the perceptual symptoms experienced during use. Macropsia and micropsia, halos surrounding objects or people, and intensified or flashes of colour may all be reported and cause distress.

Mood disorder

Hallucinogens and PCP, and related substances, may similarly engender a *mood disorder* within 1 or 2 weeks of substance use, and persisting for more than 24 hours following cessation of its use. An enveloping depression, elevated or expansive mood provides the predominent problem and, as with delirium, delusional and hallucinatory disorders, requires a history of substance use to enable award of this diagnostic category, due to the same features being displayed in relation to a number and variety of different aetiological factors.

SUMMARY

The previous pages have provided an outline of the major diagnostic categories used within the DSM-IV system of classification. There are others, relating to more specialist areas of practice, for example, sex and gender difficulties and sleep disorders, but the outline offered will provide some insight into the terms that may be used within general psychiatry.

It must be noted that a wide variety of aetiological factors will generate similar symptoms and problems for the individual. A cerebral tumour, schizophrenia and psychoactive substance use may all generate hallucinatory experiences. It is the responsibility of the health care professional to ensure that scrupulous history taking and clear and objective observation of clients and the manifestations of their ill health result in the correct diagnosis, care and treatment.

The chapters outlining the characteristics and fallibility of human perception are as important to the professional's functioning as to that of the client, for there is a tendency to see only what we expect to see, and to disregard other material and information that does not fit into the scheme within our minds. As professionals, we need to look beyond the label, and see the reality of the person's problems.

FURTHER ACTIVITIES

1. Read clients' case notes and care plans to ascertain the specific problems that each is experiencing across the domains of affect, behaviour and cognition.
2. Explore the ways in which care and treatment are directed at problems within each domain.
3. Take the opportunity to discuss with other care professionals the relative value of diagnostic criteria within mental health care, and of the specific criteria in use in the care environment.

REFERENCES

DSM-IV (Diagnostic and statistical manual of mental disorders, 4th edn) 1995 American Psychiatric Association, Washington DC

ICD-10 (International classification of mental and behavioural disorders, 10th edn) 1992 World Health Organization, Geneva

Part II
Interventions in mental health practice

The six chapters of Part II extend biopsychosocial thinking into intervention. They range from one that provides a detailed consideration of biological aspects of treatment and intervention to another that explores various social, economic and political factors associated with mental health promotion. Three chapters explore interventions based primarily on psychological or psychosocial insights (Chapters 8–10) and the last one considers spiritual care.

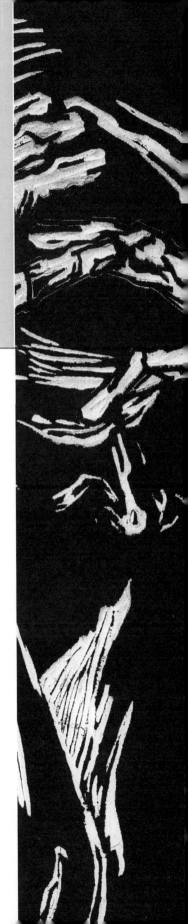

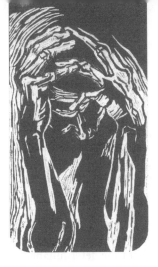

Chapter Seven

Mental health promotion

Gary F McCulloch   Judy Boxer

AIMS

- ◆ For practitioners to draw upon evidence and good practice in mental health promotion
- ◆ To identify their role and contribution in collaboration with agencies, programmes and service users to promote health
- ◆ To highlight opportunities for individual, community and social regeneration

KEY ISSUES

There is a mental health promotion (MHP) theory and evidence base to draw upon and a range of resources and support material available

The new regeneration agenda to support communities is an opportunity for promoting mental health

Practitioners can become involved in partnership with other agencies to promote mental health

Any work requires collaboration with service users

INTRODUCTION

It has taken some time for mental health promotion (MHP) to be considered as an area of study in its own right and a way of describing an approach to mental health practice that has as much place in strategic planning and commissioning as does the recent requirement to target services for people with severe and enduring mental illness (HEA 1998). Major changes are proposed to the funding, structure and management of mental health services at all levels and MHP has a vast agenda in identifying the different types of involvement required at all levels of provision. MHP spans various approaches to the complex subject of mental illness; it attempts to address the mental health needs of individuals, communities and society as a whole. It places the notion of health in a socio-political–cultural domain and in encourages a comprehensive approach to meeting the needs of mental health service users in statutory, voluntary and private provision. Collaboration is essential to effective MHP. The need to plan within an identified framework of interagency provision is a major requirement in the move toward intensive family and community support. This increases the need for an identified plan of care within a specific locality, and a coordinated approach to avoid the obvious problems associated with multiagency involvement in the care of someone with a diagnosis of serious mental illness. The need to provide 24-hour support for those who have the most serious problems perhaps provides a long-awaited opportunity for mental health workers to become more involved in mental health-promoting activities. This is clearly identified in the Health Education Authority (HEA 1997) 'Quality framework' for MHP. This chapter provides many examples of what is happening in the field of MHP. For other examples and discussion on the skills required and the theoretical basis to the study of mental health promotion, both the book we wrote (McCulloch & Boxer 1997) and Tudor 1996) provide an up to date account.

HEALTH PROMOTION

The World Health Organization (WHO) describes health promotion as the process of enabling people to increase control over and to improve their health. This places the promotion of health into a social as well as medical dimension. Health promotion incorporates three main elements within the broad context of a social model of health consisting of:

- ◆ *Health education*—informing, influencing and empowering individuals and groups, communities and policy makers about the determinants of health and ways in which health may be preserved and improved.
- ◆ *Prevention*—programmes and activities aimed at preventing ill health, disease, and accidents.
- ◆ *Health protection*—encompassing a range of environmental, legal, fiscal, political, economic and social measures that promote health.

This has been reflected in the definition in Box 7.1. This definition also begins to suggest methods that can be employed including work in the areas of: communication, education, legislation, fiscal measures, organizational change and community development.

Well-being in the context of MHP includes both mental and social well-being. This concept of well-being can be considered as comprising three elements: needs, skills, and feelings and beliefs (HEA 1997). Needs include basic needs, social support and security, which are affected by the provision of healthy structures. Emotional skills include communication, relationships and psychological survival. These skills are influenced by our social

---

Box 7.1 Sheffield Health's (1996) definition of health promotion

The promotion of health is concerned with maximizing individuals' and communities' involvement in improving and protecting their quality of life and well being. Health promotion aims to address equity in health, the risks to health, sustainable environments conducive to health, and the empowerment of individuals by contributing to health public policy, advocating for health, enabling skills development and education.

world. Feelings and beliefs are expressions of our inner, psychological selves. They are affected by early experience and influence our ability to deal with the inner world. Therefore, health promotion is about more than information giving and education. It is the pursuit of structural as well as individual change. This is clearly reflected in the theory and evidence base of MHP, which we will now discuss.

THEORY AND EVIDENCE FOR MHP

It is important that would-be practitioners do not engage in an endless and fruitless debate on the merits or otherwise of MHP. A significant body of theory and research evidence provides more than adequate direction if not a detailed 'street map'. The following list identifies key work in MHP and a brief outline is given for each:

◆ MHP paradigms and practice
◆ Society of Health Education and Health Promotion Specialists
◆ conceptualizations of mental health and MHP
◆ how we feel
◆ MHP in high risk groups
◆ collaboration with service users
◆ a quality framework.

Paradigms

In a comprehensive study, Tudor (1996) argues that a separation between mental illness and mental health is required, but this should not neglect the mental and emotional well-being of people diagnosed with mental illness, as it has tended to in the past. His historical survey of MHP and its development highlights how it has been drawn into a community care agenda. This has clear implications for practice and the 'division of labour' between clinicians and others. Tudor considers the paradigms that inform the theory of mental health promotion. These span the functionalist, structuralist and humanist approaches to understanding health and social interaction. The theoretical basis of mental health practice is also

considered from a broad social science perspective and especially what effects the impact of class, race and gender have on physical, emotional and social well-being. The need to consider anti-oppressive practice as a core requirement is not as explicitly addressed by Tudor as it has been by other theorists and practitioners (Dominelli 1997, McCulloch & Boxer 1997).

Society of Health Education and Health Promotion Specialists

MacDonald & O'Hara (1998) set out the Society of Health Education and Health Promotion Specialists' (SHEPS) position on MHP. This largely theoretical discussion sets out a robust argument and evidence for prioritizing work in this area. It also provides a map of 10 key elements for promoting or demoting mental health. It stresses the importance of addressing societal, organizational and environmental issues as well as interventions focusing on the individual.

Mental health and MHP

In a review of the literature, Secker (1998) alerts us to the tensions between definitions of mental health and MHP principles and practice. An examination of the literature on positive health, working at structural levels and the use of participatory methods, suggests an overall focus on individual approaches is the norm. A call is made for further work in the following three areas:

1. focus on quality of life and potential for health rather than on symptoms and deficits
2. forging links with the antipoverty movement to address inequalities
3. needs assessments that reflect service users' concerns.

Feelings

Gordon & Grant (1997) report on a study in secondary schools throughout Glasgow of adolescents aged $13\frac{1}{2}$–$14\frac{1}{2}$ years. Over 1500 anonymous questionnaires were completed and analysed. They asked what it felt like to be a young person developing psychologically, intellectually, socially and spiritually. The focus was on mental health rather than mental illness. The collected data give a valuable insight into the emotional world of teenagers. They also provide valuable information from an adolescent rather than an adult view of feelings, needs and aspirations. This in turn can inform interventions, which can assist the transition from childhood to young adult, when there is a higher risk of experiencing a range of mental health and social problems or being diagnosed as mentally ill. Picking up on the study's findings, Bryce (1997) recognizes the modest effect health services can have on the quality of mental health in a community. Instead there is a call for establishing a network of services that are flexible and adaptable, as the needs of young people change. The participants in the study identified stimulating and positive school experiences, a supportive family and, most importantly, friends and friendship as essential to their mental health and well-being.

High risk groups

The Health Care Bulletin published by the NHS Centre for Reviews and Dissemination (1997) provided a survey on the effectiveness of health service interventions. It focused on people who are likely to be at higher risk of developing mental health problems and included health promotion and prevention models. It identified the effective contribution of social support, training as well as problem solving and cognitive behavioural approaches. The survey also identified general characteristics of people who are at risk and is further confirmation of the correlation between dis-

advantage, stress vulnerability and the life cycle. These are listed in Box 7.2.

Service users

Collaboration with service users and their participation in key aspects of the planning and delivery of mental health services continue to improve (Rose et al 1998). The current government has made a commitment to supporting individuals who are mentally ill by providing extended services to cover a 24-hour period and in identifying the importance of intensive home support and assertive outreach initiatives. There is also a continued tension between the needs of people in crisis and the legislation that has to exist to protect both individuals and the public. Keeping people in hospital for extended periods is still considered to be detrimental to their overall well-being, but equally this provides some security for people who cannot manage to look after themselves in the community where they live. There are many examples of innovative and creative approaches to coping with mental illness and mental health problems. These are still too often considered within a medical framework and this places an enormous burden and role for voluntary and more informal organizations to cope with the demand that exists for support and therapy of some kind.

Quality framework

The HEA MHP Quality framework (HEA 1997) draws on existing evidence and presents a framework for measuring success to enable practitioners

---

Box 7.2 Some characteristics of people at high risk

Children

- ◆ Living in poverty
- ◆ Exhibiting behavioural difficulties
- ◆ Experiencing parental separation and divorce
- ◆ Families experiencing bereavement

Adults

- ◆ Undergoing divorce or separation
- ◆ Unemployed
- ◆ At risk of depression in pregnancy
- ◆ Experiencing bereavement
- ◆ Long term carers of people who are highly dependent

Box 7.3 Summary of effective interventions for MHP

◆ Promoting good social relationships, for example, through social skills and assertiveness training, as well as communication and relationship skills
◆ Developing effective coping skills, such as problem solving, cognitive skills and parenting skills
◆ Providing social support and making social changes: examples include changing school attitudes regarding bullying, home visits from health workers to support new parents, supporting bereaved families, supporting widows and carers
◆ Mass media campaigns supported by community activities can be a measurable impact on knowledge, attitudes and behavioral intentions

(HEA 1997, p 17)

to identify priorities and plan effective interventions. It provides selected references on effectiveness for programmes directed at preschool and school age children and adults. A summary of the available evidence drawing on the work collated by Tilford, Delaney & Vogels (1997) is set out in Box 7.3.

MAINSTREAM PRACTICE

Practitioners now need to assist in the process of integrating MHP into mainstream practice in key areas. There are some common features to draw on from an existing body of knowledge identified in this framework. There is a need to consider the potential for health gain that lies beyond the realm of the individual, to the social, organizational and environmental dimensions alluded to previously. This is still often unfamiliar territory for practitioners and one they will be increasingly expected to participate in, if the notion of collaboration with service users is more than rhetoric. At the level of primary care and mental health provision, primary care groups (PCGs), which include nurses

as equal participatory members with GPs, will be required to work at the front line of health care. The government has invested heavily in identifying 'health action zones' and single regeneration budget areas because there has for a long time been enough compelling evidence that links poverty, deprivation and unemployment as key indicators in mortality and morbidity and in terms of the underlying factors relevant to the incidence of mental illness and suicide.

The new practitioner is also in a position to assist in the development of appropriate evaluation tools and to enable research and evidence-based practice where it can be best targeted. MHP needs to be integrated more clearly in the models of care and case management being used and as a way of considering both consistent and creative approaches to care, treatment and rehabilitation (keys). The creation of a national standards framework for health care intervention and a Centre for Clinical Excellence provides another opportunity to clarify how best to care and provide treatment for people experiencing mental illness. Hopefully this will not obscure the problems, at national level, in terms of joint working arrangements between health and social services as this is an integral part of planning quality mental health services and interventions such as psychosocial assessment and care (DOH 1998c).

DEFINITIONS

There are a range of definitions, underpinned by theoretical analysis and evidence from practice. These are valuable starting points for the practitioner in attempting to understand and incorporate a MHP approach into practice. There is no one definition of mental health or its promotion and there are numerous examples to consider. Definitions of mental health are 'value loaded' and, as such, they determine the philosophy and practice of prevention, education and health promotion (MacDonald 1994). Similarly, the choice of a MHP definition will reflect the focus of personal, professional style and influence the choice of interventions (McCulloch & Boxer 1997).

A possible working definition is as follows:

Mental health promotion aims to enable people to manage life events, both predictable and unpredictable, by increasing self-esteem and a sense of well-being. It involves working directly with individuals, groups and communities, and also trying to influence the social, economic and environmental factors that can have an impact on mental health.
HEA website 1998

It may be more appropriate to modify a definition over time in view of local circumstances and priorities. This is a process that has to include dialogue with your constituency: client group, carers, peers and other disciplines. This should ensure a comprehensive definition, which can enable practical action in a specific locality. A clarification of roles

and contributions in implementing MHP can also assist in evaluation processes. Through the process of formulating definitions and working with them, it is important to consider community-orientated interventions as well as individual focused activity.

It would be relatively easy to take a solely preventive definition and view of the world as part of MHP. For example, another HEA definition describes MHP as 'a kind of immunisation, working to strengthen the resilience of individuals, families, organizations and communities' (1998). This notion of MHP as a form of 'coping inoculation' is not new. Protecting the individual and community from the threats of stress is a key component of psychosocial interventions. Likewise, identifying and developing coping strategies with at-risk groups can have significant impact on

Table 7.1 Approaches to health promotion: the example of mental health

Approach	Aims	Methods	Worker/client relationship
Medical	To identify those at risk from disease	Primary health care consultation, e.g. detection of depression	Tends to be expert led with passive, conforming client
Behaviour change	To encourage individuals to take responsibility for their own health and choose healthier lifestyles	Persuasion through one to one advice Information, e.g. medication, compliance	Expert-led Dependent client May have victim-blaming ideology
Educational	To increase knowledge and skills about healthy lifestyles	Information Exploration of attitudes through small group work Development of skills, e.g. postnatal depression group	May also be expert led May also involve client in negotiation of issues for discussion
Empowerment	To work with clients or communities to meet their perceived needs	Advocacy Negotiation Networking Facilitation, e.g. user group running an employment initiative	Health promoter is facilitator Client becomes empowered
Social change	To address inequalities in health based on class, race, gender, geography	Development of organizational policy, e.g. hospital policy, on advocacy Legislation, e.g. on welfare entitlement for user involvement	Entails social regulation and can be a top-down approach

admission and relapse. However, a broader view is required to consider the role and influence the practitioner can have at the social and economic levels. Having looked briefly at theory and definitions, the different approaches to promoting health are clearer. This can be demonstrated in more detail utilizing the work of Naidoo & Wills (2000).

APPROACHES TO MHP

Table 7.1 lists some approaches to health promotion. For the sake of brevity the table does not take into account some of the more complex areas practitioners engage with. For example, we would acknowledge that medication compliance is managed by drawing on a range of approaches, some of which have inherent conflict. Empowerment for a voice hearer support group may not sit easily with demands for medication under the legislative framework of the Mental Health Act. However, many of the approaches, aims and methods described are familiar to those in practice. Indeed information giving, negotiation skills and empowerment all feature highly as core competencies for mental health practitioners. Such skills are also valuable in the field of health promotion and in the pursuit of MHP. Thus, practitioners are already engaged and involved in activity that, if taken further, can contribute to promoting mental health. A step in this direction is to look at the bigger picture. To do this we will examine the policy context for MHP to help identify opportunities for influencing the social change agenda.

THE REGENERATION POLICY CONTEXT

Boxer & McCulloch (1996), in a review of mental health policy, consider it as a potential vehicle for change and diversity. This is truer several years on with even greater changes and opportunities for practitioners. There is a range of relevant policy with regeneration at its focus. Much of this is captured in the Social Exclusion Unit's recent report: Building Britain together: a national strategy for neighbourhood renewal (DOH 1998a). This sets out a range of interventions to reduce poor housing, crime, social division and exclusion. The report provides a range of good practice examples where integrated approaches have had positive effects on employment, training, housing and community safety. Essentially it is an 'area-based' agenda to improve opportunities in pockets of deprivation, ill health and social and economic inequality. There is a specific reference to people suffering from mental health problems with emphasis on supported accommodation and assertive outreach. It describes some key 'structural tasks' including:

- investing in people, not just in buildings
- involving communities, not 'parachuting in' solutions
- ensuring mainstream policies work for the poorest neighbourhoods through integrated approaches.

This bottom-up approach envisages a partnership arrangement between government policy and its local implementation by agencies and locally inspired solutions to problems. Much of this calls for a community development approach to tackling deep-rooted social problems. Such themes were also raised in the previous administration's Variations in health report (DOH 1995). However, this provided guidance on interventions solely within the NHS to address differences in health. There is now a new ideological position, to refer to them as inequalities in health status and to look further than health services to meet them. To achieve this, a series of national programmes are to be to implemented. These are aimed at tackling the causes of social exclusion and include:

- *unemployment*—a 'New Deal' programme to provide training and employment opportunities
- *benefits*—welfare reform to target benefits and offer incentives for training and employment
- *crime and drugs*—establishing a national 10-year drugs strategy
- *young people*—establishing education action zones (EAZ) to improve educational attainment

◆ *housing*—the release of capital receipts for new projects
◆ *sustainable economic development*—supporting the role of regional development agencies
◆ *public health*—Our healthier nation (OHN) (DOH 1998b) has a key emphasis on reducing health inequalities.

All of the above are relevant to the client group of specialist mental health services and to the overall mental health of the general population. Social exclusion is a key issue for people with mental health problems and for their fellow citizens living in areas of deprivation. Practitioners need to get to understand what these policies and programmes will mean to their local community and clients and see how they can make some impact in the area of social action as well as in 'therapeutic' partnerships. Exclusion and isolation also occur in the peripheral estates of towns and cities and in rural communities. These have not been spared the same problems and social conditions of their urban counterparts. The problems may be on a smaller scale but they remain just as significant. The example of the regeneration agenda described below is very 'urban', yet there are lessons for us all in how we can become involved.

URBAN REGENERATION AND MENTAL HEALTH

The King's Fund (1997) report on London's mental health identified significant pressures on mental health services in the capital. The call was for more resources and targeting them on the care and treatment of the most severely mentally ill. One of the potential consequences of this is the low priority given to prevention and MHP. To resolve this and maximize opportunities in the new policy environment a review of urban initiatives was commissioned by the King's Fund. The review, Urban regeneration and mental health in London (Hogget et al 1997) examined how community regeneration schemes can play a key role in addressing social and psychological well-being. Social well-being is defined as concern for the

quality of the social fabric, the strength and diversity of local social networks and the health of the social environment.

In order to tackle social and economic problems previous administrations have established a range of regeneration support schemes. The most recent is the Single Regeneration Budget (SRB). This is allocated to regions on formulae based on indicators of deprivation. Schemes run over 5 to 7 years and tend to cover projects such as employment and retraining, improving housing stock, developing new businesses and community projects. Increasingly community development methods and approaches are being seen as crucial to the implementation of schemes if they are to be 'owned' by local people. So far, there has been limited health input to SRB nationally. The report calls for mental health to become part of the wider regeneration agenda. A variety of strategies, which can promote the well-being of communities with a clear mental health dimension, are suggested. These include:

◆ promoting community safety schemes
◆ antipoverty campaigns
◆ bottom-up community economic regeneration
◆ prevention—dealing with bullying, parenting skills, recovery from abuse, stress and anxiety management
◆ training and employment opportunities for people with mental health problems
◆ reducing teenage pregnancy
◆ tackling drug and alcohol misuse.

Note the similarity between these suggested strategies and the 'high risk groups' identified by the Health Care Bulletin (1997). Similarities in the evidence base and the regeneration agenda are starting to become clearer. What is also evident is that planning of interventions should not take place in a clinical vacuum. The key to them all is partnership working. Action in the field of MHP and drawing on the regeneration agenda require the support and cooperation of other groups and agencies. The practitioner should sustain and maintain a range of contacts. For example, inpatient services should forge links with black and ethnic minority groups and organizations. Community mental health teams should be well versed in interagency community forums and tenants' groups and have good contacts with housing and supported-housing schemes. In order to highlight the opportunities that regeneration and other significant policy can bring to MHP, examples of possible interventions are set out in Table 7.2.

There is also scope within other policy such as that developed by drug action teams and youth offending teams. The role of PCGs cannot be overlooked. They too must be assisted in engaging with a regeneration agenda; it has significant implications for people who use primary care. We suspect they would be keen on looking at methods and interventions that assisted them in their management of people with lower levels of psychiatric morbidity and the emotional distress of their practice population. We will now discuss what resources are available to help support MHP interventions.

INFORMATION AND RESOURCES

Information is not simply the handing out of leaflets or advice. Information needs vary and issues of age, race, culture and gender need to be considered. The process by which information is developed, organized, controlled and disseminated is equally important. Information produced with, rather than for, users and carers will be valued in different ways. Also, its very ownership, production and distribution can be an MHP intervention. For example, drawing on the regeneration policy previously discussed we could, in collaboration with users, establish a user group website, user or carer magazine, or user guidelines for housing services on discharge. This could pull on resources available through the SRB, New Deal and local healthy-living centre. As well as the obvious outcome of credible information, choice and empowerment, it could also provide a forum

Policy	MHP intervention
Education action zones	Work with schools on antibullying policy; emotional literacy; help other professionals support parents, e.g. in managing difficult behaviour Encourage use of the school space out of hours for self-help and user groups
Health action zones	Involve users and carers in need assessment and quality review Work with black and ethnic community groups to ascertain their mental health needs Influence the mental health components of healthy-living centres
New Deal	Check out the possibilities and put forward proposals for employment and training schemes in day services Identify training opportunities with adult education and service users
Our healthier nation	Devise practical guidelines for supporting self-help Contribute to community safety: make buildings and venues women and child friendly Ensure there are positive images of black and minority ethnic groups, sexuality, disability in your public areas and services Propose joint training with community groups, user groups, carers and professional staff
Single Regeneration Budget	Ensure schemes address the needs of homeless and rootless Work with other agencies on antiracist policy and support for victims, e.g. with housing services Support community groups to develop projects that address 'at risk' groups; support credit unions and community enterprise

Table 7.2 MHP intervention policies

for individuals to be more involved in service development, commissioning and allocation of resources. Partnership with community forums on community safety, women's groups, training and enterprise could all become available. This normalization approach to information is also important so as not to ghettoize mental health to minority issues. This process would ensure that partnership meant inclusion and not tokenism.

What would be the practitioner's role in this process? There is a range of possibilities. There would be a need to become familiar with local opportunities, policy and health strategy. The practitioner could access this via local community workers or existing projects. Options would have to be discussed with the practitioner's client group to avoid an expert-driven agenda. Practitioners would need to check out what they have got in mind, what possibilities they are aware of. This would draw on their strengths and resources. Practitioners could also secure approval, champion credibility and identify practical support such as venues and contacts. Practitioners could also access research and evaluation through their own service, the health authority, local authority or universities. If client groups decided on a course of action, practitioners could offer contacts, meetings and suggest they involve their service at management level, to increase the likelihood of success and support. Finally, practitioners could link other clients into the process and look at how the venture could be replicated in other parts of the service. This facilitation role does not have to be intensive. The ideal of partnerships is that skills, resources and time are shared. The outcome is a benefit for all partners and in this example could result in a user-led resource.

One area in which specific information in relation to MHP has been developed is that produced as part of World Mental Health Day. Practitioners could see this as a positive step toward bringing the information and regeneration agenda together.

World Mental Health Day—'Positive images, positive steps'

World Mental Health Day (WMHD) was established by the World Federation for Mental Health and is cosponsored by WHO. It takes place on 10 October each year and the HEA coordinates a campaign in England on behalf of the Department of Health. The 1998 campaign 'Positive images, positive steps' followed its predecessor with themes of challenging discrimination and increasing social inclusion. Four target groups particularly likely to experience discrimination and be excluded were highlighted:

1. older people
2. mental health service users
3. black and minority ethnic groups
4. lesbians and gay men.

Mental health practitioners need to employ antidiscriminatory and antioppressive approaches with the client group they serve. They also need to recognize the wider picture in terms of the overall population and the impact that negative views and stereotypes can have on the groups listed above. Practitioners have a valuable role to play in taking forward the key campaign messages. However, this role needs to be seen as long term rather than as limited input to a once a year event. A plan of action is required that is coordinated and takes place in partnership with other groups and organizations for a genuine and sustained commitment to MHP throughout the year.

The key campaign messages of WMHD are:

◆ Mental health concerns everyone.
◆ Challenging discriminatory attitudes (ageism, racism, homophobia and myths and stereotypes about mental health service users) is a positive step for mental health.
◆ Everyone can take positive steps to improve their mental well-being and that of others.
◆ People with mental health problems have a valuable contribution to make.

To assist the practitioner, as well as other professionals, community groups and the general population, a range of resources for WMHD have been developed. The range of material and support material available, is designed to be used all year round. They include posters, postcards, books and various fact sheets to photocopy. As well as information on problems, these resources suggest different ways of working and provide contact details for national organizations. Practitioners should familiarize themselves with such material, adapting them to local circumstances. As discussed previously this approach should include the ideas, views and input of the groups they are aimed at.

MHP fact sheets

Fact sheets are available for:

◆ mental health service users
◆ older people
◆ young people
◆ sexual identity
◆ black and minority ethnic groups.

The service user fact sheet provides information on stigma and discrimination and suggests a range of ways to work with users of services to promote mental health. These include a set of principles, policy change and supporting skill development and community involvement. Ideas to challenge stigma include: forming a group to challenge negative media reporting (see the Schizophrenia Media Agency in Further Reading), seminars and debating forums, use of positive images and the use of writing, theatre and drama workshops to combat discrimination.

The older people fact sheet provides statistical information on the health and social needs of older people. It addresses the effects of stereotyping, isolation, reduced income, physical ill health, carers and caring as well as depression and dementia. Strengthening social support networks is seen as key to promoting mental health for older people.

The fact sheet for young people provides information about three broad age groups: 4–11 years, 12–16 years and 16–24 years. As well as basic facts on mental health and social problems in young people, it provides a range of approaches to take. These include: personal and social education, positive policies for behaviour and bullying, peer support, mentoring, volunteering schemes, clubs and activities, youth counselling, creative activity, support for families and work with the media. There are also specific worksheets available for young people to increase understanding

and awareness of their own feelings and those of other people.

The fact sheet on MHP and sexual identity provides advice and information on 'coming out'. It also highlights the importance of services and organizations not assuming heterosexuality as the norm. Training, development and education of staff, particularly within mental health services is seen as one way of tackling prejudice and discrimination.

There are four fact sheets on MHP for African–Caribbean, South Asian, Irish, and Chinese and Vietnamese people. There is a general call for health and social care professionals to gain better insight of these specific communities as well as the need to support self-help and social support. There are clear training implications for practitioners and a need to understand how perceptions of health and mental health are culturally determined.

Community action for mental health

Another valuable resource for practitioners is the case study approach of 21 innovative projects working with a range of groups on mental health in England, Scotland and Wales. This was produced for WMHD by the HEA (1998). Examples range from developing a district wide interagency strategy for MHP to a women's mental health and well-being event. Guidelines about consulting locally, working in partnership and methods of measuring the impact of projects are set out. Contact details about the individual projects are provided to share good practice. The headings below are used to describe the existing projects and can be used to assist in evaluation. They can also be used as a preintervention checklist to inform thinking and establish a case:

◆ *Background to MHP project/initiative*—what is the policy context nationally and locally, why and how has the idea come about? Who drives it?
◆ *Rationale*—what is the evidence base, what does local health strategy/policy say about this aspect of need?
◆ *Target group*—what and who are the initiative or intervention aimed at?

◆ *Consultation, partnership and alliances*—what team of players are involved, what will they offer?

◆ *Principles and aims*—what are the MHP principles that guide the initiative, what will it set out to do?

◆ *Timescale*—over what period will it take place and are there any specific milestones?

◆ *How it works and activities undertaken*—description and résumé of progress.

◆ *Evaluation, success and feedback*—methods used, quantitative–qualitative, dissemination of findings and outcomes.

Other resources

Internet and MHP

The Internet can offer an inexhaustible range of views and information and is increasingly being used by the user and voluntary sector. Another interesting link is how information technology features highly in the range of new government policies. Here is further opportunity to exploit such policy and resources for MHP. A good example of a user-focused website is that produced by MadNation. This is a mental health user website for people working together for social justice and human rights in mental health. It aims to present the 'creativity and thoughtfulness' of users worldwide. Content ranges from essays, reports, personal stories and research as well as a message link and chat room. It also has a mailing list, which can be subscribed to. MadNation describes itself as prohuman and prosocial justice rather than antipsychiatry. As its information sheets explain, the belief and opinions within the mental health activist community are very diverse. This is an important point and user sites should not be deemed antipsychiatry and dismissed accordingly by practitioners and the mental health mainstream.

It is important to look creatively and laterally in terms of other information and good practice resources. Health promotion and education departments and agencies can be a useful source. There is also considerable material from the voluntary, user and carer sector. Valuable lessons can be learned from public information campaigns in areas such as substance misuse, sexual health and public safety programmes. It is important for practitioners not to limit their information and resource needs to mental illness information.

> **Practice Point: How would you organize an activity for WMHD, who would you involve, how would you involve them and what would the focus be?**

Having looked at regeneration, the policy context and resources to support MHP we will now examine the more familiar territory of prevention.

PREVENTION

Mental illness prevention and suicide prevention have been highlighted as a target by the World Health Organization (WHO 1991), Health of the nation (DOH 1993) and its successor, Our healthier nation (DOH 1998b). All targets tend to focus on people with an established mental illness, although the measures to reduce mental illness and suicide reside in social as well as the psychiatric domain. WHO defines prevention as to 'equip people to deal with the distressing conditions associated with cultural and social change in society' (WHO 1991).

> WHO target 12—Reducing mental disorder and suicide
>
> *By the year 2000, there should be a sustained and continuing reduction in the prevalence of mental disorders, an improvement in the quality of all people with such disorders, and a reversal of the rising trends in suicide and attempted suicide.*

The WHO sees the target being achieved through a range of measures including:

◆ tackling unemployment and social isolation
◆ measures to equip people with coping strategies to deal with distressing or stressful events and conditions
◆ formal and informal support for carers

- a focus on improving access to measures that support carers, both formal and informal
- development of comprehensive community-based mental health services with a greater involvement of primary health care.

There are also calls for an improvement in the quality of service provision to maintain the human rights and quality of life for people with a mental illness. More specifically a request is made for educational programmes to strengthen coping skills and preventive intervention for people facing crisis, unemployment or social isolation. WHO also sees initiatives to strengthen formal and informal social networks and living and working environments that break down social isolation. The specific needs of vulnerable groups including the unemployed are highlighted.

Much of what was proposed under WHO target 12 is within the mental health target as part of Our healthier nation (DOH 1998b). As well as a specific target on reducing suicide it also proposes a national contract to improve mental health at three levels: what government and national players can do, what local players and communities can do and finally what people themselves can do. Newton (1988, 1992) in a comprehensive review highlights three areas to address in the prevention of mental illness. These are:

1. targeting vulnerable individuals—a medical model for prevention
2. helping people to take control over their own lives
3. making maximum use of natural, voluntary and community support networks.

The first of these is clearly a role of good quality mental health services. Yet, we can go beyond a medical model of prevention. The practitioner could look at an existing client group and identify some of the risk factors associated with them. For example, are they going through some life crisis such as unemployment or bereavement? In this case, the client may need some practical welfare rights advocacy. Part of the practitioner's role is to have developed a good range and high quality of community contacts to make this happen. This can also move us away from faceless referrals on

to unknown and untested groups and organizations. Knowing and trusting the credibility, flexibility and limitations of a range of crisis alternatives provides a useful toolbox for the practitioner. Time invested in establishing such contacts will be well rewarded. This is also true of the other two areas described by Newton (1998, 1992). The second can lead to interventions that empower people, through self-help and self-determination. This requires a degree of risk taking and in some respects deskilling by the practitioner. The final area calls for an infrastructure of social support. It is because the latter has been so damaged over the past decades that we feel this is where effort should be placed.

Suicide prevention

The National Confidential Inquiry (Appleby 1997) study of 479 cases found that 26% of people who commit suicide have been in contact with mental health services in the year before death. The majority of cases were judged to be at no or low immediate risk at the time of their contact with services. The inquiry highlights the importance of compliance, not just in terms of medication compliance. Rather, the relationship between patients and services and patients' view of what their main problems are should be a priority. One avenue for work here is on the social support and network structures, the social assets people may have at their disposal and increasing these assets. Another is the development of protocols and tools for services and agencies that meet people when they are at a 'no or low immediate risk'. One mechanism is through primary care to detect mental health problems before they become more serious.

THE PRIMARY CARE TOOLKIT

Compiled by Armstrong (1997) the Primary mental health care toolkit is a flexible resource to assist non-specialist staff such as practice nurses improve the assessment and management of people with depression and anxiety within primary care. It provides a systematic approach to a range of mental health problems featuring templates on depression, anxiety, schizophrenia, dementia and alcohol. There are a range of validated assessment and screening tools, management advice, an audit mechanism and set of resources for further help. Practitioners should become familiar with the material and look at how it could be adapted and used with voluntary and self-help groups. A local example is the Dealing with depression resource pack developed by Young & McCulloch (1996), which is designed for generic health workers, individuals and members of support groups.

Having looked at prevention we now need to consider the role and good practice within the voluntary, user and educational sector to the promotion of mental health. This should help the practitioner identify routes in to joint endeavours at the levels previously discussed.

MHP AND THE VOLUNTARY SECTOR

The Sainsbury Centre report Down your street (1998) examined models of extended community support services for people with mental health problems. It looked at five services that provide social and practical support to people with severe mental illness in their own homes. The report highlighted several features that are relevant to MHP for practitioners:

◆ Practical, emotional and social support by voluntary sector services can relieve pressure on specialist services.
◆ The subjective improvements in the quality of life for users is an important outcome.
◆ The voluntary sector should be recognized as 'professional' rather than 'amateur' service providers.

These aspects are also crucial to the way in which practitioners can enhance their work in the field of MHP. Partnership working, respect for alternative approaches and an appreciation of quality of life outcomes for users are all vital prerequisites. The practitioner can respect and support the voluntary sector contribution and share this with colleagues and other disciplines. The days of territorial boundaries are over, and such an approach can only hasten their demise.

USER-FOCUSED MONITORING

Users and carers can play a significant role in the quality monitoring of services, the development of strategies and policy change in mental health. One recent example is The Sainsbury Centre's study, In our experience (Rose et al 1998). It illustrates how people with a mental illness can have more of a voice in decisions about the mental health services that they experience. Through training and support users acted as evaluators and interviewees in the study. It concludes: 'We took as our starting point the view that interviews with people with serious and enduring mental health problems can give rise to fruitful and valid findings which have implications for policy' (Rose et al 1998, p 5). The overall results revealed a high percentage expressing satisfaction with mental health professionals, especially community psychiatric nurses (CPNs) and social workers. There are useful lessons in terms of the process and for agencies to take user-focused monitoring seriously.

As with many initiatives in this field, the potential strengths and opportunities for skill development have been employed. A deficit model of mental illness can further exclude service users and lose a valuable contribution to service changes. Leader (1995) provides an example of a strengths model for people who want to develop their own care plans and support networks. He has developed an information pack for service users to enable them to develop their support networks and a personalized plan of care. As well as a range of useful checklists to inform discharge planning there are pointers for practitioners to encourage empowerment.

Users and research and information

The Mental Health Foundation's 'strategies for living' project is a 3-year programme. It aims to document and disseminate people's strategies for living with mental distress. It is run and staffed by service users and ex-users. It is undertaking a qualitative research study about user views and experiences of different therapies and treatments. A user-led resource will be developed to encourage users to undertake their own research locally. This will be backed up with support, information and training. The project also provides a newsletter and has established a network of professional allies to the project.

Users have helped shape a needs assessment tool developed by Smith (1998) called DISC (developing individual services in the community framework), which identifies components of comprehensive mental health services. This provides a framework to identify what needs to be in place to meet a range of health and social care needs. As she points out, 'the multifaceted nature of people's needs means that mental health care is only partly about statutory services. Many of the factors that contribute to an individual's well-being—good housing, a job, adequate income—are not, or cannot be provided by mental health services alone' (Smith 1998, p 154). This makes a more rounded assessment of need all the more important and one the practitioner should consider when looking at more traditional accounts.

Users and advocacy

The United Kingdom Advocacy Network (UKAN) is a federation of independent patients' councils, advocacy projects and user forums for mental health service users. There are 10 UK regions offering advice, networking, training, lobbying and providing education and a national voice to promote user issues and equal opportunities.

MHP EDUCATION AND TRAINING

It is not clear how any changes proposed to the role of mental health practitioner will impact on an educational and training agenda, as an increased role by health authorities in leading and funding nurse education might increase the chance of some cohesion, from primary to forensic care. There are many ways of accessing health and social care education and common sense has to

prevail, rather than continued arguments about nursing's position in academic study. Approaches that can link health and education, with a community focus, is a necessity. In the book we wrote (McCulloch & Boxer 1997), one chapter was devoted to an examination of an education and training framework for MHP. The idea that lifelong or inclusive learning was essential to positive mental health has two strands, one being the notion of social action and social inclusion and the other the idea that therapeutic relationships or partnerships do not occur in a vacuum but require commitment to a user-focused perspective that is underpinned by antioppressive practice.

MHP PRACTICE

It is important to differentiate two possible methodologies (Table 7.3) available for practitioners (McCulloch & Boxer 1997). The first of these is a standard approach drawing on existing structures and systems to implement mental health policy hidebound by a medical and legislative tradition. The second is an MHP methodology in which these boundaries are broadened to a role that includes social action as part of good mental health practice (Dominelli 1997). The emphasis is to increase the scope of practice rather than a call for significant resource shifts to the field of health promotion and prevention. A further movement would be to engage non-psychiatric services in the approach, thereby contributing to the broader structural and social dimensions that can influence the capacity of all citizens, not just those with mental illness.

What does this mean at the practical level? It is about taking those few positive steps from the familiar territory of practice and widening horizons. For example, Copsey (1997) studied the multifaith communities in the London borough of Newham. 'Faith communities' refers to a range of world religions such as Christian, Jewish, Muslim, Hindu, Buddhist, Sikh and others. One key issue was the perception of mental health workers. Many of them saw religious beliefs as too complex to deal with and beliefs themselves actually contributing to mental health problems. Putting

Table 7.3 Traditional and MHP methodologies

Method	Traditional method	MHP
Assessment involving the clients and their carers	Inviting to meetings Professionally led and focused Literature produced by professionals	Actively involving advocacy services Supporting user-focused approaches Development of information by and for users/carers
An understanding of the needs and perceptions of the local community and positive efforts to promote awareness	Mapping out the high profile groups and organizations Public meetings Professional/voluntary forums Literature produced by professionals	Mapping out all mental health stakeholders Focus groups Community-led assessment of needs, recommendations and solutions Community inspired/produced resources
A conscious effort to deal sensitively with issues of race, creed and gender	Training for staff on culture and race Equal opportunity policy Use of interpretation and translation services	Antioppressive training for all staff Proactive attempts to involve marginalized individuals and communities in methods described above Encourage support groups for minority ethnic users

such assumptions of personal beliefs and spiritual practice aside, practitioners have to acknowledge there are significant religious communities throughout the UK. Moreover, the range of non-Christian faiths is inevitably higher within multicultural areas. These tend to be in areas of poverty and deprivation with higher psychiatric morbidity—the very areas of economic and social exclusion we have been discussing.

Copsey found that the Western worldview and medical model of psychiatry do not sit comfortably with the world and belief systems of faith communities. There was also concern that people found hospitals and day services centres to be places in which it was made very difficult to express their faith. Many of the people and faiths understood the more severe mental health problems as having a spiritual cause and therefore required a religious response. The recommendations included: an improved dialogue between mental health professionals and the different faith communities to break down taboos on both sides, meeting with communities of different faiths in their territory and on their terms, and workers learning and appreciating the belief systems of the clients they support. There is a clear training

element for the services here. Community development approaches would also support improvements in this area.

Practice Point: Often it is a simple matter of a ward or service being sensitive to religious festivals and events. This has practical implications for attendance at clinics, case conferences and appointments.

Action in the above example is not about an immediate intervention, nor does it require the wholesale switch of scarce mainstream resources to the general community thereby missing out on the most mentally needy. Instead it requires a commitment to contact and a willingness to learn from different facets and viewpoints of the community. Inpatient services do not leave social 'structures' and processes behind when they close their doors. For example, Williams & Lindley (1996) emphasize the importance of social inequalities, power and powerlessness within 'expert' mental health services. They describe how they tried to gain the trust of patients in establishing a patients' council

DISCUSSION QUESTIONS

1. Construct a series of counter arguments to accusations of MHP being a low priority or not relevant to clinical work.
2. What interagency partnerships would you need to plan, run and evaluate a programme of events for World Mental Health day?
3. How could you work with service users and the voluntary sector to identify vulnerable and at risk groups for prevention and mental health promotion?
4. Think about how you and your colleagues could influence the regeneration of communities. How could you get mental health on that agenda, what help would you require?
5. Would a mentally healthy community deal better with mental ill health than an 'unhealthy' one?

FURTHER READING

McCulloch G F, Boxer J 1997 Mental health promotion: policy, practice and partnerships. Baillière Tindall, London
A practice-focused introduction to MHP offering a range of examples and options to test out.

Naidoo J, Wills J 2000 Health promotion: foundations for practice, 2nd edn. Baillière Tindall, London
An overview of health promotion theory, influences on practice and effectiveness.

Read J, Wallcroft J 1995 Guidelines on equal opportunities and mental health. MIND, London
An examination of oppression, its relationship with mental distress and a range of recommendations with a focus on mental health service delivery.

The Clifford Beers Foundation was established in 1996. This international charity publishes a journal, organizes conferences and has a website:
http://www.soc.staffs.sc.uk/~cmtrmk/cbfl.htm

The HEA website provides details of the world mental health campaign and a set of frequently asked questions to justify action in this area. Contact:
http://www.1stWebSite.com/hea/mentalhealth.

The Schizophrenia Media Agency campaigns to ensure people with a diagnosis of schizophrenia get a fair deal from the media. It offers training, information and guidelines for media coverage. Contact:
SMA@hector4.demon.co.uk

in a secure psychiatric hospital. If we are to be genuine in our commitment to MHP then the social inequalities both within services and beyond them need to be challenged and changed. The recent inquiry into inequalities in health (Acheson 1998) makes a range of recommendations. The measures and policies required to meet these recommendations span structural change and action at the individual level. MHP and the mental health practitioner can contribute to this new agenda.

SUMMARY

The HEA and the DOH have high expectations for what MHP and WMHD can achieve: reducing the incidence and severity of mental health problems, reducing the cost of mental health to individuals, carers, employers and communities, supporting healthy lifestyle choices and adopting 'effective roles in society'. We would endorse such an endeavour. Unfortunately, not everyone wants to adopt an effective role in society. We have generations of people in poverty and social and economic exclusion. This is the context within which

we are expected to address an MHP agenda. This makes work at the structural as well as individual levels so important. This focus is not an easy one. It is safer and more tested to work on preventive programmes. However, for long term changes we need to address the social process and structural factors. This is a more messy business. Roles may not be as clear cut and our contribution appear diluted in the process of partnership working. Here, though, lies a strength rather than a weakness. Time is a scarce resource for an overstretched profession. You cannot be expected to tackle MHP alone and so should invest as much energy in collaborative working as is possible. Sometimes you may be on the edges of an initiative or activity, sometimes your role will be more integral; each is valuable and necessary to the promotion of mental health.

REFERENCES

Acheson D 1998 Independent inquiry into inequalities in health report. The Stationery Office, London

Appleby L 1997 National confidential inquiry into suicide and homicide by people with mental illness progress report. HMSO, London

Armstrong E 1997 The Primary mental health care toolkit. Department of Health, London

Boxer J, McCulloch G 1996 Mental health policy and practice In: Gastrell P, Edwards J (eds) Community health nursing frameworks for practice. Baillière Tindall, London

Bryce G 1997 Caring for teenagers in the 21st century: young voices matter. In: Gordon J, Grant G (eds) How we feel: an insight into the emotional world of teenagers. Jessica Kingsley, London, ch 21

Copsey N 1997 Keeping faith: the provision of community health services within a multi-faith context. The Sainsbury Centre for Mental Health, London

DOH (Department of Health) 1993 Health of the nation: mental illness key area handbook. HMSO, London

DOH (Department of Health) 1995 Variations in health: what can the Department of Health and the NHS do? HMSO, London

DOH (Department of Health) 1998a Building Britain together: a national strategy for neighbourhood renewal. HMSO, London

DOH (Department of Health) 1998b Our healthier nation. The Stationery Office, London

DOH (Department of Health) 1998c Modernising health and social services: national priorities guidance 1999/00–2001/02. HMSO, London

Dominelli L 1997 Anti-racist social work. 2nd edn. BASW Macmillan, London

Gordon J, Grant G (eds) 1997 How we feel: an insight into the emotional world of teenagers. Jessica Kingsley, London

Health Care Bulletin 1997 Effective health care, mental health promotion in high risk groups. NHS Centre for Reviews and Dissemination 3(3): University of York, York

HEA (Health Education Authority) 1997 Mental health promotion: a quality framework. Health Education Authority, London

HEA (Health Education Authority) 1998 Community action for mental health. Health Education Authority, London

Hogget P, Stewart M, Razzaque K, Barker I 1997 Urban regeneration and mental health in London. King's Fund, London

King's Fund 1997 London's mental health: the report to the King's Fund 1997 Commission. King's Fund, London

Leader A 1995 Direct power: a resource pack for people who want to develop their own care plans and support networks. Pavilion Publishing/MIND, London

McCulloch G F, Boxer J 1997 Mental health promotion: policy, practice and partnerships. Baillière Tindall, London

MacDonald G 1994 Promoting mental health? Health Education Authority, London

MacDonald G, O'Hara K 1998 Ten elements of mental health, its promotion and demotion: implications for practice. Society of Health Education and Health Promotion Specialists, Glasgow

MadNation http://www.madnation.org/FAQMN.htm

Naidoo J, Wills J 2000 Health promotion: foundations for practice, 2nd edn. Baillière Tindall, London

Newton J 1988 Preventing mental illness. Routledge, London

Newton J 1992 Preventing mental illness in practice. Routledge, London

Read J, Wallcroft J 1995 Guidelines on equal opportunities and mental health. MIND, London

Rose D, Ford R, Lindley P, Gawith L and the KCW Mental Health Monitoring Users' Group 1998 In our experience: user-focused monitoring of mental health services in Kensington and Chelsea and Westminster Health Authority. The Sainsbury Centre for Mental Health, London

Sainsbury Centre 1998 Down your street. The Sainsbury Centre for Mental Health, London

Secker J 1998 Current conceptualizations of mental health and mental health promotion. Health Education Research 13(1):57–66

Sheffield Health Promotion 1996 Policy paper on health promotion. Sheffield Health, Sheffield

Smith H 1998 Needs assessment in mental health services; the DISC framework. Journal of Public Health Medicine 20(2):154–160

Tilford S, Delaney F, Vogels M 1997 Review of the effectiveness of mental health promotion interventions. Health Education Authority, London

Tudor K 1996 Mental health promotion: paradigms and practice. Routledge, London

WHO 1991 Health for all targets: European health for all, series 1, p 53. WHO, Geneva

Williams J, Lindley P 1996 Working with mental health service users to change mental health services. Journal of Community and Applied Social Psychology 61:14

Young S, McCulloch G 1996 Dealing with depression: a resource pack for working with people who suffer from depression. North Derbyshire Health Authority Chesterfield.

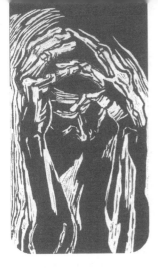

Chapter Eight

Cognitive behavioural interventions

Sue Marshall

AIMS

- ◆ To put cognitive behavioural therapy (CBT) into a context reflecting the move toward clinical governance and the promotion of evidence-based practice.
- ◆ To outline the historical origins of the therapy and show how it developed into an integrated approach to understanding human behaviour
- ◆ To illustrate the core themes of CBT by describing the nature of some of its essential components
- ◆ To outline how to carry out an assessment and how to structure ongoing therapy, describing some of the 'tools' that may be used when using CBT as an approach to working with people

KEY ISSUES

Collaborative, active, problem-centred and educational process

Techniques developed from the behavioural and cognitive schools of therapy

Theoretical underpinnings of cognitive behavioural therapy

Assessment as a critical first step

Enabling the client to overcome a range of mental health difficulties

Providing individuals with an 'inoculation'

INTRODUCTION

A first class service (DoH 1998) describes an NHS in which clinicians are urged to adopt routinely those practices that have an evidence base that demonstrates effectiveness. 'Cognitive behavioural therapy' or CBT has become a generic name for a group of therapies that have such a base.

A national review of psychological therapies showed CBT to have demonstrable effect with a range of both physical and mental health difficulties (DoH 1996)

Prior to this review the efficacy of CBT had been demonstrated in connection with a range of psychological difficulties, for example in helping adults and children who experience self-control problems (Meichenbaum & Goodman 1971, Novaco 1975), helping those who have suffered a traumatic event that has left them with difficulties in coping (Foa, Rothbaum & Murdoch 1991), those who suffer with depression (Biram & Wilson 1981), or those who suffer with anxiety-related difficulties (Salkovskis & Warwick 1986). It has been shown to be more effective than alternative therapies in the treatment of these and other psychological difficulties (Foa, Rothbaum & Murdoch 1991, McCullough 1991, Morse et al. 1991, Rush et al 1977).

More recently this therapeutic approach has been used in working with people with severe and enduring mental illness (Fowler, Garety & Kuipers 1995), working with people who suffer chronic pain (Turk 1996) and with children and families (Johnson 1996).

A DEFINITION OF COGNITIVE BEHAVIOURAL THERAPY

Cognitive behavioural therapy has been variously described (Blackburn & Davidson 1990, Dryden & Golden 1986, Meichenbaum 1977, Moorey 1996, Newell & Dryden 1991). A definitive description is elusive but the underpinning and definitive characteristic for all types of CBT is that cognitions are the mediating factor in human behaviour and that people are constructivists who think actively about the world. It is best viewed as

representing a theoretical approach that encompasses a range of specific techniques.

Today the term 'cognitive behavioural therapy' is used generically to describe a large number of therapies, all of which share the characteristics identified above. Three broad schools exist.

Ellis described rational emotive therapy (RET) in the early 1960s (Ellis 1962). This approach focuses on the irrational appraisals individuals make in response to events and the beliefs people have about their appraisal. These beliefs give rise to the difficulties experienced by the client.

Meichenbaum (1977) developed self-instructional training under the influence of RET. This therapy involves individuals learning to use a range of problem-solving skills in order to overcome the negative self-statements they make to themselves.

Also in the 1970s Beck (1976, 1989) described his cognitive therapy, which focuses on the errors in logic individuals make in response to a set of events. His form of cognitive therapy differs from Ellis' RET in the emphasis placed on the content of the thoughts about events. Ellis places more emphasis on the emotional response that is elicited as a result of the belief the person holds about the events.

This chapter will describe CBT from a Beckian perspective, with some references to Meichenbaum's self-instructional training.

THE PURPOSE OF THIS CHAPTER

The heterogeneity of CBT means that a whole text would be needed to describe its various types, and the range of techniques used by cognitive behavioural therapists. What follows is an overview that illustrates the core themes of the approach. It provides an insight into the theory and methods associated with cognitive behavioural approaches to therapy.

However, this chapter is not intended as an inclusive review of all the techniques used by cognitive behavioural therapists or of the related literature but, rather, its purpose is to sensitize readers to the depths and diversity of CBT. It is not a procedural manual and should not be used in isolation from other texts. The reader should not think that they can read this and 'have a go at CBT'.

A number of other texts are available that give an overview of how to use CBT with individuals who present with particular difficulties (Birchwood & Tarrier 1992, Blackburn & Davidson 1990, Dryden & Rentoul 1991, Hawton et al 1989, Stern & Drummond 1991).

The chapter will provide material that may inform practitioners already skilled in the use of cognitive behavioural approaches. For those yet to develop those skills it will give some insight into the background and efficacy of this approach when working with people who have, or are vulnerable to the development of, mental health difficulties. Like other therapies, CBT requires supervision by someone experienced in its practice and should not be attempted just on the basis of reading this introduction.

Before embarking on a description of the elements of the practice of CBT, an insight into the theoretical concepts and the historical developments that underpin the therapy will be given.

A glossary of terms is provided at the back of the book to help both in deciphering the jargon associated with CBT and as a reference resource.

HISTORICAL AND THEORETICAL DEVELOPMENT OF COGNITIVE BEHAVIOURAL THERAPY

The Institute of Psychoanalysis was founded in 1919. It offered the first psychological treatments. As its name suggests these treatments were psychoanalytic in nature and were available only to a very small minority of people. The opening of the Tavistock Clinic followed soon afterwards. It too offered psychoanalytic psychotherapy to those who could afford to pay. Only with the birth of the NHS in 1948 did psychological treatments become more readily available and accessible to the general public. These continued to be largely psychoanalytical in the early days of the NHS and

it was only during the mid 1960s that behavioural treatments began to emerge.

Central to behavioural approaches to therapy are stimulus response models. The seminal work of Pavlov with his description of classical conditioning was published in 1927 (Pavlov 1927). Thorndike (1898) had previously described the Law of Effect and Watson & Rayner (1920) demonstrated the practical application of these new theories. In 1938 Skinner published 'The Behaviour of Organisms', in which he identified the role of operant conditioning in learning.

These non-mediational theories of learning (Skinner 1953) propose that the exhibition of behaviour is based on learning that is founded on the development of a bond between a particular stimulus event and a particular response. This bond is developed and maintained simply by a process of reinforcement. If an activity is reinforced the likelihood of it occurring again will be increased. Conversely, if it is not reinforced then it will ultimately disappear from that person's repertoire of behaviours.

By the 1950s and 1960s these theories began to be incorporated into clinical work and to form elements of behavioural therapy. This work proliferated in the 1960s and by the 1970s operant and classical techniques of behavioural therapy had become firmly established. Behavioural therapy was the treatment of choice for a whole range of difficulties, from simple phobias to sexual dysfunction. It gained credence beyond the field of mental health and showed itself to be effective in working with people with mental handicaps (Ayllon & Azrin 1968).

The appendix to this chapter (p. 229) contains an overview of some of the fundamental aspects of behavioural approaches to therapy and is designed to be read at this point by those new to the approach.

Behavioural theories of learning do not allow for the interjection of any kind of cognitive processes. It is the response-strengthening effect of the behaviour that is primary in promoting learning, not the information conveyed in the event. Thorndike (1898) first describes this as the Law of Effect. It describes how the likelihood of a behavioural response reoccurring depends on whether it produces a pleasing or irritating state of affairs for the individual. Thorndike argued that behaviours that elicit a pleasing response are more likely to be repeated. How should 'pleasing' be defined? What is pleasing or irritating for one individual need not be so for another individual. Whilst there may be evidence for the Law of Effect in purely theoretical terms, in practice the assertion is problematic because the notion of pleasure is subjective and value laden. Reinforcement should not be equated with reward. What is reinforcing for one individual need not be so for another.

According to the behavioural stimulus response model of learning, the individual who is described as socially anxious will behave in a particular way because reinforcing consequences act directly and automatically to strengthen overt responses. They will therefore avoid situations that, through a process of association, have become linked with unpleasant sensations and feelings. The model proposes that the link between stimulus and response is direct; there is no mediating thought interpreting these events. Yet if we accept that pleasure and irritation are both subjective then the stimulus response model begins to lose its power as an explanatory model for considering complex human behaviour. What is the explanation for why some individuals, on entering a crowded room, feel perfectly at ease, whilst others hover outside with their hand tentatively on the door handle summoning up the courage to sneak into the room as unobtrusively as possible? What accounts for the two quite different responses to what is apparently the same stimulus? Is it possible to construct an argument that highlights a difference in individual learning history that accounts for these differences (Wolpe 1982)?

An approach that accommodates individual differences in behavioural response is what is needed. Such a model could integrate behavioural approaches to therapy with a model that explains individual differences more fully. Blackburn & Davidson (1990) describe cognitive and behavioural approaches to therapy as sharing much in common but highlight how the cognitive approach utilizing a mediational model can accommodate for individual differences.

Cognitive mediation in learning arose from the early work of Tolman (1932) although the so-called 'cognitive revolution' in academic psychology did not really get underway until the 1960s. Tolman's experimental work with rats led him to postulate that cognitive factors are important in the development and maintenance of new behaviours. Tolman argued that internal representations of events are crucial when considering the person's behaviour. An example of this is Novaco's cognitive or mediational model of anger (Novaco 1975). He proposes that individuals perceive events as being aversive and respond in an angry way in response to a set of assumptions. It is these assumptions that mediate between the event and their behaviour. If individuals have an expectation that an event is likely to be frustrating, threatening or insulting, this expectation will mediate between their thoughts and feelings in such a way that their behaviour will reflect their expectation. It is the information conveyed to the individual by the event that is primary in promoting learning.

A mediational model maintains there is an interaction between the way individuals think, feel and behave. Individuals' observable behaviour is the result of the way they construct events in their environment. Kelly paved the way for this when he developed his personal construct theory (Kelly 1955). In this he described people as scientists who interpret events that go on around them. These interpretations are based on personal templates, which act as blueprints used to impose meaning on the world. Construction occurs through a process of cognitive mediation.

If the mediation model is used to explain behaviour then a whole range of explanatory variables, including the role of expectation and anticipation, become important. Take again an example of people who are fearful in social situations. These individuals are likely to report that they dread some terrible disaster befalling them when they are in a public place. For example, they will often report how they think they are likely to faint or lose control in some way and as a result make a fool of themselves in front of a crowd of people. It is their anticipation of what may happen that is critical in the maintenance of their difficulties. Their thoughts mediate between events and their behaviour or response to those events.

S - R
Stimulus   **Response**
A crowded room   Walking away

S - - - - - - - - - - - M - - - - - - - - - - R
Stimulus   **Mediation**   **Response**
A crowded room   'will lose control'   Walking away

Fig. 8.1 A representative of mediational and non-mediational models for describing behaviour.

This relationship is illustrated in Figure 8.1, which contrasts the traditional behavioural model, in which there is no mediation between stimulus and response, with a representation of Tolman's model, in which cognitive variables intervene between the stimulus and the response. Figure 8.1 illustrates how, through a process of mediation, the behavioural response to a stimulus is formed. That response will be different across individuals but will also be different within individuals if the circumstances change.

Rotter & Hochreich (1975) refer to this intra-individual difference as the person's psychological situation. They argue that it is not enough to know details of the situation or settings in which the stimulus occurs; in addition we need to know how the person interprets the stimulus before we can make sense of the observable response. Knowing about people's psychological situation may help to make some sense of how they respond and to explain why individuals behave in a particular way. Individuals' behaviour patterns will become established because, over the course of events, they observe the differential consequences of different types of response. Through this process of observation they are encouraged to engage in particular responses.

Rotter & Hochreich (1975) refer to this as reinforcement value. This concept allows for recognition of the subjective nature of reinforcement. Take again Novaco's model of anger: individuals who anticipate that another person is intent on threatening their security are likely to model their response on their observations of others, if they consider that this model has successfully achieved their goal via this behaviour. More recent develop-

ments in CBT have identified the importance of personal histories in working with clients.

Although mediational models of learning appear to have more commonsense appeal, it is important to consider if there is sufficient theoretical evidence for them. Any critique of the theoretical basis of a new development in psychology will focus on the experimental methodology used in its development: how the data have been gathered and interpreted. Depending on the perspective of the critic, what is acceptable as data varies. For some, the data of self-report and introspection are not substantive and should therefore not be allowed. A radical behaviourist is likely to consider using 'mediating processes' as data as unscientific and nonsensical. Indeed Wolpe (1982) describes a cognitivist view as a demonstration of 'loose thinking'. Such a dismissive approach to alternative perspectives should be treated with caution; a critical approach is called for in respect of evidence both for and against a particular perspective. Ericsson & Simons (1981) present a detailed historical account in which they argue cogently for cognitions to be accepted as valid data.

It is essential that the practitioner has a grasp of what underlies the theory of any particular therapy. It may be argued that this is particularly the case when considering CBT. CBT is essentially an educative process, its aim being to enable the client to use the skills demonstrated by the therapist. Without a good grasp of the underlying theory the practitioner will not be able to engage fully in this educational element of the therapy.

AN INTEGRATED APPROACH TO UNDERSTANDING BEHAVIOUR—THE COGNITIVE BEHAVIOURAL MODEL

The cognitive revolution in academic psychology in the late 1960s and early 1970s emphasized the importance of cognitive processes. The human information-processing model along with Bandura's (1977) social learning theory emphasized that individual patterns of behaviour arise because of an interaction between people and their environment. The individual is considered to play an active part in processing information.

The human information-processing model has become very influential. It proposes a model that accounts for all aspects of human cognition. The model argues that from an investigation of cognitive processes evidence will be forthcoming that will advance our understanding of behaviour. There are many excellent introductory descriptions of the human information-processing model (Baddeley 1976, Reed 1981).

The major tenet of the human information-processing model is that cognitive processes occur as a series of events. Information from the environment passes through a series of stages before being stored into long term memory. Given the plethora of information in the environment, some selection is necessary. This selection is proposed to take place in response to a range of processes; the selection results in individuals focusing attention and heeding particular bits of information from their surroundings. This process of selection occurs automatically and it is this that accounts for differences in the way the same event is 'seen' by two different people in two different ways. Social learning theorists, typified by Bandura (1977), recognize that people can symbolically represent and manipulate situations and images in their heads. This allows individuals to anticipate the possible outcomes of a situation and to decide on a course of action.

These developments in academic psychology coincided with an increasing recognition that behavioural therapy did not always lead to a successful treatment outcome. It became increasingly apparent that behavioural therapy, even if delivered competently, did not always achieve the success that was anticipated. Foa & Emmelkamp (1983) edited a book concerned with treatment failures. This work highlighted failures across a range of difficulties including obsessions, phobias, problems of addiction, sexual dysfunction and relationship problems.

Foa & Emmelkamp (1983) identified several types of failure. These were relatively small in number and could be put under several headings; amongst these failures were inaccurate diagnosis of the problem, which resulted in the inappropri-

ate application of a treatment, inaccurate application of the selected technique and poor generalization of the newly acquired behaviour to settings beyond the 'treatment room'. They argued that part of the difficulty was the attempted imposition of a homogeneous technology, namely behavioural therapy, upon a heterogeneous group of psychological difficulties. They suggested practitioners were trying to use a standard technique to help people who have a range of difficulties. People presenting with problems were being fitted into the treatment, rather than the treatment being designed to fit the presenting problem. The authors highlighted the explicit need to use an integrated model.

Wolpe (1982) described how many cognitive therapists utilize behavioural techniques but fail to recognize their importance. Meichenbaum (1977), in describing work done by Wolpe in the area of systematic desensitization, highlights how Wolpe appears to fail to take full account of the cognitive elements in a behavioural approach to therapy. Blackburn & Davidson (1990) claim that a major difference between cognitive therapy and behavioural therapy is that behavioural approaches use behavioural techniques exclusively, whereas cognitive therapy uses both behavioural and cognitive techniques. They demonstrate how these artificial distinctions are still influential today. It is important to acknowledge both elements in therapy and their respective utility and evidence base.

THE NATURE OF COGNITIVE BEHAVIOURAL THERAPY

The core theme of CBT is that individuals experience difficulties because of the way they are interpreting events. Beck et al (1979) identified errors in logic in people suffering from depression. These errors include arbitrary inferences, catastrophizing, personalization, selective abstraction and overgeneralization. They inform the person's view of the world and as a result they have a mediating effect on behaviour. Although Beck highlighted these errors in people suffering from depression, similar errors have been found in other groups of people—for example, those suffering from anxiety-related problems and relationships difficulties can often display similar errors in the way they interpret events (Beck & Emery 1989). He also identified them as occurring in the healthy population; automatic thoughts need not have a negative content but they become problematic at the point at which they have a negative effect on behaviour and affect.

The crucial issue in the practice of CBT is that the therapist assists clients in the identification of the errors of logic that they persistently engage in. These may not fit neatly into Beck's categories but it will be possible to detect a cognitive style that is affecting the way a client interprets events.

Some essential components of cognitive behavioural therapy

CBT can be used for a wide range of difficulties and the literature has consistently demonstrated its comparative efficacy. It also has utility in offering inoculation against the recurrence of future difficulties. Meichenbaum has shown that by learning the techniques of CBT some individuals can be enabled to recognize and avoid situations that may cause them difficulties (Meichenbaum 1986). It may be used when working with groups and with individuals. There is evidence for its efficacy in the treatment of children, adults, older adults and people with learning disabilities (Kendall & Braswell 1985, Lindsay 1986, McCullough 1991, Reeder 1991, Stern & Fernandez 1991, Zerhusen, Boyle & Wilson 1991).

CBT is problem centred; it deals with the here and now, with the current difficulties that the client is experiencing. It is undertaken in a spirit of collaboration in which the client has a central role to play, not only revealing the nature of the problem, but also in the completion of the tasks, which the therapeutic encounter identifies as being important. Without a commitment by the client to therapy there is unlikely to be any change in the nature of the client's difficulties. The therapy is aimed at influencing the underlying pathology, which is causing the distress to the individual. The nature of this pathology relates to the way individuals interpret their world and how they behave in it. Individuals who persistently think that events in

their life happen because they are unable to influence them positively, who then withdraw from social contact, are likely to suffer a whole range of psychological problems. Such people may start to feel depressed, they may be anxious about social contact, they may behave aggressively when they are in anxiety-provoking situations or feel quite unable to cope with the everyday demands of living. By engaging in CBT they may be enabled to cope with these demands.

CBT is in part an educational process and in part an insight-oriented therapy. It is concerned with identification of difficulties with clients and the development of skills to help them deal with their difficulties in an adaptive way. It is way that does not have them resort to behaviour that isolates them from their peers or affects their self-esteem, preventing them from engaging in ordinary social activities.

It is structured and time limited, with the client being aware of both the intended structure and format. The expectations in respect of the time commitment are explicit. Unlike other psychotherapeutic techniques, there is no 'hidden agenda' or use of paradoxical techniques (Cade 1979). Such techniques would be contrary to the ethos in which CBT should be conducted.

Some essential skills in cognitive behavioural therapy—establishing a therapeutic alliance

As has already been highlighted, amongst the necessary basic skills that are important for carrying out CBT is an understanding of the theoretical background of the approach to therapy. Without such an understanding it would not be possible to engage in a therapeutic alliance with a client, which is vital to the participation in CBT. In addition to knowing the theory behind the practice of CBT, it is essential that therapists have the necessary skills to enable clients to make the changes they identify as important to them.

These skills will include those identified many times before in other texts (Rogers 1951, Truax 1963); they are genuineness, warmth and empathy. Rogers (1961) considers these qualities as affording the 'mainspring of change'. In addition,

Rogers describes 'unconditional positive regard' as central to client-centred therapy in ensuring change for the client. This could not readily be ascribed to therapists who adopt CBT as their model for treatment. Although CBT is client centred in that it aims to address and explore issues that are identified by the client, it is more directive and challenging than Rogerian therapy. This directive element of CBT is made apparent in its goal-directed nature. The way this change is achieved is via a process of engagement in a series of tasks that are identified in collaboration with the therapist. In order for clients to achieve these goals it will be necessary for therapists to challenge clients and to ask them explicitly to provide evidence for constructing their world in a particular way.

In some situations it will be prescriptive. During the course of CBT goals and outcome are identified; these will include aspects of behaviour or cognition which the client seeks to change. In challenging the client, the therapist aims to encourage change. The notion of unconditional positive regard as described by Rogers (1961) does not sit easily with this more challenging approach. That is not to say that the role of the therapist is to disregard what clients report or to make them feel foolish because of what they report, as clearly such behaviour would be unacceptable. Despite some apparent differences between Rogerian and CBT, however, the essential skills of warmth, positive regard and genuineness have been identified as essential elements in establishing a working relationship with a client.

What follows is an overview of the practice of CBT. It may read as though it were a cookbook offering a quick and easy way to deal with a range of difficulties, but this is a misperception and it cannot be overemphasized that, as with any therapy, there must be a complete assessment. Only after the assessment processes have been embarked upon can any therapeutic intervention be considered.

Aspects of assessment in cognitive behavioural therapy

Assessment should be the first stage of any thera-

peutic intervention; it should not been seen as a 'one-off' but as a continuous and integral part of the therapeutic process. The material gathered during assessment will inform therapy and changes may be made in response to the findings of the evaluative aspects of assessment. The main object of the initial stages of assessment is to get a broad overview of the problem, as the client perceives it, the focus of which becomes increasingly narrowed as primary difficulties are identified.

In addition to assessing the nature of the problem the initial assessment session should be used to ascertain the client's suitability for a cognitive intervention. Safran et al (1993) describe a number of factors that are predictive of people's capacity to engage in short term cognitive therapy. These include willingness to accept personal responsibility for change, their capacity to differentiate emotional states, their capacity to maintain a problem focus during the session and the accessibility of automatic thoughts. Where these features are absent and the problem is chronic a person is less likely to be able to engage immediately in a cognitive behavioural intervention.

Cognitive therapy is essentially collaborative; in the spirit of collaboration it is important that the therapists seek clients' view and description of the problem. This process may highlight several difficulties that clients are currently experiencing and it may be that they have to identify which of these difficulties is a priority for them. On occasions this primary difficulty will not be what has been identified by the referring agent. This presents an early challenge to the therapist's commitment to working in collaboration and partnership with the client. Often this can be overcome and therapy can proceed using the priorities identified by the client. Occasionally, however, there may be a dilemma for the therapist. Individual clients may be referred because they are engaging in a behaviour that is potentially damaging, yet they may seek to highlight another problem as being the primary problem in their view. For example a young woman may be referred because of an eating problem that has reached such a stage as to cause concern about her physical and psychological well-being. However, she may consider that her tension headaches are the primary difficulty. On further questioning it may become apparent that these headaches are unrelated to the eating difficulties. She may admit to them being infrequent and unrelated to exacerbation in her eating problem. Despite this she may insist that before she can address the issue of eating she needs to overcome these tension headaches. The therapist must deliberate between working on the problem for which the person has been referred and working on the problem the client identifies as of primary concern. Such debates are particularly problematic when the therapist is attempting to establish a therapeutic alliance that has collaboration as a central theme.

In such cases it will be necessary to negotiate and in some cases compromise. Where there is a refusal to address major problems, particularly those in which clients are damaging themself, therapists must question if an approach that is firmly grounded in collaboration and requires full participation is the therapy of choice. It is these issues that should be addressed during the course of supervision. This highlights an ethical dilemma in therapy. In pursuing a treatment path, therapists must take account of clients' right to have their autonomy respected. Autonomy in this case means one's capacity to think, decide and act freely and independently. When a decision is taken about what problem to tackle there is a danger that the client's autonomy will be compromised. Because a therapy may appear to be prescriptive and directive that does not mean that therapists should disregard the ethical dilemmas that will face them during a course of cognitive therapy (Allison 1996).

Once an agreement has been reached about which problems to tackle and in which order to tackle them, the therapist needs to elicit some information about the nature of the problem. The therapist will need to gather information that allows a cognitive behavioural formulation to be made. This will include information about how the problem effects the person's everyday life. Questions about the frequency, intensity and duration of the problem will need to be answered (Herbert 1987).

Using these headings as guidelines for gathering material the therapist will gain information that relates not just to the observable aspects of the problem—the behaviour—but also that related to the cognitive aspects of the problem. Clients will be asked what sense they make of the problem, what they think about the problem, and also what they think about when the problem is manifest. It may be that eliciting this material is challenging for therapists and they may have to work hard to engage clients in this process. Some clients may misunderstand the purpose of this line of questioning and may begin to take a pseudopsychoanalytical line offering explanations related to their unconscious. Such misunderstandings offer therapists the opportunity to educate clients, both about the nature of CBT and about the proposed link between thoughts, feelings and actions.

In addition to information about the difficulties, the therapist should spend time gathering material related to the individual's living and working circumstances. This should include an exploration of who else is involved with the maintenance of the problem—would anyone benefit from the continuance of this difficulty; what are the secondary gains for the individual? If clients are being reinforced for engaging in this behaviour for which they now seek help then there will be a conflict of interests, which may interfere with the motivation to change. If other people do appear to be directly involved then they may need to be involved in some aspects of therapy at some stage of the process.

Information about individuals' early life and their school history should also be gathered. Details of any significant or traumatic events, in terms of both their emotional and physical health, will be important. Once these broad areas of information have been elicited, more detailed assessment of the current problem should be undertaken.

By the end of the first session therapists should have gathered material related to the primary problem that clients identify as the area where they would like to attempt change. Additionally, therapists will have material in relation to the problem in respect of its frequency, intensity, nature, duration and the sense clients make of their problem and the symptoms they experience. Material related to demographic details, to work and home life will also have been gathered. Therapists should have also taken time to describe CBT and to identify for clients what expectations they have for the therapy. Finally, therapists should close with a review of the session, including their understanding of what work is to be undertaken. They should ensure some agreement from clients that they are willing to participate in the therapy and have an understanding of the commitment in terms of time and effort. CBT requires clients to make changes, many of which may provoke discomfort and anxiety, but unless clients are prepared to engage in these changes the therapy will not be successful.

The task of assessment is to both gather and give information. These tasks may be summarized as follows:

◆ Gather material related to clients':
 — developmental history
 — vocational history
 — family and social relationships
 — significant events
 — significant traumas
 — medical history
 — how they cope with their problem.

◆ Gather material, in behavioural terms, related to the presenting problem:
 — frequency of their symptoms
 — intensity of their symptoms
 — nature of their symptoms
 — duration of the presenting problem
 — sense that they make of the problem.

◆ Gather material, in cognitive terms, related to the presenting problem:
 — content of the automatic thoughts
 — core beliefs about themselves
 — rules they apply to themselves.

◆ Gather information to assess clients' suitability to engage in CBT.

◆ Give material related to the nature of CBT:
 — collaborative

 — active
 — problem centred
 — educational.

The purpose of assessment is for the therapist to begin to identify the cognitive distortions that are contributing to the client's difficulty. In addition, through assessment the therapist will identify what behavioural patterns are associated with the difficulty.

At the end of the assessment therapists should be able to summarize for clients how they conceptualize the problem. This should be done in terms of both the cognitive and behavioural aspects of the problem. It is important that this formulation of the problem is agreed with clients because it is this that will inform the process of therapy. It may not be possible to elicit all the information in one session; often during ongoing therapy clients will give additional information that alters the therapist's formulation. It is, therefore, standard practice that at the end of each session the therapist reformulates the problem for the client.

THE STRUCTURE FOR ONGOING THERAPY SESSIONS

Each session should follow a similar structure. Usually the structure would look something like this:

◆ Check how the person is feeling.
◆ Check out how the person got on with the homework tasks that were set at the last session.
◆ Set an agenda for the work of this session.
◆ Discussion of these agenda items.
◆ Reformulate the problem based on any new information.
◆ Set a homework task based on the agenda and check that the person knows what is required.
◆ Summarize the session.
◆ Seek feedback from the client about the session.

TECHNIQUES USED DURING THE COURSE OF COGNITIVE BEHAVIOURAL THERAPY

The initial stage of assessment will highlight the problems the client wants to work on. If there are several problems it may be necessary to prioritize them and to agree, with the client, which problem should first be addressed. After this the therapist will need to select from a whole range of techniques which fall under the rubric of CBT. The techniques should be chosen to match problems that have been identified during assessment. The basis of selection will be that the essence of CBT is to challenge the assumptions and expectations that currently inform individuals' behaviour and to teach individuals a range of techniques, both behavioural and cognitive, that will enable them to do this. The techniques chosen will match the problem that has been identified. In making this choice the practitioner must be mindful of the complex nature of mental health difficulties and should be flexible in selection.

The techniques may be cognitive or behavioural in nature. Listed below are some of the more commonly applied techniques.

Behavioural	Cognitive
Activity monitoring	Evaluating automatic thoughts
Behavioural experiments	Labelling cognitive distortions
Relaxation exercises	Cognitive rehearsal
Assertiveness training	Imagining feared consequences
Distraction techniques	Evaluating core beliefs
Exposure to feared events	Modifying images
Graded task assignment	Problem solving
Time management	Self-instruction

These and other techniques would be used to challenge the cognitive errors that have been identified during the assessment and to test the reality of the assumptions the client is making.

This is achieved during therapy sessions using a technique called Socratic questioning. This technique is undertaken in a collaborative way, the client and therapist jointly working to uncover the errors of logic present in the client's thinking. The therapist asks questions to identify what evidence there is for the client's interpretation of events. The goal of this is to illustrate the self-defeating nature of the client's line of thinking.

For example, through a process of assessment and ongoing self-monitoring, it may become apparent that clients who are fearful in social situations are consistently searching their environment for evidence to reinforce their core belief that they are useless and ineffectual. Such people will concentrate on small and often trivial details from all the incoming material and in doing so they may misinterpret the meaning of events. This process would be analogous to Beck's description of selective abstraction. In this case clients should be helped to consider the evidence for their core belief. This can be done using a behavioural experiment in which the person tests out the reality of this belief. This would be complemented with cognitive restructuring of the core belief.

An example of a behavioural experiment would be agreeing with clients that they put themselves in a situation that they consider they cannot be in because they will not cope with it—yet they have no evidence for this being the case. For instance where no one has spoken to the person at coffee time because the client does not go to the coffee room, or takes coffee at a different time. The probability is that colleagues are not ignoring the person, but simply have not had an opportunity to talk with the client. Where this is the scenario therapists can develop a behavioural experiment that will test out clients' hypotheses that no one talks to them. In this case they should be encouraged to think of one person they could ask one question of. Therapists need to carefully work through with clients who they will speak to, what question they should ask and how to ask a follow-up question. Therapists should role play the situation to help clients feel more confident about their social skills.

In addition to the behavioural experiment the therapist and client should identify the cognitive errors that are being made in the situation. Therapists should work with clients to discover what evidence there is for them to think in the way they do about the situation. The process of Socratic questioning is described below.

Cognitive restructuring can be achieved through the implementation of the following techniques:

◆ self-monitoring via a thought diary to enable clients to identify errors of logic
◆ training in using Socratic questioning to challenge these identified errors in logic.

Throughout the process there would be education of the client regarding the nature of the link between thoughts, feelings and behaviour.

Self-monitoring will be used to provide the material for the therapist and client to work with. It is also essential in providing material with which to demonstrate the link between thoughts, feelings and behaviour. The recognition of this link is a critical first step in the whole process of CBT. In order for cognitive therapy to be successful, the client must recognize this link. If that recognition comes through working on the client's own thoughts and feelings elicited by self-monitoring it will be more meaningful than if the link is hypothetically illustrated by the therapist.

Self-monitoring as a tool in the practice of cognitive behavioural therapy

Self-monitoring can be achieved through various means. The principal method is through the use of some kind of diary. In order for this to be of any use it is important for it to be structured. Ensuring the client uses a structured approach serves a learning function beyond the client's immediate needs and can assist in the inoculation process. If clients need to use their newly acquired skills at some point in the future they will readily recall the structure that was previously used if it has been used consistently—they will have gone through a process of overlearning and the skill will become relatively automatic.

The diary need not be written—for some clients this will not even be an option if they have limited literacy skills. An alternative is that the client use some kind of audiotape—for example, a hand-held Dictaphone. The content and structure of the diary will vary depending on the nature of the client's difficulties. It is also likely to vary at different stages in the therapy. The structure of the diary should allow for the recording of some specific material but this will invariably be centred on a structured analysis of the individual's difficulties.

As has already been highlighted, information related to frequency, intensity, nature, duration and sense of the problem should be obtained both during the assessment session and as an ongoing process through the diary. The diary should be structured in such a way as to access material related to these parameters. The frequency of episodes will be readily available if a record is kept each time an episode is experienced. Obtaining this information will, therefore, be relatively straightforward.

The individual must then be enabled to record material related to the other parameters. The intensity of the difficulty needs to be defined in some way so as to make recording as objective as possible. This objectivity should be viewed as important only in terms of the individual—it is not meant to be a reliable measure that can be used across a group of people. The therapy is about individual change and as such all measures, unless they are those of standard questionnaires, relate to the individual.

In measuring intensity, it may be possible to employ one of several measures; these include visual analogues or, as a variation on that theme, bar charts can be used (Fig. 8.2). The labelling of

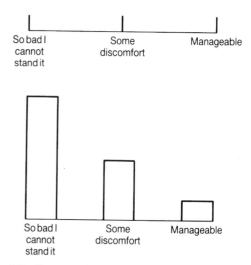

Fig. 8.2 Two examples of methods of recording the intensity of the problem.

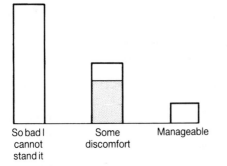

Fig. 8.3 An example of how to introduce finer detail into the recording of intensity of the problem.

the points on the scale should be altered to suit the needs of each client; they should be written using the words the client uses to describe the intensity of the problem. More than three points on the scale can be used if it is thought necessary. The bar chart can be used to enable the client to give some degree of differentiation within each category. It may be that clients feel a good deal of discomfort but not enough to place them in the 'so bad I can't stand it' category. In this case the middle box can be shaded to represent the level of intensity. Additionally, the height of the shading can vary according to the relative degree of intensity; in this way each category could be viewed as having an internal axis (Fig. 8.3).

It may be helpful to use a standard questionnaire to elicit detailed information about the relative intensity and nature of the individual's difficulties; for example, the Beck Anxiety Inventory (Beck 1990) measures the severity of anxiety in adolescents and adults. It evaluates both cognitive and physiological symptoms of anxiety. It is useful in that it gives both reliable and valid information in relation to an individual's condition and in doing so augments the material gathered through self-report. Such information is particularly important when writing reports in that it is objective and can be used as comparative data. Such questionnaires are commercially available.

The nature of the problem refers to what the problem is like. It is about the observable behaviour and the related cognitions. If, for example, the person is having self-control problems then the

nature of the problem will be concerned with actions such as banging doors, changes in body posture and tone of voice. It will also relate to what the person is thinking about before, during and after the incident. Self-monitoring via thought diaries has an implicit problem-solving element. The structure of the diaries should reflect the Socratic questioning that the therapist uses during the therapy session.

For therapists to help the clients access their automatic thoughts and the core beliefs which underlie them clients will be asked to keep a thought diary in between sessions. There is a variety of ways in which the thought diary is constructed. The instruction to clients is that they should complete the thought diary whenever they notice their mood changing, or when they become aware that the physical symptoms of their problem are present. In Beck's model of cognitive behaviour therapy, the diary will include the columns shown in Box 8.1. For each of these columns clients are given some prompt questions to help them complete the thought diary.

The questions, which relate to generating an alternative interpretation of the event, will be similar to the Socratic questions used in therapy sessions. Examples of such questions are:

◆ What is the evidence for my automatic thought being true?
◆ What is the evidence for my automatic thought being false?
◆ What is the effect of my believing the automatic thought?
◆ What could the effect be if I changed the interpretation I have made of the situation?
◆ What is the most realistic interpretation of the event?
◆ Am I confusing a thought with a fact?
◆ Am I blaming myself for something that cannot be my fault?
◆ Am I worrying about the way things ought to be instead of accepting how they are?
◆ Am I using double standards?

If the diary is taped then the verbal reports should be structured in the same way so that the material can be used in the therapy sessions. The diary should be used from the assessment sessions

Box 8.1

Date/time	Situation	Automatic thought	Emotion	Alternative interpretation	Outcome
	What actually happened that led to the unpleasant emotion?	What went through your mind? How much did you believe this?	What emotion did you feel? How intense was the feeling?	(see Box 8.2)	How much do you now believe each automatic thought? What emotions do you now feel? What will you do?

Box 8.2

Date/time	Situation	Automatic thought	Emotion	Alternative interpretation	Outcome
	Walking down the road I saw my friend—she ignored me	'I must have done some thing to upset or offend her.'	Worried, sad This was a very strong feeling	Maybe she didn't see me. Maybe her mind is on something else—she has been really busy lately	I think that is the most likely explanation. I saw her last week and she was fine with me I do not feel so worried that I have done any thing to upset her

throughout the contact. It represents a baseline record and can be used at various stages as a way of evaluating progress and change and on the basis of this evaluation any alteration in therapy may be embarked upon.

For the diary to be effective practitioners must give clients sufficient information to enable them to keep a record of behaviour, thoughts and feelings. Without adequate information clients may be made to feel deskilled and foolish. Some clients may even default on their appointments or withdraw because they feel unable to complete the task. Behavioural techniques such as shaping and

offering positive reinforcement should be used to guide clients in their early efforts at diary keeping. It is important to be sensitive to clients when asking them to complete a diary and to recognize what a difficult task it may be. It should be borne in mind that there is always a potential danger in asking clients to keep diaries; they may think they have to record what you as the practitioner want to read, and they may think that there are 'right' answers. This good subject effect has been shown to influence the outcome of experiments performed in the psychology laboratory and it should be considered when asking individuals to keep accounts of their thoughts, feelings and behaviour (Rosenzweig 1986). An example of a diary entry is given in Box 8.2.

During the initial assessment session, clients should receive instruction on how to keep a diary so that by the time they return for the second interview they will have some material from which to work. This material gathered before this second session will act as a baseline because it will have been gathered before any therapeutic intervention has begun.

The early stages of self-monitoring help to sensitize the clients to their internal dialogue. For many this will come as an important revelation, for some it will be something akin to a religious conversion experience in which they suddenly recognize the power they have to influence their own behaviour. For others it will merely confirm what they had suspected. Importantly for many clients, it will legitimate a process that they have already engaged in—that is, trying to talk themselves into a positive frame of mind by challenging their negative assumption, in order to influence their behaviour.

Once clients have begun to make the link between internal dialogue of automatic thoughts and behaviour then they need to go through a process of challenging and restructuring their cognitive style. They should be encouraged to do this though a process of self-talk, during which they recognize the negative self-talk, challenge its underlying assumptions and substitute positive self-talk.

There are many examples of the various ways that thought diaries can be kept (Blackburn 1987, Kirk 1989, Rakos 1991, Stern & Drummond 1991, Twaddle & Scott 1991).

Relapse prevention through self-regulation and self-instruction

Relapse prevention can be achieved through the proactive and continued use of a range of skills including self-monitoring, self-instruction and self-reinforcement. The potential for inoculation highlights how CBT can be used to promote mental health as well as offering methods for coping with current difficulties.

For change to be maintained clients should be encouraged to use positive reinforcement with themselves. Bandura (1969) argued that self-regulation is especially important in cases where change is attempted of a behaviour that is maladaptive but reinforcing for the client. If the newly acquired adaptive behaviour such as Socractic questioning is practised in an environment in which there is only weak reinforcement then change is less likely to occur. An example of such a situation could be the individual who engages in obsessive behaviours 'behind closed doors'. Here naturally occurring reinforcement from the environment is limited. Clients may report that before they can leave their home they feel compelled to engage in rituals. These rituals may include obsessively washing, checking doors and windows, dressing and redressing. The person who engages in such behaviour gets very little obvious positive reinforcement for engaging in such behaviour. They will describe a feeling of relief of anxiety if they do engage in the ritual. They will often be able to keep their problem hidden away from significant others who potentially can provide feedback to them. The relief of anxiety on completion of the ritual will be a naturally occurring reinforcement, increasing the probability of the ritual being repeated. In these circumstances self-regulation via self-reinforcement is particularly important for any change to be maintained. Other examples may be people who suffer with bulimia but hide it from the people around them, or people who are dependent on alcohol.

Self-instructional training occupies a central role in CBT as described by Meichenbaum (1977). It is a broad term that describes a technique in which individuals are trained to talk to themselves in a way that decreases their maladaptive behaviour and increases their adaptive behaviour. Meichenbaum (1977) refers to this as learning to engage in 'healthy talk'. It is the basic technique that is elaborated in other aspects of CBT; for example, the process of cognitive restructuring, challenging negative assumptions and engaging in self-reinforcement all take place via self-talk.

Self-instructional techniques are based on the experimental work of the Soviet psychologists Luria and Vygotsky (Luria 1961, Vygotsky 1962).

They demonstrated verbal control over motoric behaviour, arguing that internal dialogue influences behaviour. Self-instruction techniques exploit this proposed relationship, providing the individual with a dialogue, which will effect behaviour in such a way as to ensure positive outcomes. By altering the content of the internal dialogue the client can influence not only behaviour but also affect. Monitoring and altering one's internal dialogue in such a way promotes adaptive rather than maladaptive behaviour and can be an effective tool in ensuring relapse prevention.

Self-instruction has been demonstrated to be effective in enabling generalization of change (Meichenbaum 1977). Generalization refers to the process whereby skills that are acquired in one specific area can be used to guide and inform behaviour in other situations. This is particularly important when considering complex and pervasive mental health difficulties. Examples include individuals who suffer with social anxiety that pervades a whole range of situations and clients who have a pervasive depression that is not reactive to any particular situation. These clients will need to be enabled to use skills across a range of situations. They will benefit from being taught skills, which have demonstrable advantages, in that they generalize more readily.

The issue of generalization has been closely studied during investigations into methods of behavioural change with people with learning disabilities. This group of people presents the practitioner with major difficulties in ensuring the maintenance and generalization of newly acquired skills. There is a great deal of evidence to demonstrate that training people with learning disabilities to use self-instructional techniques overcomes problems of maintenance and generalization (Whitman, Spence & Maxwell 1987). The importance of these findings is not only in highlighting the utility of self-instructional training, but also to demonstrate that as a therapeutic technique self-instructional training need not be limited to individuals who have well-developed verbal skills. Indeed Meichenbaum has proven the utility of self-instructional training with a group of people with schizophrenia (Meichenbaum 1969). However, as with any technique, practitioners should not assume it will be effective in all cases. Although the weight of evidence is such that it suggests self-instructional training has broad utility, there are examples of treatment failures (Oei, Lim & Young 1991).

A course of CBT will last a variable length of time depending on a number of factors, for example the nature of the problem, the frequency of contacts and the opportunities available to clients to practise their newly acquired skills. During the course of therapy the client and the practitioner should continue to work in a collaborative way in an effort to overcome the difficulties identified by the client. If the initial assessment and formulation of the problem are accurate then the practitioner should be confident that CBT will assist clients in overcoming their difficulties and in addition it will help them to avoid similar difficulties in the future.

SUMMARY: RECENT DEVELOPMENTS IN COGNITIVE BEHAVIOURAL THERAPY

Recently CBT has begun to be used with people with severe and enduring mental illness. It has been shown to have particular utility for people who suffer with schizophrenia (Birchwood & Tarrier 1992, Fowler, Garety & Kuipers, 1995). There are also studies which illustrate its effective-

---

DISCUSSION QUESTIONS

1. How does nursing practice reflect elements of CBT? (Is it relevant to nursing as a problem-solving activity?)
2. What are the ethical implications of a therapy which seeks to challenge individuals' core beliefs about themselves?
3. To what extent is CBT a set of tools rather than an approach to therapy? (In thinking about this focus on what the therapy process would be like if the practitioner did not have a 'constructivist' view of people.)

ness with people with borderline personality disorders (Lineham 1993). These developments offer promising ways forward in working with client groups who have traditionally been considered to be resistant to psychotherapeutic interventions.

FURTHER READING

Beck A T 1976 Cognitive therapy and the emotional disorders. Meridian, New York

Blackburn I M, Davidson K 1990 Cognitive therapy for depression. Blackwell Scientific, Oxford

Dryden W, Golden W L 1986 Cognitive-behavioural approaches to psychotherapy. Harper & Row, London

Hawton K, Salkowskis P, Kirk J, Clark D 1989 Cognitive behaviour therapy for psychiatric problems. A practical guide. Oxford University Press, New York

Meichenbaum D 1979 Cognitive-behaviour modification. An integrative approach. Plenum, New York

Persons J 1989 Cognitive therapy in practice: a case formulation approach. W W Norton, New York

REFERENCES

Allison A 1996 Ethical issues in cognitive behaviour therapy. In: Marshall S, Turnbull J (eds) Cognitive behaviour therapy. An introduction to theory and practice. Baillière Tindall, London

Ayllon T, Azrin N 1968 The token economy: a motivational system for therapy and rehabilitation. Appleton-Century-Crofts, New York

Baddeley A 1976 The psychology of memory. Harper & Row, New York

Bandura A 1969 Principles of behaviour modification. Holt, Rinehart & Winston, New York

Bandura A 1977 Social learning theory. Prentice Hall, Englewood Cliffs, NY

Beck A T 1976 Cognitive therapy and the emotional disorders. Meridian, New York

Beck A T 1989 Cognitive therapy and the emotional disorders, 2nd edn. International University Press, New York

Beck A T 1990 The Beck anxiety inventory. The Psychological Corporation, Sidcup, Kent

Beck A T, Emery G 1989 Anxiety disorders and phobias: a cognitive perspective. Basic Books, New York

Beck A T, Rush J A, Shaw B F, Emery G 1979 Cognitive therapy for depression. Guilford Press, New York

Biram M, Wilson G T 1981 Treatment of phobic disorders using cognitive and exposure methods: a self-efficacy analysis. Journal of Consulting and Clinical Psychology 49:886

Birchwood M, Tarrier N 1992 Innovations in the psychological management of schizophrenia. John Wiley, Chichester

Blackburn I M 1987 Coping with depression. Chambers, Edinburgh

Blackburn I M, Davidson K 1990 Cognitive therapy for depression. Blackwell Scientific, Oxford

Cade B 1979 The use of paradox in therapy. In: Walrond I, Skinner R (eds) Family and marital psychotherapy: a critical approach. Routledge & Kegan Paul, London

Department of Health 1996 NHS Psychotherapy Services in England: a review of strategic policy. NHSE, London

Department of Health 1998 A first class service: quality in the new NHS. DoH, London

Dryden W, Golden W L 1986 Cognitive-behavioural approaches to psychotherapy. Harper & Row, London

Dryden W, Rentoul R 1991 Adult clinical problems: a cognitive–behavioural approach. Routledge, London

Ericsson K A, Simons H A 1981 Sources of evidence on cognition: an historical overview. In: Merluzzi T V, Glass C R, Genest M (eds) Cognitive assessment. Guilford Press, New York

Ellis A 1962 Reason and emotion in psychotherapy. Lyle Stuart, New Jersey

Foa E, Emmelkamp P 1983 Failures in behaviour therapy. John Wiley, New York

Foa E, Rothbaum B O, Murdoch T B 1991 Treatment of post traumatic stress disorder in rape victims: a comparison between cognitive-behavioural procedures and counselling. Journal of Consulting and Clinical Psychology 59(5):715

Fowler D, Garety P, Kuipers E 1995 Cognitive behaviour therapy for psychosis: theory and practice. John Wiley, Chichester

Hawton K, Salkovski P, Kirk J, Clark D (eds) 1989 Cognitive behaviour therapy for psychiatric problems. A practical guide. Oxford University Press, New York

Herbert M 1987 Behaviour treatment of children with problems: a practice manual. Academic Press, London

Johnson C 1996 Addressing parent cognitions in interventions with families of disruptive children. In: Dobson K, Craig K (eds) Advances in cognitive behaviour therapy. Sage, California

Kelly G 1955 The psychology of personal construct theory. Plenum, New York

Kendall P C, Braswell L 1985 Cognitive-behaviour therapy for impulsive children. Guilford Press, New York

Kirk J 1989 Cognitive-behavioural assessment. In: Hawton K, Salkovski P, Kirk J, Clarke D (eds) Cognitive behaviour therapy for psychiatric problems: a practical guide. Oxford University Press, New York

Lindsay W R 1986 Cognitive changes after social skills training with young mildly handicapped adults. Journal of Mental Deficiency Research 30:81

Lineham B M 1993 Cognitive behaviour treatment of borderline personality disorder. Plenum, New York

Luria A 1961 The role of speech in the regulation of normal and abnormal behaviours. Liveright, New York

McCullough J P 1991 Psychotherapy for dysthymia. A naturalistic study of ten patients. Journal of Nervous and Mental Disease 179(12):734

Meichenbaum D 1969 The effects of instructions and reinforcement on thinking and language behaviours of schizophrenics. Behaviour Research and Therapy 7:101

Meichenbaum D 1977 Cognitive-behaviour modification. An integrative approach. Plenum, New York

Meichenbaum D 1986 Stress inoculation training. Pergamon, New York

Meichenbaum D, Goodman J 1971 Training impulsive children to talk to themselves: a means of developing self control. Journal of Abnormal Psychology 77:115

Moorey S 1996 Cognitive therapy. In: Dryden W (ed) Handbook of individual therapy. Sage, London

Morse C A, Dennerstein L, Farrell E, Varnavides K 1991 A comparison of hormone therapy, coping skills training, and relaxation for the relief of premenstrual syndrome. Journal of Behavioural Medicine 14(5):469

Newell R, Dryden W 1991 Clinical problems: an introduction to the cognitive–behavioural approach. In: Dryden W, Rentoul R (eds) Adult clinical problems: a cognitive–behavioural approach. Routledge, London

NHS Psychotherapy Services 1996

Novaco R 1975 Anger control: the development and evaluation of an experimental treatment. Heath & Company, Lexington

Oei T P, Lim B, Young R 1991 Cognitive processes and cognitive behaviour therapy in the treatment of problem drinking. Journal of Addictive Disorders 10(3):63

Pavlov I 1927 Conditioned reflexes. Oxford University Press, New York

Rakos R F 1991 Assertive behaviour: theory, research and training. Routledge, London

Reed S K 1981 Cognition: theory and application. Brooks Cole, Monterey

Reeder D M 1991 Cognitive therapy of anger management: theoretical and practical considerations. Archives of Psychiatric Nursing 5(3):147

Rogers C R 1951 Client-centred therapy: its current practice, implications and theory. Houghton Mifflin, Boston, MA

Rogers C R 1961 On becoming a person: a therapist view of psychotherapy. Constable, London

Rosenzweig R 1986 Freud and experimental psychology: the emergence of idiodynamics. Academic Press, New York

Rotter J B, Hochreich D J 1975 Personality. Scott Foreshaw, Glenorew

Rush A J, Beck A T, Kovacs M, Hollon S D 1977 Comparative efficacy of cognitive therapy and pharmacotherapy in the treatment of depressed out-patients. Cognitive Therapy and Research 1:17

Safran J D, Segal Z V, Vallis M T, Shaw B F, Samstag L S 1993 Assessing patient suitability for short-term cognitive therapy with an interpersonal focus. Cognitive Therapy and Research 17(1):23

Salkovskis P M, Warwick N M 1986 Morbid preoccupations, health, anxiety and reassurance: a cognitive–behavioural approach to hypochondriasis. Behavioural Research and Therapy 24:597–602

Skinner B F 1938 The behaviour of organisms. Prentice Hall, Englewood Cliffs, NJ

Skinner B F 1953 Science and human behaviour. Macmillan, New York

Stern R, Drummond L 1991 The practice of behavioural and cognitive psychotherapy. Cambridge University Press, Cambridge

Stern R, Fernandez M 1991 Group cognitive and behavioural treatment for hypochondriasis. British Medical Journal 303:1229

Thorndike E L 1898 Animal intelligence: an experimental study of associative processes in animals. Psychological Monographs 2:223

Tolman E C 1932 Purposive behaviour in animals and men. Appleton, New York

Truax C B 1963 Effective ingredients in psychotherapy: an approach to unravelling the patient–therapist interaction. Journal of Counselling Psychology 10:256

Turk D 1996 Cognitive factors in chronic pain and disability. In: Dobson K, Craig K (eds) Advances in cognitive behaviour therapy. Sage, California

Twaddle V, Scott J 1991 Depression. In: Dryden W, Rentoul R (eds) Adult clinical problems: a cognitive behavioural approach. Routledge, London

Vygotsky L 1962 Thought and language. Wiley, New York

Watson J B, Rayner R 1920 Conditioned emotional responses. Journal of Experimental Psychology 3:1

Whitman T, Spence B H, Maxwell S 1987 A comparison of external and self instructional teaching formats with mentally retarded adults in vocational settings. Applied Research in Developmental Disabilities 8:371

Wolpe J 1982 The practice of behaviour therapy, 3rd edn. Pergamon, New York

Zerhusen D, Boyle J, Wilson W 1991 Out of darkness: group cognitive therapy for depressed elderly. Journal of Psychosocial Nursing and Mental Health Services 29(9):16

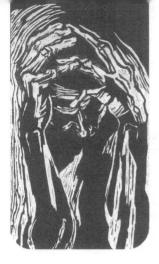

Appendix

Behavioural aspects of therapy

Sue Marshall

AIMS

- To provide a brief overview of fundamental aspects of behavioural approaches to therapy
- To serve as an introduction to Chapter 8 on cognitive behavioural therapy

KEY ISSUES

Origins of the behavioural approach

Classical conditioning

Operant conditioning

Reinforcement

Behavioural programmes

Before an individual can consider using cognitive behavioural therapy he or she must have a working knowledge of both behavioural and cognitive elements in therapy. The major thrust of this appendix is to give a relatively detailed account of how used together, these two approaches to therapy can offer a powerful tool in enabling some people with mental health difficulties to overcome their problems successfully. What follows is a brief overview of some of the fundamental aspects of behavioural approaches to therapy; it is given in order that the worker may be made aware of the complexity of using a behavioural approach in therapy and not consider it an easy option when working with people with mental health problems.

Behavioural approaches to therapy are based on the laboratory work of Pavlov (1927) and Skinner (1953). They are concerned with observable events and assessment of behaviour is made by considering only what can be observed. Radical behavioural approaches take no account of unconscious desires, or of individuals' thoughts and feelings about what is going on around them. The focus of this appendix is to suggest that such radical approaches should be replaced by integrated therapy which takes account of the individuals' thoughts about their difficulties. Integrated approaches do, however, use techniques that originated in the seminal work of the early behaviourist and it is important to recognize these origins.

Pavlov identified a process of learning based on reinforcement. What he described as classical conditioning demonstrated that through a process of association it is possible to establish a link between events that would under other circumstances be quite unconnected. Pavlov established such a link between the sound of a bell and salivation as a physiological response in preparation for food. This link was established by presenting food to a dog immediately after ringing a bell. Over a period of time and a number of such events the dog learned to associate the sound of the bell with the presentation of food. Once the association had been learned by the dog the sound of the bell alone would be sufficient to elicit salivation. This response would continue for a certain period of time but in the continued absence of the presentation of the food then the salivation response would eventually disappear.

A whole set of terminology has developed around conditioning. This terminology is used to describe the various elements that are necessary for classical conditioning to occur. In the example given above the conditioned stimulus is the bell, the unconditioned stimulus is the food and the conditioned response is salivation on ringing of the bell.

For classical conditioning to be possible there are several conditions that must be met, one of which is that there must be temporal contiguity between the stimulus to be conditioned and the unconditioned stimulus. This means that the sound of the bell must be followed almost immediately by the presentation of food. If this does not happen then the link will not be formed.

The role of classical conditioning in mental health difficulties is not clearly identified. It has been argued that classical conditioning is an element in the development of phobias (Eysenk & Rachman 1961), although this is not entirely clear and other workers would argue that the process involved in the development of phobias is a more complex matter involving processes other than classical conditioning.

Operant conditioning offers more in terms of both an explanatory framework and a therapeutic tool when working with people with mental health difficulties. Operant conditioning was first described by Skinner (1953).

Within the field of mental health, behavioural techniques that rely on aspects of both operant and classical conditioning can be used to enable people to cope with a whole range of difficulties. Assessment forms a crucial aspect of such work and focuses on identifying the function of an individual's behaviour and what is responsible for maintaining the maladaptive behaviour. To complete an assessment can be a lengthy and complex process, the nature of which is the subject of other texts. Only some aspects of the process can be covered here.

Much of Skinner's early work was done with animals (Skinner 1953). Through his experimental laboratory work he identified that actions in animals could be learned because of the effect those actions have on the environment. He found that if an animal is reinforced for an action it performs, then there is an increased probability of the action being performed again. Skinner went on to identify various 'schedules of reinforcement'. These have particular importance for workers using behavioural techniques therapeutically. He discovered that if reinforcement is offered intermittently then the strength of the learned association between an action and the response elicited by that action is greater than if reinforcement is offered each time the behaviour is performed. Therefore the link is more difficult to break than if reinforcement has been offered on each occasion that the behaviour has been performed. In practical terms this means that when behavioural programmes are designed the role of intermittent reinforcement has to be carefully considered during the assessment phase of work. The aim of many programmes will be to decrease the frequency of an identified target behaviour and to increase the frequency of the adaptive behaviour using a system of offering positive reinforcement for exhibition of the adaptive behaviour and offering nothing for the maladaptive behaviour. Under such conditions if the individual is able to elicit some positive reinforcement for engaging in the maladaptive behaviour intermittently, then the outcome of the programme may be unpredictable. This source of reinforcement may be difficult to control and has a potential for undermining what may otherwise be an adequate behavioural programme.

An example of the role of intermittent reinforcement may be the case of an individual who is depressed and as a result of this is not doing very much. This person may be passive and withdrawn and as part of treatment could be started on a behavioural programme aimed at increasing levels of engagement in those activities that have been previously identified as adaptive. The success of this programme depends on many things, one of which is the absence of intermittent reinforcement for relative inactivity. If, therefore a neighbour intermittently offers to take on the responsibility for doing the shopping, because the person is not feeling well, then this may be sufficient to prolong that individual's difficulty and in doing so may undermine the programme.

Within an institutional setting the potential sources for intermittent reinforcement are legion and need to be carefully considered and identified before any programme is embarked upon. Intermittent reinforcement can, however, establish strong links when used therapeutically—it need not always be something that creates difficulties for the practitioner.

This issue of potential for intermittent reinforcement highlights a whole range of important aspects of using behavioural approaches when working with individuals, with consistency in approach being amongst them. In order for behavioural techniques to be used effectively to describe maladaptive behaviours and to increase adaptive behaviours a programme must be written in such a way that it can be applied consistently. Without consistency in the delivery of reinforcement there will be limited potential for developing the link between a stimulus and a response. If it has been identified that a target behaviour should be responded to in a particular way then that should be the case invariably or intermittently if that is the requirement of the programme. A programme should specify under what circumstances a reinforcer should be delivered. These circumstances may change as the programme is evaluated and reviewed.

When designing a behavioural programme it is important to give consideration to the nature of the reinforcement that is being offered and to embark upon a process of surveying potential reinforcers. This can be done in a variety of ways, the most obvious being by simply asking individuals what they enjoy doing, who they like doing things with, and under what circumstances they find various activities pleasurable. It is essential that consideration be given to who will be delivering the reinforcer because this may affect its potential power. If, for example, we enjoy walking with a particular member of our family or a friend then the attention that we are receiving from that individual during the walk will be a variable in making the activity reinforcing. On the other hand, if we are given the opportunity of engaging in the same activity with another person then that element of the activity is changed and the reinforcement value of the activity may be significantly altered. Where it is not possible to get the information from the individual then the practitioner will need to conduct a reinforcement survey. This may be the case when working with someone who is depressed or who has long-standing mental illness that has resulted in the person being withdrawn and passive. A reinforcement survey is a process whereby a sample of potential reinforcers is presented to the individual and an assessment of their relative value is made based on the person's reaction to them. The reinforcers are not all presented at the same time, but over a period of time and over a number of trials. The hypothesis would be that individuals respond favourably to those reinforcers they rate most highly. They would be offered access to the reinforcer for engaging in a target behaviour. Their engagement or otherwise would serve as an indication of the value they attach to a particular reinforcer. It may, of course, also be possible and less time consuming to gather this information from someone who knows the person well.

The recognition of the role of the deliverer of the reinforcer has been illustrated by work examining the role of the various elements of a token economy system (Ayllon & Azrin 1968). A token economy is a method of structuring an environment in order to reinforce individuals for engaging in identified target behaviour. It has been used with people suffering with long term mental health difficulties who, as a result of these difficulties, have lost some skills in performing activities of daily living, for example they may have stopped taking care of their personal hygiene. In such a case the target behaviour may be washing or cleaning teeth. The individual would be reinforced for engaging in the target behaviour. The reinforcer would be a token which could be exchanged at a later time for a range of other things. Each target behaviour would have a value given to it and each token would represent a particular value. At face value it would appear that the success of a token economy is based on the individual acquiring tokens to be exchanged for other objects, usually consumable. However, recent work has demonstrated that the efficacy of

token economy is based on the social interaction that takes place during the handing over of the tokens. The most powerful aspects of token economy are suggested to be the feedback, guidance and social contact that individuals get as a result of the system (Falloon, Boyd & McGill 1984, Hall & Baker 1986). These are important findings because they demonstrate that behavioural techniques can be effective by simply using existing human resources and furthermore that the nature of relationships within an environment can have a demonstrable effect on the behaviour of individuals.

This has implications not only for the use of behavioural therapy as an intervention but also as a proactive or health-promoting technique. If individuals are offered reinforcement in their daily lives then it influences their ability to respond to their environment. In the absence of reinforcement, it has been argued that the individuals are at risk from developing learned helplessness—a state which some workers identify with depression (Brown & Harris 1978, Seligman 1973). Negative reinforcement refers to a situation where, if a desired behaviour is demonstrated, an unpleasant stimulus is removed.

Negative reinforcement has been particularly associated with learned helplessness. Seligman (1973) has argued that learned helplessness is a common feature of depression. It arises from individuals' persistent inability to avoid unpleasant events. Negative reinforcement is not accessible to them from their environment. Over time they give up trying to elicit reinforcement from their surroundings. This leads to a person who is apathetic, passive and withdrawn. In a situation where individuals had been given reinforcing feedback from their environment then, Seligman argues, they would be less likely to develop learned helplessness. They would be better able to elicit reinforcement from their environment.

The manipulation of the environment is a crucial element of behavioural work. This is a relatively new development in the therapeutic use of behavioural theories although the early laboratory work of Skinner clearly showed how by manipulating the environment the experiment could observe different responses from the individuals.

Traditionally, workers have considered the consequences of events as being of primary importance (Lyttle 1986), and have paid little attention to the antecedents of the behaviour. This preoccupation can result in a narrow focus for behavioural therapy and the potential to blame the individuals for their own difficulties. If a practitioner is working with someone who persistently behaves in a particular way and that assessment of the behaviour focuses on the results or consequences of the behaviour, then material related to what may have prompted the behaviour will not be available during the assessment and analysis stage of the intervention. The setting events may not be considered and aspects of the environment may go unconsidered. It could be that individuals are engaging in behaviour that is entirely adaptive given the circumstances in which they live. An example might be individuals who are misusing drugs. They could be responding to a set of circumstances that are causing them distress. The only strategy available to them may be to misuse drugs. Similarly, self-control and anger management problems will be assessed as the result of some individual difficulties. The outcome of an assessment which concerns itself entirely with the individual will inevitably identify the source of the difficulties as being located within the individual. An assessment that takes account of the setting events has the potential for recognizing the role of the environment in effecting and promoting maladaptive behaviours which may become part of a mental health problem.

Setting events and cues to behaviour can be manipulated and offer a rich source of interventions for the worker. Take as an example an individual who describes suffering from panic attacks which affect his or her capacity to do everyday things like go to the shops. When assessing the individual's needs it will be important to identify exactly what happens before, during, and after the panic attack. This will be done by using the procedures of functional assessment, that is, making an assessment of antecedents and consequences of the behaviour as well as gathering detailed information about what happens during the panic attack. Information related to the antecedents will yield information about the setting events of the behaviour, for example the individual may describe the preparation for going out on the shopping trip. The preparation may be elaborate and include a whole range of behaviours which make the person feel secure and safe and able to go out. It may be that these preparations merely serve to heighten anxiety and in fact increase the probability of a panic attack. By manipulating these preparatory routines it may be possible to enable the person to go out without having to rely on these props, thereby increasing feelings of personal control and also to reduce the anticipatory anxiety which the person experiences and which may translate into a panic attack.

There may be occasions when the setting events for a particular behaviour may not be clear. There is increasingly a recognition that antecedents may be both proximal and distal. This means that a behaviour may be prompted by events that are closely linked in terms of time, that is, proximal. Other behaviours may be prompted by events that are more distant in time, that is, distal. In the case of distal antecedents it may be difficult to use a strictly behavioural approach in assessment of the person's behaviour and it would be appropriate to consider additional elements in the assessment process, for example cognitive aspects of the behaviour.

REFERENCES

Ayllon T, Azrin N 1968 The token economy: a motivational system for therapy and rehabilitation. Appleton-Century-Crofts, New York

Brown G W, Harris T 1978 Social origins of depression. A study of psychiatric disorder in women. Tavistock, London

Eysenck H J, Rachman S 1961 The causes and cures of neurosis. Routledge & Kegan Paul, London

Falloon L R, Boyd J L, McGill C W 1984 Family care of schizophrenia. Guilford, New York

Fao E B, Rothbaum B O, Murdock T B 1991 Treatment of part traumatic stress disorder in rape victims. A comparison between cognitive-behavioural procedures and counselling. Journal of Consulting and Clinical Psychology 59(5):715

Hall J N, Baker R D 1986 Token economies and schizophrenia: a review. In: Kerr A, Snaith R P (eds) Contemporary issues in schizophrenia. Gaskell, London

Lyttle J 1986 Mental health and disorder. Baillière Tindall, London

Pavlov I 1927 Conditioned reflexes. Oxford University Press, New York

Reber A S 1987 The penguin dictionary of psychology. Penguin Books, Harmondsworth

Salkovskis P M, Warwick H M C 1986 Morbid preoccupation, health anxiety and reassurance: a cognitive behavioural approach to hypochondriasis. Behavioural Research and Therapy 24:597–602

Seligman M E 1973 Helplessness. Freeman, New York

Skinner B F 1953 Science and human behaviour. Macmillan, New York

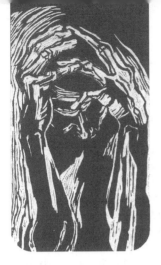

Chapter Nine

An introduction to psychosocial interventions in services

Kieran Fahy   Mike Dudley

AIMS

- ◆ To provide an overview of a contemporary view of psychosis
- ◆ To provide the background to the development of psychosocial interventions
- ◆ To show how such interventions might be incorporated in the service context

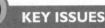

KEY ISSUES

Psychosocial interventions for serious mental illness have a well-established evidence base for their efficacy

Psychosocial interventions are not widely available within routine services

Service configuration of mental health services in the UK and elsewhere hinder the implementation of these approaches

INTRODUCTION

Understanding schizophrenia

Schizophrenia is a major mental illness with estimates of prevalence ranging from 2 to 6 per thousand of the population and an incidence between 0.1 and 0.5 per thousand. The illness is typified by symptoms consisting of hallucination (usually auditory, but it can also affect somatic, olfactory and visual modalities), delusional beliefs and interference with thinking. These symptoms are described as positive symptoms. In addition poor motivation, apathy and social withdrawal affect patients. These symptoms are described as negative symptoms.

There are many factors involved in the outcome of psychosis, especially when applied to schizophrenia. Even those that first described the illness 100 years ago recognized that a minority appeared to have a better outcome. Kraepelin (1919, 1986) believed that schizophrenia had a poor prognosis, finally succumbing to dementia, but still described patients who did rather better. However, it was probably Bleuler (1950) who noticed different patterns of illness with apparently different effects on the individual. Before discussing the contemporary view of serious mental illness in general and schizophrenia in particular, it is worth mentioning the human experience of this illness. This can be understood from the perspective of those who early in the illness experience: How would it be if we were to reconstruct your life? Think of your ambitions and your aspirations, think of the things that society expects for young adults in industrialized societies, such as occupational, social and educational goals—what if something occurred in your life that turned many of these things around ... and the help you received from services you were in contact with gave you little hope of recovery and even less hope of returning to your previous construct of how you thought your life would be? This reconstruction would be similar to the experience of someone suffering their first psychotic episode: the beginning of the illness is often insidious, beginning perhaps with low grade anxiety and intrusive thoughts, and subtle changes in behaviour as the person attempts to make sense of new and bewildering psychological experiences. The person may become confused, find it difficult to concentrate and attempt to cope with the situation by avoiding the situations that are most anxiety provoking; unfortunately for most people these are the complex social situations we encounter every day and without which we would find it hard to function. Slow withdrawal may follow in an attempt to control social stimuli. The fear that they may be going crazy could even cross their minds, and early hallucinatory experiences may occur, stimuli appearing intense.

After many months may have passed the intensity of arousal increases; the person's experiences are still difficult to explain; however, they may begin to form early delusional explanations, and these may be of a paranoid nature. The person may feel suspicious of others' intentions, and this is reinforced by the feelings of anxiety and low mood. The person may also be confused by the reactions of others who do not seem to understand what is *really* going on. The feelings of confusion and mental deterioration continue, the person is less able to process information, attention is adversely affected and the person is unable to filter out stimuli that require less attention from those that require full attention. The person may withdraw completely from social interactions; this situation may continue for weeks or months until the drift into psychosis is complete.

Acute psychosis

The acute phase itself is typified by the core symptoms of the illness; hallucinosis and delusions, severe anxiety and/or depression may be present, and disorders of thinking affect concentration. This may be almost a 'road to Damascus' experience, or a frightening experience, depending on the conclusions the person has come to and how much evidence has been gathered to support these beliefs along the way. Rational thought is difficult; insight has slowly disappeared. This is usually the time the person is in contact with psychiatric services. The world becomes even more confusing as the person may be admitted to hospital, and may be asked to comply with treatment by people who do not understand what is really going on. Within a short time negative symptoms may emerge affecting the person's ability to achieve social and self-care goals.

COURSE AND PROGNOSIS

Much of our understanding of serious mental illness in terms of outcome is illuminated by the long term follow-up studies. There have been many studies that attempt to report the natural history of illnesses like schizophrenia; however, until more recent studies results were difficult to compare owing to differences in methodology used by the researchers involved. None the less, broad themes begin to emerge that challenge the rather negative view of outcome commonly portrayed by other commentators such as the media. In particular the inevitability of chronicity is shown to be only one possible outcome of many.

Studies such as that of Shepherd et al (1989), although being of shorter duration than other studies, take more robust measures of outcome and suggest that schizophrenia sufferers follow one of four possible outcome 'tracks'. It is important to note that a distinction is made between 'social outcome' and the remission of the main symptoms of the illness; this is because many people with schizophrenia maintain or improve social functioning despite suffering residual positive symptoms of the illness. If these four main outcomes are looked at against a backdrop of the stress vulnerability model (see later) an intriguing possibility emerges. If this were the natural history of the illness for a person receiving 'routine care' then the introduction of invulnerability factors such as supportive psychosocial interventions would move people into better outcome tracks.

Legislation in the UK has indicated that services to the seriously mentally ill need to supply a comprehensive service that recognizes the needs of both patients themselves and their families and carers (DOH 1989, 1990). The emergence of case management models in the USA has also served to refocus the work of mental health professionals on those with serious mental illness. These models emerged as a result of the poor conditions many found themselves in once discharged from large institutions. These models have informed the development of the care programme approach (CPA) in the UK. Case management aims to (Onyett 1992):

- get a clear picture of the individual's needs and strengths
- develop a plan that meets the individual needs, with a clearly specified outcome
- implement the plan with the involvement of users and carers
- monitor progress towards the specified objectives
- undertake reviews with the involvement of all interested parties.

All the above are delivered (depending on the model adopted) through an identified 'care coordinator' who is involved not only in the coordination of care, but also in its delivery. Case management normally includes the assertive follow-up of people with serious mental illness, especially those who would otherwise 'slip through the net'. A good CPA system will incorporate many of these approaches (see later). The role of the mental health workers and especially community psychiatric nurses (CPNs), has changed from the early beginnings in the 1950s, where much of their work would have been with people suffering schizophrenia and similar illnesses, to more of a primary care focus and patients with less serious difficulties (Woof, Goldberg & Fryers 1988). Even as this transition of service provision was occurring, pockets of research were beginning to point to the efficacy of what were to become known as psychosocial interventions. The majority of this work has its roots in social psychiatry and psychology; however, as the evidence base continued to grow it became obvious that if these approaches were to be implemented they would need a large, dedicated staff group. It was nurses themselves who began to explore the possibility of using psychosocial interventions within routine services and to suggest that schizophrenia should once again be the priority of services (Brooker, Barrowclough & Tarrier 1992).

WHAT ARE PSYCHOSOCIAL INTERVENTIONS?

Psychosocial interventions for serious mental illness have developed over the past 40 years or so, largely due to the following five seminal developments in our understanding of serious mental illnesses such as schizophrenia.

The role of medication

The first was probably the development of the neuroleptic medications in the mid 1950s and their introduction in the late 1950s. These drugs, such as chlorpromazine and haloperidol, act as dopamine agonists, blocking the uptake of this neurotransmitter. The result was to offer some control over the positive symptoms of illnesses like schizophrenia (hallucinations, delusions, thought disorder) although these drugs have been less effective at dealing with the negative symptoms (apathy, withdrawal, amotivation). These drugs have been largely credited with the closure of large psychiatric hospitals because they offered the first real effective treatment for these illnesses. However, others have challenged this view, suggesting that the large hospitals were contracting prior to this period (Bentall 1990). Despite this there have been numerous studies demonstrating the effectiveness of these drugs (e.g. Birchwood, Hallett & Preston 1988). Our present understanding of drug treatment seems to point to some problems; for instance, there is the issue of treatment adherence (Piatkowska & Farnill 1992) and further that many individuals still suffer significant symptoms despite receiving optimum treatment (Birchwood, Hallett & Preston 1988) Newer drugs have been introduced (known as atypical neuroleptics) that have an affinity with receptors other than dopamine and yet have been demonstrated to be more efficacious. This has challenged the assumption that dopamine is the only neurotransmitter implicated in psychosis and has paved the way for the development of newer, albeit more expensive, drug treatments that are more effective and have fewer anticholinergic side-effects, which are associated with patient discomfort and non-adherence.

Stress vulnerability

The second pivotal development was that of stress vulnerability models (Zubin & Spring 1977). The introduction of stress vulnerability models has helped the understanding of psychosis and unified research and treatment. Before the introduction of these models an unhelpful division of opinion in treatment and research existed, which meant that many strands of research into serious mental illness were quite separate. This may explain why, despite the plethora of research into illnesses like schizophrenia, our conceptualization of the illness is 100 years old and stems from the work of early workers such as Kraepelin and Bleuler.

The stress vulnerability model suggests that a person has a predisposition to developing schizophrenia (most likely biochemical), which, when triggered by a stressful life event, will result in an acute episode. Zubin & Spring (1977) make a distinction between *vulnerability to* schizophrenia, which they regard as relatively permanent, and *episodes* of a schizophrenic illness. Following the first episode, it is suggested that there is a complex interplay between psychosocial factors and internal and external stressors, which can precipitate further episodes. The stress vulnerability model implies that if suitable interventions, together with medication, are available then relapse may be to some extent controlled. It is further suggested that further relapse increases intrinsic vulnerability (Birchwood et al 1994).

It also provides a rationale for many of the psychological, social and biomedical interventions for this client group, including family intervention, medication and the psychological approaches to symptoms. Stress vulnerability models also provide a conceptual framework of how services might be configured to best support clients with psychosis. A potential course of the illness is postulated and factors are identified that may contribute to outcome and, of course, relapse.

Family studies and family intervention studies

The third important development was the family studies in the late 1950s that dispelled commonly held beliefs that the family, and more particularly mothers of people with schizophrenia, were somehow causative agents in the development of the illness (Barrowclough & Tarrier 1992). The role of the family in the outcome of schizophrenia has also received much attention over the years, with a renewed emphasis on the family as being both the most useful potential resource and as a potential stress-maintaining factor. This work began with the finding of George Brown and his colleagues some 40 years ago.

Previous work on families had focused on family members being the cause of the illness; however, none of this work was based on research findings and has since been discredited (Barrowclough & Tarrier 1992). Much damage was caused to the reputation of families in whom a person with schizophrenia was produced and of course a greater feeling of burden and stress was experienced by family members who were told they were the cause of their relative's distress.

Researchers in the late 1950s began to follow up those patients discharged from a large psychiatric hospital in London (Brown et al 1962). George Brown and his colleagues found that those patients who returned from hospital to live with a family or relative fared worse in terms of relapse than those patients who lived alone or in supported accommodation; this was perhaps a surprising finding at the time as the prevailing view was that patients would do better with their families. The research continued and it was found that patients who returned to live where there was an emotional climate of high expressed emotion (HEE) were likely to relapse quicker than those who returned to live with families where the emotional climate was one of low expressed emotion (LEE). The dimensions of HEE found to be important were the degree of hostility and criticism expressed to the client and the degree of emotional involvement (Brown, Birley & Wing 1972, Brown & Rutter 1966). Another important finding was that both the contact time between the patient and relatives within HEE households and the patient's compliance with medication were factors that influenced outcome. Clients who spent fewer than 35 hours per week in face to face contact with a HEE relative and who adhered to their medication regimen

relapsed less than those who had a high degree of face to face contact (above 35 hours per week) and did not adhere to their medication (Vaughn & Leff 1976).

A semistructured interview, the Camberwell Family Interview (CFI), was developed as a method of rating the relatives of people with schizophrenia by rating the number of critical comments they made about the patient, their overall hostility to the patient and their emotional overinvolvement with the patient. By assessing EE within the family of a number of recently discharged clients, it was possible to predict relapse. Of those clients returning to a HEE home 58% relapsed; of those returning to a LEE home only 16% relapsed (Brown, Birley & Wing 1972, Vaughn & Leff 1976). A large number of EE studies have been carried out since, in a number of different countries, that confirm EE as a robust predictor of relapse.

The finding that HEE is associated with significantly greater relapse rates has been found to be consistent (Kavanagh 1992). As a result family interventions have developed and been shown to decrease relapse in intervention studies (Lam 1991).

Family intervention studies have largely been aimed at helping reduce sources of stress and distress within the family unit. Sources of stress include the functional knowledge the relative and client have about the illness, relatives' beliefs and attributions about client behaviours and other stressors including those that impinge on the family from outside sources (Barrowclough & Tarrier 1992). It is important to note that the description of HEE and of course LEE in no way suggests that the family are causal agents of the illness, but rather that these responses typify a range of normal responses that any family member might experience as a result of having a relative suffer an episode of serious mental illness. From the family studies came family intervention studies, where carefully designed and controlled studies were completed to discover whether stress within families could be reduced and therefore the stress experienced by the sufferer reduced; as a result many intervention approaches were developed. Common to most family intervention strategies was their effect on relapse rates; the approaches that emerged to have most therapeutic value were cognitive behavioural in orientation. The most well-known approaches are those of Barrowclough and Tarrier (1992) and Falloon et al (1984). Although these two approaches differ quite largely they have at least two fundamental things in common; the first is the behavioural or cognitive behavioural components and the second is a focus on the reduction of stress within the household. Therefore, in line with stress vulnerability models, it can be seen that the rationale for this intervention is to reduce the stress of the relatives to help them cope, but also to reduce the level of ambient stress in the household and its effect on the sufferer of the illness.

Information processing

Fourthly, the developing literature on cognitive deficits in schizophrenia has further informed our understanding of the illness. Information processing refers to the underlying mechanisms thought to generate psychotic phenomena. This is seen as a biochemical deficit, which involves the arousal and other systems of the central nervous system. The net effect of information-processing deficit is demonstrated most commonly when an individual with schizophrenia is faced with processing complex social situations. Individuals with unaffected information processing are able to shift the focus of attention from one set of stimuli to another with relative ease. This is a vital function because without it we would be at the mercy of a bombardment of stimuli competing for attention. Very soon we would be in a position where the capacity for attention and processing would reach overload and it is not difficult to imagine the resulting anxiety that this would provoke (Neuchterlein & Dawson 1984).

A useful illustration of this is the common experience of meeting a group of friends in a public house that is quite busy. In this situation there are literally thousands of pieces of information to process. In particular there are the complex social verbal and non-verbal behaviours of others and ourselves in the environment. In addition there are others having conversations nearby, music playing and activities going on outside the building that we may be able to see and/or hear. Somehow we are able to direct attention and focus our attention on particular things out of this plethora of stimuli. Even with those unaffected by psychosis a level of anxiety in social situations may be present, and maybe a degree of vigilance for potential threat, especially in the company of strangers.

In psychosis, however, it is suggested that the activity of the arousal system is not so controlled. In ordinary circumstances when a threat presents itself the arousal system kicks in briefly, rather like a single shot from a gun with a rather stiff trigger, allowing us to deal with the threat using the flight or fight response. In psychosis the gun is more like an automatic machine gun with a hair trigger; hypervigilance biases may be heavily coloured by delusional material and the person is subject to a stream of information, all of it demanding equal attention. The result is a feedback loop culminating in further activity of the arousal system and further information-processing difficulty.

Psychological interventions in psychological management of symptoms

The fifth major influence has been the upsurge of research activity in the development of interventions to help sufferers with the residual symptoms they often endure despite optimal doses of medication. These interventions are targeted either at coping with resistant symptoms level or are in fact directed to modify the symptom itself. Although the weight of research evidence at present demonstrates the utility of family interventions, the evidence for psychological management of symptoms is less well established (see Haddock et al 1998 for a review).

Although cognitive behavioural approaches to psychotic symptoms had been described as early as the late 1950s and early 1960s, it was not until the 1980s that renewed interest began to gather momentum. What is common to all psychosocial interventions in serious mental illness is their basis in cognitive behavioural models; indeed, much of the evidence for the efficacy of these interventions comes from psychological research completed in the UK and the USA.

These interventions have been developed to help sufferers from psychosis to cope with the various changes in their illness by targeting either the psychotic symptoms themselves, or the thoughts and behaviours associated with them, even when on optimal levels of treatment (see The role of medication above) or both. The results of this have been the common practice of dealing with patients suffering acute or residual psychotic symptoms by using a variety of distraction techniques of variable quality, or ignoring the patient's delusional talk because of the fear of reinforcing the delusion. We have all witnessed the spectacle of mental health staff being asked by a patient about a delusional belief which is clearly important to them or even distressing, only to be told 'Come and have a cup of tea'! It is partially as a result of the family intervention work, which demonstrated considerable successes, that the work with individual treatments has found a new impetus. The approaches are best divided into those that can be applied to hallucinosis and those that can be applied to delusions and other approaches aimed at enhancing the individual's response to symptoms without directly targeting the symptoms themselves. However, even in this situation some stage in the psychotic symptom itself should be observed as it rarely exists in isolation from other thoughts and feelings an individual may have.

Hallucinations and their management have been of particular interest to researchers and clinicians alike. Clearly they can be one of the more obvious symptoms and therefore the source of considerable distress to the patient in a lot of cases. The key here, as with all of the approaches outlined in this chapter, is that any intervention has to be based upon sound assessment material; as a result of the assessment a careful formulation, which is shared with the patient, is constructed. The preferred approach is one of guided discovery, where patient and therapist set out on a journey to understand, give meaning to and intervene with the symptoms. The assessment of the individual (as with family interventions) begins with a thorough assessment of all of the present symptoms. A useful tool to help do this is the Psychiatric Assessment Scale (also known as the Manchester Scale or the KGVM—from Krawiecka, Goldberg

& Vaughan 1977, revised by Lancashire, unpublished work, 1994). This scale examines 14 symptom items via a detailed interview schedule coupled with detailed observations of non-verbal behaviour. The results of such an interview allow the therapist to gather detailed information about the symptoms in each area covered by the scale; this in turn allows the formation of an outline formulation through which specific symptoms are targeted for intervention. The KGVM is primarily a measure of frequency intensity and duration and so it describes behaviour. The useful thing about carrying out such an interview, apart from the context we are discussing here, is that it is likely that this will be the first time patients have been asked in detail about what they actually experience. Further assessments can then be utilized to focus down on particular symptoms (for instance, delusions). From this information a detailed formulation (which may take various guises depending on the patient) is drawn up and fed back to the client; only when an agreement has been reached as to what areas should be worked on can the therapy proceed.

The approaches used with hallucinosis can be broadly divided into those that employ distraction (basic distraction techniques are widely used by patients, such as using Walkmans) and those that use focusing. Focusing, as its name suggests, goes against traditional models and approaches and encourages patients to pay more attention to their voices rather than trying to suppress them. Several focusing approaches have been described, but perhaps the best described is by Haddock & Slade (1996). They describe four stages of the focusing process:

- describing the physical characteristics of the voice, the antecedents and consequences
- describing the content of the voices, recording exactly what the voice says, shadowing the voice and examining the content; concurrent self-monitoring of the voice in vivo
- describing related thoughts, thoughts that result from the voice-hearing experience and thoughts that might precede the voice
- ascribing meaning to the voice, and self-challenging.

Most focusing approaches have the aim of getting

patients to own the voice as their own thoughts and thus render them open to challenge like any other thoughts we may have. With practice clients can manipulate the voice in order to reduce distress, by modifying their belief about the voices.

The work on delusions, as you might expect, also calls into question the previous distraction approaches described above. Distraction of troublesome thoughts may still be of use to patients themselves, especially if the belief is a particularly painful or unhelpful belief. Other approaches are more directed at obtaining patients' acceptance and understanding of their beliefs and opening up the possibility that they may be open to self-challenge.

It is important to state here that, as described in Chapter 8, cognitive behavioural approaches do not allow the therapist to challenge patients' beliefs directly; indeed, this type of approach has been demonstrated to be very unhelpful to patient and therapist alike; rather it is the use of Socratic questioning techniques (see Chadwick 1997 for a practical guide on the approaches). The aim may be that, through demonstration, reality testing and gathering actual evidence, patients may modify their own belief system through the experience of therapy. Although these approaches do have less evidence to support them, there is about to be released a number of large scale well-designed studies and trials of these approaches that show a deal of promise. We are about to see a revolution in the way we interact with our clients.

EARLY INTERVENTION AND EARLY PSYCHOSIS

Actively learning from the experiences of people requiring treatment for the first time may assist service providers, managers and policy makers within the psychiatric system to purposefully plan for more visible, constructive and generally efficacious pathways to mental health services.
Lincoln, Harrigan & McGorry 1998

There is also evidence that delaying the initiation of neuroleptics in early psychosis (which is in fact the standard treatment) will have a detrimental effect on clinical outcome (see Birchwood, Todd & Jackson 1998 for a review). It follows also that prodromes have recently stimulated interest from researchers and clinicians alike. Prodrome refers to a period before the acute phase of the illness, where subtle changes in the client's psychological well-being and behaviours may herald an acute relapse of the illness. The word 'prodrome' is a term from descriptions of tropical diseases that refers to a period of low grade symptoms before the acute phase of illness (Ashok, Malla & Ross 1984). Prodromes appear to be typified by nervousness, poor appetite, concentration and sleep disturbances, but may also include prepsychotic signs such as suspiciousness and mild feelings of paranoia. Very little work examining prodromes can be identified before 1980, except for single case reports (Ashok, Malla & Ross 1984). Investigations since 1980 have been more systematic in their approach, but have used various methods that confound much in the way of comparison (Beiser et al 1993). The Herz & Melville (1980) study included 145 people with a diagnosis of schizophrenia and 80 of their relatives. The authors discovered that 70% of patients and 93% of relatives reported changes that heralded relapse into an acute episode. In this study, frequently reported prodromal symptoms included sleep problems, fright, tension and anxiety, depression and withdrawal, poor appetite and aggression. Subotnik & Neuchterlein (1988) found that anxiety and depression and thought disturbance were raised prior to relapse; using the Brief Psychiatric Rating Scale to identify these symptoms they reported they could predict 59% of relapses.

Pharmacological early intervention has also been an area of interest to researchers and the speedy introduction of these drugs. Those adopting the low or targeted dose approach include Falloon et al (1993) and Kane (1987). Jolley et al (1989, in Birchwood & Tarrier 1992) compared early drug intervention with a placebo during an identified prodrome and discovered that those receiving intermittent medication relapsed most (all patients were medication free prior to the study). More recently psychological interventions during the so-called critical period have been postulated; the most invasive symptoms and an even greater risk of suicide typify this period (Birchwood 1995, 1996).

The first prodromal phase is often a confusing presentation of cognitive, behavioural and social changes (Birchwood, Todd & Jackson 1998). The greatest variability in morbidity appears to be within the first few years after onset; after 5 years the disorder is less likely to display major fluctuation in symptom and social function. A plateau effect has been observed following this period that appears to be highly predictive of social outcome (Shepherd et al 1989).

Studies following clients prospectively suggest that time to treatment for subsequent episodes, together with length of stay in hospital, are predictive of subsequent episodes (Johnstone et al 1986). Many of these conclusions are drawn from natural history follow-up studies of schizophrenia. The role of social functioning as a measure of outcome has emerged to have little correlation with residual symptoms; however, baselines taken at 6 months posthospitalization is predictive of social function over the coming 5 years (Shepherd et al 1989). In addition, the tragic loss of young lives through suicide is particularly pertinent within the critical period (Drake & Cotton 1986, Westmeyer, Harrow & Maringo 1991). The barriers to treatment that presumably have an effect on treatment lag have not been fully understood, but efforts to improve the reliability of identification have been made (Beiser et al 1993, Johnstone et al 1986, Larsen, Johannessen & Opjordsmoden 1998, Linszen et al 1998), although notions such as the tolerance of men behaving badly (that is, the greater tolerance of young men's behaviour over young females' behaviour in our society), poor education of primary health care, etc. have been postulated as factors in delaying identification. Family, gender, service and socioeconomic factors may also have a part to play (Shepherd et al 1989). Flaherty & Jobe (1990), in a review of gender and expressed emotion and outcome in schizophrenia, suggest that there may be evidence pointing to toxicity in inner city areas, whereas more stable environments may exist in rural areas. The conclusion may be drawn that sociocultural and economic variables may affect outcome.

It is suggested that pathways to care are inconsistent for those with early psychosis (Lincoln et al 1998). Hogman & Pearson (1995), when describing a survey carried out by the National Schizophrenia Fellowship in the UK, refer to the great diversity in terms of contact with agencies, even in those that were previously established within services. This does not bode well for clients and their families who are new to psychiatric services and related services. There is now sufficient circumstantial evidence to suggest that time to treatment is a vital area that demands further study.

Treatment lag, or time to treatment, has been estimated to vary tremendously between subjects, from a number of weeks to at least a year (Johnstone et al 1986) with one study identifying time to treatment of 11 years for one individual (Beiser et al 1993). A longer time to treatment has been associated with increasing complications of frank psychotic experiences, including behavioural disturbances and family difficulties often against a backdrop of multiple attempts by the family to access appropriate care. If we are able to understand more about what stands in the way of clients and their families being able to access appropriate services quickly, the potential impact in terms of outcome could be immense. Less importantly, although arguably, a compelling argument is the potential cost saving to health and social care providers; schizophrenia in particular incurs a heavy cost in terms of inpatient stays.

Evidence from retrospective studies (Beiser et al 1993, Johnstone et al 1986, Shepherd et al 1989) appears to suggest that time to treatment may be a robust predictor of outcome, both in terms of symptoms and social function. The longer the time to treatment the poorer the outcome (Linzen et al 1998). Thus, a pattern of illness that includes overlapping phases emerges along which clients may or may not have opportunities for contacting services and embarking on a pathway to care. This includes time from first changes in behaviour to the emergence of frank psychotic symptoms and the time from frank psychotic symptoms to treatment initiations.

Donlan & Blacker (1975), in their description of early decompensation in schizophrenia point to overlapping phases of the early psychosis experience.

◆ stage 1—the feeling of excitement and loss of control
◆ *stage 2*—transition to overt psychotic symptoms—the interface between early phenomena
◆ *stage 3*—a developing psychotic process
◆ *stage 4*—symptomatic resolution within the acute phase.

Donlan & Blacker (1975) suggest that these stages take several months or years to develop, the early stages having the potential to be the longest; they identify the presence of prehallucinosis experiences as early as stage one. This work is in agreement with contemporary views of the early development of psychosis.

The role of non-prescribed illicit drugs in early psychosis and the effect this may have on treatment lag have been poorly understood, although there is the suggestion that the use of these drugs may potentiate psychosis earlier in those who are vulnerable. It seems worthy then to include changes in the pattern and use of drugs and alcohol as a possible variable in measuring treatment lag. Further evidence is drawn from psychological management of psychosis literature, which describes building on the client's present coping repertoire, which may include the use of illicit substances and alcohol (Barrowclough & Tarrier 1992). In a climate where such substances are readily available to the young and where there is significant pressure to use illicit drugs from peers, it may be no accident that many of those in early psychosis have adjusted their intake of these drugs accordingly, long before the first episode itself becomes known (see stages of early psychosis above).

FROM ROBUST RESEARCH TO PRACTICE

Follow-up studies of trainees who have completed psychosocial interventions courses suggest that there is presently a large gap between providing training and producing workers who will implement these approaches. Two studies demonstrate that a small number of the trainees account for a large part of the clinical work at follow-up. Of the outcome studies completed only the University of Manchester Thorn (COPE) programme shows a good outcome in terms of both patient outcome and implementation of skills (Lancashire et al 1996). Only the University of Sheffield programmes demonstrate that course content affected students' attitudes and beliefs about the illness in a positive way (Milne et al, unpublished work, 1998).

Some of the difficulties outlined by these studies include lack of support by managers, service configuration difficulties and lack of support amongst peers for the approach. These issues are consistent with barriers to implementation of behavioural therapy in general (Corrigan, Kwartman & Pramana 1992). However, these problems need to be seen in the wider context of the particular service system in which they are placed (Woof 1992). Services are configured along traditional views of outcome in schizophrenia. Birchwood & Macmillan (1993) have suggested that the management of schizophrenia is dominated by two philosophies.

1. *Crisis management and medication for prophylaxis*—this treatment can be described as 'routine treatment': no attempt is made to predict possible crisis and there is an overreliance on medication. An example of this may be the patient attending a depot clinic but having no other contact with the service.

2. *Rehabilitation*—traditional rehabilitation models have their roots in institutional practice and focus on occupational and social skills.

They suggest a *third* approach involving early intervention targeted at young vulnerable people in an effort to reduce deterioration. It is this group who may be able to benefit most from early intervention strategies as many will have suffered few relapses and hence will not have the same degree of secondary disabilities as more chronically affected individuals As a result this group may become marginalized, because they are not ill enough for rehabilitation!

It will be surprising to many that, despite the presence of good quality, methodologically sound scientific enquiry validating psychosocial interventions, especially in schizophrenia, comparatively few of these approaches find their way into the training of professionals involved with the care of people with schizophrenia and their families. Also suprising is the long term effect of some of the earlier theories about the illnesses, which leaves relatives feeling blamed and sufferers feeling that their beliefs and experiences are being ignored by those who are meant to care for them, and sufferers themselves feeling there is little that can be done for them. However it appears that the future will see more innovative approaches developed in order to help sufferers and their families. It is clear that these approaches can be delivered within ordinary service settings, provided that the service has clear objectives about its remit.

Service provision for schizophrenia sufferers: strategic psychosocial intervention

Management and managers are not popular in mental health. Management jobs are far the least secure, and managers are frequently held to blame by clinicians when things go wrong. Training for mental health managers is virtually non-existent—most seem to settle for degrees or diplomas in business management. Sadly, there seems to be no clear opportunity for managers to drive their services from a clinical perspective. The idea of doing so (i.e. configuring the service, deriving policies and structuring management around severe and enduring mental illness) we call strategic psychosocial intervention. Our work with over 50 NHS trusts, and survey work such as Sainsbury's, makes it clear that there is no service blueprint in use in the UK; there are large regional differences. Furthermore, there is very little in the way of research addressing the effect of service configuration, management structures and training strategy on clinical outcome. The conclusions drawn in this section, therefore, are based on the following:

1. Close observation of a benchmark service widely acknowledged for its quality, particularly the comment of Shepherd (Director, Health Advisory Service 2000) who wrote in his executive summary, 'the … service was clearly very impressive. It probably has the best developed joint planning and management structure in the country and this, combined with very rigorous targeting on those with severe and enduring problems, a highly developed CPA (Care Program Approach) and monitoring process, and excellent levels of user involvement, make it an outstanding service.' (HAS Report Tameside and Glossop, Community and Priority Services NHS Trust).

2. Some awareness of the things that go wrong for services, based upon our long history (10 years) of providing consultancy.

3. Making logical assumptions about the necessary shape of services, given what we know of the course and treatment of severe mental illnesses.

What can research about schizophrenia tell us about the sort of services we should offer? The research is far more enlightening than many planners are aware. In Table 9.1, we have laid out elements of the research (which you will have found out about in the earlier part of this chapter) and their implications for service shape.

None of these could be called, 'rocket science', and yet many of those who commission or manage services are unaware of the salient areas of the literature. What follows is an effort to show how services can be configured so as to make the above service activities commonplace for all clients with severe and enduring mental illnesses. To make sense of this, we will start with a survey of issues that seem to us to be common trouble spots, which are:

◆ The discharge of people from hospital, especially from acute admission wards, is frequently mishandled.

◆ Equity of opportunity and provision across sector community teams is a very common problem. Frequently the practice of the sector community teams has more to do with the team and team leader than it does with any central trust direction.

◆ The maintenance of a clinically relevant CPA database presents a challenge. Clinicians will tend

Table 9.1

Information from research	Implications for services
Long term illness with varying need level	Stay in touch with the person so you're there if needed
Sufferers can find it hard to engage with services	Don't take 'no' for an answer; never give up attempts to engage the person
Sufferers get into difficulty (with health, suicidal tendencies and the law) especially when they are in chaos and the service does not offer a continuous service with a care coordinator to be responsible for coordinating care and engagement	Never discharge people from any care system without being certain that everyone involved knows what to do
Depression is very common in schizophrenia; suicide rate is very high in young schizophrenic men	Keep a very close eye out for depression; be ready to provide intense support and monitoring for those at risk
Relapse is often predictable and it may be that relapse can be averted by rapid intervention (called early intervention)	Make sure that relapse indicators are recorded for every client, and that this information is known by the client and all formal and informal care givers
Family work has substantial effect on clinical outcome	Make sure families are engaged fast, before relations have so far deteriorated that the client has left/been thrown out of the family home, making family work much harder
Many clients have the same level of disability at year 10 of the illness as they do at year 2	Make efforts to identify new patients quickly and offer intensive intervention

to regard the CPA as a mere bureaucratic exercise if the data lack clinical utility. This impression is reinforced when clinicians are not party to feedback from the database.

◆ The allocation of clients to various levels or tiers of the CPA is, apparently, fraught with difficulty. Trusts vary in the number of levels they recognize, some having only two levels and some as many as five. It is unlikely that all these systems make sense, given that the objective of the CPA was the prioritization of severely mentally ill clients for case-managed service. An additional difficulty is that frequently the allocation of cases to CPA levels is controlled by local definitions of 'severe mental illness' that are often very broad indeed, or can be interpreted as such. This means that operational differences between services for clients on different levels are neither reliable nor helpful, thus further enhancing the CPA's image as an ineffective administrative exercise. Finally, even if the above problems are resolved, if the CPA levels do not link to distinct service units, it is likely that confusion will result.

◆ Community teams are often overloaded by referrals from general practitioners, often cited as the reason for spending little time with clients suffering serious mental illness (SMI). It is rare that a trust-wide screening and allocation system for newly referred clients is implemented, which compounds the problem, leaving too much to individual workers' judgement and the pressures they feel influenced by at the time.

◆ The care of clients who have SMI and are reputedly 'stable', often because of high levels of medication, is inadequate. These patients are often in receipt of low levels of service contact and commonly display poor social function. It is not uncommon for these clients to be unrecognized as severely mentally ill, and may not even be registered on the CPA.

◆ Many trusts have found it difficult to establish effective links with Social Services and with 'user' agencies such as Mind. We have not formed a view as to the common causes of this problem, but suspicion and philosophical difference appear to be influences.

◆ The impact of service confusion on the chances of SMI clients receiving an equitable and effective service should not be underestimated. In chaos (i.e. the absence of policy and procedure), SMI clients will probably lose out to louder voices.

Any attempt to make services more effective must sort out all these problems, because, as will become clear, unresolved difficulties come back to haunt you! Although it would be difficult to lay down a blueprint for services, it is possible to offer a reasoned argument for a sequence of steps that could address these problems.

SOLUTIONS

Getting the bedrock right

Rather like the 'final solution' to the problem of the leaning tower of Pisa, intervention at the base is required in services. The only sound footing that one can build on for mental health services is case management. Not only is the approach well supported by the literature (see above), it offers a system of interagency and multidisciplinary communication and accountability. To begin with, health and social services must establish channels of communication, at a senior level that ensures the joint development and complete integration of the CPA and care management. Thus, services must address the CPA, which means making it do the prioritization job it was intended for, which in turn means that the definition of the priority group, severely mentally ill people, be defined. Pretty well the only definition that can target services is one that leaves few or no 'grey' areas— that is, severe mental illness applies only to those clients suffering from primary psychoses (schizophrenia, bi- and unipolar disorders, schizoaffective disorder, drug-induced psychosis), severe depressive illness and anyone on section 117 of the Mental Health Act. This definition leaves it clear that all other clients of the service occupy level 1 and SMI clients level 2. A subgroup of SMI clients who are deemed particularly at risk can be assigned to level 3. Such a system ensures that those who require a case-managed service

(i.e. SMI clients) get one, and that the other clients who do not need, and might even be damaged by, a case management service do not get one.

Having got a definition into place, the next step is to ensure that the organization of the service reflects the CPA levels 1 and 2. This means having two community services: one secondary service exclusively for psychosis patients (which would also cater for level 3) and the other, a primary service, almost exclusively for level 1 clients. The primary service also provides a screening function, so that only clients who have mental illness (or substantial mental health problems) are offered a service. Clients with common mental disorder are referred to appropriate counselling services such as Relate or GP-based counsellors, or to computer-based self-help or other self-help programmes. Usually this will require the psychosis service to be the larger of the two, probably with higher grades of staff and more advanced skills to reflect the more demanding work. Having established a CPA-level-based service, it is then necessary to provide clinically relevant paperwork to help clinicians and their clients and which also collects data, which can be analysed and fed back as needed to planners and clinicians via a computerized database. Finally, an audit system must be created that allows the CPA coordinator to ensure the procedure is being used correctly.

Strategic clinical objectives

Objectives for the service can be derived from the literature. As far as SMI goes, these are fairly clear: all clients who present a relapse risk must have an early intervention plan in place that must include all carers, both professional and informal, who are involved. Clients in the first 3 to 5 years of their illness must be targeted for intense support and intervention so that in years to come chronicity risks are reduced and the overall service burden from so-called 'revolving door' clients is also reduced. This will enable, in the future, current chronically ill clients to receive the specialist help they need (i.e. the remediation of cognitive deficit to enable them to engage with evidence-based psychological assistance).

DISCUSSION QUESTIONS

1. What principles would help to decrease family stress and distress?
2. How might stress vulnerability models affect how you work with people with psychosis?
3. How might you work differently with early psychosis patients?
4. What effect is your knowledge about information processing going to have on your future practice?
5. What should a service for people with psychosis look like?

SUMMARY

Whilst very few services are configured rationally to meet the needs of SMI clients, some are, thus demonstrating that it is possible. It should be understood, though, that because of the widespread developments most organizations would have to undergo to focus properly on SMI clients it would be hard to do this on a 'bottom-up' or 'clinician-led' basis. However, while the NHS culture continues to undervalue management by frequent exhortation to reduce management costs, by making management posts more vulnerable than most to redundancy, and by failing to provide a coherent and strategically focused training pro-

FURTHER READING

Barrowclough C, Tarrier N 1992 Families of schizophrenic patients: cognitive behavioural intervention. Chapman & Hall, London.
Although showing its age by now, this remains the definitive text on family interventions. It describes in some detail the background to the development of the authors' formulation-driven approach; however, it assumes prior knowledge of CBT approaches and can be difficult to follow if you do not have this background.

Bentall R 1990 Reconstructing schizophrenia. Routledge, London.
A first class text that challenges our views of schizophrenia and psychosis in general: very detailed, meticulously described and a good read.

Chadwick H, Birchwood M, Trower P 1996 Cognitive therapy for delusions, voices and paranoia. John Wiley, New York
Excellent text describing some of the latest approaches to tackle residual psychotic symptoms; again assumes prior knowledge of CBT.

Falloon I R H, Laporta M, Fadden G, Graham-Hole V 1993 Managing stress in families. Routledge, London

Another seminal book on family interventions; describes the authors' 'behavioural family management' approaches in detail, a more flexible approach than at first it looks. Some of the approaches are described in rather 'mid-Atlantic' terms, but it is well worth reading.

Kingdon D, Turkington D 1994 Cognitive behavioural therapy of schizophrenia. Lawrence Erlbaum, New York
Probably one of the most useful books to come out in the past decade (at least as far as clinicians are concerned). It is readable, helpful and obviously written by people working at the 'sharp end' and is therefore a must.

Nelson H 1997 Cognitive behavioural therapy with schizophrenia, a practice manual. Stanley Thornes, Cheltenham
Another trail-blazing text that makes no assumptions about the reader's level of knowledge and describes in detail very practical approaches that can be used with residual symptoms, again very easy to read, written from experience and again a must.

gramme for mental health managers, it is not likely that aspiring, high quality personnel will be attracted by managerial jobs. Hopefully, readers will not take this as yet another example of management bashing. Rather, it is our intention to suggest that most services are not well led (witness the widespread failure to implement the CPA properly or develop fully joint strategies between health, social services and user organizations) and that we need to invest in managers.

ACKNOWLEDGEMENTS

The authors would like to thank Sheila Dudley of Tameside and Glossop Mental Health Services for providing a service model and guidance which forms the basis of our comments on service systems.

REFERENCES

Ashok K, Malla A K, Ross M G N 1984 Prodromal symptoms in schizophrenia. British Journal of Psychiatry 164:487–493

Barrowclough C, Tarrier N 1992 Families of schizophrenic patients: cognitive behavioral intervention. Chapman & Hall, London

Barrowclough C, Tarrier N, Watts S, Vaughn C, Bamrah J, Freeman H 1987 Assessing the functional value of relatives' reported knowledge about schizophrenia. British Journal of Psychiatry 151:1–8

Beiser M, Erickson M A, Flemming J A E, Iacono W G 1993 Establishing the onset of psychotic illness. American Journal of Psychiatry 150(9):1349–1353

Bentall R 1990 Reconstructing schizophrenia. Routledge, London

Birchwood M 1995 Early interventions in psychotic relapse: cognitive approaches to detection and management. Behaviour Change 12(1):2–19

Birchwood M 1996 Early intervention in psychotic relapse. Cognitive approaches to detection and management. In: Haddock G, Slade P (eds) Cognitive-behavioural interventions with psychotic disorders. Routledge, London

Birchwood M, Macmillan F 1993 Early intervention in schizophrenia. Australian and New Zealand Journal of Psychiatry 27:374–378

Birchwood M, Tarrier N 1992 Innovations in the psychological management of schizophrenia: assessment, treatment and services. John Wiley, New York

Birchwood M, Hallett S, Preston M 1988 Schizophrenia: an integrated approach to research and treatment. Longman, Harlow

Birchwood M, Smith J, Macmillan F, Hogg B, Prasad R, Harvey C, Bering S 1989 Predicting relapse in schizophrenia, the development and implementation of an early signs monitoring system using patients and families as observers. A preliminary investigation. Psychological Medicine 19:649–656

Birchwood M, McGorry P, Jackson H, Edwards J, McGarry A 1994 Early intervention in psychosis: opportunities and prospects. Keynote address at the first National Early Psychosis Conference, University of Melbourne, Australia

Birchwood M, Todd P, Jackson C 1998 Early intervention in psychosis, the critical period hypothesis. British Journal of Psychiatry 172(suppl 33):53–59

Bleuler E 1950 Dementia praecox or the group of schizophrenias (trans Zinkin J), (original work published 1911). International Universities Press, New York

Brooker C, Barrowclough C, Tarrier N 1992 Training community psychiatric nurses in psychosocial interventions: evaluating the impact of health education for relatives. Journal of Clinical Nursing 1:19–25

Brooker C, Tarrier N, Barrowclough C, Butterworth A, Goldberg D 1993 Skills for CPNs working with seriously mentally ill people: the outcome of a trial of psychosocial intervention. In: Brooker C, White E (eds) Community psychiatric nursing: a research perpective, vol 2. Chapman & Hall, New York

Brown G W, Rutter M L 1966 The measurement of family activities and relationships. Human Relations 19:241

Brown G W, Monck E M, Carstaires G M, Wing J K 1962 Influence of family life on the course of schizophrenic illness. British Journal of Preventive and Social Medicine 16:55–68

Brown G W, Birley J L T, Wing J K 1972 Influence of family life on the course of schizophrenic disorders: a replication. British Journal of Psychiatry 121:241–258

Chadwick H 1997 Cognitive therapy with schizophrenia, a practice manual. Stanley Thornes, Cheltenham

Corrigan P W, Kwartman W Y, Pramana W 1992 Staff perception of barriers to behaviour therapy at a psychiatric hospital. Behaviour Modification 64 (Jan): 132–144

Creer C, Wing J 1974 Schizophrenia at home. National Schizophrenia Fellowship, London

DOH (Department of Health) 1989 Caring for people. HMSO, London

DOH (Department of Health) 1990 The care programme approach for people with a mental illness referred to the specialist psychiatric services. HMSO, London

Donlan P T, Blacker K H 1975 Clinical recognition of early schizophrenic decompensation. Diseases of the Nervous System June:323–327

Drake T, Cotton T 1986 Relationship between psychosis and suicide amongst schizophrenics: a comparison of attempted and completed suicides. British Journal of Psychiatry 149:784–787

Falloon I R H, Boyd J L, McGill C W, Razani J, Moss H B, Gilderman A 1982 Family management in the prevention of exacerbations of schizophrenia: a controlled study. New England Journal of Medicine 306:1437–1440

Falloon I, Boyd J, McGill C 1984 Family care of schizophrenia. Guilford, London

Falloon I R H, Lapporta M, Fadden G, Graham-Hole V 1993 Managing stress in families: cognitive behavioural strategies for enhancing coping skills. Routledge, London

Falloon I R H, Coverdale J H, Laidlaw T M, Merry S, Kydd R R, Morosoni P and the OTP collaborative group 1998 Early intervention for schizophrenic disorders, implementing optimal treatment strategies in routine clinical services. British Journal of Psychiatry 172 (suppl. 33):33–38

Flaherty J A, Jobe T H 1990 Gender, expressed emotion and outcome in schizophrenia. Current Opinion in Psychiatry 3:23–28

Haddock G, Slade P (eds) 1996 Cognitive–behavioural interventions with psychotic disorders. Routledge, London

Haddock G, Tarrier N, Spaulding W, Yusupoff L, Kinney C, McCarthy E 1998 Individual cognitive-behavior therapy in the treatment of hallucinations and delusions: a review. Clinical Psychology Review 18(7):821–838

Hatfield A 1990 Family education in mental illness. Guilford Press, London

Herz M, Melville C 1980 Relapse in schizophrenia. American Journal of Psychiatry 137:801–812

Hogman G, Pearson G 1995 The silent partners: the needs and experiences of people who provide informal care to people with a severe mental illness. NSF National Office, Kingston-upon-Thames, February

Johnstone E C, Crow T J, Johnson A L, Macmillan J F 1986 The Northwick Park Study of first episode schizophrenia: I Presentation of the illness and problems relating to admission. British Journal of Psychiatry 148:115–120

Kane J 1987 Low dose and intermittent neuroleptic treatment strategies for schizophrenia (interview). Psychiatric Annals 17(2 February)

Kavanagh D J (ed) 1992 Schizophrenia: an overview and practical handbook. Chapman & Hall, New York

Kraepelin E 1919 Dementia praecox and paraphrenia (trans Barclay R M). E & S Livingstone, Edinburgh

Kraepelin E 1986 Dementia praecox. Psychiatrie 5th edn. Translated in: Cutting J, Shepherd M (eds). The clinical roots of schizophrenia concept. Cambridge University Press, Cambridge, pp. 426–441

Krawiecka M, Goldberg D, Vaughan M 1977 A standardised psychiatric assessment scale for chronic psychotic patients. Acta Psychiatrica Scandinavica 55:299–308

Lam D 1991 Pschosocial intervention: a review of empirical studies. Psychological Medicine 21:423–441

Lancashire S, Haddock G, Tarrier N, Baguley I, Butterworth A, Brooker C 1996 The impact of training community psychiatric nurses to use psychosocial interventions with people with severe mental health problems. Psychiatric Services 48:39–41

Larsen T K, Johannessen J O, Opjordsmoden S 1998 First episode schizophrenia with long duration of untreated psychosis: pathways to care. British Journal of Psychiatry 175 (suppl 33):45–52

Leff J, Vaughn C 1985 Expressed emotion in families. Guilford Press, London

Leff J P, Kuipers L, Berkowitz R, Sturgeon D 1985 A controlled trial of social intervention in the families of schizophrenic patients: two year follow up. British Journal of Psychiatry 146:594–600

Lincoln C V, McGorry P 1995 Who cares? Pathways to psychiatric care for young people experiencing a first episode of psychosis. Psychiatric Services 46(11):1166–1171

Lincoln C, Harrigan S, McGorry P 1998 Understanding the topography of the early psychosis pathways. An opportunity to reduce delays in treatment. British Journal of Psychiatry 172 (suppl 33):21–25

Linszen D, Lenior M, De Haan L, Dingemans P, Gersons B 1998 Early intervention, untreated psychosis and the course of early schizophrenia. British Journal of Psychiatry 172(33):84–89

Neuchterein K H, Dawson M 1984 Information processing and attentional functioning in the developmental course of schizophrenic disorders. Schizophrenia Bulletin 10:160–203

Onyett S 1992 Case management in mental health. Chapman & Hall, London

Piatkowska O, Farnill D 1992 Assessment of family interaction with a schizophrenic member. In: Kavanagh D J (ed) Schizophrenia: an overview and practical handbook. Chapman & Hall, New York

Shepherd M, Watt D, Falloon I, Smeeton N 1989 The natural history of schizophrenia: a five year follow-up study of outcome and prediction in a representative sample of schizophrenics. Psychological Medicine: Monograph suppl 15. Cambridge University Press, Cambridge

Subotnik K I, Neuchterlein K H 1988 Prodromal signs and symptoms of schizophrenic relapse. Journal of Abnormal Psychology 97:405–412

Vaughn C E, Leff J P 1976 The influence of family and social factors on the course of psychiatric illness. British Journal of Psychiatry 129:125–137

Westmeyer J F, Harrow M, Maringo J T 1991 Risk of suicide in schizophrenia and other psychotic and non-psychotic disorders. Journal of Nervous and Mental Diseases 179:259–269

Woof K 1992 Service organisation and planning. In: Birchwood M, Tarrier N (eds) Innovations in the psychological management of schizophrenia: assessment, treatment and services. John Wiley, New York

Woof K, Goldberg D P, Fryers T 1988 The practice of community psychiatric nursing and mental health social work in Salford: some implications for community care. British Journal of Psychiatry 152:783–792

Zubin J, Spring B 1977 Vulnerability—a new view of schizophrenia. Journal of Abnormal Psychology 86(2):103–126

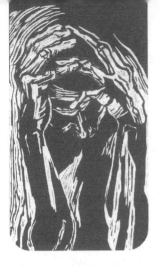

Chapter Ten

Social skills training

Mike Musker

AIMS

- ◆ To describe components of social skills
- ◆ To examine models of communication and the training cycle
- ◆ To describe the set-up and tools required for a social skills programme
- ◆ To assess, implement, and evaluate a social skills programme
- ◆ To provide information about verbal and non-verbal components of communication within a social skills model

KEY ISSUES

Components of the communication cycle

Molecular and molar skills

Setting up a social skills group

Evaluating an individual's progress

Exercises for developing social skills

INTRODUCTION

Many of us will take our own social competence for granted, but even mental health professionals are known to be poor at communicating with others. Social skills can be described as the way two or more humans interact in a variety of situations. The way we interact with each other can be broken down into specific behaviours, which will be referred to as *molecular skills* (Pope 1986). The subunits of communication are made up of small nuances from our everyday socialization such as eye contact, smiling and handshakes. We learn to mix with others just as we learn any personal skill. Behaviours can be grouped together into schemas, which allow us to use learnt behaviours in new situations. These grouped behaviours are referred to as *molar skills*. Every new social situation is likely to be different from the last and the brain remembers the way we dealt with similar situations through schematic processing (Atkinson et al 1996). This is an efficient form of remembering how to behave in social arenas. People who have mental health problems have difficulties in learning and remembering how to use even the most basic social skills for a variety of reasons, which will be explored. Even when people are fully conversant with the theory of a skill, they may have difficulty in practice because of anxiety or because they have had a bad experience when dealing with others. Social skills training is known to be effective when juxtaposed with other forms of treatment and it has reduced the risk of relapse in some people diagnosed with schizophrenia (Hayes, Halford & Varghese 1995, Hogarty et al 1986). This is supported by a 2-year study on social skills training, which proved more effective than other supportive therapies (Marder et al 1996). This chapter will help mental health practitioners examine social skills in more detail and then describe a social skills training programme that can be implemented in most settings.

COMPONENTS OF SOCIAL SKILLS

The basic model of communication involves a sender, receiver, message, feedback, and context (Stuart & Laraia 1998). Argyle (1978) expanded this model of interaction to explain how people usually have a goal, which provides an initial stimulus to achieve a desired response. We then modify our behaviour in accordance with changes in the other person's reaction. Any subtle changes have to be perceived correctly, translated and a new response given for the interaction to be successful. From early childhood we learn acceptable ways of behaving through classical conditioning, operant conditioning, habituation and complex learning. So we learn social skills from those around us, our parents, role models at school and from television. Some human behaviours can be considered innate and have been shown to be consistent across cultures and even species (Ekman 1982). An example of cross-cultural behaviour is facial expressions such as smiling with happiness, baring teeth in anger and frowning in fear. These are fairly spontaneous reactions and are closely related to how we feel—so close, in fact, that the facial feedback hypothesis suggests that we can make ourselves feel better by smiling more often (Tompkins 1962). Many social responses are innate and relate back to some survival function: smiling inferring submission, baring the teeth signalling aggression. If we analyse these signals more closely we begin to see the importance of each component. On average talking takes up only 10 minutes of our day, the rest being filled with other forms of communication (Hargie & McCartan 1986). Most of our behaviours can be broken down into their most simple parts including social distance, gaze, posture and the way we dress. These small components are the molecular skills (Pope 1986). As we grow older we experience new situations and learn to group molecular skills in the most effective way, these grouped behaviours are the molar skills. New social skills are reinforced through operant conditioning in the form of internal and external positive rewards (Dickson, Saunders & Stringer 1993). We also learn to copy others through modelling and role play. This may be through imitating a person we like and respect, but may include faulty role models that we see on television. Albert Bandura demonstrated how children will mimic adult behaviour, including verbal and non-verbal behaviour (Atkinson et al 1996).

UNDERSTANDING THE COMPONENTS OF A SOCIAL SKILLS MODEL

Every social situation we enter into is different and how we perceive this experience is combined with an individual's memory of learnt behaviours. This interplay has been referred to as the 'person situation context' (Hargie, Saunders & Dickson 1994). We can examine this more closely by working through a model of social skills using the following example. Imagine you see someone across a crowded room and want to talk to them. Some of the dynamics that should be considered when understanding this basic interactive process are illustrated in Figure 10.1.

Sender—initiator of interaction

Perception

You have to be alert enough to look around the room, demonstrating how communication is closely related to neocortical abilities and brain function. You also have to recognize from memory the person to whom you wish to speak. To do this you utilize the five senses when analysing the social environment.

Motivation

You have to want to speak to the individual concerned and you may have a specific goal to achieve by talking to them. There are a variety of ways to think of motivation and desired goals. For example, Maslow's hierarchy of needs (1954) is useful in describing goals of interaction, such as the need for love and belongingness. Eric Berne (1985) identified the fact that interactions are often moti-

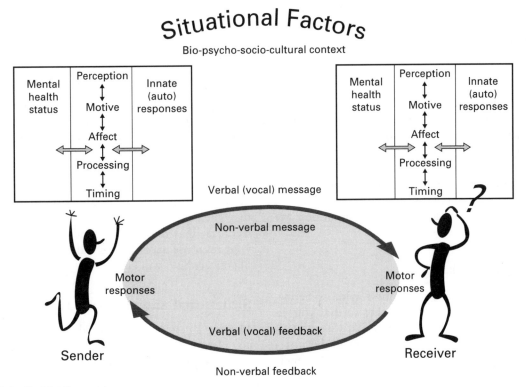

Fig. 10.1 Social skills model.

vated by complex interpersonal games in the form of hidden agendas. He used transactional analysis to describe the importance of ego states during interaction. A complementary transaction, for example, means that two people are using the same ego state, such as adult to adult.

Affect

Your mood will affect your desire to talk to other people and the way you will greet them. It will also have an effect on all other factors. It is common that people who lack social skills have low self-esteem and lack the motivation to seek the pleasure of mixing with others (anhedonia). This is made worse by a depressed outlook on life. Once people have experienced a loss of control or fear during an interaction, they may learn to associate this with helplessness. A lack of social skills has been compared with learned helplessness, whereby a person becomes almost phobic about being with others (Power & Dalgleish 1997). Such powerful influences are accumulated during childhood experiences with parents or significant others and these are ingrained into our behavioural schemas.

Processing

Your brain has to process all this information by assessing your previous experiences with the individual you are about to meet, recall and process earlier experiences of similar situations, and then choose which motor responses you will display in order to achieve your goal. As you can imagine, the possible combinations between knowledge, emotional experience and social situations are almost infinite.

Timing (meshing)

When you have a conversation with someone, your timing has to mesh together so that you do not both speak at the same time. This is an intricate skill that requires feedback from all the aforementioned processes and signalling cues. Timing is a combination of the flow of themes in a conversation, appropriate pauses between speakers and spontaneous turn taking (Trower, Bryant & Argyle 1978).

Motor responses

These are the observable aspects of human interaction and therefore are easily measured. You will display a set of molecular skills such as waving, smiling and approaching the other person, which make up the more complex molar skills such as greeting or initiating a conversation. The verbal and non-verbal behaviour are both considered as motor responses.

Messages

The behaviours you display will send a message to the other individual. This can be verbal (including paravocal cues such as volume, pitch and speed) and non-verbal. Remember that the message is highly dependent on the context, and much of it is lost in transfer. Some speech contains metamessages, which can completely alter the verbal information. Examples include altering the pitch and tone of your voice to infer hostility or sexual attraction (McKay, Davis & Fanning 1995).

Receiver—respondent of interaction

Other people will also use all of their five senses to perceive your message and then go through the same set of cognitive and behavioural processes to interpret it (Dickson, Hargie & Morrow 1989). Once they have spotted you from across the room, they will decide whether they want to meet you or not and go through all the above mechanisms, as they then become the sender. Depending on the feedback that the receiver sends, you will adjust your response accordingly, and the two-way flow of conversation will begin.

Situational and contextual issues

Meeting a person across crowded rooms may be a completely new situation for you personally, or you may hate meeting people in public situations. You may not be very confident and your self-esteem may be low to the point where you have developed a social phobia. Previous experience will have informed you how to behave. All of the following attributes are examples of contextual factors that may affect how you perform in such a social situation:

◆ biological factors including the temperature, how you feel physically and gender
◆ psychological factors including anxious, tense, and hostile situations
◆ social factors including class, location, family and social relationships
◆ cultural factors including behavioural practices, rituals and language barriers.

Your mental health status will also affect how you respond to others, as people with mental health problems are known to be poor receivers (Trower, Bryant & Argyle 1978). You may feel so tired or be too distracted that you do not see the other person waving to you. More serious symptoms may affect social skills significantly. People who are hallucinating may perceive a wave as a threat, or a paranoid person may misinterpret the way you look at them. Non-verbal behaviours can be ambiguous and are culturally based. The way we use interactive signals is important in communication and these can be divided into four parts. 'Emblems' include behaviours such as waving and can replace the need to say hello. These are usually key messages specific to a culture. 'Illustrators' can be used to support something you are saying, such as length and height. 'Regulators', such as nods, hand movements and eye contact, help an individual to gauge their timing and support language. Finally, 'adaptors', such as crossing the legs, tapping the feet, scratching the head, and even use of objects in the environment, are all ways of supplementing messages (Hargie 1997). Social skills training will involve helping individuals to relearn and become more sensitive to such cues.

A depressed person may have difficulty in responding to others, lacking the motivation to react to even the warmest invitation of conversation. They are likely to avoid eye contact, and have limited hand movements (Hargie & McCartan 1986). Someone suffering from schizophrenia may be experiencing unusual thought processes and may provide you with an incongruous response. A common example used is knight-move thinking, whereby the person makes unusual sideways leaps in conversation. By examining the model of normal interaction, we can begin to understand how the complexities of mental health can affect every component of social skills, particularly perception, cognitive processing and the way we feel during a conversation.

DEVELOPING A SOCIAL-SKILLS-TRAINING GROUP

Social skills training is a unique area of health where interdisciplinary team working can prove very effective. The referral process should seek the views and support of the multidisciplinary team. A referral form should be completed by the care team, which should also provide permission to use audiovisual equipment during the training. An explanation of what will be done with the recordings, and who will be allowed to view the material, should be discussed as part of the referral process. If within a hospital setting it may be necessary to approach the ethics committee for permission to use video-recording equipment as part of your programme. The assessment and practising elements of the programme will require support from the individual's caseworker. The caseworker will be expected to help trainees with their homework assignments, which will be set for completion between sessions. They will also be asked to complete a social skills assessment document at the beginning and following the final group, which is a subjective measurement of the person's skills. As mental health practitioners we can use social skills training as a form of mental health promotion with the aim of improving the trainees' ability to perform within social settings (Downie, Tannahill & Tannahill 1996). This acts as a form of enablement, allowing individuals to act more autonomously, reducing their dependence on the psychiatric system and in some cases allowing them to mix better with their family members, reducing high expressed emotion (HEE) (Davison & Neale 1998). A training programme should have a minimum of two facilitators, preferably of the opposite sex to enable the trainees to practise their skills with either gender (Littrell & Freeman 1995). This is because men and women tend to behave differently in conversation. Men try to dominate a conversation, whereas women are more polite and ask more questions. There are also more obvious differences, as in pitch and vocabulary (Argyle 1992). The following social skills programme is based on the cybernetic model, which means the training uses a cognitive behavioural method of teaching incorporating four critical stages of guidance, demonstration, practice and feedback (Ellis & Whittington 1981). This process can be broken down into identification and acquisition of skills. The main focus of training is in the psychomotor domain and improvement in this area can be measured by observing changes in molecular and molar behaviours. The following assessment method is provided as a guide in measuring improvements in the trainee's social skills. This type of assessment is essential for providing feedback to the care team and the person taking part in the programme, and for setting outcome measures for future groups (Collins & Collins 1992).

ASSESSMENT

Some consideration should be given to the level of training being provided and the expected outcomes in the provision of a social-skills-training group. The main focus of this programme is to get service users talking to each other and functioning within their community, even at the most basic level of interaction. Many individuals with mental health problems are left to just sit around wards or at home and hardly ever get the opportunity to practise communicating with other people (Rosenhan 1973). They may be so ill, or anxious, that the lack of practice of basic interaction skills has been extinguished or the fear of meeting people has become too great. Advanced social-skills-training programmes are available, for example, to assist those having difficulties with job interviews, or who require specific assertion training. Such specialized programmes are not to be confused with the training described here. Facilitators should be aware of the difference in skill levels

within their group. The first focus should be in attempting to match the level of skill when setting up the group. Where this is not possible, consider how you will use the individual differences to the group's advantage, possibly enlisting the more able participants as role models for the rest of the group (Trower, Bryant & Argyle 1978).

The assessment form is divided into three key areas: molecular skills; molar skills; and specific situational skills (Box 10.1). This should be tailored to follow the agenda and skill level of the group. Facilitators will ask the caseworker, or a member of the care team who knows the trainee well, to complete an assessment form prior to week 1 (baseline) and following week 10 (outcome measure). This information will provide a baseline toward outcome measures and evidence-based practice. There are two scales of measurement that can be used, which are the Likert Scale and the Semantic Differential Scale. The Likert Scale uses five headings such as very poor, poor, average, good and very good. The Semantic Differential Scale is a scale between two extreme poles such as 'not competent = 0' and 'highly competent = 10' (Depoy & Gitlin 1994). The latter is the preferred scale because it focuses on the positive aspect of people's progress rather than their deficits. It is also useful in graphing individuals' progress across the 10 weeks that a programme can take. The accumulated information is beneficial when discussing improvement in skills with the participant, and care team. It is important that the same facilitator continues as the assessor throughout the 10-week programme, so variation in skill measurement will not be affected by interrater reliability. There are specialized social skills assessments, but these will not have the same relevance to your group and participants, but rather will provide greater validity and reliability for research. You may want to consider completing standardized questionnaires in conjunction with the progress assessment provided here, and it is worth consulting the team psychologist about this. Notes should be taken about each individual's general performance and specific deficits immediately following each session. This will enable you to write an accurate summary report to feed back to the person's care team.

Box 10.1	Social skills assessment					
	Week 1 - Score	Week 2 - Score	Week 3 - Score	Week 4 - Score	Week 5 - Score	Up to week 10
Molecular skills						
Observing others						
Listening skills						
Voice clarity and volume						
Eye contact						
Gestures and touch						
Head nods						
Paravocal cues (aha, etc.)						
Posture						
Facial expression						
Smiling (specific training)						
Proximity and orientation						
Timing (meshing)						
Appearance						
Confidence						
Use of daily diary						
Molar skills						
Greetings						
Initiating a conversation						
Maintaining a conversation						
Joining a conversation						
Questioning others						
Terminating a conversation						
Asking for help/refusal						
Apologizing						
Asserting yourself						
Situational skills	*Comments about progress in group*			*Comments about progress on day out*		
Using the telephone to set up a meeting						
Making an appointment with care team member						
Using a bank or post office or public transport office						
Purchasing and asking a question about retail goods						
Getting information—e.g. from an information centre						
Ordering a meal and a drink in a restaurant						
Setting up a date with a friend						

(use scale of 0–10: 0 = not competent 10 = highly competent)

SETTING UP A SOCIAL SKILLS PROGRAMME

With the advancement of modern technology the resources required for social skills training are accessible to most areas of practice. Where necessary, social skills training can be provided on a one to one basis or in a very small group and feedback can be given verbally. The equipment suggested here is for the ideal set-up. The main requirements are:

◆ a large room and chairs
◆ a tape recorder (for homework practice)
◆ a video camera and remote
◆ a video recorder and remote
◆ a television
◆ pens and paper
◆ A3 pads and pens or
◆ dry marker boards and pens
◆ cue cards (scripts) developed by the facilitator
◆ video examples of good and bad social skills
◆ daily diaries
◆ props where available, such as newspapers and an empty box.

The reason the audiovisual equipment and other items are needed is to provide reflective information to the trainees as a form of microteaching. This allows the facilitators to supply clear, honest feedback, allowing the participants to criticize their own practice and alter their behaviour accordingly. The amount of people in a group should be about six to nine. Any larger a group would make it difficult to work through the video feedback, and any smaller provides fewer models for others to learn from. Setting up the room is important and two variations are proposed. A common set-up is to have the audiovisual equipment in a separate room with a one-way mirror separating the practice and the feedback. If these facilities are available, you may prefer to use them; however, a less laboratory-style set-up is preferred. In this style, all the equipment should be in one large room and the participants should be encouraged to get involved in working the equipment to reduce their anxieties and fear about being on film. It also enables the facilitators to focus on the participants rather than on the equipment—see Figure 10.2.

Week 1: Warm-up and introducing social skills

Anyone who has problems with social skills will undoubtedly find the first week anxiety provoking and challenging. The assessment completed by the caseworker should be examined and an awareness gained of the skill deficits for each individual prior

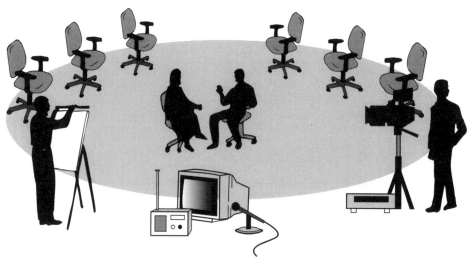

Fig. 10.2 Room layout for a social skills group.

to the group meeting. A vague strategy should be developed of how you will identify compatible pairs and threesomes within the group. The main objective of the first week is to get the participants comfortable with each other and being part of a group, relaxing with the equipment in the room, and introducing some information about social skills. Another important aspect of the first group is to set the ground rules. Some of the group may smoke or like a drink during the session, so it would be productive to provide a drink and smoke break in the middle of each session. Others may be concerned about how often they have to attend, how long the group will last and if anyone else will be joining the group. Once a social skills group has been formed it is usually a closed group with the same facilitators for all sessions. A closed group means that no new members may join. It is important that individuals attend every session if possible, as skills are usually graduated from basic to more complex skills. Sessions should last between 1 and 2 hours, and the group should meet between once and twice per week, allowing enough time to practise and develop skills. Every effort should be made to gain consensus about such issues prior to the group starting. Consensus about ground rules, attendance and homework assignments can be strengthened through a written contract. The facilitators will introduce themselves and provide a brief explanation of what the social skills group is about and then move toward explaining the aims and objectives of the first session. Supplying nametags for the whole group would be helpful for those who have difficulty in remembering names. Handouts are useful, allowing participants to follow the session and in providing information about specific skills. We then move to the first exercise, which is known as an icebreaker.

Exercise 1: icebreaker

The group is seated in a semicircle. A beanbag or cushion is used to throw to another person in the room. The person throwing the beanbag states 'my name is … what's your name?'. This can be developed into '… has just thrown the beanbag to … and I am throwing it to …' and this allows

the facilitators to assess concentration, memory, general eye contact, facial expressions, body postures and listening skills.

Information giving: body language

Part of each session will involve some didactic teaching about the social skills being learnt. It is up to the facilitators to gauge the level and pace of their discussion. So you may want to use the first week to find out how much the group knows about specific molecular skills. An information handout should be provided and the items discussed as a group. Here is a brief introduction to non-verbal skills.

Molecular skills

Observing others. It is necessary to observe others so we can study the non-verbal communication from all the five senses. It is calculated that around 7% of what is being communicated is expressed in words, 38% in paravocal cues and 55% in non-verbal cues (Stuart & Laraia 1998). Non-verbal behaviour is seen as more honest than verbal messages and this is because we find it difficult to suppress 'leakage'. Leakage are non-verbal clues to what a person really feels and can indicate when someone is lying—for example, when they place their index finger horizontally below their nose, using the rest of the hand to cover up what they are saying (Trower, Bryant & Argyle 1978). Non-verbal aspects of communication, or body language, are occasionally referred to as kinesics (Birdwhistell 1970).

Listening skills. Active listening takes a lot of concentration and it is suggested that we encode only about 50% of what is communicated. Listening is about acquiring the information, being able to process it and being able to interpret it in the context of what is being said (Hargie 1997).

Voice clarity and volume. There are many aspects to the voice including tone, pitch, fluency and accent. This can alter the meaning of a word or sentence. Using volume is particularly evident in demonstrating submissiveness and assertion. Excessive use of volume can indicate aggression.

Some individuals may talk too quietly or too quickly making it difficult for others to hear, resulting in others' avoidance of that person in the future.

Eye contact. It is often said that the eyes are the windows to the soul. We use eye contact to see whether a person is interested in what we are saying, whether they are sincere, and to empathize with how they feel. Eye contact is sometimes used to intimidate another person by staring too long, but some people go to the other extreme of avoiding eye contact completely. We use eye contact in turn taking during conversation. While listening we look 75% of the time; whilst talking 40% and mutual glances take up around 30% of the time (Trower, Bryant & Argyle 1978). Glances last approximately 3 seconds and mutual glances last half that time.

Gestures and touch. A person who is shy or reluctant to mix with people may have great difficulty in using touch with others. Even shaking someone's hand can prove to be an ordeal. This is noticeable with a person who is anxious, thought disordered, or phobic. The way we use our body to express ourselves is important in effective communication. You may notice that a depressed person may hardly move at all when talking, whilst others may overgesticulate. Pointing and use of the hands is useful in expressing an idea or how you feel and can be an effective indicator in turn taking (illustrators). Learning about touch between genders is significant because there are socially acceptable norms in the level of touch and this gradually increases as relationships become more intimate (Hargie & McCartan 1986).

Head movements and nods. Nodding the head during conversation shows acceptance of what is being said, and interest in maintaining the conversation; it can also be used along with facial expressions to communicate a query or disagreement (regulators). Movement of the head can be very effective in telling the other person you are puzzled, trying to think, wanting to be defiant or dominant, and if you are sad (Hargie 1997).

Paravocal cues (umm's, etc.). Paravocal cues include aspects of the voice and volume mentioned earlier; other cues include the use of non-words such as umm's and ahh's. Some individuals may have a nervous cough or stammer and this can interfere with effective communication. We need utterances such as umm's and ahh's to provide feedback that we are listening to the other person and that we wish them to continue with their train of conversation. 'Prosodic' sounds are also used to affect timing, including intonation, pauses and stress (Trower, Bryant & Argyle 1978).

Posture. Your posture is a good clue to how you feel. Slouched shoulders can infer that you are unhappy (adaptors). It also tells the other person if you are interested in them and may also reflect the status of the company you are with. For example when interested in another person you lean toward them and mirror their posture. You are unlikely to slouch in a chair if you are in an interview with your boss or if an important visitor is with you, and hence you are communicating a level of respect.

Facial expression. When trying to understand another person we look to their facial expression. There are seven key facial expressions, and most others are variations of these: happiness, anger, surprise, fear, disgust, sadness and interest (Hargie 1997). Practising the use of facial expressions and understanding their use by others is a key part of social skills training.

Smiling (specific training). Although smiling is part of a facial expression, it is an important aspect when greeting others. People with mental health difficulties, particularly depression, may have difficulty with smiling and their mouths are often turn downward. Individuals with schizophrenia sometimes have a mask-like expression when talking to others (this may be a side-effect of medication). Another symptom is incongruity of affect, which is grimacing at the wrong time during a conversation. Expressing oneself and appearing warm to others is an essential part of interaction, so the importance of smiling must be indicated early on in the programme.

Proximity and orientation. Edward T. Hall, an anthropologist, described differences of interpersonal distances, referred to as 'proxemics' (1990).

There are four main zones, which are: intimate (0–50 cm, or 0–18 inches), personal (0.5–1.3 m, or 1.5–4 feet), social (1.3–4 m, or 4–12 feet), and public (4–6 m, or 12–20 feet). People who are shy, anxious or aggressive may prefer more personal space than others (Hargie & McCartan 1986). Also, when we talk to someone we usually orientate ourselves toward a 90-degree angle. Orientation and proximity are related in that the closer we get to someone the more side on we move. The tendency is to move from a face to face position on the approach to a side-on position as we meet (Hargie, Saunders & Dickson 1994). This is useful when considering how you will place chairs during social skills practice. Different cultures have different 'comfort zones', which is the comfortable distance for general conversation, and this may be relevant for your client group (McKay, Davis & Fanning 1995).

The way we position the limbs and body can send messages about our interest in the conversation, and how comfortable we feel with the other person. These can be generalized into open and closed posture. Crossing your arms and legs for example is a closed posture, which indicates that you are not comfortable and that you are protecting your intimate self (adaptors). Try to encourage a relaxed and open posture.

During the 'information-giving' process, it is worthwhile introducing the verbal skills that will be worked through in later weeks, explaining their importance as components of a conversation. Timing (meshing) and appearance issues are easier to demonstrate than describe. As you develop the social skills programme, graduate the difficulty of the tasks, which will help participants enjoy successful experiences.

Molar skills

These include:

◆ greetings
◆ initiating a conversation
◆ maintaining a conversation
◆ joining a conversation
◆ questioning
◆ terminating a conversation
◆ asking for help/refusal

◆ apologizing
◆ asserting yourself.

Exercise 2: Getting to know you (pen and paper required)

It's time to split the group into pairs. Participants will tell their partners a bit about themselves. They will also express one anxiety they have about the group. Once they have exchanged this information, their partners will then feed back the information to the group. Problems may occur at this point where trainees are too anxious to talk; ask them to think about it a bit longer and move on to the next person. Watching other participants may inspire them with the confidence needed. Some people may not be able to read or write, so changes to the exercises will be necessary, and extra support provided by the group facilitators. Any difficulties of this nature should be identified in the assessment phase through the referral document. For those who are particularly shy, preparatory sessions should be arranged.

Many individuals are anxious about being on video or audiotape so the use of the equipment must be introduced sensitively. You may prefer to leave this exercise for the second week.

Exercise 3: Getting familiar with video feedback

An explanation should be provided about why the equipment is being used to provide feedback for the exercises during the training programme. In order to get participants comfortable with the video equipment and what they look like and sound like, it is necessary to film each person stating a simple phrase. A chair is seated in front of the video at the range that will be used during the role-play exercises. The video camera should be set up on a tripod prior to the group session and operation usually involves pressing the button on and off (most modern video cameras can be operated by remote control and digital video cameras allow the option for analysis and storage on computer). It is helpful to get a different trainee to do the recording and another to do the video playback. This participation should reduce the anxiety about the machines being used. The exercise involves the person sitting in the chair and saying 'my name is … and I am from …'. The trainees are then played the video recording and most people are very surprised at how they look and sound on tape. Once the initial anxiety is tackled, the exercise becomes more fun.

Homework assignment

At the end of each session a homework assignment will be set, which usually involves the participants practising what they have learnt. Trainees should go through the assessment list with their caseworker or a friend and identify which areas they would like to practise or improve on. The group must be informed that they will be expected to provide feedback from their daily diaries at the beginning of the next session for each homework assignment. This should be part of a written contract to encourage participation (Trower, Bryant & Argyle 1978).

Use of daily diary

Each week a daily diary should be provided for each person. This is in the form of headed paper with the days of the week. As part of the homework assignments the trainees will be asked to identify any difficult situations they have had in practising their social skills. These can be shared with the group as part of the homework feedback, or discussed with a facilitator. Experience with difficult situations can be re-enacted as part of the exercises. A summary at the end of each social skills session should be provided, reflecting on what has been discussed, together with time allocated for questions.

Week 2: Learning from others

The group is welcomed back. The aims and objectives of the day's session should be discussed. The first item on the agenda of each week is reflection on the homework assignment and daily diaries. Participants should be informed that this will happen at the beginning of every session.

Exercise 4: A favourite soap

The facilitators need to record excerpts from tele-

vision programmes and capture good and bad examples of the interactions that you want to discuss for that day. Using characters that the trainees can identify with, and respect, helps in picking up specific social cues. Use this exercise to reflect on the information about molecular skills given in the previous session, particularly aspects of non-verbal communication. Ask the group to focus on a specific non-verbal skill, then examine it more closely. Most modern videos have a freeze frame and slow motion, so use these to the group's advantage. This exercise can be used each week at the level the group has achieved. Modelling by the facilitators should support the use of videotaped role models.

Information giving: components of conversation

As the weeks go by it will be time to consolidate how we use non-verbal and verbal communication in a structured way during a conversation and in varying situations. The first task will be to practise the molar skill of starting a conversation. Each aspect of non-verbal interaction is important at this stage including approach, posture, eye contact and facial expression. We often form an opinion about a person when we first meet, so the first encounter with a stranger will effect the future of that relationship (Hargie & McCartan 1986). Skills training is very specific and the phases of interaction should include how we behave at a distance, during the approach and at the actual meeting. If we consider the cybernetic model described earlier, it is important to go through each phase carefully. The stages are guidance, demonstration, practice and feedback. The guidance is in the form of information and knowledge provided about elements of a conversation and how to perform each component part. It also involves answering questions and concerns about each exercise. The guidance and demonstration will involve the facilitators acting as role models. The trainees need to empathize with the facilitator, so examples should be aimed at the level of competence of the participants on the course. Rather than demonstrating the execution of perfect social skills, the facilitator should aim their performance as if they were one of their trainees, gradually shaping demonstrations to an acceptable level of social competence (Trower, Bryant & Argyle 1978). A bad example should be used to show how the skill should not be performed, followed by criticism from the audience, and then the correct example provided. For each exercise there will be a demonstration and guided practice session. Then, once candidates are comfortable with their performance, it is time to video the skills practice. The video is then played back to the audience and the feedback process begins. The group is asked the following three 'reflective questions':

◆ What did you do well?
◆ What do others think you did well?
◆ What do you think you would like to have done differently?

Feedback should invariably be positive; however, problems need to be identified and acknowledged so improvement can take place. Most trainees will have the basic social skills within their behavioural repertoire, but the lack of opportunity for practice and a lack of confidence results in self-isolation and a reluctance to mix with others (Musker 1992). Each exercise is used to provide this opportunity to practise and to build up confidence through operant conditioning in the form of positive feedback and the experience of success.

Exercise 5: Greetings and terminating a conversation

The participants are paired together and the facilitators demonstrate the competent skills of starting and terminating a brief conversation. Guided role play is used to ensure successful completion of the skill. The trainees are then asked to imagine they are walking along a corridor when they bump into a friend. Even this limited interaction will make some trainees anxious and one way of overcoming this is to use cue cards. The facilitators will have typed out a script for each trainee to follow and this will be used for many of the situational exercises. The script will include non-verbal messages like when to look at the person, when to smile and other supportive comments like the importance of

nodding to continue the conversation. Using a script reduces the anxiety of thinking about what to say, which is often the main concern when initiating a conversation. Prior to the video recording, the group will have practised enough to perform the task without the script cards. Here is a simplified example of a script, but facilitators will need to design their own according to the level of skill of their group and the intricacy of the exercise involved. A demonstration of how to use the scripts should be performed by the facilitators each time:

An example of conversation scripts:

Speaker card 1
Look at the person to show you want to talk.

Say: 'Good afternoon' and support this with a smile. Look at the other person as they greet you. Offer a handshake.

Then say: 'I'm fine thanks, how are you?' Look at the other person to show you have finished speaking and wait for response.

Then say: 'It was nice meeting you again—goodbye'.

Speaker card 2
Meet the look of the other person as they make eye contact—raise your eyebrows in recognition.

Look and wait for a response.

You say: 'Good afternoon. How are you?' Look at the person to show you have finished and give a positive smile.

You say: 'I'm OK.' Look and wait for a response.

You say: 'Goodbye.'

When you have worked through the video playback of this exercise, you then obtain the positive feedback for each pair using the three 'reflective questions' described earlier. At the end of the session, the homework assignment should reflect what has happened during the group, such as practising the skills on the ward with peers. Experiences should be recorded in the participant's daily diary provided and used as feedback at the beginning of the following week. You will need to gauge the pace of each session and the amount of material you wish to cover per week.

The guidance, demonstration, practice and feedback model must be used for every exercise, as described earlier, to ensure that successful and transferable learning takes place. Each week a key exercise should be used focusing on a specific theme of social skills. The facilitators will need to gauge how fast the group progresses over the 10-week period.

Other useful exercises (using video feedback)

What's in the box?

The group is asked to identify different facial expressions from cuttings you have made from a magazine. The A3 pad or marker board is used to identify and discuss the seven facial expressions described earlier. Later an empty box is passed around the group and the trainees open the box imagining what it may contain. Each member is then prompted to display one of the seven facial expressions, and the group is asked to interpret what type of expression they are attempting to display. The trainee reports back to the group what they had imagined and to describe the actual facial expression they were using.

Initiating a conversation

Use an extension of the example put forward in exercise 5 described earlier (Greetings and terminating a conversation), but focus on beginning the conversation, which may involve trainees practising the use of some short phrases like: 'How have you been over the past few days?', 'Are there any activities planned for today?', 'How are you getting on with …?' and 'Would you like a game of…?'

Maintaining a conversation

It is often easy to say hello and give initial short responses, but maintaining a conversation is one of the most difficult aspects of social skills training because it requires spontaneity. A useful exercise here is to ask the candidates to read some articles from the newspaper or watch the news before the

following week's session as part of their homework assignment so that they can discuss it with the group in detail. Alternatively, suggest a television programme or topic area that they can think about, such as football, cooking, politics, religion or a personal hobby. The following week, pairs are organized to allow a practice discussion. A similar exercise is to organize a debate between two sides of the group.

Joining a conversation

Here the group is divided into threesomes and, whilst two are asked to go through the previous exercise of maintaining a conversation, another person has to come and join them. This should be a positive experience, whereby another member immediately welcomes the new arrival into the group, introductions are made and the person is updated about the previous conversation.

Questioning others

This is an easier exercise in that it has a specific goal. Role reversal can be used, where one participant is asked to play a particular care team member and the facilitator takes the role of the participant, demonstrating different ways to ask a question. Ask the client group which type of questions are important to them and whom they would like to ask these questions. Attempt to role play each suggested situation, such as approaching a care team member about side-effects of medication, or about a problem with a relative. After role playing the scenario in the group, the real life situation can be set as a specific homework assignment and recorded in the daily diary for feedback to the group the following week, as can each of the following assignments.

Asking for help/refusal

Requesting the assistance of others may be an obvious recourse for some, but people with mental health problems are likely to endure their difficulty rather than seek help. Trainees are asked to imagine they are doing a crossword for which they need some help. They have to approach their partner, introduce their difficulty and ask for support. The reverse can then be used whereby they are doing the crossword when they are approached by their partner who offers their help. A polite refusal can then be offered with an explanation. Another example that can be used is in seeking directions, or asking a shop assistant about a product. It is important to identify the difference between open, closed and rhetorical questions and how this can affect a response. (A closed question is usually answered with 'yes' or 'no'.)

Apologizing

If you have problems with your mental health, there may be times when you want to offer an apology for earlier behaviour and to help mend relationships. If the person has difficulty apologizing the problem can go on unresolved. The role play should involve an experience that the person is able to share with the group and then the way to apologize can be designed together. A few ideas should be worked through first. Examples include: you have spilt someone's drink, you have shouted at someone earlier, you panicked and left the room, and you offended a friend with your behaviour.

Asserting yourself

Although assertion training is a specialized form of training in itself, it is worth practising being assertive as part of a social-skills-training programme. Assertiveness is about defending your rights without impeding the rights of others. Essentially this is usually saying 'no' to a person without being aggressive or hostile. An example could be refusing to take medication that is being offered to you, whilst providing an explanation. In hospitals there are cases where individuals find it difficult to say no to others who want to borrow items such as tobacco and other personal property. This then leads to hidden frustration, which in turn can lead to violence because the person found it difficult to express themselves by saying 'no' at the appropriate time. Assertion training should involve adding diplomacy and positive responses to difficult situations. Examples might include:

refusing to lend items, defending yourself against intimidating comments and standing up for yourself when you know you are in the right. There are situations where being assertive may be uncomfortable, and so providing face-saving opportunities can prove useful to enable positive withdrawal from difficult situations.

CASE STUDIES OF GROUP PARTICIPANTS

Here is a description of three service users and how they benefited from a social-skills-training programme.

CASE STUDIES

George (a pseudonym)

George is a 62-year-old man who had worked all his life but used to lock himself in his room all day, lying in bed. When he did get up, he would nervously ask for things he needed and would not speak other than at essential times (for medication and meals). His verbal responses were usually tremulous and monosyllabic in nature. He did not go to rehabilitation and when care team members asked him to get involved his usual reply was a timid 'I'd rather not', followed by a quick retreat to his room. After consultation with his caseworker George was encouraged to participate on the programme and was noted to benefit from the roleplay exercises. Essentially, he had to learn how to use his basic interaction skills again within a safe and comfortable environment. These included basic skills like when to smile and how to initiate a conversation. George began to attempt to mix with others on the ward and other service users eagerly welcomed him into their company. He became more confident and his willingness to mix enabled him to be discharged back into the community.

Susan

Susan is a 26-year-old woman who, when speaking to acquaintances, would invade their personal space. When a person engaged her in conversation she would not pause to allow them to speak and would talk about the same subject to the point where the other person became bored, resulting in future avoidance of interaction. When confronted about this issue, she appeared to have no insight into her behaviour. Susan enjoyed the course and learnt about personal space. She was given some techniques in gauging her proximity and orientation, which was reinforced through video feedback. Susan was encouraged to explore a variety of topics in conversation, increasing her personal repertoire. The course also increased her self-awareness. This led to other service users being more patient toward Susan and more likely to engage her in conversation.

Ron

Ron is a 45-year-old man with an IQ of 75. He could not read or write and appeared nervous during interaction with others. His posture would go rigid and he would gaze at the person trying to engage him in conversation with a frightened stare and his extrapyramidal side-effects would worsen—for example, his hand tremor would increase. After further assessment it was established that Ron's self-esteem was so low that he felt he was not worthy of other people's attention. He would say, 'Oh, they're too important to talk to the likes of me'. As part of the course in social skills he began to initiate conversation with others, or tried tentatively asking them questions like 'What is the time?' The slight changes in his own confidence could be seen in his non-verbal behaviour, for instance, his smile was more spontaneous. Ron seemed to gain pleasure in having the courage and confidence in being able to say 'hello' or 'good morning' to others, which would lead to brief conversations.

EVALUATION

To evaluate each individual's progress, the following information should be utilized: the referral document, the baseline and post-training assessment by the case worker, the summary reports from each session and the progress assessment form. Evaluation questionnaires that seek information about the subjective experiences of the trainees will be useful for future programmes. Each group should culminate with a test of the transferability of skills into the community. A day out into town should be organized with a set agenda that will enable the trainee to employ all of the skills from the course. The excursion should include purchasing goods from a shop, which may involve seeking information from a shop assistant, such as asking questions about goods. Another useful exercise is visiting an information centre, the post office, or the local train station to ask for appropriate information. A nice way to finish the day out is by taking the group for a meal, which is an ideal informal opportunity to use the social skills training in a real situation. Transferability and maintenance of social skills is an important part of the evaluation. If skills are not practised outside the group setting they will easily be forgotten. You may consider maintenance groups for participants with long term mental health problems. Maintenance sessions help with revision of social skills and can be done in the person's home with their family's help or on the ward with their caseworker.

SUMMARY

Social skills training in mental health should be a mainstay of any rehabilitation programme. The training described here is to prevent institutionalization for people being admitted to hospital, and to support the severely mentally ill within the community. Mental health problems are likely to cause social withdrawal and this is known to exacerbate ill health. For some people, their social competence is crippled to the extent that they are unable to seek the support they need. As you can see from the three case studies provided earlier, some service users just need a little bit of encouragement to get them out of their trap of despair and self-isolation. Being unable to interact with others lowers an individual's self-esteem and removes a major personal source of help. Designing and implementing a social skills programme is an activity that can be achieved with the minimum of resources.

DISCUSSION QUESTIONS

1. How does another person effect the way we communicate?
2. What is the difference between molar and molecular skills?
3. How can social skills training help somebody?

FURTHER READING

Hargie O D W 1997 The handbook of communication skills, 2nd edn. Routledge, London.
An exploration of communication skills, which reviews the literature and theory of communication in detail.

Hargie O, McCartan P J 1986 Social skills training and psychiatric nursing. Croom Helm, London.
Another basic text to help the novice practitioner develop the art of social skills training, describing the dynamics mental health can play in this process.

Hargie O, Saunders C, Dickson D 1994 Social skills in interpersonal communication, 3rd edn. Routledge, London.
Examines interpersonal skills from a 'person situation context'.

Pope B 1986 Social skills training for psychiatric nurses. Harper & Row, London.
Another view of developing social skills training, looking at molar and molecular skills.

Trower P, Bryant B, Argyle M 1978 Social skills and mental health. Methuen, London.
Provides an in-depth look at creating and managing a social skills group.

ACKNOWLEDGEMENT

Bill Jackson – Thorn Nurse/Nurse Tutor

REFERENCES

Argyle M 1978 The psychology of interpersonal behaviour, 3rd edn. Penguin, Harmondsworth

Argyle M 1992 The social psychology of everyday life. Routledge, London

Atkinson R L, Atkinson R C, Smith E E, Bem D J, Nolen-Hoeksema S 1996 Hilgard's introduction to psychology, 12th edn. Hartcourt Brace College, Fort Worth

Berne E 1985 The games people play. Ballantine, New York

Birdwhistell R L 1970 Kinesics and context: essays on body motion communication. Ballantine, New York

Collins J, Collins M 1992 Social skills training and the professional helper. John Wiley, Chichester

Davison G C, Neale J M 1998 Abnormal psychology, 7th edn. John Wiley, New York

Depoy E, Gitlin L N 1994 Introduction to research: multiple strategies for health and human services. Mosby, St Louis

Dickson D A, Hargie O, Morrow N C 1989 Communication skills training for health professionals: an instructor's handbook. Chapman & Hall, London

Dickson D A, Saunders C Y, Stringer M 1993 Rewarding people: the skill of responding positively. Routledge, London

Downie R S, Tannahill C, Tannahill A 1996 Health promotion: models and values, 2nd edn. Oxford University Press, Oxford

Ekman P 1982 Emotion in the human face, 2nd edn. Cambridge University Press, New York

Ellis R, Whittington D 1981 A guide to social skill training. Croom Helm, London

Hall E T 1990 The hidden dimension. Doubleday, New York

Hargie O D W 1997 The handbook of communication skills, 2nd edn. Routledge, London

Hargie O, McCartan P J 1986 Social skills training and psychiatric nursing. Croom Helm, London

Hargie O, Saunders C, Dickson D 1994 Social skills in interpersonal communication, 3rd edn. Routledge, London

Hayes R L, Halford W K, Varghese F T 1995 Social skills training with chronic schizophrenic patients: effects on negative symptoms and community functioning. Behaviour Therapy 26:433–449

Hogarty G E, Anderson C M, Reiss D J et al 1986 Family psychoeducation, social skills training, and maintenance chemotherapy in the aftercare treatment of schizophrenia: 1. One-year effects of a controlled study on relapse and expressed emotion. Archives of General Psychiatry 43:633–642

Littrell K H, Freeman L Y 1995 Maximising social interventions. Journal of American Psychiatric Nurses Association 1(6):214–218

McKay M, Davis M, Fanning P 1995 Messages: the communication skills book, 2nd edn. New Harbinger Publications, Oakland

Marder S R, Wirshing W C, Mintz J et al 1996 Two-year outcome of social-skills training and group psychotherapy for outpatients with schizophrenia. American Journal of Psychiatry 153:1585–1592

Maslow A H 1954 Motivation and personality. Harper & Row, New York

Musker M 1992 Making contact. Nursing Times 88(47):31–33

Pope B 1986 Social skills training for psychiatric nurses. Harper & Row, London

Power M, Dalgleish T 1997 Cognition and emotion: from order to disorder. Psychology Press, Hove

Rosenhan D L 1973 On being sane in insane places. Science 179:250–258

Stuart G W, Laraia M T 1998 Stuart and Sundeen's principles and practice of psychiatric nursing, 6th edn. Mosby, St Louis

Tompkins S S 1962 Affect, imagery, consciousness, vol 1. Springer, New York

Trower P, Bryant B, Argyle M 1978 Social skills and mental health. Methuen, London

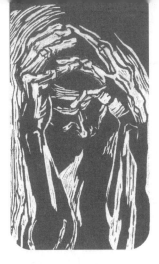

Chapter Eleven

Biological aspects of treatment and intervention

Antoine P Farine

AIMS

- To identify aspects of neurophysiology relevant to treatments and intervention
- To consider the main characteristics of schizophrenia, depression, Alzheimer's disease, Parkinson's disease, Huntington's disease and epileptic seizures and to explore the use of drugs and other biologically based interventions in each one

KEY ISSUES

Section 1: Aspects of neurophysiology

Section 2: Schizophrenia

Section 3: Depression

Section 4: Dementia of Alzheimer's, Parkinson's and Huntington's disease

Section 5: Seizures and epilepsy

INTRODUCTION

Faced with the rapid development of information technology, health professionals are at risk of losing credibility, especially if not keeping abreast of or updating themselves in their specific areas of practice, since patients/clients now have access to information via the internet and other media and can be very knowledgeable about their illnesses. It is therefore imperative that health professionals acquire relevant knowledge that can put them at the forefront of nursing and allow them to communicate rationally with clients about aspects of their illness. Thus, there is a need for health professionals to focus on aspects of anatomy and physiology, and especially psychiatry as it is often more complex and often symptoms cannot be easily explained in terms of altered physiology. For example, why do we sometimes observe a particular behaviour in a patient, when this may be absent in another patient suffering from a similar disease?

Drugs often play a crucial role in the management of clients with psychiatric disorders. Much has been learnt about possible causes of mental disorders, by understanding how drugs may interact in the nervous system and also their side-effects. For example, through observing the side-effects of neuroleptic drugs in the management of schizophrenic individuals, it has been made possible to understand the possible altered physiology that gives rise to Parkinson's disease.

This chapter is divided into five sections, each with its own aims.

SECTION 1: Aspects of neurophysiology

AIMS

- ◆ To introduce those structures of the brain thought to be involved in the pathophysiology of mental disorders
- ◆ To consider the role of neurotransmitters
- ◆ To promote an understanding of possible drug action in the brain

INTRODUCTION

The brief overview that follows will be divided into sections so as to identify aspects of neurophysiology relevant to the treatments and interventions explored in later sections of this chapter. It will focus on:

1. structures that are believed to contribute to the pathophysiology of mental disorder and also of physical disorders that may require psychiatric intervention and
2. related neurotransmitters and their receptors and pathways.

For more in-depth or detailed anatomy and physiology of specific structures in the brain, you may wish to consult the appropriate textbooks (see Further reading). Other chapters in this book, particularly Chapter 4, also consider biological aspects of health and disorder and refer to the basal ganglia, the limbic system and neurotransmitters.

Here the basal ganglia and their connection to other parts of the brain will be discussed, a brief section on the limbic system will be included and some basic properties of neurotransmitters will be considered.

BASAL GANGLIA

There is increasing evidence that the basal ganglia are involved in many disorders of the central nervous system, either through the loss of specific groups of neurons affecting the concentration of neurotransmitters or through malfunctions that alter their metabolism. In order to understand how and why an individual may be affected, a grasp of the essential anatomy and physiology of the basal ganglia is important.

The basal ganglia are found in a core of grey matter deeply seated in each cerebral hemisphere (see Fig. 11.1). They consist of several nuclei that are interconnected—the caudate nucleus, putamen, globus pallidus, subthalamic nucleus and substantia nigra. The caudate nucleus and the putamen form what is known as the corpus striatum. The caudate nucleus is C-shaped and lies in proximity to the lateral ventricle. It consists of three parts: the head, which is adjacent to the anterior horn of the lateral ventricle in the frontal lobe, the body, which runs along the lateral wall of the lateral ventricle, and the tail, which runs in the roof of the inferior horn of the lateral ventricle. The globus pallidus lies medial to the putamen and lateral to the internal capsule. The globus pallidus and putamen are often referred to as the lentiform nucleus.

The nuclei of the basal ganglia, especially the corpus striatum, have an intricate network of neuronal circuits. They receive afferent neurons from the cerebellum, the cerebral cortex (mainly the premotor cortex) the substantia nigra and the thalamus. The basal ganglia do not have direct afferent or efferent connections with the spinal cord. Their motor functions are mediated by the frontal cortex.

Functions of the basal ganglia

The neuronal connections of the basal ganglia are extremely complex and, since they are not easily accessible, explanations of their functions have been possible mainly through studying postmortem brain specimens of patients with specific diseases and also by studying the effects of medications in specific diseases. Since diseases of the basal ganglia produce abnormal motor responses in the form of tremor, athetosis (slow, writhing movements of the fingers and hands), chorea (rapid, flick-like move-

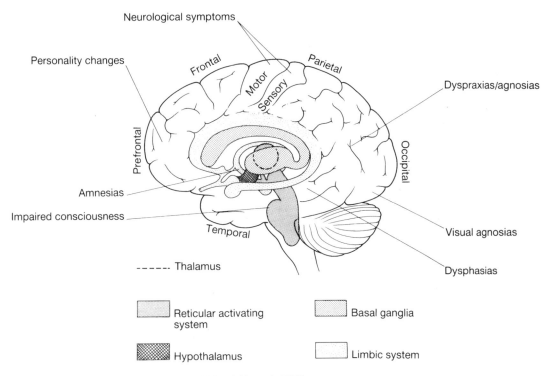

Fig. 11.1 Brain structure and function (from Weller & Eysenck 1992).

ments of the limbs and facial muscles) and ballism (uncoordinated swinging of the limbs and jerky movements), it has been deduced that their normal functions must be associated with coordination of the fine motor movements and these are dependent on specific neurotransmitters.

Neurotransmitters that are important in maintaining a balance between the many neuronal pathways in the basal ganglia, and thus contribute to the coordination of motor movements, are dopamine, gamma aminobutyric acid (GABA) and acetylcholine. Disturbances in their concentration (i.e a lower concentration) as indicated by postmortem brain studies may affect movement in a variety of ways (see Chapter 4, and later sections in this chapter).

Neurotransmitters interrelate in an excitatory or inhibitory nature and it is unlikely that a specific neurotransmitter will be the sole agent responsible for a particular function. So, until more elaborate studies are undertaken in situ in live patients with specific basal ganglial disease or

in healthy volunteers, the precise role of the nuclei in the basal ganglia and their neurotransmitters is likely to remain rather unclear.

LIMBIC SYSTEM

The limbic system is derived from the word 'limbus', which means 'border'. In fact, it forms a circle on the medial side of each hemisphere (see Fig. 11.2). The limbic system is a very complex structure consisting of cortical areas, nuclei and major connecting tracts and connections. The cortical areas consist of the parahippocampal gyrus, the hippocampus of the temporal lobe, and the cingulate gyrus which overlies the corpus callosum. The hippocampus is a C-shaped structure that gives rise to the fornix and mamillary body (Fig. 11.2).

The nuclei-forming parts of the limbic system are the amygdaloid nucleus, which lies deep within the temporal lobe, and the septal and hypothal-

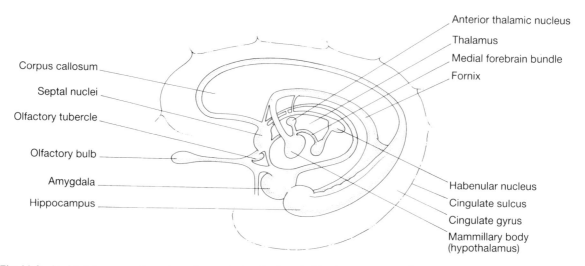

Fig. 11.2 Limbic lobe connections: the major cortical and subcortical brain structures implicated in the limbic system (from Hinchliff & Montague 1988).

amic nuclei. The amygdaloid nucleus is thought to be involved in the control of emotional behaviour such as fear and rage.

Functions of the limbic system

The extensive interconnections between structures forming the limbic system have made it very difficult for neurophysiologists to identify specific functions of this complex system. For example, the exact pathways that control the emotions and motor behaviours are not clearly understood, but it is believed that the limbic system works in association with the autonomic nervous system and the spinal cord. Thus, it allows for coordination of blood pressure, heart rate and pupillary size. The limbic system also influences all of the endocrine systems of the body by controlling the release of hypothalamic hormones. The hippocampus is believed to play an important part in the retention of memory (see Chapter 5).

Stimulation of the septal nucleus can produce aggressive behaviour in animals, while tumours within that area can give rise to irritability and emotional instability in humans. Stimulation of structures such as the amygdala, hypothalamus and cingulate gyrus can also produce behavioural disturbances. In some studies it has been observed that the destruction of the cingulate cortex in

monkeys increases tameness. There are reports that psychological processes involving the cingulum or the cyngulate gyrus can control intractable fears, anxiety, hostility and obsessional states.

The limbic system plays a vital role in the control and modulation of emotion, but it is still difficult to understand abnormal behavioural responses as a result of faulty connections within the limbic system. In terms of psychiatric illness, as long as the pathways forming the limbic system and their functions are not clearly understood, a dilemma will remain as to how best to manage affected individuals and help them choose the most appropriate or effective therapy.

NEUROTRANSMITTERS, RECEPTORS AND PATHWAYS

To appreciate altered physiology and its effects on the brain, it is essential to understand the normal interactions of neurotransmitters and their specific receptors in the nervous system. Through the understanding of these specific physiological functions, it has been possible to produce drugs that either mimic neurotransmitters (agonists), or block the receptors or release of the transmitters and therefore prevent the neurotransmitter functioning (antagonists). Such drugs have revolution-

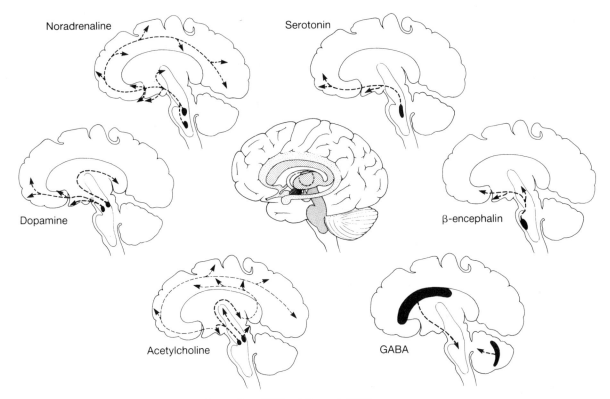

Fig. 11.3 Principal neurotransmitter pathways (from Weller & Eysenck 1992).

ized the treatment of some mental disorders and have also made it possible for researchers to begin to understand the possible associated physiological changes.

An increase, reduction or absence of neurotransmitters will affect brain functions. Neurotransmitters are low molecular weight substances released across the synaptic cleft in response to an action potential passing down the nerve axon (Fig. 11.3). They interact with specific receptor sites on the postsynaptic region of the receiving neuron. Neurotransmitters are distributed throughout the brain but are localized in specific clusters of neurons whose axons project to other highly specific brain regions (see Fig. 11.3). Neurotransmitter receptors are transmembrane glycoproteins and their function is to allow communication between cells. The receptors have parts sticking out above and below the membrane like floating icebergs. The surface of the neurotransmitter receptor is precisely tailored to match the shape and configuration of the transmitter molecule, so that the latter fits into the former with the precision and specificity of a key entering a lock.

Many transmitter receptors have two functional components: (i) a binding site for the transmitter molecule, and (ii) a pore/channel passing through the membrane that is selectively permeable to certain ions.

The binding of the transmitter to the receptor alters its three-dimensional shape so that the pore is opened and ions inside and outside the cell membrane flow down their concentration gradient, resulting in either an excitatory or an inhibitory effect. There are two basic types of transmitter receptor: those reacting rapidly through mediating the transfer of information by controlling the permeability state of an ion pore and those that are long-acting receptors that cause the formation of a second messenger chemical, which then triggers a series of physiological events.

There are specific receptors for specific neuro-transmitters; some examples are: muscarinic and nicotinic acetylcholine receptors, dopamine D_1, D_2 and D_3 receptors, adrenergic receptors, GABA receptors, and serotonin and opioid receptors.

Neurotransmitters that help transmit excitatory impulses in the main include: dopamine, nor-adrenaline (norepinephrine), serotonin and acetyl-choline, whereas GABA has an inhibiting effect. Other amino acids and polypeptides may also act as neurotransmitters, or in some way affect trans-mission of impulses. The principal neurotransmit-ter pathways illustrating how neurotransmitters are localized into clusters of neurons are shown in Figure 11.3. The ideas and concepts included in this section will find application in the remaining sections of this chapter.

DISCUSSION QUESTIONS

1. Giving a rationale for your answer, discuss the reasons why psychiatric disorders have not always been fully understood as compared with physical disorders.
2. Based on symptoms that occur in the pathophysiology of the basal ganglia (think of two to three disorders), suggest the normal functions of the basal ganglia in healthy individuals.
3. Discuss the possible pharmacological actions of drugs in relation to the receptors and neurotransmitters in the brain.

FURTHER READING

Doane B K, Livingstone K F (eds) 1986 The limbic system: functional organisation and clinical disorders. Raven Press, New York

Hinchliff S, Montague S 1988 Physiology for nursing practice. Baillière Tindall, London

Holmes O 1990 Human neurophysiology. Unwin & Hyman, London

Siegel G, Bernard A E, Albers R W, Molinoff P 1989 Basic neurochemistry. Molecular, cellular and medical aspects, 4th edn. Raven Press, New York

Weller M, Eysenck M 1992 The scientific basis of psychiatry. W B Saunders, London

Wilkinson S 1992 Neuroanatomy for medical students. Butterworth/Heinemann, Oxford

Tortora G J, Grabowski S R 1996 Principles of anatomy and physiology, 8th edn. HarperCollins, London

SECTION 2: Schizophrenia

AIMS

◆ To promote an understanding of the possible causes of schizophrenia based on research studies

◆ To summarize the main characteristics of schizophrenia

◆ To examine the use of drugs in the treatment of schizophrenia

INTRODUCTION

Schizophrenia is one of the commonest psychiatric disorders accounting for approximately one-half of first admissions to the psychiatric hospitals. It is classified as one of the functional psychotic disorders and its incidence in the population is approximately 1% (8–10 per 100 000 of the population) (Kallman et al 1938). This figure is believed to be fairly uniform throughout the world (with the exception of Ireland, North Yugoslavia and parts of Scandinavia, which have slightly higher rates) even though different definitions of schizophrenia are used by clinicians in different countries. The onset is most common in the 15–35 years group (Kendler, Ernenberg & Tsuang Ming 1985).

Since its classical definition by Eugen Bleuler in 1911 in Switzerland, there have been several attempts to elaborate the definitions and classification of schizophrenia. The current criteria of schizophrenia require that a patient be continually ill for at least 6 months and that one or more of the following groups of symptoms be present:

◆ auditory hallucinations (hearing voices)
◆ bizarre delusions, often of a paranoid nature
◆ disorder of thought consisting of marked poverty of speech, loss of normal association of ideas
◆ passivity of feelings (loss of emotional responsiveness).

It is also possible to group symptoms of schizophrenia into catatonic, paranoid, hebephrenic and simple subtypes (Snyder 1982). Crow (1980) has postulated the existence of two discrete disease syndromes: type I and type II. Type I corresponds to acute schizophrenia and is associated with the 'positive' symptoms of hallucinations, thought disorder and delusions; patients have a good prognosis and excellent response to neuroleptics as well as normal cerebral ventricles. Type II is associated with 'negative symptoms', which include flattening, poverty of speech and loss of drive; patients respond less well to neuroleptics and tend to have enlarged ventricles. On the basis of response to treatment Crow suggests that type I schizophrenia involves abnormalities in the neurotransmitter dopamine whereas type II schizophrenia is associated with organic brain changes.

The search for pathophysiology of schizophrenia has been one of the most fascinating areas of study in psychiatric illness. Several lines of investigation have been undertaken and, whilst for some there is evidence for the basis of pathology, others clearly lack such evidence. The lines of investigation have focused on: (i) chemical neurotransmitter systems in the brain (dopamine hypothesis), (ii) altered functional structures in the brain, (iii) infection and (iv) genetics.

Genetics is an area that is being rigorously pursued in an attempt to determine the precise cause of schizophrenia. Several studies have indicated that schizophrenia may be genetically linked, but so far there has been no conclusive evidence for this. Family, adoption and twin studies have so far not explained the precise genetic basis of schizophrenia. However, some studies (adoption studies) show that schizophrenia is familial, and the reason must be that family members share the same environment. In one investigation, it was found that the frequency of schizophrenia in adopted offspring of schizophrenic mothers was high when compared with adopted children of unaffected parents.

The parameter usually measured in twin studies is 'concordance' and it is defined as 'the percentage proportion of identical twins who both suffer from a disease or exhibit a phenotypic trait when that disease or trait occurs in one member of the pair'. Since monozygotic or identical twins are genetically identical and dizygotic twins share only 50% of their genes, the risk of one individual of a monozygotic pair suffering from a particular disease if the other is affected would be greater. In monozygotic twins, environmental factors play a significant role in the development of diseases. In schizophrenia, twin studies show that the concordance percentage is 44% whereas it is only 16% in dizygotic twins.

Investigations into genes associated with schizophrenia have not yet yielded conclusive results. Some studies suggest that a region of chromosome 6 carries a gene involved in schizophrenia. However, other studies have failed to detect any such linkage whilst yet others have suggested that other genes on other chromosomes could be involved. Obviously, these discrepancies show the complexities of schizophrenia genetics, but the search goes on for the elusive gene or genes.

Perhaps the most compelling evidence for the involvement of the neurotransmitter system is that of the introduction of the drug Largactil (known to block dopamine receptors) in the 1950s, which completely revolutionized the treatment of schizophrenia, and also the discovery that drugs such as mescaline and LSD can cause hallucinations and other disruptions of normal mental function resembling those in schizophrenia.

With the development of several neuroleptic drugs that could ameliorate the symptoms of acute schizophrenia, research has tended to focus on the neurotransmitters.

DRUGS IN THE MANAGEMENT OF SCHIZOPHRENIA

Drugs which are used in the treatment of symptoms of schizophrenia are commonly referred to as neuroleptics or antipsychotics. The very first drug synthesized was chlorpromazine (Largactil) in 1950 by Charpentier. Chlorpromazine was first used in 1951 in the treatment of schizophrenic patients at the Val-de-Grace hospital in Paris (MacKay 1982).

Neuroleptic drugs can be divided into three main groups: phenothiazines (i.e chlorpromazine, thioridazine, trifluoperazine), butyrophenones (haloperidol) and thioxanthenes (thiothixene).

Pharmacological effects of neuroleptics

There is general agreement that neuroleptics block dopamine D receptors in certain parts of the brain, mainly in the nigrostriatal and mesolimbic pathways (Bartolini 1976, De Belleroche & Neal 1982). This is in accordance with what is known as the 'dopamine hypothesis' in the causation of schizophrenia. The dopamine hypothesis suggests that, in the brain of the schizophrenic individual, there is either an increase in dopamine and its receptors or there is a decrease in the level of the enzyme that is essential for its metabolism.

Neuroleptics have effects on other neurotransmitter systems and can block alpha adrenergic, serotonin and cholinergic receptors. GABA is also affected. Neuroleptics can produce severe extrapyramidal side-effects (to be discussed later) and this is due to their anticholinergic properties. Neuroleptics with the least anticholinergic properties (thioridazine) have the most extrapyramidal effects, whilst those with the most anticholinergic properties have the least extrapyramidal side-effects. It would appear that extrapyramidal side-effects occur because the balance mechanism between cholinergic and dopamine neurons in a particular part of the brain (the striatum) is affected when dopamine receptors are blocked.

It would appear that neuroleptics are much more effective in the treatment of the so-called 'positive' symptoms of schizophrenia (e.g. delusions, hallucinations).

Neuroleptic drugs in the treatment of resistant schizophrenia

There is a proportion of schizophrenic patients who may not response to neuroleptic drugs; this is referred to as treatment resistant or treatment refractory schizophrenia (Kane, Hongfeld & Singer 1988, Turkelsen et al 1990). These patients respond to clozapine (an atypical neuroleptic) and a new antipsychotic drug known as olanzapine. Olanzapine (licensed in UK in October 1996) has shown efficacy against positive and negative symptoms of schizophrenia, with minimal extrapyramidal effects (Martin et al 1997). Another atypical antipsychotic is Seroquel (Quetiapine) (Arvanitis et al 1997).

Most neuroleptics are predominantly effective against the positive psychotic symptoms of schizophrenia, but are only partially effective or ineffective against the negative symptoms.

Side-effects of neuroleptics

Neuroleptics can produce many side-effects, but the most common ones are those involving the extrapyramidal system. They include tardive (late) dyskinesia, bradykinesia, akathisia and dystonia. These side-effects occur as a result of a reduction of dopamine in the extrapyramidal pathway and they are similar to the effects of Parkinsonism.

Dyskinesia

Dyskinesia is a disorder of movement. It is characterized by resting tremor and may present as an acute reaction. Tardive or late dyskinesia involves involuntary movements of the tongue, mouth and face, which may present as grimacing or chomping (Weller 1981). The patient is often largely unaware of these buccal–lingual–masticatory movements. Tardive dyskinesia is more common in older patients who have been treated with high doses of neuroleptics for many months or years. The basic mechanism is thought to be the development of supersensitivity to dopamine in the extrapyramidal system (especially the nigrostriatal system). The symptoms are made worse by the use of anticholinergic drugs. A neuroleptic such as thioridazine that has greater affinity for the mesolimbic pathway may be less likely to induce tardive dyskinesia.

The management of tardive dyskinesia is difficult and there is much controversy as to the earlier use of anticholinergic drugs, since there is a suggestion that anticholinergic drugs may themselves predispose to tardive dyskinesia.

It has even been suggested that tardive dyskinesia may be an aspect of schizophrenia itself and not the result of a neuroleptic alone.

Bradykinesia

Bradykinesia leads to symptoms that affect normal spontaneous movements such as the swing of the arms when walking. More severe bradykinetic effects are similar to symptoms in Parkinson's disease, such as a mask-like, expressionless face and sometimes excessive salivation.

Akathisia

Akathisia is an increased motor restlessness, which prevents the individual from sitting still for more than a few minutes. It takes the form of persistent rocking from one foot to the other, or stamping alternative feet. It is believed that the mechanism of this side-effect is as a result of the involvement of the mesocortical dopamine pathway (Marsden & Jenner 1980).

Dystonia

Dystonia (persistent pathological change in muscle tone) occurs in the first few days of treatment and is more common with the more potent neuroleptics such as haloperidol and piperazine phenothiazines. Symptoms may be expressed as torticollis (affecting the neck muscles), trismus (affecting the jaw muscles), contraction of the tongue, opisthotonos (spasm affecting neck, back and legs) and occulogyric crises (affecting eye muscles). Passive movements of the limb may be prevented by persistent resistance, which is referred to as lead-pipe rigidity and later gives rise to the so-called 'cogwheel rigidity'.

Other side-effects

Many of the other side-effects of neuroleptics are due to antimuscarinic activity in the peripheral nervous system. This may produce dry mouth, blurred vision, constipation and difficulty in micturition. Hypotension can occur especially if neuroleptics such as haloperidol or piperidine-type phenothiazines are given intramuscularly.

Allergic (contact) dermatitis used to be common in nursing staff handling phenothiazine syrups. Toxic effects such as agranulocytosis can also occur. Agranulocytosis has been associated with chlorpromazine and thioridazine. Patients on maintenance therapy should have differential blood counts every 6 months.

Patients on chlorpromazine may become sensitized to the effects of sunlight and the use of suncreams may be helpful. Long term exposure to neuroleptics sometimes gives rise to abnormal melanin deposits in skin exposed to sunlight and the skin appears metallic grey. Opacities can occur in the cornea and the lens.

Some of the possible side-effects that may occur with the newer antipsychotic drugs such as Seroquel may be: nasal congestion, a slight increase in weight, mainly in the first weeks of treatment, tachycardia, especially when the drug is first taken, fast breathing, sweating, muscle stiffness and reduced consciousness. In rare cases, fits and seizures have been reported.

Other uses of neuroleptics

Neuroleptics can be used as sedatives, anxiolytics and some of them (metoclopramide and prochlorperazine) are effective as antiemetics. Gilles de la Tourette syndrome and tics also respond to neuroleptics.

SUMMARY

Neuroleptics have revolutionized the management of schizophrenia since the 1950s, and the most important benefit has been that of allowing patients to be treated in their own home and their early discharge from psychiatric hospitals.

Despite the introduction of newer neuroleptics, they are in the main prophylactic drugs and therefore reduce symptoms, but they do not offer a cure for schizophrenia.

The obvious severe side-effects of the neuroleptics pose serious concern amongst psychiatrists, as, for example, whether or not to use anticholinergic drugs (WHO 1990) to prevent extrapyramidal side-effects.

It is known that most neuroleptics block dopamine receptors in the mesolimbic and nigrostriatal pathways. The latter is responsible for the extrapyramidal side-effects. Other neurotransmitters are also involved and it is a combination of those other pharmacological effects that obscures the precise efficacy of neuroleptics. Thus, until more specific neuroleptics are developed, and the precise pathways of the various neurotransmitters are mapped out and their physiological functions clearly identified, the treatment for schizophrenia will remain in the status quo.

However, such biochemical studies are extremely difficult unless precise techniques are developed that can allow in vivo studies to be carried out on the brains of patients. Obviously this poses a very big ethical question.

DISCUSSION QUESTIONS

1. Based on relevant research studies, discuss the possible causes of schizophrenia. To answer this question, you would need to review the literature, and the areas that you might consider could be as follows: infection, genetic, neurotransmitter hypotheses, and abnormal structures within the brain.
2. Discuss how brain structures may be affected in schizophrenia.
3. With reference to specific drugs, discuss some of the advantages and disadvantages in their uses for clients with schizophrenia.

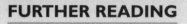

FURTHER READING

Crow T J 1982 The biology of schizophrenia. Experentia 38:1275–1282
This is an interesting paper and discusses the biology of schizophrenia sensibly and in a manner that the reader will find very stimulating. Although it appears outdated, schizophrenia has not changed in its presentation.

REFERENCES

Arvanitis L A, Miller B G, the Seroquel Trial 13 Study Group 1997 Multiple fixed doses of 'Seroquel' (Quetiapine) in patients with acute exacerbation of schizophrenia: a comparison with haloperidol and placebo. Biological Psychiatry 42:233–246

Bartolini G 1976 Differential effect of neuroleptic drugs on dopamine turnover in extrapyramidal and limbic system. Journal of Pharmacy and Pharmacology 28:423–429

Bleuler E 1911 Dementia praecox or the group of schizophrenics (transl Zirkin J 1950). International Universities Press, New York

Crow T J 1980 Molecular pathology of schizophrenia: more than one disease process. British Medical Journal 280:66–68

De Belleroche J S, Neal M J 1982 The contrasting effects of neuroleptics on transmitter release from the nucleus accumbens and corpus striatum. Neuropharmacology 21:529–537

Kallman F J 1938 The genetics of schizophrenia. Augustus, New York

Kane J M, Hongfeld G, Singer J 1988 Clozapine for the treatment resistant schizophrenic: a double-blind comparison with chlorpromazine. Archives of General Psychiatry 45:789–796

Kendler K S, Ernenberg A M, Tsuang Ming T 1985 Psychiatric illness in first degree relatives of schizophrenic and surgical control patients. A family study using DSM-III criteria. Archives of General Psychiatry 42:770–779

Mackay A V P 1982 Antischizophrenic drugs. In: Tyrer P J (eds) Drugs in psychiatric practice. Butterworth, Sevenoaks, Kent

Marsden C D, Jenner P 1980 The pathophysiology of extrapyramidal side-effects of neuroleptic drugs. Psychological Medicine 10:55–72

Martin J, Gomez J C, Garcia-Bernardo E, Cuesta M, Alvarez E, Gurpegui M 1997 Olanzapine in treatment-refractory schizophrenia: results of an open label study. Journal of Clinical Psychiatry 58:479–483

Snyder H S 1982 Neurotransmitters and CNS disease. Schizophrenia. The Lancet ii:970–973

Weller M P I 1981 Schizophrenic neuroleptics and Parkinson's disease. In: Rose F C R, Capildeo R (eds) Recent advances in neurology. Pitman Medical, London

WHO 1990 Prophylactic use of anticholinergics to patients on long-term neuroleptic treatment: a concensus statement. British Journal of Psychiatry 156:412

SECTION 3: Depression

AIMS

- To explore the biological basis of depression
- To examine the use of drugs in the treatment and management of depression
- To promote an understanding in the choice of drugs used in the management of individuals with depression

INTRODUCTION

Depression is a very common psychiatric disorder and may be described as reactive or endogenous. Reactive depression usually occurs as a result of a loss or any other major stressful events in an individual's life, whilst endogenous depression (the most severe form) occurs without any apparent cause. The type of depression to be described here is the endogenous type.

Depression is classified as an affective disorder, marked by distinct symptoms that in their most severe form can lead the patient to commit suicide. Fifteen per cent of depressed patients commit suicide.

Over the last 20 years depression has also been described as unipolar (UP) or bipolar (BP). The unipolar type is characterized by periods of depression only whilst the bipolar type coexists with episodes of hypomanic mania (less severe than mania), which is manifested as euphoria in which the individual appears elated. This may also be accompanied by hostility, irritability and sudden irrational decisions. In extreme cases delusions and hallucinations may be present. Women are affected about two to three times more often than men in unipolar depression. In bipolar both sexes are affected equally. Unipolar illness may be endogenous or reactive (Aubelas 1987).

Depression covers a wide spectrum of symptoms such as:

- insomnia, giving rise to morning awakening (3 a.m. is not unusual); loss of appetite (although, as reported by Young et al 1990, some women have increased appetite and weight gain)
- negative self-concept in which there is severe lack of confidence and self-worth and the individual may be unable to maintain personal cleanliness
- unresponsiveness to normal stimuli, which is preceded by depressed mood
- changes in motor activity, poverty of movement, lack of motivation, restlessness, slowing down of thoughts, difficulty in concentrating and persistent repetition of tasks.

The pathophysiology of depression is still obscure, although several biochemical theories have been postulated that include changes in neurotransmitter activity and neuroendocrine abnormalities. There is also perhaps a very strong gender predisposition for the development of endogenous depression. Some studies also show a link between seasonal variation and depression.

DRUGS IN THE MANAGEMENT OF DEPRESSION

Although various therapies may be used in the management of depression, only drugs (e.g. antidepressants, lithium) and electroconvulsive therapy (ECT) will be described here.

Antidepressant drugs fall into two main groups: the tricyclics and the monoamine oxidase inhibitors (MAOIs). The precise mechanism by which those two types of drug work is not clear, but the result is an increase in postsynaptic neurotransmitter, either through blocking of the reuptake of neurotransmitter from the presynaptic bouton or prevention of its degradation by the enzyme monoamine oxidase. As a result, more neurotransmitter is available for the postsynaptic bouton and its receptor sites. Thus the levels of noradrenaline (epinephrine) and serotonin are raised.

Tricyclics

Tricyclic antidepressants are the most widely pre-scribed antidepressants and they have been found to be beneficial in about 70% of depressed patients (Klein & Davis 1969).

It is believed that most tricyclic antidepressants exert their effects by blocking alpha$_2$ adrenocep-tors (autoreceptors) on the presynaptic bouton (Raisman, Briley & Langer 1979). In so doing, they cause increased neuronal firing of the bou-tons and hence release of neurotransmitter. In the intact system (absence of depression) alpha$_2$ adrenoceptors inhibit the release of neurotrans-mitters. Several studies have suggested that there is an excess of alpha$_2$ adrenoceptors during depres-sive illness.

Another mode of action of tricyclic antidepres-sants is to blockade the reuptake of neuro-transmitters. For example, imipramine and amitriptyline, which are tricyclic antidepressants, inhibit the uptake of serotonin (5-hydroxytrypta-mine, or 5-HT). Tricyclic antidepressants also act as antagonists at the cholinergic muscarinic recep-tors and this accounts for some of the side-effects such as dry mouth, urinary retention, constipa-tion, blurred vision and even confusion. Postural hypotension can also occur as a side-effect and this is as a result of adrenergic blockade. Other side-effects that can also occur, especially in the elderly, are: cardiac arrhythmias, tachycardia, weight gain, sweating, epilepsy and aggravation of glaucoma.

Many drugs belong to the tricyclic antidepres-sant group, including amitriptyline, nortriptyline, mianserin, trimipramine, oxaprotiline, alapro-clate, fluoxetine, citalopram, talsupra, nomifen-sine, bupropion and maprotiline.

Monoamine oxidase inhibitors

MAOIs cause irreversible inhibition of the enzyme monoamine oxidase A and thus block deamina-tion of the neurotransmitters 5-hydroxytrypta-mine and noradrenaline in the nerve terminals. They therefore increase the level of neurotransmit-ters available to be released from the presynaptic bouton or terminal. MAOIs also act upon the walls of blood vessels.

MAOIs may be useful in depression combined with anxiety, including phobic anxiety, and hyper-somnia.

MAOIs can give rise to several side-effects such as urinary retention, dry mouth, blurred vision, failure of ejaculation, liver damage, postural hypotension and epilepsy. One of their most unde-sirable side-effects is the so-called 'cheese effect', which gives rise to such symptoms as hyperten-sion, headache, hyperpyrexia and possibly stroke. This occurs because of the accumulation of tyra-mine, a chemical substance found in many foods and drinks such as cheese, yeast extracts and Chianti wine. Tyramine is usually metabolized by MAO but, in the absence of the latter, it binds with presynaptic vesicles and causes the release of noradrenaline and, since it is also a sympath-omimetic agent, this accounts for the symptoms mentioned above.

Patients on MAOIs should carry an information card indicating the foods that they should not drink or eat and foods that they should also avoid (see Box 11.1, adapted from Weller & Eysenck, 1992). Because MAOIs can often cause insomnia, they are usually prescribed to be taken no later than noon. There are several drugs belonging to the MAOIs group:

Generic name	Trade names
phenelzine	Nardil
isocarboxazid	Marplan
iproniazid	Marsilid
tranylcypromine	Parnate

Other antidepressants

Over recent years many newer compounds have been used as antidepressants, although their actions are not very clear. Some of the newer com-pounds are: mianserin, anoxapine, maprotiline and flupenthixol.

Lithium

Lithium is a drug that has been used successfully to treat manic depressive illness since 1979 (Cade 1980). It exerts a prophylactic effect (Souza, Mander & Goodwin 1990) although its pharma-

---

Box 11.1   Information card for users of monoamine oxidase inhibitors

Monoamine oxidase inhibitor

What you need to know
Carry this card with you always. Show it to any doctor who may treat you, to your dentist if you require dental treatment, and to the pharmacist when you buy any medicine for yourself.
Please read carefully.
While taking this medicine, and for 10 days afterwards, you must follow these instructions.

Do not eat or drink anything that contains:
Cheese, beef extract or beef extract cubes, or similar meat or yeast extract.
Pickled herrings.
Broad bean pods (the long green envelope that contains the beans), though you can eat the beans themselves.

Avoid
Chianti wine completely, and drink no more than a little alcohol of any kind.
Game, or meat that has not been well preserved.
Other foods cause no problems.

Do not take other medicines:
(including tablets, capsules, nose drops, or suppositories) whether bought for you or previously prescribed by your doctor without consulting your GP.
NB Cough and cold cures, pain relievers, tonics and laxatives are medicines.
These drugs are safe if the above precautions are observed. You may use plain aspirin BP or plain paracetamol BP if necessary.
If you need something for constipation ask your pharmacist for a bulk laxative.
Report any severe symptoms to your GP and follow any other advice given.

Adapted from Weller & Eysenck 1992

---

cological action is still unclear. There is a delay of 2 to 3 weeks before any clinical improvement is observed, once treatment is started.

Lithium is administered as lithium carbonate; it has a low therapeutic index and thus can give rise to many side-effects arising from toxic concentrations. It is therefore important that serum lithium is monitored regularly following its administration, for example after 7, 14, 21 and 28 days and thereafter at 3–6 weeks. Mild neurological side-effects may occur and they include mild lethargy and fine tremor. More serious side-effects at toxic levels are coarse tremor, drowsiness, vomiting, dysarthria, ataxia and eventually convulsions, coma and death. Long term side-effects can occur following several months of treatment, for example hypothyroidism, polyuria and polydipsia.

Permanent renal glomerular and tubular damage may also occur. It has been reported that lithium toxicity can occur in the presence of diminished renal function. It is also suggested that patients who are on diuretics and thus can lose sodium are more at risk, since the renal tubules cannot distinguish between sodium and lithium. Therefore when the kidneys need to conserve sodium then lithium will be also reabsorbed, which will increase blood lithium levels. But, despite toxic effects, lithium continues to play an important role in the management of the bipolar form of depression.

Recent advances

There is increasing evidence that valproate or valproic acid (Depakene or Depakote) and carbamazepine (Tegretol) are effective in manic depressive individuals who are not tolerant to lithium, because of side-effects.

The side-effects of carbamazepine are: sedation, nausea, a drunk-like sense of clumsiness and, more rarely, aplastic anaemia. Carbamazepine has recently been associated with a set of birth defects.

The side-effects of valproate are: nausea, vomiting, indigestion and, in rare cases, liver toxicity.

ELECTROCONVULSIVE THERAPY

ECT has been used for a very much longer period of time than the above in the treatment of major unipolar and bipolar depression. It can produce full remission or marked improvement in about 90% of patients suffering from severe depression.

Although the mechanism of ECT therapeutic action is still not understood, it is believed that it may well cause changes in aminergic receptor sensitivity. (It should be remembered that changes in amine concentration in the brain are thought to be associated with depression.) ECT is given under anaesthesia with complete muscle relaxation. It induces a generalized seizure. A series of 4–12 treatments is usually administered (average 6–8) at 2-day intervals over a 2–4-week period and this usually produces remission of symptoms.

In the history of psychiatry, ECT is the one treatment that has caused and continues to cause much controversy. Since its application in psychiatry by Laslo Meduna in 1935, there have been various modifications, for example the use of anaesthesia and muscle relaxants. ECT is opposed by many advocacy groups and the one issue of concern is the memory impairment that is an adverse effect of ECT.

However, many psychiatrists (Royal College of Psychiatrists 1987) recognize the efficacy of ECT in the management of depression and other medication refractory disorders.

Evidence for usefulness of ECT in the management of depression

There is conclusive evidence (Abrams 1988, Fink & Ottoson 1980) that ECT is effective in the management of depression. To show that ECT has a therapeutic action, many studies have been undertaken in the United Kingdom (Brandon et al 1984, Freeman 1978, Gregory, Shawcross & Gill 1985, Johnstone et al 1980, Lambourn & Gill 1978, West 1981) by comparing real and simulated ECT (anaesthesia and muscle relaxant only) in the treatment of depression. All the studies but one demonstrated that ECT is indeed effective in the treatment of depression (Table 11.1).

The recommended treatment is the administration of a moderately superthreshold amount (100–150% above initial threshold), which must be adjusted to age and sex (Sackeim et al 1987).

The technique of ECT involves the use of electrodes that can be applied bilaterally (for bilateral treatment, BL) or unilaterally (for non-dominant treatment, ULND). There is much debate in the choice of ULND versus BL treatment, although it is generally accepted that ULND electrode placement significantly reduces memory impairment (Weiner et al 1983). It is therefore recommended that ULND ECT be the treatment of choice unless the patient does not respond and therefore BL is then applied. McAllister et al (1987) suggested that twice and three times weekly schedules of ULND ECT is effective, whilst Lerer et al (1990) believe three times weekly treatment induces a significantly more rapid antidepressant effect, although it is associated with more memory impairment.

Health workers (such as nurses) who are closely involved in the management of patients undergoing ECT therapy must be aware of the emotive issues and should be familiar with the observations that should be undertaken before and after ECT treatment. It is paramount that the patient is given as much information as possible prior to consenting to ECT treatment.

Pharmacological manipulation of seizure duration

There is a significant increase in seizure threshold

Table 11.1 Studies comparing real and simulated ECT[a]

Study	No. of subjects	Stimulus parameters	Anaesthesia	Outcome
Lambourn & Gill (1978)	Real = 16 Simulated = 16	UL Brief pulse 6 treatments	Methohexital Suxamethonium	No difference
Freeman et al (1978)	Real = 20 2 Simulated + real = 20	BL Sine wave Treatment no. variable	Pentothal Suxamethonium	Real superior More ECTs in similar group
Johnstone et al (1980)	Real = 31 Simulated = 30	BL Sine wave 8 treatments	Methohexital Suxamethonium	Real superior
West (1981)	Real = 11 Simulated = 11	BL Sine wave 6 treatments (with cross-over)	Althesin Suxamethonium	Real superior
Brandon et al (1984)	Real = 43 Simulated = 34	BL Sine wave 8 treatments	Methohexital Suxamethonium	Real superior
Gregory et al (1985)	Real (UL) = 23 Real (BL) = 23 Simulated = 23	UL or BL Sine wave 6 treatments	Methohexital Suxamethonium	Real UL and BL superior

[a]All treatments administered twice weekly.
UL, unilateral; BL, bilateral.

and reduction in seizure duration when patients are undergoing a series of ECT treatment. To remedy this situation, the clinician usually increases the stimulus intensity, although the latter is associated with increased cognitive adverse effects.

In an attempt at resolving such a problem, Shapira et al (1985) have demonstrated that the use of intravenously administering caffeine sodium benzoate (500–2000 mg) 10 minutes before ECT did increase seizure duration. Other studies (Coffey et al 1990) have demonstrated that caffeine administration was equivalent to increased stimulus intensity in maintaining seizure duration.

Mechanism of action

The precise mechanism of action of ECT is not known, but there are suggestions by various authors that it may interact with different neurotransmitters in different syndromes. Thus, ECT may enhance serotoninergic and noradrenergic systems in the alleviation of depression. Adverse side-effects of ECT such as impairment of memory may be attributed to the effect of ECT on the cholinergic system (Lerer 1987). The antiparkinsonian effects of ECT have also been observed (Grahame-Smith, Green & Costain 1978) and may be attributed to the enhancement of the dopamine nigrostriatal pathway.

There are suggestions that ECT may perhaps have a direct effect on the hypothalamus and therefore may enhance release of specific hypothalamic peptides that have effective neurophysiological effects, as for example in the control of depression (Fink & Ottoson 1980). Further studies are needed to establish its precise neurobiological effects.

ECT remains a controversial issue, but as more research is undertaken to demonstrate the scientific basis of this treatment it may become universally accepted and may even be applied in other medical fields. Until then, the main reason in support of ECT treatment is that it does alleviate the symptoms of depression and thus can contribute to the quality of life in the affected individuals.

then, the best model remains that of amine involvement.

DISCUSSION QUESTIONS

1. Based on research evidence of amines involvement, discuss how they may contribute to endogenous depression. Give a rationale for your answer.
2. Discuss the use of ECT in the management of endogenous depression. Your arguments should focus on evidence of the effectiveness of ECT and the ethical issues surrounding its use.
3. Choose two types of antidepressant drug used in the management of patients with endogenous depression and, for each one, discuss its possible action in the brain and also its side-effects.

FURTHER READING

Aubelas A 1987 Life-events and mania—a special relationship? British Journal of Psychiatry 150:235–240
A thorough account of depression is given and is clearly presented and makes interesting reading.

SUMMARY

Several theories based on the reduced activity of amines have been put forward as to the aetiology of depression. There is evidence for some of the theories, but many are still unclear. Tricyclic antidepressants and MAOIs through their pharmacological actions, either in blocking reuptake of amine or in reducing their degradation, give some indications of amine involvement in depression. However, the precise nature of the pharmacological actions is still unclear, for it takes 2 to 3 weeks from the time of the drug administration for the depressed individual to feel any improvement of the condition. These hypotheses are continuously being reviewed.

Another pitfall in the hypothesis is that administration of drugs such as lithium, and the use of ECT, control depression effectively and yet they do not behave as tricyclic depressants or MAOIs.

The search for the precise mechanism for the aetiology of depression will continue but, until

REFERENCES

Abrams R 1988 Electroconvulsive therapy. Oxford University Press, Oxford

Aubelas A 1987 Life-events and mania—a special relationship? British Journal of Psychiatry 150:235–240

Brandon S, Cowley P, McDonald C, Neville P, Palmer R, Wellstood-Eason S 1984 Electroconvulsive therapy: results in depressive illness from the Leicestershire trial. British Medical Journal 228:22–25

Cade J F J 1980 The story of lithium. In: Ayd E J, Blackwell D (eds) Discoveries in biological psychiatry. J B Lippincott, Philadelphia

Coffey C E, Figiel G S, Weiner R D, Saunders W B 1990 Caffeine augmentation of ECT. American Journal of Psychiatry 147:579–585

Fink M, Ottoson J O 1980 A therapy of convulsive therapy in endogenous depression. Significance of hypothalamic functions. Psychiatric Research 2:49–61

Freeman C P L 1978 The therapeutic efficacy of electroconvulsive therapy (ECT). A double blind controlled trial of ECT and simulated ECT. Scottish Medical Journal 23(1):71–75

Grahame-Smith D G, Green A R, Costain D W 1978 Mechanism of the antidepressant action of ECT. Lancet i:245–256

Gregory S, Shawcross C R, Gill D 1985 The Nottingham ECT study. A double blind comparison of bilateral, unilateral, and simulated ECT in depressive illness. British Medical Journal 146:520–524

Johnstone E C, Deakin J F, Lawler P, Frith C D, Stevens M, McPherson K, Crow T J 1980 The Northwick Park ECT trial. Lancet ii:1317–1320

Klein D F, Davis J M 1969 In: Klein D F, Davis J M (eds) Diagnosis and drug treatment of psychiatric disorders: a review of mood stabilising literature. Williams & Wilkins, Baltimore

Lambourn J, Gill D 1978 A controlled comparison of simulated and real ECT. British Journal of Psychiatry 133:154–159

Lerer B 1987 Neurochemical and other neurobiological consequences of ECT. Implications for the pathogenesis and treatment of affective disorders. In: Meltzer H Y (ed) Psychopharmacology, the third generation of progress. Raven Press, New York

Lerer B et al 1990 Optimising ECT schedule—a double blind study. American Psychiatric Association 43rd annual meeting, New York

McAllister D A, Perri M G, Jordan R C, Rauscher F P, Sattin A 1987 Effects of ECT given two versus three times weekly. Psychiatric Research 21:63–69

Raisman R, Briley M, Langer S F 1979 Specific tricyclic depressant binding sites in rat brain. Nature (Lond) 281:148–150

Royal College of Psychiatrists 1987 Memorandum on the use of ECT. British Journal of Psychiatry 131:261–272

Sackeim H A, Decina P, Kanzler M, Kerr B, Malitz S 1987 Effects of electrode placement on the efficacy of titrated low-dose ECT. American Journal of Psychiatry 144:1449–1455

Shapira B et al 1985 Potentiation of seizure length and clinical response to ECT by caffeine pretreatment. Convulsive Therapy 1:58–60

Souza F G M, Mander A J, Goodwin G M 1990 The efficacy of lithium in prophylaxis of unipolar depression: evidence from its discontinuation. British Journal of Psychiatry 157:718–722

Weiner R D 1984 Does ECT cause brain damage? Behavioural Brain Sciences 7:1–53

Weller M, Eysenck M 1992 The scientific basis of psychiatry, 2nd edn. W B Saunders, London

West E D 1981 ECT in depression: a double-blind controlled trial. British Medical Journal 282:355–357

Young M A, William A, Scheftner J F, Klerman G L 1990 Gender differences in the clinical features of unipolar major depressive disorder. Journal of Nervous Mental Disease 178(3):200–203

SECTION 4: Dementia of Alzheimer's, Parkinson's and Huntington's disease

AIMS

◆ To distinguish between Alzheimer's disease, Parkinson's disease and Huntington's disease

◆ To explore the biological basis and treatment possibilities for each condition

◆ To appreciate research studies so as to keep abreast of new developments in the aetiology of Parkinson's disease, Alzheimer's disease and Huntington's disease

INTRODUCTION

Dementia is one of the most distressing conditions of the nervous system and its prevalence may be as high as 10% in people over 65 years, rising to 20% in those over 80. It is a progressive illness leading to severe mental impairment and physical changes whereby sufferers are unable to lead independent lives and may be a danger to themselves.

Although there are many causes of dementia, for example Alzheimer's disease, Parkinson's disease, Huntington's disease, vascular disorder of multi-infarcts (accounting for about 25% of patients with dementia), hypothyroidism and alcoholic dementia, only the first three will be described here, since the individuals affected are likely to require admission to psychiatric units at some stage.

Dementia is defined by the Diagnostic and statistical manual of mental disorders (DSM-IIIR, APA 1987) as loss of intellectual ability with resulting occupational and social handicaps and is accompanied by one or more of the following: impaired thinking or judgement, aphasia, agnosia, constructional difficulties and changes in person-

ality. Verbal skills may be affected but show least decline. The most common cause of dementia is Alzheimer's disease.

ALZHEIMER'S DISEASE

Alzheimer's disease (AD) was first described by Alois Alzheimer, a psychiatrist and neuroanatomist, in 1907 in a woman patient who died following a progressive disorder with loss of memory and language ability.

AD is the most common cause of dementia in the elderly, accounting for almost two-thirds of cases of senile dementia. It may be a genetically linked disorder; for example, 15–20% of sufferers fall into the category of familial AD, which is an autosomal dominant, inherited condition (St George Hyslop et al 1989). Other evidence of genetic linkage is based on the observation that most people with Down's syndrome (trisomy 21) eventually develop features of AD. Studies confirm that proximal chromosome 21 is likely to be the locus (St George Hyslop et al 1987). The twin concordance values for Alzheimer's are 58% in monozygotic twins and 26% in dizygotic twins.

Several physical changes have been observed in AD, brain atrophy (weight from 1200 g and 1350 g to 1000 g less), enlarged ventricles, and usually symmetrical cortical atrophy, especially of the frontal and temporal lobes. In postmortem studies using the whole temporal lobe of normal elderly and matched demented patients, Bowen et al (1977) found that about one-third of nerve cell components are lost from the temporal lobe. Histological studies also show loss of large pyramidal cells (up to 60% in the cortex) from the temporal cortex and occipital region, as well as from the hippocampus and amygdala.

Pearson et al (1985) observed that AD spreads along projection neurons from the olfactory cortex to association areas, but spares the occipital and motor cortex. Talamo et al (1989) confirmed that the olfactory neurons showed pathological changes in AD patients. Neuronal loss, neuritic plaques (NP) and neurofibrillary tangles (NFT) are common pathological changes. Alzheimer's disease is characterized by loss of neurons in

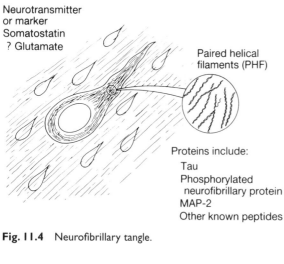

Neurotransmitter or marker
Somatostatin
? Glutamate

Paired helical filaments (PHF)

Proteins include:
 Tau
 Phosphorylated
  neurofibrillary protein
 MAP-2
 Other known peptides

Fig. 11.4 Neurofibrillary tangle.

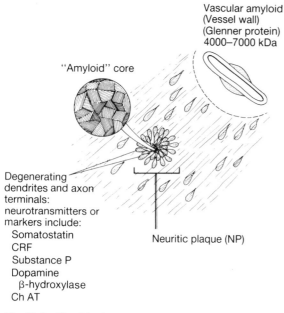

Vascular amyloid
(Vessel wall)
(Glenner protein)
4000–7000 kDa

"Amyloid" core

Degenerating
dendrites and axon
terminals:
neurotransmitters or
markers include:
 Somatostatin
 CRF
 Substance P
 Dopamine
  β-hydroxylase
 Ch AT

Neuritic plaque (NP)

Fig. 11.5 Neuritic plaque.

certain areas of the brain and the presence of NFTs and NPs in association areas of the cortex, hippocampus, amygdala and with certain subcortical nuclei.

NFTs are abnormal neuronal soma in which the cytoplasm is filled with filamentous structures arranged in paired helical fashion (Fig. 11.4). In the cortex, tangles are found in clusters in the pyramidal neurons of layers III and V. Other pathological brain changes found in Alzheimer's

are accumulation of products derived from the proteolysis of amygdaloid (Beyreuther et al 1988) in arterioles, in meninges and cerebral cortex. NPs consist of clusters of degenerating nerve endings, both round and dendritic, with a central core (Fig. 11.5), which resembles an amyloid protein (Katzman & Thal 1989).

Cholinergic involvement in Alzheimer's disease

It is believed that there is reduced activity of the brain as reflected in studies in which labelled deoxyglucose is used and its utilization measured and shown on positron emission tomography (PET) scans. NPs are easily detected using a fluorescent thioflavine stain. Many plaques are acetylcholine positive. It has been discovered that the degree of dementia in AD patients measured during life is highly correlated with the number of NPs in the cerebral cortex. It has been found that the number of NPs in the cerebral cortex is correlated with the level of enzyme acetyltransferase.

Several studies on postmortem AD brains have confirmed a decrease in the enzyme choline acetyltransferase in the cerebral cortex and hippocampus (Davies & Maloney 1976). The greatest loss of cholinergic activity was in the temporal and parietal cortex, hippocampus and amygdaloid nucleus. Surgical biopsy samples taken from the cerebral cortex of Alzheimer patients in the first year of symptomatology show a reduction in acetyltransferase. Bowen et al (1977) also found a reduction in choline acetyltransferase activity, which correlated with the degree of pathological damage to the temporal lobe. On the other hand, Perry and colleagues (Perry & Perry, 1980, Perry et al 1977) demonstrated a decrease in acetylcholinesterase activity in parallel with an increase in NP density and premortem intellectual impairment. Sims et al (1983) also showed that choline acetyltransferase activity, choline uptake and acetylcholine synthesis were significantly reduced within a year of the onset of the disease.

It is believed that AD may also be associated with loss of muscarinic receptors, but as yet data are sparse and much of the work needs to be confirmed. However, as a result of muscarinic receptor loss, there are claims that there is loss of presynaptic cholinergic terminals (Mash, Flynn & Potter 1985).

Noradrenaline (norepinephrine) and serotonin in AD

It would appear that there is a reduction in the number of neurons in both the locus coeruleus and raphe nuclei in AD. Postmortem Alzheimer brain examination has also revealed reduction in levels of both noradrenaline and serotonin. Bowen et al (1983) also demonstrated reductions in serotonin uptake in brain biopsies.

Glutamate, somatostatin and corticotrophin-releasing factor in AD

There is some evidence that glutamate may be reduced in AD. Hyman, Van Hoeson & Damasio (1987) demonstrated an 80% reduction of glutamate in some of the cortical pyramidal cells, which are usually destroyed in AD.

Davies, Katzman & Terry (1980) and Beal et al (1986a) have shown that the concentration of somatostatin was reduced in the neocortex and hippocampus in Alzheimer's brain. Ferrier et al (1983) also demonstrated that levels of somatostatin were reduced in the temporal, frontal and parietal cortex but increased in the subtantia innominata in AD. It is not clear as to the significance of somatostatin decrease in AD.

It has also been found that corticotrophin-releasing factor is lowered in several brain areas of patients with AD (Bisette et al 1985). Larger reductions of approximately 80% were found in the occipital cortex.

Nerve growth factor (NGF)

The absence of a nerve growth factor (NGF) may be responsible for the degeneration of cholinergic neurons in AD. Evidence for this has been demonstrated in studies in which NGF was infused into the brain of aged rats with spatial memory impairment and they recovered spatial memory as observed in a water maze test. It should be remembered that acetylcholine may be responsible for memory storage in the brain.

Drugs in the management of AD

Most of the drugs used in the treatment of AD have so far proved to be ineffective. The search continues in finding a drug that will be able to improve memory of the patient. The approaches to drug therapy have been to:

◆ increase synthesis and/or release of acetylcholine (use of choline phosphatidylcholine)
◆ reduce the metabolism of acetylcholine by inhibiting the enzyme acetylcholinesterase (use of physostigmine, tetrahydroamino acridine)
◆ increase the release of acetylcholine (use of aminopyridine)
◆ use of muscarinic agonists (arecoline)
◆ increase glucose and oxygen utilization.

Use of choline

Choline in the form of lecithin (phosphatidylcholine), which is a natural source of choline found in foods such as eggs and fish, has been administered to patients in many studies in the hope of improving memory (Smith et al 1978); however, the results have been negative.

Sitaram, Weingartner & Gillin (1978) found that a single 10 g dose of choline significantly enhanced serial learning of lists of words as compared with subjects on placebos. Mohs & Davis (1982) have also reported that subjects who were given choline, but had also received physostigmine previously, showed a slight improvement in memory.

Anticholinesterases

Kaye et al (1982) have reported that there were small improvements in memory on word recall test in AD patients who were given the anticholinesterase tetrahydroamino acridine (THA) together with lecithin. Other studies have used the drug physostigmine, but in general the results are still very poor.

Cholinergic agonists

There are reports indicating that intravenous infusion of arecoline (an agonist at both nicotinic and muscarinic receptors) did improve recognition memory in patients with AD. Use of arecoline has also been shown to enhance learning in both normal young volunteers and elderly monkeys.

Increasing the release of acetylcholine

Since it is known that there is a significant decrease in the level of acetylcholine produced in AD, it is reasonable to speculate that any drug that can increase its release might improve the memory of patients with AD. Drugs like 4-aminopyridine and THA have been reported to show improvements in tests of orientation and memory in patients with AD. There were also marked improvements in everyday behaviour in patients who had been taking the drug for 12 months.

Increasing glucose and oxygen utilization

There is some evidence in animal studies that the drug Hydergine (co-dergocrine mesylate) can promote glucose metabolism under conditions of ischaemia. Another drug considered to be a metabolic stimulant, piracetam, has been shown to improve learning in animal studies.

Summary

It would appear that more studies need to be undertaken to establish the exact pharmacological properties of many of the drugs currently in use. As yet, the evidence for efficacy of the drug in use is still not very clear. It is reasonable to assume that many drug trials will go on, in the hope of helping existing patients with AD.

In search of the factors that may contribute to AD, it is important to realize that environmental factors may also play a role, for example aluminium (Duckett 1976). Aluminium has been found in excessive concentrations in the plaques of some patients with AD.

PARKINSON'S DISEASE

Parkinson's disease (PD) is one of the commonest progressive degenerative conditions of the central nervous system. It occurs predominantly in those over 55 years, affecting at least 1% of the population. Forty per cent of those suffering from PD progress to dementia.

James Parkinson, a GP from Shoreditch, described some of the signs and symptoms as (Parkinson 1817):

◆ slowness and poverty of all movements (bradykinesia, akinesia)
◆ muscle stiffness, which is referred to as 'cogwheel' rigidity
◆ tremor of the limbs mainly at rest
◆ dementia/depression.

Another feature of the disease is the shuffling gait that is observed in all of the patients.

The breakthrough as to the pathophysiology of Parkinson's disease came about in the 1960s, with reports that there was a decrease in concentration of dopamine in the basal ganglia of postmortem brains of PD sufferers. This is now universally accepted, but the aetiology is still obscure.

However, there is some speculation that PD may be the result of a viral infection or a particular toxic substance that affects the basal ganglia. This is based on the evidence that many people developed PD following a worldwide pandemic of encephalitis around 1920. Also an outbreak of Parkinsonism occurred amongst Californian heroin addicts in 1982. Research has indicated that 1-methyl-4-phenyl-1,2,3,6 tetrahydro-pyridine (MPTP) can actually induce symptoms identified as PD, if injected cutaneously or through inhalation. It has been reported (Langston et al 1983) that, in an attempt to synthesize heroin illegally, MPTP was present in the chemical used.

Other distinct pathology in PD is the absence of the dark pigment in the substantia nigra (SN). Cell bodies of neurons that project from the SN to the corpus striatum contain melanin granules pigment. It is not known why the pigments are lost, but MPTP does show selective toxicity for the nigrostriatal neurons. Are there perhaps other toxic substances that may be the causation of PD? Studies by Hornykiewicz (1982) also show that many types of neurons are lost.

There is general agreement that patients with PD lack dopamine in the basal ganglia, for patients treated with neuroleptic drugs, which reduce dopamine level, develop symptoms analogous to PD. It is therefore not surprising that patients with PD respond to drugs that raise the level of dopamine.

Treatment of PD

L-dopa or levodopa

Treatment has focused mainly on the use of dopamine precursors such as L-dopa, which is a naturally occurring amino acid. But because the drug is absorbed mainly in the duodenum and the jejunum, thus causing dopamine formation in the circulation, it gives rise to many unwanted side-effects: postural hypotension, nausea, vomiting and involuntary movements. L-dopa is decarboxylated to dopa in the circulation but not in the brain. Less than 1% reaches the brain unchanged. Side-effects such as vomiting can be reduced if levodopa is combined with benserazide or carbidopa (Sinemet). Other effects of levodopa in advanced states of PD are mild visual hallucinations, toxic confusional states and frank paranoid psychosis. Patients on long term treatment can also develop the so-called 'on–off effects' (patients alternately freeze and go hypotonic) and also end of dose akinesia (in which stiffness towards the end of the dose becomes a problem). Some patients can develop severe orofacial dyskinesia, which occurs as a result of overstimulation of dopaminergic receptors.

Bromocriptine

Bromocriptine, a dopamine receptor agonist, has also been used in the treatment of PD. It is often given in association with levodopa. It has been reported that patients treated with bromocriptine do not experience the abnormal involuntary movements seen in those treated only with levodopa.

Selegiline

Selegiline is a selective inhibitor of the monoamine oxidase (MAO) isoenzyme type B found in platelets and also in the striatum. It can be given with levodopa, and there is no need for diet restriction. Its function is to increase dopamine concentration by preventing its breakdown via MAO. Side-effects such as euphoria, insomnia and hallucinations may occur.

In conclusion, evidence still strongly suggests that lack of dopamine is responsible for the symptoms of PD, but as yet it is unclear as to the aetiology. Drugs currently in use may arrest the progression of the disease and reduce symptoms short term, but are not effective in the long term.

Recent studies indicate that treatment may be successful by grafting fetal tissue in the affected area of the substantia nigra. There have been some positive reports from Mexico of clinical trials (surgical fetal tissue transplants) on patients with PD. This could well be the preferred choice of treatment in the future, but there are moral and ethical dilemmas.

HUNTINGTON'S DISEASE

Huntington's disease (HD), first described by George Huntington in 1872, is an autosomal dominant disorder, affecting approximately 6000 individuals in the UK. It is speculated that 50 000 individuals are at risk of developing the disease. Men and women are affected with equal frequency—about 5 per 100 000 population. The onset of the disease occurs in most cases in the fourth to fifth decade of life. Each child of an affected parent has a 50% chance of inheriting the disease.

The HD gene was cloned in 1993 and it is located near the telomere on chromosome 4. The mutation that causes the disease is known as a trinucleotide repeat expansion. Nucleotides are the building blocks of deoxyribonucleic acid (DNA) and contain the bases adenine, thymine, cytosine and guanine. Adenine pairs with thymine and guanine pairs with cytosine in DNA. The arrangement of the bases gives each of us our unique characteristics. The bases are indeed our genes. Bases code for specific amino acids and the coding system consists of a group of three bases, referred to as a 'codon' or 'triplet code'.

In relation to HD, it has been found that there is a repeat of the triplet CAG to 36 or more, as opposed to only 15 repeats in normal individuals. CAG encodes the amino acid glutamine, and if there is an increase in the repeats of CAG then more glutamic acid will be found in the protein coded. The coded protein is referred to as huntingtin, but its function is not known. Longer repeat lengths of CAG are associated with juvenile onset and more severe symptoms.

George Huntington observed four characteristics of this disease:

◆ its heritability
◆ the presence of chorea
◆ the development of dementia
◆ the occurrence of death after 15 or 20 years.

The signs and symptoms are many, and they include irritability, depression, fidgeting, clumsiness, sudden falls and absent-mindedness. The prominent feature of the disease is uncontrolled involuntary choreiform movements. These involuntary movements disappear during sleep.

Speech is also affected. It is slurred at first, but later becomes incomprehensible and finally it ceases altogether as facial expression becomes disturbed and grotesque. Mental functions deteriorate. The whole body may also be affected by exhausting dyskinesia. Some individuals may have outbursts of excitement or temper and suicidal tendencies.

The pathophysiology of HD as revealed through postmortem studies and also by CAT scan shows atrophy and shrinkage of the basal ganglia and loss of cortical neurons. There is loss of a specific set of cholinergic neurons and neurons that synthesize GABA in the striatum. There is also marked decrease of both choline acetyltransferase and the enzyme glutamic acid decarboxylase required for GABA. Some peptides, such as substance P, methionine enkephalin and dynorphin are also reduced. The degree of loss of cortical neurons is associated with the severity of the dementia that occurs.

The mechanism by which neurons are lost is unknown, but an animal model in which kainic acid is injected in the striatum created symptoms similar to those in HD. Because of the striatal involvement in HD, it is postulated that an endogenous neurotoxin like kainic acid might be involved in the pathophysiology of HD.

Treatment

Most drugs used in the treatment of HD are to alleviate symptoms, thus helping the individuals to cope with life. Drugs that can increase GABA concentration, such as the GABA agonist baclofen, have given satisfactory results in clinical trials.

Until the pathophysiology of HD is clearly understood, specific drugs for the management of HD remain in the distant future.

DISCUSSION QUESTIONS

1. There are several causes of dementia. Identify three causes of dementia and for each one explore how the brain and its structure may be affected. Your arguments must focus on research studies.
2. Discuss the genetics of Huntington's disease to include some of the emotive issues surrounding screening.
3. In relation to drugs, discuss the management of clients with Alzheimer's disease. You should identify the possible actions of the drugs and their side-effects.

FURTHER READING

Sanger D J, Blackmore D E (eds) 1984 Aspects of psychopharmacology. Methuen, London

Siegel G J (ed) (1982) Basic neurochemistry, 3rd edn. Little, Brown, New York
Both books provide relevant scientific investigations and are indeed suited for those wishing to enhance their understanding of brain functions and drug interactions.

REFERENCES

APA (American Psychiatric Association) 1987 Diagnostic and statistical manual, 3rd revision. American Psychiatric Association, Washington DC

Beal M F et al 1986a Somatostatin: alterations in the CNS in neurological diseases. In: Martin J B, Barchas J D (eds) Neuroleptics in neurologic and psychiatric disease (Association for Research in Nervous and Mental Disease, vol 64). Raven Press, New York, pp 215–258

Beal M, Kowall N W, Ellison D W, Mazurek M F, Swartz K J, Martin J B 1986b Replication of the neurochemical characteristics of Huntington's disease by quinolinic acid. Nature 321:168–171

Beyreuther K et al 1988 Molecular pathology of amyloid deposition in Alzheimer's disease. In: Henderson A S, Hendersin J H (eds) Aetiology of dementia of Alzheimer's type. John Wiley, Chichester

Bisette G et al. 1985 Corticotrophin releasing factor-like immunoreactivity in senile dementia of the Alzheimer's type. Reduced cortical and striated concentration. Journal of the American Association 254:3067–3069

Bowen D M, Smith C B, White P, Flack R H, Carrasco L H, Gedye J L, Davison A N 1977 Chemical pathology of the organic dementias. II. Quantitative estimation of cellular changes in post-mortem brains. Brain 100:427–453

Bowen D M et al 1983 Biochemical assessment of neurotransmitter and metabolic dysfunction and cerebral atrophy in Alzheimer's disease. In: Katzman R (ed) Banbury report 15: biological aspects of Alzheimer's disease. Cold Spring Harbor Laboratory, New York, pp 219–223

Davies P, Maloney A T F 1976 Selective loss of central cholinergic neurones in Alzheimers disease. Lancet ii:1403

Davies P, Katzman R, Terry R D 1980 Reduced somatostatin-like immunoreactivity in cerebral cortex from cases of Alzheimer's disease and Alzheimer's senile dementia. Nature 288:279–280

Duckett S 1976 Aluminium and Alzheimer's disease (letter). Archives of Neurology 33:730–731

Ferrier I N, Cross A J, Johnson J A et al 1983 Neuropeptides in Alzheimer type dementia. Journal of Neurological Science 62:159–170

Hornykiewicz O 1982 Brain neurotransmitter changes in Parkinson's disease. In: Marsden C D, Fahn S (eds) Movement disorders. Butterworth, London

Huntington G 1872 On chorea. Medical and Surgical Reports 26:317–321

Hyman B T, Van Hoeson G W, Damasio A R 1987 Alzheimer's disease: glutamate depletion in the hippocampal perforant pathway zone. Annals of Neurology 22:37–40

Katzman R, Thal L 1989 Neurochemistry of Alzheimer's disease. In: Siegel G J et al (eds) A basic neurochemistry. Raven Press, New York

Kaye W H, Sitaram N, Weingartner H, Ebert M H, Smallberg S, Gillin J C 1982 Modest facilitation of memory in dementia with combined lecithin and anticholinesterase treatment. Biological Psychiatry 17:275–280

Langston J W, Ballard P, Tetrud J W, Irwin I 1983 Chronic Parkinsonism in humans due to a product of meperidine–analog synthesis. Science 219:979–980

Mash D C, Flynn D D, Potter L T 1985 Loss of M_2 muscarine receptors in the cerebral cortex in Alzheimer's disease and experimental cholinergic denervation. Science 228:1115–1117

Mohs R C, Davis K L 1982 A signal detectability analysis of the effect of physostigmine on memory in patients with Alzheimer's disease. Neurobiology of Ageing 3:105–110

Parkinson J 1817 An essay on the shaking palsy. Sherwood, Neely & Jones, London

Pearson R C A, Esiri M M, Hiorns R W, Wilcock G K, Powell T P 1985 Anatomical correlates of distribution of the pathological changes in the neocortex in Alzheimer's disease. Proceedings of the National Academy of Sciences USA 82(13):4531–4534

Perry E K, Perry R H 1980 The cholinergic system in Alzheimer's disease. In: Roberts P J (ed) Biochemistry of dementia. John Wiley, Chichester

Perry E K, Gibson P H, Blessed G, Perry R H, Tomlinson B E 1977 Neurotransmitter enzyme abnormalities in senile dementia—choline acetyltransferase and glutamic acid decarboxylase activities in necropsy brain tissue. Journal of Neurology and Science 34:247–265

Perry E K, Tomlinson B E, Blessed G, Bergmann K, Gibson P H, Perry R H 1978 Correlation of cholinergic abnormalities with senile plaques and mental test scores in senile dementia. British Medical Journal 2:1457–1459

St George-Hyslop P H, Tanzi R E, Polinsky R J et al 1987 The genetic defect causing familial Alzheimer's disease maps on chromosome 21. Science 235:885–890

St George-Hyslop P H, Myers R H, Haines J L et al 1989 Familial Alzheimer's disease: progress and problems. Neurobiology of Aging 10(5):417–425

Sims M R, Bowen D M, Allen S J et al 1983 Presynaptic cholinergic dysfunction in patients with dementia. Journal of Neurochemistry 40:503–509

Sitaram N, Weingartner H, Gillin J C 1978 Human serial learning: enhancement with arecoline and choline and impairment with scopolamine. Science 201:274–276

Smith C M, Swash M, Exton-Smith A N, Phillips M J, Overstall P W, Piper M E, Bailey M R 1978 Choline therapy in Alzheimer's disease. Lancet ii:318

Talamo B R, Rudel R, Kosik K S, Lee V M, Neff S, Adelman L, Kauer J S 1989 Pathological changes in olfactory neurons in patients with Alzheimer's disease. Nature 337:736–739

SECTION 5: Seizures and epilepsy

AIMS

- To describe the main features and characteristics of epileptic seizures
- To identify drugs that can be used in the management of epileptic seizures
- To understand some of the major diagnostic procedures for detecting epilepsy

INTRODUCTION

Epilepsy seizures can occur in many diseases that may directly or indirectly involve the brain; these may include disorders of carbohydrate, amino acid and lipid metabolism, ionic and electrolyte imbalance, infections, brain tumours, brain trauma, and fever in the young when no known causes are identified—a type referred to as idiopathic.

Symptoms of epileptic seizures vary in individuals according to the type of seizure (discussed below), but they include a prodrome, which is a gradual build-up of change in emotions, behaviour or alertness for several hours or days before a seizure, and an aura or warning sign, which is experienced at the beginning of a seizure and may be a motor or sensory sensation depending on the part of the brain where the abnormal electrical seizure begins. If electrical activity continues or spreads, the seizure attack or 'ictus' occurs. During the ictus period the individual may exert a degree of disturbed consciousness, which may be followed by stiffness and jerking of the limbs or engagement of purposeless movements called 'automatism'. Ictus is followed by the postictal or recovery period, when the patient quickly regains normal function or may be confused, irritable or may fall into a deep sleep.

PATHOPHYSIOLOGY— METABOLIC HOMEOSTASIS

There has been much debate as to the causes and altered physiological processes that take place in epilepsy, but so far no specific factors have been identified. However, there are indications that abnormal neurotransmitter function or abnormal neuronal membrane properties may be major factors in the production of seizure. Both can alter ionic concentration of various ions such as calcium and potassium. For example, it is known that, at the onset of the hypersynchronous discharge, extracellular calcium concentration falls and then rises later. Repetitive neuronal firing may cause the release of large amounts of excitatory neurotransmitters at synapses and thus promote seizures. Membrane properties may be altered in the presence of hypoxia, alkalosis, hypoglycaemia and respiratory poisons affecting adenosine triphosphate (ATP) production. All of these may give rise to seizures.

The neurotransmitter GABA (an inhibitory transmitter) has been implicated in the causation of seizure. The normal physiological function of GABA is the opening of membrane ion channels permeable to chloride. The influx of chloride ions in the neuronal membrane causes hyperpolarization, thereby producing an inhibitory postsynaptic potential. Thus GABA plays an important role in controlling neuronal excitation, and when there is a decrease or absence of GABA then neuronal excitation can increase and hence lead to seizures.

There are many lines of evidence for the involvement of GABA in seizures. For example, a deficiency of pyridoxine (vitamin B_6), a substance that is essential for the functioning of the enzyme glutamate decarboxylase (GAD) in the synthesis of GABA, may give rise to seizures. The concentration of GABA in the cerebrospinal fluid of epileptic individuals was found to be at a lower level than normal. Other evidence is the reduction of GAD that has been observed in human temporal lobe cortex that has been removed during neurosurgery for focal seizure. It has been observed that drugs that impair the synthesis of postsynaptic action on GABA can also cause seizures (Meldrum 1975, 1979).

I Partial seizures (seizures beginning locally).
  A Partial seizures with elementary symptomatology (generally without impairment of consciousness).
    1 With motor symptoms (includes Jacksonian seizures).
    2 With special sensory or somatosensory symptoms.
    3 With autonomic symptoms.
    4 Compound forms.
  B Partial seizures with complex symptomatology (generally with impairment of consciousness) (temporal lobe or psychomotor seizures).
    1 With impairment of consciousness only.
    2 With cognitive symptomatology.
    3 With affective symptomatology.
    4 With 'psychosensory' symptomatology.
    5 With 'psychomotor' symptomatology (automatisms).
    6 Compound forms.
  C Partial seizures secondarily generalized.

II Generalized seizures (bilaterally symmetrical and without local onset).
  A Absences (*petit mal*).
  B Bilateral massive epileptic myoclonus.
  C Infantile spasms.
  D Clonic seizures.
  E Tonic seizures.
  F Tonic–clonic seizures (*grand mal*).
  G Atonic seizures.
  H Akinetic seizures.

III Unilateral seizures (or predominantly).

IV Unclassified epileptic seizures (due to incomplete data).

From Gastaut 1970

Physiological disturbances that occur during seizure are: (i) increase in cerebral blood flow, (ii) increase in cerebral metabolic rate for glucose and oxygen in all regions that participate in seizures (Baldy-Moulinier, Ingvar & Meldrum 1983) and (iii) changes in the lipid composition of membranes in the brain.

CLASSIFICATION OF SEIZURES

Owing to the variations in the types of seizure and the way in which they affect individuals, it has been necessary to classify seizure according to electroencephalography (see Box 11.2). Generally the classification of seizure falls into two groups: partial (local) seizure (where seizure begins in a specific localized area) and generalized seizure (bilaterally symmetrical and without local onset). Both groups are further divided into subgroups. Partial seizures are described as elementary (simple), with motor, somatosensory or autonomic symptoms in which there is no impairment of consciousness, or complex, where consciousness is impaired.

Partial seizures

Partial seizure (elementary) with motor symptoms

This type of seizure is characterized by clonic or tonic movements that occur in one extremity or on one side of the face. The seizure often starts in the thumb and mouth, on account of the large representation of the hand and the mouth in the motor area of the brain. When the seizure starts focally and sequentially involves body parts it is called a Jacksonian seizure. A focal seizure can be followed by temporary paralysis (Todd's paralysis) of the involved part and may last minutes or hours but does not exceed 24 hours. In adults, but not in children, the presence of Todd's paralysis is indicative of a structural lesion.

Partial seizure (elementary) with somatosensory symptoms

The symptoms here depend on the location of the seizure focus in the brain. For example, if the seizure focus is in the parietal lobe the symptoms may range from vague to specific sensations such as warmth or numbness. If the seizure focus is in the occipital lobe, senses of sight, hearing, smell or taste may be affected. Feelings of dizziness may also be experienced.

Partial seizure (elementary) with autonomic symptoms

Symptoms that affect the autonomic system arise from deep in the brain cortex and the upper part of the brain. Individuals may therefore experience sweating, palpitations, dilation of pupils, pallor or flushing, excessive salivation and nausea.

Partial seizure (complex) with impaired consciousness only

The cognitive and affective seizure symptoms are thought to arise from the limbic system of the brain, in part of the frontal lobe and the anterior and medial parts of the temporal lobes (Svoboda 1979). The cognitive symptoms are a result of disturbance in thought or memory. Individuals may experience the so-called '*jamais vu*' situations— situations that may seem new although, in fact, they are familiar.

The affective symptoms are associated with brief episodes of emotions and/or behaviour unrelated to the patient's immediate environment. Sensations may be those of pleasure, fear, anger, anxiety or displeasure. In cases where individuals break into meaningless laughter, this is referred to as 'gelastic seizure' (Chen & Forster 1973, Gascon & Lombroso 1971).

Partial seizure (complex) with psychomotor or psychosensory symptoms

This group comprises one of the commonest types of seizure, which is also referred to as psychomotor or temporal lobe seizures. These seizures usually last 1–2 minutes and are often preceded by an aura. Patients frequently exhibit automatisms (repetitive, purposeless behaviour) such as scratching, chewing or lip smacking. The affected individual may stare blankly and is not responsive to verbal stimulation and often not aware of the sur-roundings. Confusion can occur postictally, as can amnesia for event prior to the seizure. The EEG during the ictus may show spikes, sharp waves or rhythmic temporal waves.

Psychosensory seizure symptoms are not as common as psychomotor symptoms. Individuals affected usually experience hallucinations, illusions, unpleasant taste or smell, or dizziness.

Generalized seizures

In comparison to partial seizure, generalized seizure affects the whole body and many body functions at once. There is marked impairment of consciousness during all types of generalized seizure. It is believed that the seizure activity arises from areas beneath the cortex and in deep centres of the brain. EEG patterns are bilaterally synchronous and symmetrical.

This type of seizure is rarely preceded by an aura. Affected individuals fall at the onset of the seizure if they are standing. Some of the manifestations of generalized seizure are abnormal body movements, no movement, loss of muscle tone, and staring. Postictal symptoms may vary.

Absence seizure (previously known as 'petit mal')

This is one of the commonest types of seizure occurring in children usually between 4 and 13 years of age (Currier, Koci & Saidman 1963, Livingston et al 1965). This seizure is not preceded by an aura and usually lasts 10–30 seconds, but the individual may suffer from a brief lapse of consciousness that is associated with staring, eye fluttering and sometimes twitching of the hands and mouth. Individuals may not be aware of the seizure and usually resume their activity before the seizure. The frequency of seizure ranges from several a day to as many as 200 per day. Some individuals may exhibit automatism and some degree of confusion.

The EEG shows a bilateral synchronous symmetrical 3–3.5 per second spike and wave pattern. The EEG and seizure can be precipitated by hyperventilation for 3 minutes.

Myoclonic seizures and infantile spasms

Myoclonic seizure is similar to infantile spasm, but the latter occurs more frequently in male babies between 3 and 8 months of age. The typical myoclonic seizure in adults and young children is sudden, and without warning, comprising brief, involuntary movements of the trunk and extremities.

Babies with infantile spasms may show marked intellectual and motor development (Jeavons, Harper & Bower 1970, Millichap et al 1962). Infantile spasm may last no more that a few seconds and is preceded by a cry or colour change, followed by a flexion spasm, which varies from involving nodding of the head only to doubling up of the entire body.

The EEG shows hypsarrhythmia, which is a specific wave pattern denoted by slow waves of high voltage, and with multifocal spikes. After a few years an affected child will develop myoclonic seizures where the EEG will show multiple spike foci, single foci and wave complexes at a rate of 2–2.5 per second.

Clonic, tonic, tonic–clonic seizures

According to specific symptoms, individuals can be grouped either under clonic or tonic seizure or both. A clonic seizure occurs when there are only rhythmic repeated jerking movements. A tonic seizure is said to exist when there is stiffness of the extremities and arching of the back.

In the tonic–clonic seizure, the so-called *grand mal* seizure, which lasts from one to a few minutes, the individual may cry or yell at the beginning of the seizure, then lose consciousness and fall to the ground. In the tonic phase, the body becomes rigid with the back arched and the extremities extended. There may be apnoea and cyanosis. This phase is followed by the clonic phase, where there is rhythmic contraction and relaxation of the trunk and extremities. The individual may be incontinent with respect to urine, faeces or both, may vomit, bite the tongue and have excessive salivation. After the seizure the individual may be quite confused and sleep deeply for several hours and may complain of headache upon awakening.

EEG tracings during seizure show bilaterally synchronous spiking.

Atonic and akinetic seizures

Atonic or 'drop attack' can often be observed in children with absence seizures. This type of seizure occurs frequently in drowsy states when the child has just woken up in the morning. There is momentary loss of consciousness, movement is arrested and the individual falls as normal muscle tone and tension are lost.

Akinetic seizure differs from atonic seizure in that there is no loss of muscle tone and the individual does not fall.

DIAGNOSIS

Apart from the history and a thorough physical examination of the affected individual, several non-specific tests may have to be carried out to detect any abnormality responsible for the seizure; for example, blood and urine tests may reveal kidney and liver malfunction. Various tests for detection of infection should be carried out.

Specific tests on the nervous system in the diagnosis of epilepsy include: electroencephalography (EEG), skull radiography, echoencephalography and CAT.

Electroencephalography

EEG is very useful in detecting abnormal spikes and waves, which could help to locate a seizure focus in particular areas of the brain. If possible, an EEG should be recorded during a seizure. The patient can also be monitored by EEG over a 24-hour period.

Skull radiography

Radiographs of the skull may be useful in the detection of a tumour, congenital defects, raised intracranial pressure, calcification or abnormal blood vessels. All of these abnormalities may give rise to seizures.

Echoencephalography

The use of high frequency sound waves to produce a picture of the individual's head may reveal abnormality such as asymmetrical shifting of the midline of the ventricles, which can occur as a result of haemorrhage, a tumour or atrophy of the brain.

Computerized axial tomography

CAT scans may show abnormal brain structures, thus indicating the possible reason for epilepsy.

DRUG TREATMENT IN THE MANAGEMENT OF EPILEPTIC SEIZURES

Although there are other approaches in the management of epileptic seizures (e.g. stress reduction, behavioural strategies and neurosurgery) only drug therapy will be discussed here. An overview of drug reactions will be discussed first and examples of various drugs will be referred to.

Once diagnosed, individuals with epileptic seizures must be treated promptly so as to prevent the development of status epilepticus.

The objective in management is to find the most effective way of controlling or stopping the seizures (reducing their frequency and severity) through the use of antiepileptic or anticonvulsant drugs, minimizing the risk of side-effects so that patients are able to function at optimal levels. Because of the long term treatment needed some patients may develop adverse drug reactions. These can be classified as dose-dependent adverse reactions, non-dose-dependent adverse reactions, and drug interactions.

The dose-dependent adverse reactions occur as a result of rapid accumulation of the drug in the body. The reactions, mostly related to the central nervous system, include drowsiness, irritability, vertigo, diplopia and dysarthria. The non-dose-dependent adverse reactions may give rise to minor skin rashes, which may be localized or widespread. The symptoms may appear immediately or within hours or days of the drug administration.

Drugs interactions result when two or more drugs are administered.

Drugs used in treatment are known as antiepileptics or anticonvulsants. There are different types of antiepileptics and their usage depends on the specific type of seizure. Examples of some antiepileptic drugs are:

◆ phenytoin (Epanutin, Pentran)
◆ phenobarbitone (Gardenal)
◆ primidone (Mysoline)
◆ carbamazepine (Tegretol)
◆ ethosuximide (Emeside, Zarontin)
◆ sodium valproate (Depakene, Epilim, Orlept)
◆ clonazepam (Clonoprin, Rivotril)
◆ acetazolamide (Diamox, Diamox SR)

Although the precise mechanism of action of anticonvulsant drugs is not known, it is postulated that they enhance the GABA neuronal system (increasing inhibitory actions) through promoting opening of chloride channels at postsynaptic neurons. They may also promote cationic movements, for example sodium and potassium, which may have an effect on both the pre- and postsynaptic membranes.

Phenytoin

Phenytoin was first synthesized by Biltz in 1908 and was first used as an anticonvulsant in 1938. It is one of the most common drugs used in epileptic treatment. It belongs to the group hydantions. The daily dose administration is approximately 4–6 mg/kg. Peak plasma level is reached in 8–12 hours. The biological half-life of the drug varies from 4 to 72 hours. Initially a loading dose is given as peak level is not reached until 5–7 days.

Side-effects of phenytoin include nystagmus, ataxia, drowsiness, diplopia, blurred vision, dizziness, dermatitis, measle-like rash and lupus erythematosus. Blood complications can occur and they may include thrombocytopenia, agranulocytosis and different types of anaemia. Gingival hyperplasia may occur, so good oral hygiene is essential.

Phenobarbitone

Phenobarbitone is a long-acting barbiturate and is used especially in the generalized tonic–clonic seizure. Adults may require 2–3 mg/kg. When administered intramuscularly, it should be given deeply into a large muscle to reduce tissue necrosis. Intravenous administration may give rise to respiratory depression, apnoea, laryngospasm and vasodilatation leading to a fall in blood pressure.

The side-effects include a lack of concentration, or inability to perform selected motor skills, slowness, ataxia and decreased level of consciousness. Various allergic reactions may occur in the form of urticaria, fever, rash, and Stevens–Johnson syndrome.

Primidone

Primidone is a structural analogue of phenobarbitone and therefore behaves similarly. It is used for generalized tonic–clonic seizures and complex partial seizures.

Side-effects are similar to phenobarbitone, although psychiatric or psychological problems may occur in individuals who are so predisposed (Hughes 1980).

Carbamazepine

Carbamazepine has been used especially in individuals with temporal lobe epilepsy. Hughes (1980) reported that 85% of patients with temporal lobe epilepsy would benefit from this drug. It can also be used in patients with generalized seizures.

Side-effects include blurred vision, nystagmus, dizziness, nausea and vomiting. Aplastic anaemia may also occur occasionally.

Ethosuximide

Ethosuximide is the drug of choice in absence seizures. The dose is approximately 20–30 mg/kg per day. Peak value is reached 3 hours following oral administration. Side-effects include nausea, anorexia, vomiting and dizziness. Systemic lupus erythematosus can occur.

Sodium valproate

Sodium valproate is used in individuals who have bilaterally synchronous and symmetrical three per second spike and wave complexes in their EEG with absence attacks. It has been found useful in patients with atonic, akinetic and myoclonic seizures.

Administration is every 6 to 8 hours. Side-effects are few and may include weight loss, weight gain and temporary hair loss. If taken with meals, nausea and vomiting may be prevented.

Clonazepam

Clonazepam belongs to the group benzodiazepines. It is often used in treating individuals with myoclonic, akinetic types of seizure. Clonazepam is a very powerful drug amongst the anticonvulsants. Side-effects may include drowsiness on account of its sedative action. Clonazepam may give rise to the development of tolerance.

Acetazolamide

This drug is used frequently for women whose seizures increase prior to or during their menstrual cycles. It is believed that the excess water that is present during the menstrual cycle is responsible for the changes in frequency of seizures. Acetazolamide assists in the removal of excess water and it appears to have direct anticonvulsant effect.

When caring for individuals who experience epileptic seizures, all health workers should be able to observe for any symptoms that may occur as a result of side-effects of the drug being used. They should be able to give advice with regards to the importance of drug compliance in the affected individuals. They should also promote education with regards to self-care so that the individual can lead and enjoy a full active life.

REFERENCES

Baldy-Moulinier M, Ingvar D H, Meldrum B S 1983 Current problems in epilepsy; cerebral blood flow, metabolism and epilepsy. John Libbey, London

DISCUSSION QUESTIONS

1. Based on research studies, discuss the classification of seizures.
2. Discuss the appropriate drugs that may be used in the management of specific types of seizure. For each drug also identify the possible side-effects.

FURTHER READING

Porter R J 1989 Epilepsy: one hundred elementary principles, 2nd edn. Baillière Tindall, London

Scambler G 1989 Epilepsy. Routledge, London
Both books give a thorough account of epilepsy and are easy to read.

Chen R C, Forster F M 1973 Cursive epilepsy and gelastic epilepsy. Neurology 23:1019

Currier R D, Koci D A, Saidman L J 1963 Prognosis of 'pure' petit mal. A follow-up study. Neurology 13:959

Gascon G G, Lombroso C T 1971 Epileptic (gelastic) laughter. Epilepsia 12:63

Gastaut H 1970 Clinical electroencephalographical classification of epileptic seizures. Epilepsia 26:103–113

Hughes J R 1980 Medical aspects of epilepsy: an overview. In: Hermann B P (ed) A multidisciplinary handbook of epilepsy. Charles C Thomas, Springfield, IL

Jeavons P M, Harper J R, Bower B D 1970 Long-term prognosis in infantile spasms: a follow-up report on 112 cases. Developmental Medicine and Child Neurology 12:413

Livingston S, Torres I, Pauli L L, Rider R V 1965 Petit mal epilepsy; results of a prolonged follow-up of 117 patients. Journal of the American Medical Association 194:227

Meldrum B S 1975 Epilepsy and GABA-mediated inhibition. International Review of Neurobiology 17:1–36

Meldrum B S 1979 Convulsant drugs, anticonvulsants and GABA-mediated neuronal inhibition. In: Krogsgaard-Laresen P, Scheel-Kruger J, Kofod H (eds) GABA-neurotransmitters. Munksgaard, Copenhagen

Millichap J G, Bickford R C, Klass D W, Bakus R E 1962 Infantile spasms, hypsarrhythmia and mental retardation; a study of aetiologic factors in 61 patients. Epilepsia 3:188

Svoboda W B 1979 Learning about epilepsy. University Park Press, Baltimore

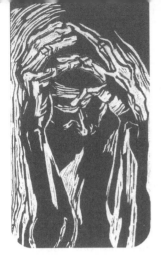

Chapter Twelve

Spiritual care and mental health competence

Aru Narayanasamy

AIMS

- ◆ To offer clarification of the meaning of spirituality
- ◆ To identify the competence required in the provision of spiritual care
- ◆ To examine the implications for nursing

KEY ISSUES

Mental health and spirituality

Spiritual well-being

Spiritual needs

Competences for spiritual care

Putting competence into action through the nursing process

INTRODUCTION

In mental health care a focus on individuals as psychosocial–spiritual beings is gaining recognition, but there is little elaboration on what is meant by spirit. This problem is further compounded by the misuse of the term 'spirituality' in that this word is equated to, or is applied synonymously with, institutional religion. Institutional religions usually refer to Protestantism, Catholicism and Judaism. At the beginning of this chapter the ambiguity concerning spirituality is addressed by clarifying what it really means. Following this and the identification of clients' spiritual needs, readers are introduced to competences required for spiritual care in the context of mental health care. In the final section competences of spiritual care are put into action through the nursing process. Several case history scenarios are provided to illuminate understanding through activity-related work.

Spiritual beliefs and practices permeate the life of a person, whether in health or illness. Certain spiritual needs tend to feature during our personal development and growth. The influence of spirituality and religion is commonly seen in the following aspects of a person's life: relationships with others, life styles and habits, required and prohibited behaviours, and the general frame of reference for thinking about oneself and the world. Our spirituality features during our development and growth.

WHAT IS SPIRITUALITY?

Recently, McSherry & Draper (1998) developed a debate in exploring the concept of spirituality as applied to nursing. In this debate these authors raised issues surrounding the complex and diverse nature of spirituality, and drew the conclusion that spirituality defies definitions.

There is no single authoritative definition of spirituality although a variety of explanations is offered in the emerging literature on this subject. When we talk about holistic approach we mean care for the body, mind and spirit. Holistic care is a popular theme, at least from a theoretical angle,

but spirituality as an aspect of nursing care is scarce. We need to understand the concept of spirituality if we are going to offer it as a component of holistic care.

Although there is an overlap between spirituality and other subject disciplines (psychology, sociology, politics and so on), it should be seen as a discipline with developing schools of theories. You will find that religious needs and spirituality are closely connected and sometimes one finds it is difficult to make the distinction between them as one need affects the other.

If you try to think about spirituality for a few minutes, several concepts may arise in your mind:

- ◆ a belief in God
- ◆ a belief affecting your life and how it relates to others
- ◆ something not necessarily religious
- ◆ a belief/concept; purpose and meaning
- ◆ faith/peace with oneself; a source of strength
- ◆ feeling of security/to be loved
- ◆ philosophy of life/death/religion
- ◆ self-esteem/inner self, inner strength
- ◆ searching/coping; hope
- ◆ an idealism, a striving to be good; a trusting relationship.

History suggests that since the beginning of humanity, spirituality has always predominated our lives in some way or another. Spirituality is one of the fashionable words in nursing, yet like so many useful and comprehensive terms, it is not easy to define. Spirituality is defined as:

Spirituality is rooted in an awareness which is part of the biological make up of the human species. Spirituality is present in all individuals and it may manifest as inner peace and strength derived from perceived relationship with a transcendent God/an ultimate reality, or whatever an individual values as supreme.

The spiritual dimension evokes feelings which demonstrate the existence of love, faith, hope, trust, awe, inspirations; therein providing meaning and a reason for existence. It comes into focus particularly when an individual faces emotional stress, physical illness or death.
Narayanasamy 1999, p. 274

In the nursing and health literature spirituality is commonly explained from the following traditions.

Christian theological traditions

In the Christian theological context an individual is seen as made up of body, mind and spirit. This belief has its origins in the book of Genesis when God breathes into Adam's nostrils to give him life. The position of Christian theological tradition is well illustrated in the writings of Bradshaw (1994), Shelly & Fish (1988) and Carson (1989) in the context of nursing. Bradshaw (1994) uses the Genesis account to develop the theological position on spirituality and illustrates that God created humanity (man and woman) in his image. Man and woman are unique and their nature is a unity, as opposed to Descartes dualism, which saw a separation of the physical body and spiritual soul.

Although the theological position emphasizes the holistic nature of humanity, there is a problem with this tradition with regard to spirituality in that it limits spirituality to being a specifically Christian phenomenon. Narayanasamy (1999) writes:

It may lead to the misconception that spirituality is equated with Christianity, hence restricting reference to the spiritual dimension and its practicalities to the context of Christian patients
(p. 277).

As an alternative to this, existentialism appears to be a promising perspective on spirituality.

Existentialism and spirituality

Contemporary existentialism (Macquarrie 1972) emphasizes that spirituality is a universal dimension; in other words, all of us possess it. Each one of us is capable of actualizing this unique potential—that is, the spiritual component.

In essence, the existential view is that humanity possesses the capacity and freedom to reach towards our potential into the roots of our beings. This potential (our spirituality) drives us to search for meaning and purpose in our lives, which may include the search for the truth, love, hope, goodness, beauty, understanding, reasons and so on. Some of the prominent existentialists who espoused spirituality are Kierkegaard (1962), Jean-Paul Sartre (1973), Heidegger (cited in Steiner 1978) and Jung (1961). As atheists, Sartre, Heidegger and Jung suggest that being atheists or agnostics:

the search for more humanistic beliefs is a way of coping with one's existence so as to make life meaningful. Therefore, in doing so, according to existentialists, turning to one's faith or otherwise ... spirituality is called into play
Narayanasamy 1999, p. 278.

However, although existentialism offers an explanation of spirituality that has a universal appeal it underplays the biological basis of spirituality. In the next section the biology of spirituality is explored.

The biological basis of spirituality

Drawing from extensive studies on spiritual experiences, Hardy (1979) and Hay (1994) postulate that spirituality is natural to human species and has evolved because it has biological survival value. Hardy (1979) related his notion of spiritual experience to those of Otto's (1950) account of the 'numinous'—that is, a direct awareness of a sacred or divine presence, and 'mystical states' (James 1902, Stace 1960). National surveys (Hardy 1979, Hay 1987) show a trend that about half of the British adult population would claim that they are spiritually aware from time to time. Hay (1990) illustrates the kind of experiences most British people intimately know, whether they are formally religious or not:

◆ being aware of an emergent unfolding pattern of life, not imposed by themselves, that links them in a meaningful way with the rest of reality
◆ being aware of the presence of God, typically in a way that helps them to relate creatively to the social context in which they find themselves
◆ feeling a unifying presence in nature

◆ feeling at one with or not different from the rest of reality.

According to Hay (1994) all of these experiences are forms of spirituality. In other words, being aware of oneself in an holistic relationship with the rest of reality, which in specifically religious experience in Western population usually implies an awareness of God.

The above understanding on spirituality has implications for nursing. Hay's qualitative research supports that individuals often experience an intensity of spiritual awareness when they are undergoing stress related to emotion, physical illness or other forms of crisis. Nurses need to be sensitive to patients' experience, otherwise patients may suppress this and remain spiritually distressed. Spiritual distress may delay the healing process.

From the above perspectives it would suffice to state that spirituality applies equally to the needs of believers and non-believers and in contexts where religious beliefs may be varied. It is not uncommon for individuals with no religious allegiance to be able to relate to some spiritual or natural force beyond the physical and self.

Spirituality is seen as an inner thing that is central to the person's being and one that makes a person unique and 'tick over' as an individual. For example, I see it as my being; my inner person. It is who I am—unique and alive. It is expressed through my body, my thinking, my feelings, my judgements and my creativity. My spirituality motivates me to choose meaningful relationships and pursuits. Sometimes we desire for personal quest for meaning and purpose in life; a sense of harmonious relationship (interconnectedness) with self and others nature, an ultimate other, and other factors that are necessary for our integrity. I would like to illustrate the points that I am making about spirituality in the case of Elsie below:

Elsie looks after her elderly mother who is suffering from senile dementia. She feels that it is her duty to care for her mother who is totally dependent on her. Elsie frequently says to the community psychiatric nurse (CPN) that it has not always been an easy task, but she learnt a lot in the last 10 years; through caring for her mother, she has become more

appreciative of the beauty and joy in life. Elsie sees each day as new opportunity to learn and grow. The CPN feels that in Elsie's presence one experiences a sense of peace and who, even in the midst of difficult and trying circumstance, affirms that life is good. Elsie says that she has done some soul-searching over the last 10 years and has come to know herself pretty well. She states to the CPN that when she felt low, she learned to 'go inside myself' and always finds guidance there and achieves a sense of relief and comfort. She also adds that she maintains close relationship with family and friends, with whom she shares love and support. Elsie is a keen gardener and when in her garden she feels close to the earth and to the Creator.
Adapted from Narayanasamy 1991, p. 4

Several of the elements of spirituality can be illustrated in the case of Elsie:

Unfolding mystery—through life's 'ups and downs' and what could be viewed as a burden, she has found meaning as peace and joy.

Inner strength—she has developed a great sense of self awareness, which she has gained by going inside herself (a process also known as introspection) for guidance.

Harmonious interconnectedness—she has loving, supporting relationships with family and friends, a sense of knowing herself.

Source of strength and hope—the garden has become a place where she is able to express a feeling of closeness to nature and to the Creator.

It appears that spirituality is essential to our well-being and is the essence of our existence. It has to do with both solitude and corporate life including the way we think, act and feel in everyday life. In essence, we can now see that it influences the whole of our lives.

Furthermore, through spirituality we give and receive love. One responds to appreciate God, other people, a sunset, a symphony, and spring. Many of us keep our spirits up in spite of adversity and it may well be because something motivates us to do so. This is because of our spirituality. Elsie's situation is a good example of spirituality as it keeps her going in spite of all the odds. We are driven forward, sometimes because of pain, sometimes in spite of pain. Spirituality permits a person to function, motivated and enabled to value, to worship, and to communicate with the holy, the transcendent.

Transcendence is a need as part of our personhood just as is the physiological or psychological. If we take this view, then we as nurses must regard all individuals as spiritual beings and not as a body with just physiological and psychological needs.

SPIRITUAL WELL-BEING

Let us now turn our attention to the concept of spiritual well-being. Spiritual well-being is an important facet of health and is considered as affirmation of our relationship with God/transcendent, self, community and environment that nurtures and keeps us as an integrated whole person. The following are features of our spiritual well-being:

◆ the belief in God that is fostered through communication with Supreme Being
◆ expression of love, concern, and forgiveness for others
◆ giving and accepting help
◆ accepting and valuing self
◆ expressing life satisfaction.

Furthermore, our spiritual well-being is usually demonstrated by our ability to find meaning and purpose in present life situations and to search for meaning and purpose in the future. We can attain spiritual well-being through a dynamic and integrative growth process which leads to a realization of the ultimate purpose and meaning in life.

MODEL FOR SPIRITUALITY

Several theorists propose that the whole person consists of body, mind and spirit, which are inseparable. Stallwood (1975) developed a conceptual model to illustrate this interrelationship

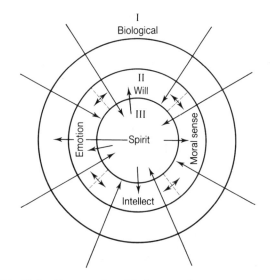

Fig. 12.1 Conceptual model of nature of person.

(Fig. 12.1). The outermost circle represents the biological nature of an individual; the middle circle depicts the mind as having four separate components—will, emotion, intellect and moral sense; the smallest, innermost circle represents the spiritual nature. Alteration to any of the three components affects the two other components, and ultimately, the whole person.

Unlike Stallwood, Gorham (1989) suggests a five-component person model. According to this model, a person is made up of five different aspects—the mental, physical, social, emotional, and spiritual. The interaction is so closely related that they are almost inseparable. The spiritual is the most difficult one to be recognized. The interaction of these five components is illustrated in Figure 12.2.

SPIRITUAL NEEDS

As previously seen in mental health care, a holistic view takes into account that we all have needs which are regarded as social, psychological, physical and spiritual. Many of us have no trouble in identifying needs that are described as social, psychological and physical, but we struggle to identify spiritual needs.

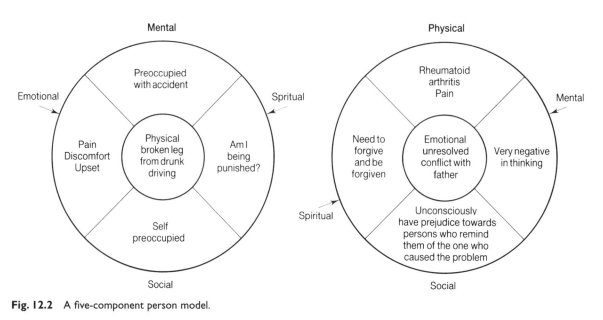

Fig. 12.2 A five-component person model.

CASE STUDY

Mary, aged 78 years and widowed, lives alone and has a history of depression following the death of her husband. She also suffers from chronic arthritis. Her daughter and two sons visit her regularly and they are her constant source of support. Mary's arthritis gives her a lot of pain and sometimes she wonders why she has to suffer and tries to find meaning in her chronic disability. However, she finds meaning and hope through her prayers as she is a devoted Christian. Mary's daughter takes her to Church whenever possible, where Mary finds the companionship of her fellow churchgoers a good source of strength and support.

Her youngest child, John, and his family have just returned to England after a long spell in Australia.

He left England for Australia 20 years ago following an argument with his father. Mary feels guilty about the unresolved conflict between her son and husband and feels that reconciliation should have taken place before her husband's death. She tries to seek forgiveness for both through her prayers. Mary is delighted to see her grandchildren from Australia whom she had missed all these years and now finds inspiration, new meaning and hope in her life as a result of this. Mary's renewed hope has given her inspiration to rework her goals and she finds a new purpose in her life. Her arthritis is no longer the dominant feature in her life and she is now able to resume painting and finds satisfaction in expressing creative talent through her artistic work.

We express our spiritual needs in a variety of ways and forms. Mary's spiritual needs may include the following:

◆ the need for meaning and purpose
◆ the need for love and harmonious relationships
◆ the need for forgiveness
◆ the need for a source of hope and strength
◆ the need for trust

◆ the need for expression of personal beliefs and values
◆ the need for spiritual practices, expression of concept of God or Deity and creativity.

Meaning and purpose

Many people tend to find themselves wrestling with the meaning and purpose in life during crisis, whether in health or illness. In the case study Mary tried to find meaning in her suffering. Meaning in this context can be defined as the reason given to a particular life experience by the individual. The search for meaning is a primary force in life. This drives us to search for meaning to life in general and discovering meaning in suffering in particular. We need to find sense out of our life and illness. Mary, in the case study above, found new meaning and purpose in her changed circumstances.

There is evidence to suggest that patients struggle with finding a source of meaning and purpose in their lives (Burnard 1990, Peterson & Nelson, 1987). Mentally ill clients often struggle with finding a source of meaning and purpose in their life. This struggle is illustrated in the following example:

CASE STUDY

George had been admitted to hospital twice in a state of despair and hopelessness. He shared his despair with staff at the hospital by saying, 'I have lost all hope'. Shortly after his last discharge he went home and killed himself.

It is suggested that people with a sense of meaning and purpose survive more readily in very difficult circumstances and these include illness and suffering. There is some truth in the expression that he who has a 'why' to life can bear with almost any 'how'.

Many of us approach the task of life in a variety of ways and so our ability to cope with a crisis varies. We can find meaning and purpose in the experience of suffering. There is a distinction between the religious and the apparently non-religious person in the way they approach spirituality, that is the religious person experiences his or her existence not merely as a task but as a mission, and is aware of a taskmaster, the source of this mission. That source is God.

In crisis such as bereavement the person experiences meaninglessness, that is, the person expresses a sense of bewilderment and loss of meaning.

For example, the person with a diagnosis of HIV infection, the survivor of a traumatic road accident, the death of a child in a family, the patient in a mental health unit, all cry out for help in search of meaning and desperately seek to talk to someone who will give attention and time in their exploration of meaning and purpose. The nurse is very often the nearest person to whom sufferers can reach out (Burnard 1990).

In a person searching for meaning and purpose there may be a need for exploration of spiritual issues. In some instances the person in search of spirituality may want to talk about religious feelings or lack of them. The person may not be asking for advice or opinions but only for an opportunity to talk about feelings, to express doubts and anguish. Such opportunity for expression can bring about clarity and a renewed sense of meaning and purpose.

People who have strong religious conviction and sense God, still need encouragement to adapt to unexpected changes. They are likely to experience hope even when their usual support systems let them down. Their experiences of God reassure them that God will never fail them. The nurse may have to act as a catalyst in providing the opportunity for finding meaning and purpose in crisis by establishing this relationship with God.

Love and harmonious relationships

Our need for love and harmonious relationships goes hand in hand with a need for meaning and purpose. The need for love is one of the fundamental human needs (Maslow 1968) which lasts throughout lifetime (from childhood to old age). A spiritually distressed person requires unconditional love, that is love that has no strings attached to it. The spiritually distressed person does not have to earn it by being good or attractive or wealthy. The person is simply loved for the way he or she is, regardless of faults or ignorance or bad habits or deeds.

Many mental health clients seek love and relationships but are unable to establish these with others because of their poorly developed social skills or deterioration of these during illness. For some, their illness, possible institutionalization, stigmatization, and even prolonged medication and its side-effects, are all damaging to their self-esteem. Many of them seek out a reason or means to value and respect themselves and thus exhibit a serious spiritual need. Mary in the illustration above met her spiritual need in this area from her family and fellow churchgoers. A further case illustrated below demonstrates this need in another client:

CASE STUDY

John, a mental health client, while attending a group dealing with feelings, shared that the last time he had been hugged by anyone was 3 years previously. When the group facilitator offered to hug him, he responded enthusiastically and even called on the facilitator the next day to describe his extreme pleasure in being hugged.

The manifestations of the need for love are self pity, depression, insecurity, isolation, and fear. These are indicators of a need for love from one-self, other people and God. The person receiving this kind of love experiences feelings of self worth, joy, security, belonging, hope and courage.

The spiritually distressed person also has a need to give love, which may include, for example, worries about financial status of family during hospitalization/separation from family and worries about separation from others during death.

Forgiveness

The need for forgiveness is commonly seen in mental health clients. Guilt and resentment are products of situations in which forgiveness does not happen. Clients often talk about having done something for which they cannot forgive themselves, or they talk about things that other people have done to them that they cannot forget or leave behind.

We saw in Mary's case the need for forgiveness and this is one of the principal causes of spiritual distress. A person who experiences spiritual distress expresses feelings of guilt and therefore

requires the opportunity for forgiveness. Mary sought forgiveness for her son and husband through her prayers. Guilt often emerges when a person experiences the realization that one has failed to live up to one's own expectation or the expectations of others. For example, we may first experience guilt as a child when our behaviour does not measure up to the standards set for us by our parents. We contradict them and do the very things we are told not to do. Guilt breeds in us in the form of regrets not only for the things we have done but for our failure in many things. Unresolved conflicts in relationships can result in feelings of guilt. Another case study below provides an example related to guilt feelings:

CASE STUDY

Leon, who was a war refugee, whilst in hospital as a client was in agony because he believed that he had caused his mother's death. In actuality his mother had been killed while trying to escape from her country. He was ridden with guilt that he was responsible for her death because as a young man he had abandoned the church and indulged in various vices. His guilt prevented him from functioning and caused him to relive horrible, painful experiences.

The feelings of guilt may be expressed as feelings of paranoia, hostility, worthlessness, defensiveness, withdrawal, psychosomatic complaints, rationalizations, criticism of self, others and God and scapegoating. Forgiveness may bring a feeling of joy, peace and elation, and a sense of renewed self worth. It seems that confession of sin is one way in which some people achieve forgiveness from God.

Hope and strength

Hope is seen by psychologists and sociologists as necessary for life and without it we begin to die (Simsen 1988). For many of us our sense of hope can be a powerful motivator in enabling an open attitude toward new ways of coping. Mary, in the first case study, achieves new hope and strength from reconciliation with her son and his family. The spiritually distressed person may experience a feeling of hopelessness. The hopeless person may see no way out; there may be no other possibilities other than those dreaded.

Earlier we saw in Mary's situation her new goals and a renewed purpose as result of her son's arrival from Australia. We strive for good relationships with others and this is another facet of our hope. This includes relationships with oneself and the world, where a person believes that what is desired is possible. According to Soeken & Carson (1987): 'Ultimate hope resides in God and belief that the Supreme Being will impart meaning to individual lives and sufferings'. Hope is also necessary for future plans. Further needs of our hope include seeking support, love and the stability provided by important relationships in our life and to put into action future plans. Mary successfully achieved all of these through her loved ones and friends in the case study. If the patient believes in God, then hope in God is important. This hoping in God is the ultimate source of strength and supersedes all aspirations that are transitional.

Hope is closely related to our need for a source of strength. A source of hope provides the strength that we may need. A source of strength gives us the courage needed to face innumerable odds in crisis. The main source of hope and strength is found by individuals who pray because of their faith in God/transcendent. Haase's (1987) study found that the subjects concurred that belief in the power of prayer helped them cope with medical interventions and opportunities to express their faith helped them to resolve the situation they described. For some, communication with God and prayer is a source of strength. For most of us a message of hope provides new energy, strength, and courage to preserve or revise goals or plan and these were apparent in Mary's situation.

Trust

We feel secure when we can establish a trusting relationship with others. The spiritually distressed person needs an environment that conveys a trusting relationship. Such an environment is one which demonstrates that carers make themselves accessible to others, both physically and emotionally. Trusting is the ability to place confidence in the trustworthiness of others and this is essential for spiritual health and to total well-being. Learning to trust in an environment which is alien could be a daunting task and not an easy skill to accomplish.

Personal beliefs and values

The opportunity to express personal values and beliefs is a known spiritual need. In this sense spirituality refers to anything that a person considers to be of highest value in life. Mary shares her beliefs with her companions at the church and expresses these through her prayers. Her spiritual needs in these areas are met easily because she has the opportunity to do so through the support of her family. Personal values that may be highly regarded by an individual include, for example, beliefs of a formalized religious path, whereas for others it may be, for example, a set of very personal philosophical statements, or perhaps a physical activity.

Spiritual practices, concept of God/Deity, and creativity

The opportunity to express our needs related to spiritual practices, the concept of God or Deity and creativity may present as a feature of spirituality. The concept of God or Deity may be an important function in the personal life of a person. The need to carry out spiritual practices concerning God or Deity may be too daunting for the person if the opportunity is not available or the environment is alien or unreceptive to this need.

Our creative needs may feature in spirituality. Mary achieves spirituality as a creative need through her paintings. A religious minister in a Connecticut Hospice uses the arts as an avenue to the Spirit in which actors, writers, musicians and artists of a university are invited to exhibit their work and give performances (Wald 1989).

COMPETENCES FOR SPIRITUAL CARE

Although a sufficient knowledge about spiritual needs and problems is necessary, competences of self-awareness, communication (such as listening), trust building, giving hope, and enabling spiritual growth need to be developed to equip the nurse to assist in meeting clients' spiritual needs.

Self-awareness

Before we instigate effective spiritual care, we must know and understand our level of spiritual awareness. An examination of our personal beliefs and values is a necessary part of spiritual care. The nurse who has a positive attitude to spiritual health is likely to be sensitive to any problem a patient has concerning spirituality. A continuous examination of one's own personal spiritual beliefs enables the nurse to appreciate that everybody does not share the same faith. An awareness of their own prejudices and bias would ensure that nurses do not impose their own values and beliefs on others, especially spiritual doctrines. Self-awareness would enable the nurse to adopt a non-judgmental approach and avoid taking any steps that would mount to the accusation that he or she is trying to proselytize. It is likely that a person who has developed self-awareness will show more tolerance, acceptance and respect for another person's spirituality.

The benefits of self-awareness are stressed here but it is a skill that has to be acquired and continuously developed. In this section self-awareness will be explained and a method for developing it will be outlined. Self-awareness is an acknowledgement of one's own feeling and behaviours, accepting and understanding or accepting to understand these. Self-awareness can be elaborated as an acknowledgement of our:

◆ values, attitudes, prejudices, beliefs, assumptions and feelings
◆ personal motives and needs and the extent to which these are being met
◆ degree of attention to others

◆ genuineness and investment of self, and how the above might have an effect on others
◆ the intentional and unconscious use of self.

It is widely acknowledged that a training in self-awareness is a fundamental process before one understands others. According to Burnard (1985), to become aware of, and to have deeper understanding of ourselves is to have a sharper and clearer picture of what is happening to others. Limited awareness of ourselves may mean remaining blind to others. The first step to being self-aware is to examine oneself as stressed earlier.

We can develop self-awareness by various means. However, the methods used for increasing our awareness must contain the facets of inner search and observations of others.

One simple method of enhancing our self-awareness is the process of noticing what we are doing—the process of self-monitoring. All that is involved here is staying conscious of what you are doing and what is happening to you. To put it another way, you 'stay awake' and develop the skill of keeping your attention focused on your actions, both verbal and non-verbal.

Assessment of our present understanding of knowledge, skills and the learning of new materials and techniques will be heavily influenced by our degree of self-awareness. We are most likely to lose control of our self-development if we remain blind to the need to increase our self-awareness. An increase in our self-awareness is not only the beginning of wisdom then, but also the growth of our personal and professional effectiveness.

Self-awareness can also be developed through introspection, through experience and through feedback.

Introspection

Meditation and yoga can be a useful way of developing self-awareness using the introspection method. Simple breathing and meditation techniques are sufficient for this purpose. Meditation and yoga serve another useful purpose in that these techniques can be useful methods of dealing with job-related stress. Becoming aware of, and consciously noting, experiences are other means of introspection. Complementing these processes the following are useful: identifying past and present prejudices; identifying past and present approaches to personal problem solving.

Experience

Self-awareness is also developed through experience. The experiential method is one useful method of learning through experience. Participation in experiential exercises brings the desirable increase in self-awareness.

Self-awareness through feedback

Self-awareness cannot be developed by adhering solely to the introspection and experiential methods alone. Introspection and experiential exercises will give us some understanding of ourselves, but a complete self-awareness requires knowledge about behaviour too; for this we require the help of others: it takes two to know one fully.

I am aware of my inner feelings (inner processes) but sometimes I cannot see my behaviour. Another person can see my behaviour, but is not aware of my inner feelings and experience. I can see the other person's behaviour, but not his inner experience. For a complete self-awareness, then, we need to strengthen the knowledge gained by introspection with knowledge obtained by feedback from others about our behaviour.

Self-disclosure involves the process of revealing information about oneself: own ideas, values, feelings that are similar to the ones experienced by those one is trying to help. There is significant clinical evidence to suggest that a carer's self-disclosure increases the likelihood of a client's self-disclosure (Stuart & Sundeen 1983). Self-disclosure results in successful therapeutic outcome. However, our self-disclosure must be handled judiciously, and this is determined by the quality, quantity, and appropriateness of higher disclosures. We must handle our disclosure sensitively so that clients feel comfortable enough to produce their own self-disclosure. A limited self-disclosure from us may reduce a client's willingness to disclose about self and conversely, too many may decrease the time available for a client's disclosure or alienate him or her.

Communication skills

Good communication skills are essential for spiritual care. The key communication skill in spiritual care is active listening without being judgmental. The points about self-awareness mentioned earlier are necessary for developing non-judgmental attitudes.

Non-judgmental means unconditional acceptance of clients. However, to have faith, trust and respect for other people despite their behaviour is often a most difficult quality to achieve, but with increasing self-awareness this can be developed. A non-judgmental approach is acceptance of an individual without any kind of judgement, without criticism, and without reservation. This also requires not only unconditional acceptance of people but respect for them without necessarily knowing what their previous behaviour has been.

As pointed out earlier, when providing spiritual care we must reserve or detach from our own personal values, ideals or beliefs. Clients must feel that we are genuinely interested, want to know them, how they think and feel, and still do not judge them. Such a relationship engenders in clients the feeling that if someone else is interested, thinks they are of worth as unique people, and cares, then they too are likely to have a positive image of themselves.

Genuineness is a quality based on people's ability to be themselves. It means being honest and open in expression of one's feelings. Again, self-awareness is a means by which this quality can be developed. It demands honesty and courage to be allowed to be seen as a real person.

Active listening is important because its purpose is to enable the client to be at ease and to make use of the listening process in such a way that the listener can help the client deal with spiritual needs and experience further spiritual growth. The active listener acts as a talking mirror, encouraging and reflecting back to the client what the listener hears, sees or senses.

The rudiments of being a good listener

The carer needs to create the right kind of climate in which the individuals requiring spiritual care feel accepted and confident enough to be able to talk about their spiritual thoughts and feelings. Clients need to feel the carer is listening to what they are saying and what they are feeling and not only listening, but accepting and understanding them. All this ties up with responding to people in ways that are helpful. Good listening is really paying close attention to what someone is saying and this is essential, but it is not easy. We need to suspend our thoughts and give the other person our complete attention.

We can demonstrate understanding by reflecting the patient's thoughts back, showing that we are listening hard, that we are making a real effort to understand what the client is thinking and feeling.

Make the clients feel it is alright to go on talking, that their feelings are being accepted. State that you are genuinely interested in what the client is saying, and respond warmly.

Trust building

Trust is necessary because confidence in the nurse–patient relationship is vital in spiritual care and, indeed, to the well-being of the patient. Trust between carer and client develops over time as the client tests the environment, risks self-disclosure, and observes the nurse's adherence to commitment. The following approach enhances initial trust:

◆ listening attentively to client's feelings
◆ responding to client's feelings
◆ demonstrating consistency, especially keeping appointments and promises
◆ viewing situation from the client's perspective.

An increasing level of self-awareness of personal feelings, along the lines suggested earlier, on the part of the nurse also enhances trust. It enables the client to disclose uncomfortable, even forbidden, feelings in safety. The carer must continue to build on the trust gained earlier and this task can be achieved by being reliable. Reliability is one other factor that strengthens and sustains a trusting relationship. Reliability is measured in terms of the carer's commitment to the spiritual needs of the client and this means promises and adherence to care plans must be carried out promptly and followed through.

Giving hope

Hope is something that we cannot easily give to another, but every effort can be made to support and encourage the hoping abilities of a patient. Mental health carers are often in ideal positions to foster or hinder hope. A caring relationship can be offered that permits, rather than stifles, the efforts of the client to develop hope. The carer can support people who are testing their own beliefs or struggling with questions of fear and faith. Further encouragement can be given to clients to talk about their fears. Helping clients to relive their memory is another way of facilitating hoping. Memories of events when life's needs were met, when despair was overcome and when failure was defeated, can all be used to take on a fresh view and face the future with confidence as part of spiritual recovery.

Herth (1990) identifies hope-fostering strategies that could be used as part of spiritual care. She defines hope-fostering strategies as 'those sources that functioned to instil, support or restore hope by facilitating the hoping process in some way'. The following can be utilized as hope-fostering strategies.

Interpersonal connectedness

A meaningful and shared relationship with close ones and others (including carers) is said to be a feature of interpersonal connectedness. For example, a harmonious and supportive relationship within the family offers the client hope and strength which are fundamental parts of a person's spirituality. The willingness of a carer to share in patients' hopes is a feature of this strategy.

Light-heartedness

The features of this are feelings of delight, joy or playfulness that are communicated verbally or non-verbally. The carer can foster light-hearted-ness among clients. The spirit of light-heartedness can provide a communication link between persons and a way of coping with deteriorations in body function and confused emotions; it can provide a sense of release from the present moment.

Personal attributes

The carer can enable clients to maximize their attributes of determination, courage and serenity. A search for a sense of inner peace, harmony and calm is one way of enabling the client to achieve serenity.

Attainable aims

A characteristic of these is the direction of efforts towards some purpose. The presence of aims often fosters hope. The carer who helps clients to search for meaning and purpose in life actually fosters hope. Helping clients to redefine their aims and channelling their thoughts on to other events or significant others are useful strategies of hope fostering.

Spiritual base

The presence of active spiritual beliefs (in God or a 'higher being') and spiritual practices is a source of hope. This may enable clients to participate in specific practices and these may include praying, corporate worship, listening to spiritual music and spiritual programmes on the radio or television, religious activities, maintaining specific religious customs, and visiting members and leaders of their spiritual community.

Uplifting memories

Recalling uplifting memories/times is another hope-fostering strategy. The carer can help clients to share happy stories from the past and to reminisce through old picture albums. Reliving positive activities from the past, such as an enjoyable holiday, significant events (birth of child, receipt of a medal) and 'sunset over mountains', can serve to renew the hoping process. It is most likely that memories of past events can serve to enrich the present moment.

Affirmation of worth

Having one's individuality accepted, honoured and acknowledged can foster hope. Carers, family and friends can be party to a client's feeling of self worth as a dignified human being. This can be very uplifting and act as a source of hope.

Enabling spiritual growth

The client needs to grow spiritually to achieve a full status of health. A good health orientation includes body, mind, spirit and additional consideration of cultural background. This can be achieved when a carer creates a relationship in which carer–client education takes place. The client may be educated to develop the hoping strategy. Trusting is another skill that can be learned and the nurse can provide opportunities for the client to develop this aspect of a relationship.

Clients need a learning opportunity to gain insights into their own spiritual awareness. They need an orientation that would help them to search for meaning and purpose. The carer as a teacher can help clients to explore this search for meaning and purpose.

The other aspects of client education may include the identification of the nature of 'right' relationship with others. Morrison (1990) asserts that caring concentration on this particular area can lead to improvements in clients' physical health. Educating clients to face up to defective relationships with others is an important aspect of spiritual care. Examples of defective relationships include the denial of the death of a loved one, a lack of social concern and an inability to accept hostility. The inability to experience the 'right relationship' is a known cause of spiritual distress (Morrison 1989).

Learning is seen as a two-way process in which the client experiences spiritual growth and the carer achieves a greater spiritual awareness as well. Millison (1988) found in his study that carers experienced heightened spirituality as a result of their work with ill people and that all carers reported that they felt they received more in terms of spirituality than they were able to give. An increasing level of knowledge, insight and coping strategies relating to spirituality can be achieved through the process of sharing as part of learning to cope with spirituality.

PUTTING SPIRITUAL CARE COMPETENCES INTO ACTION (THROUGH THE NURSING PROCESS)

The systematic approach of the nursing process can be employed to assist in meeting the spiritual needs of clients. The following four stages are included in the nursing process: assessment, planning, implementation and evaluation.

Assessment

Information obtained on religious needs alone is not enough for spiritual care. Such information does not allow us to go deeper into feelings about meaning and purpose of life, love and relationship, trust, hope and strength, forgiveness, expressions of beliefs and values. Also, this approach may lead to the assumption that a person who does not belong to a formal religion has no spiritual needs. As indicated earlier the unreligious may have spiritual needs. The person who does not express obvious religious beliefs may still struggle with guilt, or lack meaning and purpose, or with need for love and relationships. On the other hand, a person who declares as belonging to a particular religion may not necessarily abide by the beliefs and practices of that religion. Assumptions or conclusions should not be drawn about spiritual needs on the basis of clients' religious status.

The carer must remain sensitive to verbal and non-verbal cues from clients when carrying out spiritual assessment. These cues might indicate a need to talk about spiritual problems.

Assessment of clients' physical functioning may also provide valuable information for understanding their spiritual component. Such obvious status about clients' ability to see, hear, and move are important factors that may later determine the relevance of certain interventions. Also, psychosocial assessment data may serve a useful purpose in determining clients' thought patterns, content of speech, affect (mood), cultural orientation, and social relationships. All of these may provide the basis for identifying a need, or planning appropriate care, in conjunction with spiritual intervention.

CASE STUDY

George is a 56-year-old client in an acute mental health unit. Prior to his admission he was expressing feelings of despair, hopelessness and eventually became withdrawn and uncommunicative. He has been in the ward for a few weeks and now he is beginning to communicate and expresses that he wants to go to the church. At the initial assessment interview the nurse was unable to carry out a spiritual assessment of George because of his withdrawal and uncommunicativeness. Now the nurse wants to complete George's spiritual assessment.

Narayanasamy (in press) offers a useful guide for spiritual assessment (Box 12.1). The guide includes four general areas that can be appraised to derive data about spiritual concerns:

Tubesing (1980) suggests a spiritual assessment procedure in which there are five questions to assess a person's spiritual outlook. Spiritual outlook embraces a person's goal, faith, value, commitments and ability to let go and to receive forgiveness from self and others. Tubesing's assessment questions for spiritual outlook are:

◆ What is the aim of life?
◆ What beliefs guide me?
◆ What is important to me?
◆ What do I choose to spend myself on?
◆ What am I willing to let go?

The presence of religious literature, for example, the Bible or Koran gives an indication of clients' concerns about spiritual matters. Objects like religious medals, pins, or articles of clothing are sym-

| Box 12.1 | Spiritual assessment guidelines |

Meaning and purpose
What gives you a sense of meaning and purpose?
Is there anything especially meaningful to you now?
Does the patient/client make any sense of illness/suffering?
Does the patient/client show any sense of meaning and purpose?

Sources of strength and hope
Who is the most important person to you?
To whom would you turn to when you need help?
Is there anyone we can contact?
In what ways do they help?
What is your source of strength and hope?
What helps you the most when you feel afraid or need special help?

Love and relatedness
How does patient relate to: family and relatives, friends, others, surroundings?
Does patient/client appear peaceful?
What gives patient/client peace?

Self-esteem
Describe the state of client/patient's self-esteem
How does patient/client feel about self?

Fear and anxiety
Is patient/client fearful/anxious about anything?
Is there anything that alleviates fear/anxiety?

Anger
Is patient/client angry about anything?
How does patient/client cope with anger?
How does patient/client control this?

Relation between spiritual beliefs and health
What has bothered you most about being sick (or in what is happening to you?)
What do you think is going to happen to you?

If patient/client declares religious beliefs/faith the following assessment questions could added:

Concept of God or Deity
Is prayer (or meditation) important to you?
How would you describe your God or what you worship?

Spiritual practices
Do you feel your faith (or religion) is helpful to you?
If yes, tell me more about it?
Are there any religious practices that are important to you?
Has being ill made any difference to your practice of praying (or meditation) or to your religious practices?
Are there any religious books or symbols that are important to you?
Is there anything that we could do to help with your religious practices?

bolic of clients' spiritual expressions. Clients may keep a religious statue or Deity to carry out religious rituals.

CASE STUDY

Patrick, a 60-year-old client, has been readmitted to a Mental Health Unit following disordered thinking and a disruptive life style. Initially he was suspicious and hostile to his carers, but now they have gained his trust as his mental state has improved considerably. A nurse is carrying out Patrick's spiritual assessment in order to plan his spiritual care.

The observation schedules in Box 12.2 could be used to carry out spiritual assessment by observations.

Observations of the ways in which clients relate with 'significant others' (people close to them, friends, and others who matter to them) may provide clues to the spiritual needs. The quality of interpersonal relationships can be ascertained. Does the client welcome visitors? Does their presence relax the client or cause distress? Do visitors come from the church or religious community? Observations of these factors can lead to conclusions about the client's social support system. The social system enables clients to give and receive love and lack of such support may deprive clients

Box 12.2 Observation schedules for spiritual assessment

Non-verbal behaviour
1. Observe affect. Does the client's affect or attitude convey loneliness, depression, anger, agitation or anxiety?
2. Observe behaviour. Does the client pray during the day? Does the client rely on religious reading material or other literature for solace?

Verbal behaviour
1. Does the client seem to complain out of proportion to his or her illness?
2. Does the client complain of sleeping difficulties?
3. Does the client ask for unusually high doses of sedation?
4. Does the client refer to God in any way?
5. Does the client talk about prayer, faith, hope, or anything of a religious nature?
6. Does the client talk about church functions that are part of his or her life?
7. Does the client express concern over the meaning and direction of life? Does the client express concern over the impact of the illness on the meaning of life?

Interpersonal relationships
1. Does the client have visitors or does he or she spend visiting hours alone?
2. Are the visitors supportive or do they seem to leave the client feeling upset?
3. Does the client have visitors from his or her church?
4. Does the client interact with staff and other clients?

Environment
1. Does the client have a Bible or other religious reading material?
2. Does the client wear religious medals or pins?
3. Does the client use religious articles such as statues in observing religious practices?
4. Has the client received religious get-well cards?
5. Does the client use personal pictures, artwork, or music to keep his or her spirits up?

of this need and leave them distressed. The client who has faith in God or a Deity may feel estranged if cut off from this support network.

Observations of a client's environment and significant objects/symbols related to his religious practice may give evidence of his spirituality.

The other area of spiritual assessment includes attention to the three factors: sense of meaning and purpose, means of forgiveness and source of love and relationship. Observations and routine conversations with clients can lead to valuable information about each of those factors. Questions can be framed to include the following:

◆ What is your source of meaning and purpose in life?
◆ Why do you go on living?

Observations may include how clients deal with other clients, if they ruminate over past behaviours or how they have been treated by other people. How do clients respond to criticism? If clients respond with anger, hostility and blame others, these behaviours may suggest that they are unable to forgive themselves and that consequently are unable to tolerate anything that resembles criticism.

The spiritual assessment must also look at the client's ability to feel loved, valued and respected by other people.

Planning

The planning of spiritual care requires careful attention. The data obtained from assessment must be interpreted in terms of spiritual needs and a care plan should be based on this information.

CASE STUDY

Dorothy is a 40-year-old anxious client and is undergoing anxiety management therapy. She is a practising Christian (Catholic) and her spiritual care is included in the nursing care plan.

The planning of spiritual care should include respect for the patient's individuality, willingness of the carer to get involved in the spirituality of the client, use of therapeutic self, and the nurturing of the inner person, the spirit.

Assistance to meet spiritual needs should be given according to the indications of the individual, which may be unique and specific. If, for example, clients are part of a church or religious group, and the effect on them appears positive, the nurse can strengthen this contact. A client who is accustomed to practices such as meditating, praying, or reading the Bible or other religious books, should be given time and privacy. A visit by the client's religious agent (pastor, rabbi, or others) can be arranged.

The carer can make it easier for clients to talk about spiritual beliefs and concerns, especially about how these relate to their illness. The carer may need to help clients in their struggle and search for meaning and purpose in life. On the other hand, if clients are trying to find a source of hope and strength, then it can be used in planning care.

The other aspects of the care plan may include comfort, support, warmth, self-awareness, empathy, non-judgmental listening and understanding. All these measures are the essence of a therapeutic relationship. An empathetic listener can do much to support a person who is spiritually distressed by being available when needed, especially those clients suffering from loneliness, and expressing doubts, fears and feelings of alienation. The presence of another empathetic person may have a healing effect.

A powerful source of spiritual care and comfort can be prayer, scripture and other religious reading. All of these may alleviate spiritual distress. Prayers as a source of help would help a patient develop a feeling of oneness with the universe or a better relationship with God, comfort the client, and help relieve spiritual distress. A particular prayer should be selected according to the client's own style of comfort and needs. Although carers may not belong to the same faith as the clients, they can still support the clients in carrying out their spiritual beliefs.

Meditation, both religious and secular, can play an important role in enabling clients to relax, clear the mind, achieve a feeling of oneness with a Deity or the universe, promote acceptance of painful memories or decisions, and gather energy and hope that may help them to face spiritual distress.

The use of music gives an inspirational and calming effect. A wide variety of religious, inspirational and secular music may spiritually uplift a client.

Implementation

Implementation of spiritual care is a highly skillful activity. It requires education and experience in spiritual care. In carrying out nursing actions related to spiritual needs, it is imperative that carers:

◆ Do not impose personal beliefs on client or families.
◆ Respond to client's expression of need of a correct understanding of their background.
◆ Do not allow a detached scene to be used as an occasion to proselytize.
◆ Be sensitive to client's signal for spiritual support.

It is important that if carers feel unable to respond to a particular situation of spiritual need, then they should enlist the services of an appropriate individual.

Nursing intervention should be based on an action which reflects caring for the individual. Caring signifies to clients that they are significant, and are worth someone taking the trouble to be concerned about. Caring requires actions of support and assistance in growing. It means non-judgmental approach and showing sensitivity to clients' cultural values, physical preference and social needs. It demands an attitude of helping, sharing, nurturing and loving. These actions fulfil the requirement of individualized spiritual care.

An understanding of the client's unique beliefs and values or religious views is paramount in spiritual care. The carer must respect and understand the need for the client's beliefs and practices even if these are not in accord with the carer's faith. To allow a better understanding of the client's spiritual needs, the carer must establish a rapport and trust which facilitates the client to share those beliefs. The carer's own self-awareness of personal limitation in understanding these beliefs is paramount and he or she must seek outside help if necessary.

Nursing intervention should be based on a carer–client relationship that encourages the person to express views, fears, anxieties and new understanding through creative acts, writing, poetry, music or art. Time for quiet reflection and opportunities for religious practices would enable the client to develop a deeper understanding of life and a particular belief system.

The person who has no strong philosophical or religious belief may seek the opportunity to explore feelings, values and an understanding of life with another individual who is willing to give attention and time to discuss those areas of concern and share common human experiences. The carer is the person who is most immediately available and receptive to the client's thoughts and feelings. Certain clients may require close friends, family or a religious person to share those thoughts and feelings. The carer must remain sensitive to these needs and make the necessary arrangements. However, it must be remembered that spiritual growth is a lifelong process and the carer who initiates spiritual care would have been a catalyst in the client's goal to achieve eventual spiritual integrity and well-being.

Evaluation

Evaluation is an activity that involves the process of making a judgement about outcomes of nursing intervention. There are many indicators of spiritual outcomes, one of which is spiritual integrity. The person who has attained spiritual integrity demonstrates this experience through a reality-based tranquillity or peace, or through the development of meaningful, purposeful behaviour, displaying a restored sense of integrity. O'Brien (1982) comments that the measure of spiritual care should establish the degree to which 'spiritual pain' was relieved. Another view offered by Kim, McFarland & MacLane (1984) suggests spiritual care may be measured as the disruption in the 'life principle' is restored. The contents of clients' thoughts and feelings may also reflect spiritual growth through a greater understanding of life or an acceptance and creativity within a particular context.

SUMMARY

Clearly, there is no one single authoritative definition of spirituality although some authors have attempted to define it in broader terms. Spirituality refers to a broader dimension which is sometimes beyond the realm of subjective explanation. It is an inspirational expression as a reaction to a religious force or an abstract philosophy as defined by the individual. It is a quality that is present in believers, and even in atheists and agnostics, provided there is the opportunity to feel and express this inspirational experience according to the individual's understanding and meaning attached to this phenomenon.

Spiritual needs include the need for meaning and purpose, the need for love and harmonious relationship, the need for forgiveness, the need for a source of hope and strength, the need for trust, the need for expression of personal beliefs and values, and the need for spiritual practice, expression of concept of God or Deity and creativity. These are by no means exclusive, but it is commonly recognized that it is within the province of mental health nursing to incorporate them into care plans as part of the spiritual care of clients.

Competences such as self-awareness, communication (listening), trust building, giving hope and enabling spiritual growth (client education) are important prerequisites for spiritual care. These competences, together with the previous introduction to the knowledge of spirituality, offer a basis

DISCUSSION QUESTIONS

1. Discuss the reasons why it is difficult to assess spiritual needs in mental ill health.
2. Do your own spiritual beliefs, or lack of them, affect your approach to clients' spirituality?
3. Discuss why some nurses feel that they need further education to increase their awareness of spirituality and spiritual care.
4. Do spirituality and religiosity mean the same? If not, why not?
5. Identify and discuss the significance of developing spiritual care research to the care of mental health clients.

for the formulation of care plans related to spiritual care.

Effective spiritual care can be given through the systematic steps of the nursing process. Appropriate assessment strategies and tools should be employed for the purpose of assessing clients' spiritual needs. Data obtained from assessment strategies can be used for planning spiritual care. Certain pertinents outlined in this chapter should be considered when implementing spiritual care.

FURTHER READING

Bradshaw A 1994 Lighting the lamp: the spiritual dimension of nursing care. Scutari Press, London
This book provides a comprehensive review of the spiritual dimension and in-depth discussion on the history and theology of spirituality. Some of the points raised in this book would be useful material for the debate on this subject.

Carson V B 1989 Spiritual dimensions of nursing practice W B Saunders, London.
The concept of spirituality is adequately treated in Chapter one of this book.

Narayanasamy A (in press) Spiritual care: a practical guide for nurses and health care practitioners. Quay, London
This revised edition should prove to be a useful introductory reader in this subject. This updated book offers resourceful chapters on spiritual care, skills development and application of the nursing process for delivering spiritual care.

Shelly J A, Fish S 1988 Spiritual care: the nurse's role. Inter-Varsity Press, Downers Grove, IL
Although written from a Christian perspective, readers will find useful sections that explore the concept of spirituality. Chapters one to three are particularly useful and assist the reader to 'grasp' the concept of spirituality. The book also includes a workbook section that contains individual exercises for developing spiritual awareness.

ACKNOWLEDGEMENT

My thanks are due to Quay for permission to adapt material from the revised edition of my book, Spiritual care: a practical guide for nurses (in press).

REFERENCES

Bradshaw A 1994 Lighting the lamp: the spiritual dimension of nursing care. Scutari Press, London

Burnard P 1985 Learning human skills. Heinemann Nursing, London

Burnard P 1990 Learning to care for the spirit. Nursing Standard 4(18):33–38

Carson V B 1989 Spiritual dimensions of nursing practice. W B Saunders, London

Gorham M 1989 Spirituality and problem solving with seniors. Perspectives 13(3):13–16

Haase J E 1987 Components of courage in chronologically ill adolescents: a phenomenological study. Advanced Nursing Science:64–68

Hardy A 1979 The spiritual nature of man. Clarendon, Oxford

Hay D 1987 Exploring inner space: scientist and religious experience. Mowbray, London

Hay D 1990 Religious experience today. Mowbray, London

Hay D 1994 On the biology of God: what is the current status of Hardy's hypothesis? International Journal for the Psychology of Religion 4(1):1–23

Herth K 1990 Fostering hope in terminally ill people. Journal of Advanced Nursing 15:1250–1257

James W 1902 The varieties of religious experience. Fontana, New York

Jung C 1961 Modern man in search of a soul. Routledge and Kegan Paul, London

Kierkegaard S 1962 Philosophical fragments. Princeton University Press, Princeton

Kim M J, McFarland S K, MacLane A M 1984 Pocket guide to nursing diagnosis. C V Mosby, St Louis

Macquarrie J 1972 Existentialism. Penguin, Harmondsworth

McSherry W, Draper P 1998 The debates emerging from the literature surrounding the concept of spirituality as applied to nursing. Journal of Advanced Nursing 27:638–691

Maslow A R 1968 Toward a psychology of being. Van Nostrand, New York

Millison M B 1988 Spirituality and caregiver, developing an underutilised facet of care. American Journal of Hospice Care March/April:37–44

Morrison R 1989 Spiritual health care and the nurse. Nursing Standard 4(13/14):23–29

Morrison R 1990 Spiritual health care and the nurse. Nursing Standard 5(5):34–35

Narayanasamy A 1991 Spiritual care: a practical guide for nurses. Quay/BKT, Lancaster

Narayanasamy A 1999 ASSET: a model for actioning spirituality and spiritual care education and training in nursing. Nurse Education Today 19:274–285

Narayanasamy A (in press) Spiritual care: a practical guide for nurses and health care practitioners. Quay, London

O'Brien M E 1982 Religious faith and adjustment to long-term haemodialysis. Journal of Religious Health 21:63

Otto R 1950 The idea of the holy. Oxford University Press, Oxford

Peterson E, Nelson K 1987 How to meet clients' spiritual needs. Journal of Psychosocial Nursing 25(5):34–88

Sartre J P 1973 Existentialism and humanism. Methuen, London

Shelley A L, Fish S 1988 Spiritual care: the nurse's role. Inter-Varsity Press, Downers Grove, IL

Simsen B 1988 Nursing the spirit. Nursing Times 14(37):31–35

Soeken K B, Carson Y J 1987 Responding to the spiritual needs of the chronologically ill? Nursing Clinics of North America 22(3):603–611

Stace W T 1960 Mysticism and philosophy. Lippincott, London

Stallwood J 1975 Spiritual dimensions of nursing practice. In: Beland I L, Passos J Y (eds) Clinical nursing. Macmillan, New York, pp 1088–1099

Steiner G 1978 Heidegger. Fontana, Glasgow

Stuart G W, Sundeen S J 1983 Principles and practice of psychiatric nursing. C V Mosby, St Louis

Tubesing D A 1980 Stress: spiritual outlook and health. Specialised Pastoral Care Journal 3:17

Wald F S 1989 The widening scope of spiritual care. American Journal of Hospice Care July/August:40–43

Part III
Challenges for service delivery

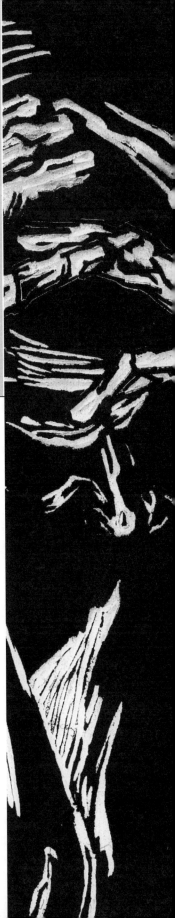

Some of the issues now considered in Part III were also of interest and significance when the previous edition of this book was published in 1994 and the new or updated chapters show something of developments since then. The chapters that deal with antiracist practice, suicide, drug abuse and work with older people reflect issues also of concern in the 1994 edition. Other chapters consider newer ideas or enduring issues that are of immediate concern for one reason or another. The chapters on social inclusion and the experience of women and mental health provision illustrate the usefulness of socioeconomic analysis and the importance of developing antidiscriminatory interventions and practice. Triumvirate nursing is a response to the challenges of working with people exhibiting personality disorder and Chapter 22 describes it in detail. Defining, predicting, understanding and managing aggression is the subject of another chapter that will be of relevance to a variety of settings within and beyond health and social care. A way of looking at the effectiveness of provision is ventured in a chapter that examines quality assurance in counselling and psychotherapy.

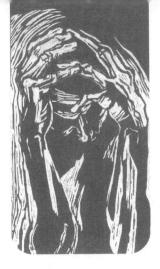

Chapter Thirteen

Developments in mental health services

Tony Thompson   Peter Mathias

 AIMS

- ◆ To identify trends in the provision of services and the implications for practitioners
- ◆ To highlight new ways of working in mental health services
- ◆ To enable the reader to appreciate the contemporary concerns which are affecting mental health policy
- ◆ To enable the practitioner to contribute towards safe, sound and supportive services for patients and users of services and to assist them in translating the principles of policy into practice at a local level

KEY ISSUES

Influences on the provision of care

Recent white papers

Creating contemporary services

Areas of weakness

Clinical governance

Service frameworks

INTRODUCTION

In the previous edition (Thompson & Mathias 1994) we drew attention to the increasing pressure on professionals and agencies to work together with a common aim of ensuring better services for those who have some form of mental disorder. Recent policy changes such as those contained in white papers from the government (e.g. The new NHS—modern, dependable (DOH 1997) and Modernising mental health services (DOH 1998), and their Scottish and Welsh equivalents) propose that a statutory duty should be placed on those commissioning and providing health and local authority services to work in partnership.

These and similar policy initiatives firmly point to a new demand that agencies and services will have to consider the need for partnership within a political and legal perspective. Since the previous edition of this textbook, the theoretical basis of interagency working has gathered momentum. However, the effective delivery of mental health services demands the operationalizing of laudable theories. In the latter part of 1998 the central administration was quite clear and explicit in its message to those who manage the services that the public and those people who utilize mental health services had lost a great degree of confidence in the ability of the main contributing agencies actually to deliver effective care, based upon the concept of community provision. It is likely that, as the pressure increases for these agencies to provide this 'joined-up' care that new and varied competencies will have to emerge from the workforce if it is to be successful in its endeavours. The essence of the new initiatives and policy formulation is that a far greater emphasis will be placed upon the delivery of services that are both responsive and match the quality that users and carers wish to see as a means of reassuring the general public.

Certain paradoxes will emerge and the contemporary practitioners will have to learn how to handle these conflicting demands. Not least of these will be the need for practitioners to play their part in delivering services that are based upon sound clinical evidence and yet are cost effective, and at the same time ensure that they cope with the emerging bureaucratic and communication processes associated with the attempt to provide a seamless service.

As we indicated in the second edition of this book, a great emphasis must be placed upon the collaboration and partnerships between the statutory organizations and the users of the services themselves. For any collaborative efforts to be generally successful, service user involvement has to be recognized at all parts of the continuum of care. Which is why it is the case that policy documents and advisory bodies are promoting partnership at every level from the strategic perspective of central administration and policy to the operational level of sound, safe and effective clinical team working.

The NHS and local authority social services have for many years been the primary form of statutory protection and support for people with a mental health problem. These historical factors are important as there is continuing significance to the lives of people with mental health problems with regard to the role of the government of the day. Certainly, for the last 20 years, successive administrations have been forced to address public perceptions and sensitivities with regard to the provision of services. The central role is an exacting and difficult one and includes the sophisticated formulation of strategy for operationalizing service delivery. These strategies have to be balanced within a framework of legislation and the constraints of overall public service resources.

As we noted in the introductory chapter, at the time of writing, a root and branch review of the 1983 Mental Health Act is being undertaken. It is going to be an extremely difficult task to try to form a reasonable match between the rights of service users to effective treatment with that of ensuring that those with more challenging conditions actually comply with the requirements of such treatment.

CREATING CONTEMPORARY MENTAL HEALTH SERVICES

In its attempt to modernize mental health services, the central administration set out the government's vision for safe, sound and supportive mental health services for working age adults. It reflected the need to introduce new strategy and this need was identified by the Secretary of State for Health, who stated that 'people who are mentally ill, their carers and the professional staff responsible for their welfare have suffered from ineffective practices, an outdated legal framework and lack of resources. We want to deal with all of these aspects to bring about a dramatic change for the better in the treatment and care of all those who are mentally ill.' Given that the role of government includes the setting of legislative frameworks, together with the allocating and prioritizing of resources and the identification of strategies and visions for changed delivery, it is not surprising that he placed great store on addressing criticisms of previous governments and the way in which mental health services work.

It would be easy to accept that the contemporary mental health services do not fulfil the expectations of everyone. It would be equally easy to accept passively that there are inequalities in the services, particularly with regard to access to proper services matched to need. In the past four decades there has been increasing evidence of unacceptable variations in performance, and outmoded practices within the services continue to raise their head occasionally, particularly through the vehicle of adverse enquiries and reports.

The latest mental health strategy draws attention to the fact that the legislative framework, which was designed when most mental health care was provided in institutions, no longer supports the delivery of care. Some commentators, and it is likely that the effect of their commentary will rebound on to a professional preparation of staff, particularly nurses and social workers, have proffered the view that community care as a concept has failed. It is still the case and it is likely to be so for a number of years that central administration is investing huge amounts of money into supporting areas of community care. It is therefore likely that the aims of producing a contemporary service will be more tuned to providing an operational framework based on a strategy for a comprehensive system of community care. If this is the case, it should come somewhere near to ensuring that the gap that occurred between the hospital closure

programme of the 1970s and 1980s and the need to have in place sound community-based facilities and resources be narrowed.

Contemporary mental health services will require a major shift in public and professional attitude, particularly in relation to the way in which staff are prepared to work together within a professional framework which might involve more risk, be exposed to a greater degree of public scrutiny and be based upon a more accountable relationship with the client population.

AREAS OF WEAKNESS

The strategic paper quite rightly points to areas of weakness that will have to be addressed both in terms of policy and within areas of professional preparation and training. These focus around the following:

◆ an outmoded and outdated legal framework that fails to support effective treatment outside hospital
◆ problems concerning the attrition rates and retention of staff working within mental health services
◆ the overwhelming burden placed upon families who have attempted to play a part in the mental health care provision of ill people
◆ problems of former patients and service users who do not comply with treatment programmes or remain in contact with the service
◆ the fact that the appropriate range of services has not always been available to provide the care and support that people need, particularly those with enduring mental health problems
◆ weak resource management and underfunding of services, which result in inadequacy of care provision.

In order to place the contemporary provision of service on a sound strategic footing, professions will require preparation. This will be aimed at ensuring the provision of services which:

◆ aim to protect the public, particularly in relation to the provision of secure hospital services; the delivery of efficient and cost effective ways of providing services based upon guidance from the body responsible for collecting and promoting information about clinical and cost effectiveness (the National Institute for Clinical Effectiveness)

◆ involve carers and service users, together with patients themselves in their specific care pathway and within the planning of services overall

◆ create systems of information that support the delivery of care and the accurate management of resources

◆ forge sound operational partnerships with education, employment, health, social care and housing

◆ integrate mental health services within primary care in order that primary care groups will work closely with specialist teams with the aim of the delivery of service within a sound planning framework

◆ accurately assess individual needs, with the aim of delivering better treatment in care, either in a domiciliary or institutional setting, but also enable 24-hour access to services; this will be aimed at ensuring public safety and more effective risk management

◆ create supportive services that work with patients and users and with their families and carers to build communities that are healthy in the widest possible context

◆ create services that promote access for patients and are comprehensive enough to facilitate the full range of provision needed when someone has a mental health problem

◆ match the provision of effective care for those with mental illness at the time that they need it, with the protection of the public and the recognition that services should be safe.

The aims listed above really do provide a tall order for practitioners within mental health services. The provision of such services represents a total of very complex interprofessional and interpersonal networks and the very nature of professions allows mixed motives to be superimposed upon the work demands. These include: seeking of

status, encouragement of professional rivalry, fear of failure and possible self-interests.

The government's white paper on the future on the NHS in England: 'The new NHS—modern, dependable' (DOH 1997) targeted deficiencies within service provision as a mechanism for identifying resources aiming for the better alignment of clinical and financial responsibilities for all practitioners within the clinical professions and line management.

CLINICAL GOVERNANCE

The above white paper on the health service requires that executive boards fashion strong partnerships and collaborate effectively with clinicians to form a more corporate accountability for the outcomes and quality of clinical care. It is somewhat unique for a government to steer an initiative such as clinical governance in such a direct manner. The initiative is quite upfront about the need for professional self-regulation, which is seen as being an essential component of delivery of quality services. The government say it is crucial that the professional standards developed nationally continue to be responsive to changing service needs and to match up to public expectations. The commitment is that the government will continue to work with the professions, the regulatory bodies and service user groups to strengthen the existing systems of self-regulation of the professions, but also to ensure that they are generally open, responsive and publicly accountable. So, the thrust of all these developments is that arrangements are to be made that allow practitioners to exercise authority and maintain control over their own practice, self-discipline, working conditions and professional affairs as they contribute to that part of the organization in which they work. The focus will be on delivering a service of a sufficiently high standard to satisfy public expectation.

Clinical governance within the health sector reflects most of the ideals described above and it really is the process of delivering quality through a model of participation and shared decision making. A new onus is placed upon chief executives and boards of trusts in relation to accountability for clinical care and the vicarious liability for the decisions made by clinical practitioners. Future practitioners and those who are intending to continue their professional development within mental health services need to be aware of the mechanisms available that form the national framework to support quality and effectiveness in the NHS. The initiatives in relation to governance fall into two main categories; those that have advisory roles such as the setting of standards, and those that have regulatory roles, which focus on ensuring performance and its monitoring in order that standards can be seen to be met.

The body responsible for collecting and promoting information about clinical and cost effectiveness will be the National Institute for Clinical Effectiveness. Its main purpose will be to:

◆ collect and appraise evidence to assess clinical and cost effectiveness of existing and new interventions
◆ examine existing services and treatments for variation and validity, alongside the identification and scrutiny of new interventions
◆ produce and disseminate clinical guidelines focused on recommended practice and the methods of auditing the treatment pathway.

NATIONAL SERVICE FRAMEWORKS

To complement the National Institute for Clinical Effectiveness, national service frameworks will be put in place. These will cover all areas of specialist treatment. They will be drawn up by expert reference groups from the best evidence of clinical and cost effectiveness and there will be user representation with regard to their perception of effectiveness. The frameworks will guide service purchasers and providers on how to ensure that specific services are provided. Each particular framework will include:

◆ information with regard to supporting programmes that will be required—for example lifelong learning, training, continuing professional development and workforce planning

◆ information to support the bench marking needed to ensure that interventions are correctly implemented
◆ identification of key interventions and practices, together with associated costs
◆ the evidence base for selected interventions.

Mental health and coronary care practices are the first areas to be subjected to a national service framework. The initiative extends to cover other areas of health through an annual programme. An expert reference group for the mental health framework is led by Professor Thornicroft of the Institute of Psychiatry. This will identify and agree the national measures of quality performance and good practice that mental health trusts would be expected to meet. The pursuance of quality services will be anchored in sound clinical practices at local level. Future practitioners will need to be competent in actively participating at all levels in relation to achieving the targets of quality clinical services. It is perhaps through lifelong learning and the preparation of the new practitioners that the main objectives will be met, associated with the need for fundamental cultural changes within mental health services and a stronger leadership by professionals to champion the total health and social care provision for this client group.

TOWARDS MENTAL HEALTH

One of the most rewarding features of professional caring within human services is being aware of skills and knowledge in a combination which helps fulfil the physical and emotional health needs of people. Although this role of fulfilment is not exclusive to nurses or social workers, these two groups particularly have to be competent in order to assist the person and their family to cope with, or prevent, life experience which impedes optimum physical and emotional health. Caring and health promotion go together when professionals strive to be effective against other factors that may hinder a person's ability to function in a well-adapted way. Professional efforts are directed towards helping people to maintain their mental capabilities, to achieve their potential and conserve their integrity.

The provision of mental-health orientated services has undergone substantial change during the past decade. The concepts of care to be undertaken by nurses and others have changed even more dramatically. Nurses working in mental health services, especially with people with a mental illness, have been expected to assume increased responsibility in the areas of (i) comprehensive assessment, (ii) development of skills and adaptive behaviour for achieving quality of life, and (iii) programme design to increase coping abilities and modify problematic or challenging behaviour. Further, they have developed sophisticated counselling services and have coordinated services in order to maximize the effectiveness of input from other agencies and disciplines. These, and other significant changes to the role and function of professionals in mental health services, have led to an expansion of the theoretical basis for practice and role expertise.

The nature of mental illness and the notion of positive mental health are always likely to be controversial. Perhaps one of the exciting aspects of training in this field is the opportunity to contribute to the controversy in an increasingly informed way. The student of mental health soon realizes that there is little consensus regarding the issues that surround present thinking and practice. One major feature of specializing in this field is its association with values tied to social and political constructs, which sometimes encourage a narrow role and function. The ideas contained in this text are those associated with liberating the professional outlook and creating a transdisciplinary view of care provision.

WHO SHAPES THE PROVISION OF CARE?

It is important to recognize that the issues and views about mental health and services are often underpinned by philosophical and political beliefs, not necessarily associated with medicine. It is this mix of ideas, proposition and theory that has shaped the present mental health services and the role and function of both the practitioner and client within these services. The concept of mental health and psychiatric illness and the way in which professional input should meet the challenge of providing an appropriate service, tend to be shaped by the prevailing or dominant views of those who influence the health care agenda.

The prevailing ideology in the UK is one of supporting community care and self-care and originates from a political view that seeks to include economic and social policy interests. Other cultures have a different view and these will be focused on briefly in other sections of this book. Historically, mental illness has confounded those with the task of providing service and preparing practitioners. One reason for this is the attempt to explain physiological illness and psychological illness using the same or similar theoretical perspectives. Whilst this is understandable as parallels can be drawn, the distance between the two remains. This may be helpful if the space between forms a testing ground for ideas which may target the person with a physical or mental health problem. The way in which problems of mental health or illness are viewed by the community as deviating from normal behaviour may make it particularly difficult for practitioners to develop a therapeutic role.

REFERENCE POINTS

Professionals who work within the field of mental health promotion and mental illness soon become aware of the fickle nature of what is considered to be a sign of mental illness. Those who have worked for over a decade within hospital settings can often reflect on the fact that behaviour associated with bizarre dress may be taken into account when confirming mental illness—yet years on may find themselves buying similar apparel for their offspring. In delusional states patients may, for example, suggest that they are affected by TV monitors or overhead electricity pylons or gases escaping from walls, symptoms sometimes taken to confirm pathological conditions and yet suddenly environmental awareness introduces us to sick building syndrome and research is initiated into the effect on people's health who are stressed by computer monitors or who live near high voltage cables!

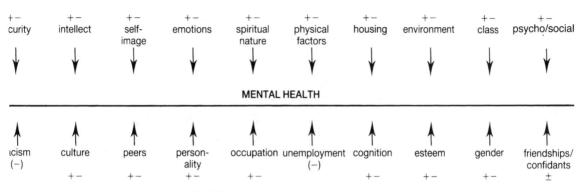

Fig. 13.1 Factors associated with mental health.

Perhaps one of the most important features of mental illness is that it is usually people close to the person exhibiting signs of irrationality who classify signs and behaviour as mental illness. They may use a change in the person's outlook, expression, thought content and rules associated with communication against a 'yard-stick' composed of 'mutual norms'. When the rationality of a behaviour or action is not understood in terms of social acceptance or boundaries, it is not unusual for lay society to deem the person mentally ill. Neither is it unusual for this view to be legitimized by a range of professionals.

A major difficulty for professionals is the fact that the so called 'norms' of expression, mood and behaviour are dependent upon the context and environment in which people function as rational human beings. On top of this is the way in which a person is able to articulate reasons for these phenomena. Society tends to ascribe the term mental illness when there is a breakdown in 'normal' or acceptable human actions. The concept of normality is rather like that of reasonableness: it is dependent to a great extent on the person who undertakes the defining. Generally speaking, our community functions with a shared reality that has constructed mutual value systems, morality, behaviour and beliefs. Figure 13.1 indicates some of the factors associated with mental health and illness. Whatever explanations are given regarding the way in which we perceive or come to understand problems of mental health, all are complex. Unfortunately, sociological explanations have themselves become abused by lay persons and professionals. Much distress can be caused to families when it is suggested that a person's mental state is simply a way in which society classifies or labels its deviant members. Whilst appearing to be acceptable to an extent in academic terms and having a value in explaining some of the experience of a person with problems of illness and ill health, the insensitive and inappropriate application of labelling theory may be of no consolation to those who see before them a loved family member disintegrating in personality and behaviour, and for whom treatment, protection and help are sought.

When considering some of these forces in the field of activity that affects the state of equilibrium in mental health, it becomes obvious that the concept is prone to ambiguity and contradiction. It is these contradictions that rest heavy on the shoulders of professional workers in mental health as psychiatry has in the past and in some cases still is seen as a form of social control. Accounts of its abuse are well recorded both in the Western world and in Eastern European and former communist bloc countries.

When judgements regarding such abstract phenomena as morality and intelligibility are made, those working in mental health have been shown to be faced with two options as to what changes mental health into a mental illness (Ingleby 1982). First, that those in psychiatry should eliminate value or moral judgements from their criteria and stick only to objective or clinical considerations when assessing or diagnosing—a tall, if not impossible, order as we all have similar forces acting on us. Secondly, we could simply regard psychiatric practice as a legitimate form of social control, like the legal or penal system. Of course, for this to be ethically and professionally acceptable the 'norms' inherent in social order would have to be fair, objective and just in their origin and maintenance. For this kind of social order to be free of all contradiction there would have to be universally constructed and accepted morality and the interests of all members of society would have to be in harmony!

When Symonds (1991) subjects these ideas to analysis he identifies that 'the reality and one of the major concerns of sociology is the nature of the conflicts and contradictions built into the social order'. It is believed, therefore, that the moral norms underpinning the social order are not objective, but 'value-loaded' and generated, transmitted and maintained in accordance with the dictates of particular interest groups. It follows, therefore, that whenever a moral judgement is made, questions must be asked regarding the nature of the person making the judgement, including their beliefs, interests and their objectives. Those working in contemporary mental health services are likely to spend time in their practice doing this not least of all in counselling sessions and team meetings. Simply put, it can be seen throughout our history that 'normality and conformity' have at times been equated with the concept of insanity. Such notions have been manipulated by the lay public particularly through the tabloid press and of course serve as a particularly powerful political slogan when used to describe deviation from policy, for example, 'the loony left'.

The major point here is that in many ways those working within mental health are vulnerable as the boundaries and imperatives of madness can so easily be associated with ideology. Therefore, history has shown us that the system has on occasions been a method of ensuring the maintenance of social order. Of course there are many other 'meanings' that account for a person's experience and behaviour and these are identified in other chapters. These cover more of the deviance theory and socially relative nature of our knowledge regarding mental health and well-being, medical

viewpoints which assume a scientific stance and the policy issues which impinge upon both care and prevention and whether this is aimed at individuals or society in general.

PROMOTION AND PREVENTION

Changes in the direction of professional practice within mental health, particularly those associated with community care, will continue to impact upon and challenge skills and knowledge associated with treatment towards those of prevention. However, we need to be aware that such notions as 'promotion and prevention' can become slogans and in-vogue words which are devalued by being euphemisms used in an attempt to reduce the stigmatizing effect of 'mental illness'. This can be seen when treatment units using legitimate ethical means to treat illnesses feel bound to include a reference to mental health in their 'logo'. The real aim in promotion and prevention is a health ethos, and the World Health Organization describes the objectives of this in explicit terms. Our mental health is in a constant flux state. It is ever changing, reflecting responses to the environment. It is intrinsically connected to our physical, emotional and social health (Ironbar & Hooper 1989).

Several contemporary approaches to the promotion of mental health and their applications have been described by Evans (1992) who draws attention to some of the possible causes of confusion within terms, including:

1. *Positive mental health*—referring to the adopting of strategies intended to enhance the existing mental health of people. The term uses the notion of maximizing human potential, emphasizing adaptive skills and draws on primary sources such as Maslow (1954) and his notion of self-actualization

2. *Mental health awareness and education*— referring to the dissemination of information aimed at dispelling myths regarding problems of mental health. Information technology and high quality, rapid desktop publishing is a good example of how the profile of issues regarding mental

health has been raised in the public arena. The range of options and resources available is included in this strategy and is particularly evident in television or radio public service announcements.

3. *Problem prevention and ill health*—the subtle difference between prevention, which is likely to be associated with biomedical approaches or interventive techniques, is contrasted with the more positive approach of promoting a 'holistic' view of health.

One of the hazards of professional work in these areas is that of confining our attention to narrow concerns of individual problems. This can in turn overemphasize people's own responsibility for their health and lead us to ignore the way in which the community or economic organization of society can adversely affect overall mental health.

A major aim of this book is to ensure that all professionals in mental health, or in therapeutic relationships with problems associated with mental illness, are aware of the wide social and political context. It is in this area of partnership that we can openly promote health and determine strategies of illness prevention. All participants in this process need to challenge both their own and others' assumptions regarding theory and practice. When this occurs we are more likely to achieve a healthy state of promoting the empowerment of those involved in the process of care, reducing the chances of controlling the communities' needs and instead adopt practices which lead to effective partnerships for the health of all as promoted by the World Health Organization for the year 2000.

SUMMARY

This chapter highlights the impetus for major changes to mental health services. It captures many of the guiding values followed by the recent external reference group who designed the national service framework and is shaped by the policy developments that have taken place in order to put those values into collaborative action. It therefore identifies the need to:

◆ promote accessibility so that people can obtain help when and where it is needed
◆ deliver high quality therapy and care that is effective and acceptable
◆ involve users of the service and those who share their care with them with regard to the planning and delivery of this care
◆ promote the safety of users of this service and the wider public
◆ offer choices that promote independence
◆ promote the coordination of services between the variety of agencies involved
◆ promote an accountable service that responds to public need.

The chapter also recognizes that the focus of mental health policy in recent years has been one that concentrates on the depopulation or deinstitutionalization programmes. It recognizes that quite often, as a result of some of these, people within the community who require the services of the specialist with mental health training and education are likely to have duel needs, be severely ill and have a greater degree of social care need.

The care programme approach is an important and essential element of the services. Many contributors to this edition stress the need for care plans that are comprehensive, multidisciplinary, dynamic and subject to regular reviews.

DISCUSSION QUESTIONS

1. What are the key features highlighted in the national service frameworks for mental health?
2. What are the major factors that have led to the central government initiative to publish the national service framework?
3. In what ways are future practitioners working within the health and social services independent sector and voluntary sectors likely to change their practices in order that they can facilitate greater integration of services for seriously mentally ill people?
4. What features have provoked the interest of policy makers with regard to interdisciplinary training in mental health?

FURTHER READING

Brooker C, Repper J (eds) 1998 Serious mental
   health problems in the community—policy,
   practice and research, Baillière Tindall, London
*This interesting and comprehensive textbook provides
an overview of current understanding about service
users who have serious mental health problems. The
authors draw together policy, research practice and
educational experts from a range of disciplines to
provide a very contemporary account of community
services, approaches, interventions and teaching
programmes for people who are disabled by serious
and on-going mental health problems. Sound
theoretical models and research findings are presented
as evidence alongside case studies and practical
examples.*

Clinical governance in the new NHS
*This significant Health Service circular of 1999 sets
out what the government programme of modernization
of the NHS is intended to achieve. It explains and
identifies quality as a driving force for the development
of health services and explains why the clinical
governance agenda is central to the quality agenda. It
sets out the principles and processes that will develop
clinical governance. It covers in a very detailed way
issues such as integrated planning; staff support and
development; workforce solutions; adopting good
practice; learning from experience; and addressing
aspects of poor performance.*

Modernising health and social services—developing
   the workforce
*This Health Service circular of 1999, which is also a
local authority circular issued in May 1999, provides
an overview of the government's key objectives and
outputs for the health and social services over the
coming years. The guidance aims to ensure that the
NHS and social services can reflect priority areas for
action in the development of strategies for education,
training and development in support of national
priorities and targets for action.*

A national service framework for mental health
*This extremely important document highlights the
modern standards and service models for mental
health. It offers comprehensive coverage of the need to
develop the national service framework for mental
health, a significant cause of ill health and disability in
England. It is centred around the mental health needs
of working aged adults up to the age of 65; it identifies
a new vision for mental health and offers explanation
of the government-wide agenda. A wide range of
evidence is synthesized in the framework and it is
graded according to the system used.*

Practice guidance—the nurses' contribution to
   assertive community treatments
*This is another important publication from the
standing Nursing and Midwifery Advisory Committee,
which is subtitled 'Mental health nursing addressing
acute concerns'. It describes assertive community
treatment as a multidisciplinary, clinically effective,
team-based approach that provides proactive, focused
and sustained care targeted at a defined group of
patients. It promotes the purposes of ensuring that
patients maintain contact with services, reducing the
extent of admissions and seeking to improve social
functioning and quality of life of service users.*

Practice guidance, safe and supportive observation
   of patients at risk
*This publication in July 1999 from the standing
Nursing and Midwifery Advisory Committee is based
around the need for professionals to recognize that
observation is an important skill, particularly in the
acute phases of mental illness. It aims to encourage
professionals to prevent potentially suicidal, violent or
vulnerable patients from harming themselves or others.
The document highlights how we assess risk and it
demonstrates signs that indicate the need for
observation. Four levels of observation are
demonstrated, which are intended to facilitate
communication, care planning and training.*

REFERENCES

DOH (Department of Health) 1997 The new NHS—modern, dependable. HMSO, London

DOH (Department of Health) 1998 Modernising mental health services, safe, sound and supportive. Department of Health, London

Evans J 1992 Healthy minds. Nursing Times 88(16):55–56

Ingleby D 1982 The social construction of mental illness. In: Wright P, Teacher A (eds) The problem of medical knowledge. Edinburgh University Press, Edinburgh

Ironbar N O, Hooper A 1989 Self-instruction in mental health nursing. Baillière Tindall, London

Maslow A H 1954 Motivation and personality. Harper & Row, New York

Symonds R F 1991 Sociological issues in the conceptualisation of mental illness. Journal of Advanced Nursing 16:1470–1477

Thompson T, Mathias P 1994 Lyttle's mental health and disorder, 2nd edn. Baillière Tindall, London

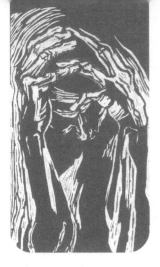

Chapter Fourteen

Social inclusion

Julie Repper

 AIMS

- ◆ To define social exclusion
- ◆ To demonstrate the extent to which people with mental health problems are socially excluded
- ◆ To discuss the impact of social inclusion on the lives of people who have mental health problems
- ◆ To consider ways of promoting social inclusion
- ◆ To raise awareness of the importance of social inclusion strategies for every mental health nurse

KEY ISSUES

Tackling social exclusion is one of the present government's priorities

On every given indicator people with mental health problems are socially excluded: they are frequently unemployed, living in poverty, in poor housing or homeless, socially isolated and in poor physical as well as mental health

Discriminatory attitudes and behaviour are probably the most serious problem facing most people with mental health problems

Social inclusion depends upon initiatives at a policy level, changes in laws, changes in public understanding and tolerance, as well as an approach to working with people with mental health problems that prioritizes access to communities

Mental health workers need to work with communities in order to support individuals, and collaborate with different disciplines, agencies and departments

INTRODUCTION

This chapter is not concerned with the development of community care over the last 50 years as this is well recorded and critiqued elsewhere (see Goodwin 1996, Rogers & Pilgrim 1996). A summary of the key policy papers published between 1952 and 1998 is provided in Box 14.1. This demonstrates a distinctive pattern: hospital closure and deinstitutionalisation began in the 1960s; the nature and timing of 'community care' were defined in the 1970s; the problems that emerged from its implementation were summarized in a number of reports in the 1980s; during the 1990s a plethora of policies and recommendations have been introduced to combat these problems. Quite apart from the specific recommendations of the recent initiatives, a number of themes run through the whole ethos of mental health policy in the past decade:

◆ prioritization of people with serious mental illness
◆ user participation in decision making at all levels
◆ evidence-based services/interventions that are routinely monitored
◆ collaborative working between disciplines and between the numerous different agencies involved in the support of people who have mental health problems
◆ increasing recognition of the impact of 'social exclusion': the effect of such factors as poor housing, poverty, lack of education and unemployment on mental health—and the impact of mental health on social status.

Whilst all of these issues have specific implications for services and the people who use them, it is the final theme, the emphasis on social exclusion, that has the greatest potential to improve the lives of people with mental health problems. Now that the majority of people with serious mental health problems exist outside institutions, the challenge for services is to facilitate their access to valued roles within society: to combat exclusionary attitudes and practices and engender acceptance and support. This not only provides a basis for change in the way that support is offered and mental

health problems are viewed; it is also very much in line with current health policy, drawing on all the themes listed above. Thus, strategies to reduce or prevent social exclusion will focus on those who are most socially disabled, whose mental health problems prevent them from living their lives as they would wish to. Social inclusion, by definition, can be achieved only by valuing the contribution that can be made by people who have serious mental health problems—giving them information, choices and decision-making power. Whilst any initiatives to reduce social exclusion must be evaluated, their effectiveness will be judged in terms of users' agendas, users' networks and changes within communities, rather than symptoms and compliance with medication. Finally, social inclusion depends upon collaboration with other agencies, disciplines, 'departments' (such as housing, education and environment), and other parts of the health service such as primary health care and acute medical services such as casualty departments.

This chapter traces the history of social exclusion, defines it in the context of a contemporary Western society, examines the evidence that people with mental health problems are excluded and proposes a number of ways in which social exclusion can be tackled at individual, service and societal levels.

A HISTORY OF EXCLUSION

People who are somehow 'different' are all to some extent excluded by societies, which, by definition, assume some form of cohesion and conformity. Yet that which is perceived as 'different', and the manner in which it is excluded, has varied considerably over time and space. Nowhere can this variation be seen more clearly than in relation to 'madness'. First, the interpretations of different symptoms of mental illness vary profoundly in different cultures; for example, in many parts of the world possession by spirits that speak or act through a person is a normative experience (Helman 1985, Romme & Escher 1993). Secondly, definitions of madness have changed dramatically over time; for example, no longer is

Box 14.1	Summary of Mental Health Policy Developments 1957–1998

1957	Report of the Royal Commission on the law relating to mental illness and deficiency
1959	Mental Health Act
1962	Hospital plan for England and Wales. Ministry of Health white paper
1975	Better Services for the Mentally Ill. DHSS white paper
1981	Care in Action. A handbook of policies and priorities for the health and personal social services in England
1983	Mental Health Act
	Care in the community. DHSS consultative document
	Common concern. Mind
1985	House of Commons Social Services Committee report on community care with special reference to adult mentally ill and mentally handicapped people
1986	Making a reality of community care. Audit Commission
1988	Community care: agenda for action. Sir Roy Griffiths
	The report of the committee inquiry into the care and aftercare of Sharon Campbell
1990	Caring for people. Community care in the next decade and beyond. White paper
	NHS and Community Care Act
	House of Commons Social Services Committee report on community care
	Community care in the next decade and beyond: policy guidance
	Care programme approach
	Mental illness specific grant
1992	Mental illness key area in Health of the nation. White paper
	DOH/Home Office review of services for mentally disordered offenders
1993	Mental illness key area handbook
	Review of legal powers on care of mentally ill people in the community
	Secretary of State's 10-point plan
1994	Guidance on establishing supervision registers
	Guidance on discharge of mentally disordered patients
	House of Commons Select Committee report on mental health services
	Ritchie report on the care of Christopher Clunis
	Working in partnership—review of mental health nursing
	Mental Health Foundation report
	Mental Health Task Force—London project
	Audit Commission—Finding a place
	Mental illness key area handbook—2nd edition
1995	Building bridges: a guide to arrangements for inter-agency working for the care and protection of severely mentally ill people
	An introduction to joint commissioning
1996	The spectrum of care: local services for people with mental health problems
	Review of purchasing of mental health services by health authorities in England
	The NHS: a service with ambitions
	Priorities and planning for the NHS: 1997–1998
	The homeless mentally ill initiative
	The National Mental Health Awards Scheme
	The Mental Health Challenge Fund
	Report of the confidential inquiry into homicides and suicides committed by mentally ill

Box 14.1	Summary of Mental Health Policy Developments 1957–1998 *(cont'd)*
	people. Royal College of Psychiatrists
	Clinical Standards Advisory Group report on schizophrenia
	Health of the nation outcome scales fully developed
1997	Housing and community care: establishing a strategic framework
	Education and training planning guidance
	Developing partnerships in mental health. Green paper
1998	Our healthier nation
	The new NHS: modern, dependable
	A first class service: quality in the NHS

homosexuality categorized as a mental illness (although it still leads to considerable social exclusion). Thirdly, the location and treatment of mental illness have changed over time, most notably with the movement of 'the mad' into large, remote and impregnable institutions, followed by the ongoing movement back into the 'community'.

Foucault's (1965) account of the treatment of 'unreason' gives some insight into the links between 'madness' and exclusion. Using the leper as an index of the regime of exclusion and confinement, Foucault points out that, throughout Europe, leprosaria proliferated in the Middle Ages, and when they were no longer needed for the treatment of leprosy they became the abode of the poor, vagabonds, the deranged, the diseased and the disorderly. Foucault argues that the isolation of the lepers was not prompted by medical concern, but as a ritual of purification and exorcism; their later inhabitation by the poorest and weakest of the area represented a widespread tactic of internment to deal with the problems of social disorder and destitution. At that time, Foucault observed that madness—or 'unreason' as he termed the disparate collection of problems that were endured by those interned—was a broad category including poverty, unemployment, transgression of sexual norms, violations of family order, insanity and sacrilege, but excluding crime and ill health. Foucault made two further points of particular relevance today. First, 'reason' or 'unreason' was taken to be an object of individual choice: it was understood that one willed to be either mad or sane. Secondly, he observed that the movement from the inhumane treatment in

the seventeenth and eighteenth centuries to the reforms of the nineteenth century might be attributed to a change in the 'perceptual framework' of the times. During the Classical Age, 'unreason' equated with non-human; therefore since only through reason did man become man, it was unnecessary to treat madmen humanely. From the end of the eighteenth century, however, madness began to be perceived as mishap rather than intention, therefore humans could be mad—and it followed that humane treatment was required. Thus Foucault explained the reformist movement in mental health care characterized by the enlightened regimes pioneered by Pinel in Paris and Tukes in York.

Although there were improvements within institutions, by the mid twentieth century conditions were poor. Overcrowding, neglect of longer term patients and the deleterious effects of total institutions were among a number of critical problems that culminated in a rejection of institutionalization for the mentally ill. The development of a number of new treatments—including medication, the success of innovative community and day-care services—and the promise of 'community care'—implying both cheaper and more libertarian regimes—led to the pursuit of a community-based system of care for people with mental illness. This move from confinement or internment is not, however, a sign of loosening perceptions of the threat that 'madness' presents to social order. For all the promise held in this utopian term, 'community care' has excluded people with mental illness just as effectively as the asylum walls did before. Lewis, Shadish a Lurigio (1989) write of the simultaneously inclusionary and exclusary nature of deinstitutionalization:

> By inclusionary, we mean a change from the mentally ill being forcibly excluded from society to their being forcibly injected back into society. ... That is they are now mostly included in [but not by] society rather than mostly excluded from it. ... [Yet] mental patients may be more of a mystery today, living among us, than they were when hidden away in the asylum. We do not know them, because they are neither outside society in a world of exclusion, nor are they full citizens—individuals who are like the rest of us.

The social boundaries of the past have become less marked in relation to certain groups. Sibley (1995) suggests that class differences have blurred, and differences between men and women and the marginalization of blacks within the UK are less pronounced, yet insidious exclusion of those perceived to threaten the social order continues:

> Clearly, the labels which signal rejection are challenged and there is always the hope that, through political action, the humanity of the rejected will be recognised and the images of defilement discarded. There is no clear picture of progress, however. Feelings of insecurity about territory, status and power, where material rewards are unevenly distributed and continually shifting over space encourage boundary erection and the rejection of threatening difference. Sibley 1995, p. 69

WHAT IS SOCIAL EXCLUSION?

The newly formed 'Social Exclusion Unit' in the Cabinet Office defines social exclusion as:

> what can happen when individuals or areas suffer from a combination of linked problems such as unemployment, poor skills, low incomes, poor housing, high crime environments, bad health and family breakdown.

Whilst this definition identifies some of the indicators of social exclusion, it throws little light on the process or outcome of exclusion. Sibley (1995, p. xi) draws on the example of a television documentary on a large shopping centre in northern England to illustrate the routine nature of exclusion as an unnoticed feature of urban life:

> Out of sight in the control room, employees of the private security firm, which polices the centre, had their eyes fixed on closed circuit television screens. They were looking for 'undesirables', mostly groups of teenage boys who did not fit the family image projected by the company. When they were located, security guards evicted them, not just from the building but from the precinct. ... There are implicit rules of inclusion and exclusion in a built form that contribute to the structuring of society and space in a way that some will find oppressive and others appealing. ... In a place dedicated to consumption by the family, there is a connection between the function and design of the space ... and the construction of one group of the population as 'deviant'.

Although this example is limited to the control of (non-consuming) adolescents in a shopping centre, it resonates of Bentham's panoptican: an architectural edifice for the segregation and observation of social undesirables in which the controller could remain invisible yet ultimately control every details of inmates' lives. Foucault (1965) developed this thesis, suggesting that the highly controlled institution 'represents a continuation and intensification of what goes on in ordinary places'. It is those who are 'different', 'imperfect', perceived to threaten the social order and fall outside the implicit rules of inclusion who are subjected to such treatment. Dahrendorf (1985) explains this in terms of the 'modern social conflict' in which the emphasis on growth and enterprise has generated a social category of people (the 'underclass') who find themselves in persistent poverty and are denied full citizenship through barriers to entitlements. Dahrendorf (1985) suggests that the real problem is that society does not need these people: 'many in the majority class wish that they would simply go away'. The relevance of this sentiment to people with mental health problems is starkly illustrated by an example of hostility described in a recent survey of public attitudes to community mental health facilities. Repper et al (1997) reported that a van parked outside a new residential facility was painted with the slogan 'Schizophrenics go home'—an ironic request, since that was precisely what those living in the house were trying to do. The same sentiment was perceived by a service user in Barham & Hayward's (1995) account of the lives of a group of people with serious mental health problems:

Virtually my whole life I've been under strain ... and when you can go forty odd years and nothing much happens to improve your lot, I mean you're virtually in the last third of your life and nothing has been done ... There might be a motive in ignoring people with illnesses. I hope the illness will go away but they hope the person will go away!

Evidently the exclusion experienced by the 'underclass' within society takes on a particular form with particular groups of people. If, as Foucault (1965) suggested, it is to do with purification, cleansing society of unwanted elements (a theme that Sibley (1995) develops in terms of the imagery of defilement and the marginalization of 'imperfect' people), mental illness is just one of a number of categories that are rejected. The exclusion of people with mental illness is, however, different from that of others because of both the particular vulnerability of the people concerned and lay understandings of madness.

People with mental health problems often have ongoing social disabilities. They need support in order to access 'entitlements', roles, facilities and opportunities within society. Exclusion from the old asylums must not, therefore, equate with exclusion from community support. Nor must inclusion within society be contingent upon 'perfection' or 'sameness'. If a person has to deny that they have mental health problems in order to be included in society, then they are excluded from positive identification as a person with special needs which must be addressed.

Since madness has been hidden away—not discussed, a 'taboo' subject—for so many years, lay understandings of mental illness are largely informed by the media, and this presents a negative and alarming picture. Philo, Henderson &

McLaughlin (1993) found that two-thirds of media coverage of mental health issues makes a direct link between mental illness and violence. The media frequently report a 'rising toll of killings' by people with mental health problems, which neglects to state that there has been no increase in homicides by mentally ill people over the past 20 years—a period over which homicides generally have more than doubled (Sayce 1998a).

Philo, Henderson & McLaughlin (1993) also reported that media coverage of mental disorder can override personal experience. Thus even if people have a relative with a mental health problem and have never witnessed any violence by people with mental health problems, they may still assume that people with mental health problems are violent because of the media imagery. 'Madness' is therefore rejected not only on the grounds of 'difference', lack of contribution to society, or 'imperfection', but also on the grounds of fear. People with mental health problems are perceived to pose a genuine threat—not just to the 'social order'—but to the safety of individuals. Yet people with mental health problems are only marginally more likely to be violent than any other member of society. The Confidential inquiry into homicides and suicides by mentally ill people in 1994 reported that 100 homicides had been committed in the previous 18 months by people who subsequently received psychiatric care (Royal College of Psychiatrists 1996); 34 of the perpetrators had been in contact with specialist services in the 12 months before the homicide, and 66 were to receive some form of treatment following the homicide, but they were not known to services before the attack. During the same period, 900–1000 homicides took place in England and Wales as whole, meaning that only 3% of homicides were committed by people known to mental health services. Furthermore, only two victims were randomly killed by strangers, all the rest were family, and in over half of the incidents the patients had refused treatment. None of the homicides was committed by a patient who had been discharged from a long stay ward. Indeed, in a separate study of violent offences among 278 people discharged from psychiatric hospital, Dayson (1993) reported only two people (0.7%) were involved in violent offences—and one of these was directly related to the research process. The risk of violence perpetrated by people with mental health problems is clearly very low, but magnified out of all proportion by the media. And it is the small number of dramatic and shocking incidents that has been reported to saturation point that has led to widespread fear of mental illness, intolerance of community care—and the recent proliferation of increasingly coercive policy responses.

THE SOCIAL EXCLUSION OF PEOPLE WITH MENTAL HEALTH PROBLEMS

Personal experiences of exclusion

Anybody who has experience of mental health problems themselves, or has worked with people who have mental health problems, need only consider basic aspects of day to day life to understand the extent to which the label, and the consequences, of mental illness lead to exclusion. A feeling of difference, of being ostracized and excluded is frequently expressed by people who have mental health problems. Although such perceptions have conventionally been interpreted as symptomatic of mental illness, they are likely to be rooted in external reality. There are numerous barriers to acceptance and inclusion when 'starting all over again' after a breakdown: rebuilding friendships when others no longer trust you, plucking up the courage to return to work or coming to terms with unemployment, struggling with feelings of depression, loss of a previous lifestyle and anxiety that the symptoms might return, negotiating the complex benefits system, maintaining any quality of life on benefits, being dependent on the support of others, and so on. Barham & Hayward (1995) provide a lucid account of these very issues from the perspectives of a small group of people who have spent time in psychiatric hospital. They describe how one 39-year-old man was moved into a flat some distance away from the town where his friends lived following his last admission; all the windows in the flat were broken, there was no furniture apart from a sideboard and a

mattress (with no bedding), and no cooking facilities. He lost all contact with services when his social worker took up a new post, his gas was cut off through non-payment of bills, his electricity meter was broken and he has been waiting for the repair man to return for several weeks. Not surprisingly he described the hospital as a relatively comfortable and companionable place:

there is nurses there to look after you all the time. Better facilities than I have here—you can watch television and listen to the radio, go for walks round the gardens, go for a pint at night which I can't afford to do whilst I'm paying the rent on this place. I can't afford to go out—only with the dog. If I were in there I could go for a drink, I could smoke a lot more than I am doing at the moment. … They've got washing facilities, like washing machines and spin dryers, and you can go out for a bath at any time you want, there's always hot water, plenty of hot water. … I was getting three meals a day which I am not doing now and am surviving mostly on sandwiches till I get my electricity on.

This is an extreme example of life on the margins of society: excluded, exiled and ignored as far as possible. Other personal accounts by people who have mental health problems describe the prejudice they have encountered in others—including mental health workers. As Chadwick (1997, p. 58) writes:

You are bound to come across people who think your mental disorder disqualifies you a priori from having anything useful or meaningful of your own to say about anything.

In a study of women with long term mental health problems, Repper et al (1998) describe the exclusion felt by one service user among her family and friends:

I just want to be normal again, you know. The way I was before I was ill … Family are a lot different towards me, my friends act differently towards me. Afraid to say the wrong thing, afraid you are going to jump down their throat. Quite different to how they treated me before … It's hard, because they don't know how you're going to react, and people have got this thing about mental health.

At the same time as wanting to be 'normal', people with mental health problems describe the strain of needing to constantly prove that they are just the same as everyone else—in much the same way as black people find that they always have to be/do better than others in order to be accepted as the same. This has given rise to literature on 'passing' as sane, which points out the need for a place where mental health problems are accepted and understood—somewhere run by and for people with mental health problems.

These personal experiences are confirmed by research. In a survey of discrimination faced by people who experienced mental health problems, Read & Baker (1996) reported that, of the 778 users responding, almost half (47%) had been verbally or physically harassed in public *because of* their mental health problems, 14% had been physically attacked (one was attacked by someone throwing stones whilst being called a 'nutter', another had dog faeces put through the letter box). Older patients frequently felt threatened by groups of young people, as one 71-year-old man said:

Various gangs in the district call me 'nutter' and spit at me. The gangs on the estate got to know I was a psychiatric patient and so I am teased and harassed.

Of the respondents, 62% claimed to have been treated unfairly by family or friends. In some cases, the whole family was ostracized—conveying a perceived threat of contamination:

Friends avoided me and would not let their children play with my children any more.

Underestimation of parenting abilities

In the same survey, of the respondents with children, 26% of men and 48% of women believed their parenting abilities had been unfairly questioned. Read & Baker (1996) quote one woman's experience:

My consultant psychiatrist told my husband and I not to have children—'they will be taken away, no doubt about it'. We now have a beautiful two and a half year old daughter; we are, to quote our GP 'excellent parents', and our care of our daughter is 'always of a high standard'.

Such routine underestimation of the parenting skills has repeatedly been reported in the literature on women with serious mental health problems. Services often operate informal policies—'in the best interests of patients'—to strongly discourage women from getting pregnant, encourage abortions, and—'in the best interests of the child'—take children into care after birth. Thus women are not permitted to have, or raise, children even where they are capable of doing so, or would be capable with supervision (Sayce 1997).

Unemployment

The impact of discrimination goes further: 62% of respondents in Read & Baker's 1996 survey had been put off applying for jobs by fear of discrimination. This may well be justified; Glozier (1998) undertook a survey of 200 personnel officers who were sent two vignettes of job applicants who had recovered from a health problem, identical except for the diagnosis of either depression or diabetes. The applicant with depression had significantly reduced chances of employment compared with the one with diabetes; discrimination was based upon perceptions of potential poor performance rather than differing expectations of absenteeism. In the UK only 21% of people with significant mental health problems are working, and only 13% are employed—a lower proportion than for any comparable groups with long term disabilities or health problems (Labour Force Survey 1995—cited in Sayce 1998a). The impact of unemployment is profound. Losing a job can be a catastrophic life event leading to depression, marital breakdown and—for people with mental health problems—relapse. Long term unemployment is stressful, isolating and demoralizing. It saps self-confidence and lowers the chances of regaining employment. In a review of over one hundred studies on the psychological effect of unemployment, Fryer & Payne (1986, p. 141) conclude:

In all cases the evidence suggests that groups of the unemployed have higher mean levels of experienced strain and negative feelings and lower mean levels of happiness, present life satisfaction, experience of pleasure and positive feelings than comparable employed people.

Poverty

For most people, unemployment means living in poverty. This automatically reduces the possibilities of social inclusion: holidays, car ownership, dining out, trips to the cinema can only be afforded if basic necessities are minimized. Poverty limits accommodation options to low cost/low rent residences, often in areas characterized by social exclusion. Thus many people with mental health problems live in housing estates ridden with problems such as crime, drugs, unemployment, 'community breakdown' and poor schools (Social Exclusion Unit website home page—www.open.gov.uk/co/seu).

Homelessness

Obviously homelessness is the worst form of housing problem and this is linked in complex ways with mental health problems. It has been estimated that between 30% and 50% of homeless people have some form of mental disorder (Allen 1993, Hitchcox, Maurin & Russell 1989, Taylor & Warren 1993, Tomlinson 1992). Although the media have repeatedly blamed the closure of mental hospitals for the increased visibility of mental illness 'on the streets', this picture is more likely to be due to the massive increase in the homeless population as a whole—estimated to have doubled between 1982 and 1992—than to an increased proportion of mental illness. The prevalence of mental illness among homeless people appears to have remained stable over this time (for earlier surveys see Tidmarsh & Wood 1972, Timms & Fry 1989). Indeed follow-up studies of discharged long stay patients indicate very low numbers becoming homeless. For example in the

TAPS study of discharged old long stay patients only 7 out of 700 patients became homeless in the 7-year follow-up period (see Leff 1997).

Nevertheless, since the proportion of mentally ill people among increasing numbers of homeless as a whole has not decreased, the numbers of mentally ill homeless people must have increased. This appears to be due to two factors: first, the shortage of low rent accommodation; secondly, the inadequacy of aftercare provided for people discharged from admission wards. During the first year of the London homeless mentally ill initiative, 544 people were identified as suffering from severe mental illness; of these only three had spent a continuous period of over 1 year in hospital (Craig & Timms 1992). The Medical Campaign Project (1990) found that two-thirds of single homeless people with psychiatric histories had left admission wards with no stable accommodation organised.

Homelessness reflects more than the mere lack of a home. It implies lack of food, clothing, social support, personal space, privacy and respect (Reisdorf-Ostrow 1989, Wadsworth 1984); once homeless many lose contact with all support services and frequently cease to claim benefits. GPs often refuse to register homeless people—denying them medical support (Dobson 1991, Royal College of Physicians 1994). Even when they are prescribed medication, homeless people will have particular difficulty taking drugs as they may have no way of tracking time, no access to a drink to wash down tablets and nowhere to keep them safely (Lindsey 1989). But not only do people who are homeless suffer the material aspects of exclusion, they are also among the most socially reviled 'deviants'. Tringo (1970) reviewed the literature on social acceptability and dimensions of difference and concluded with a 'hierarchy of preferences' for different groups, which to a large extent is defined by perceived culpability (echoing Foucault's theory of inhumane treatment for inhuman people—see above). Thus children, the elderly and retarded are most socially acceptable; ex-offenders, drinkers and drug users are least acceptable. Although homeless people, like those with mental health problems are infinitely heterogeneous, the community ascribes all the most negative attributes to this group (assuming that they are mentally ill, have a criminal history, are likely to be violent, pose a threat to children, abuse drugs and alcohol and so on).

Public attitudes

In a review of the literature on attitudes to mental health facilities, Repper & Brooker (1996) concluded that despite some evidence of growing tolerance in the postwar period (Dear & Taylor 1982, Hall et al 1993), public fears about mentally ill people living nearby had increased slightly. A survey of 2000 adults undertaken in 1993 and repeated in 1994 (RSGB 1994) indicated that over 90% of people agreed that a more tolerant attitude towards people with mental illness should be adopted, that people with mental illness deserve sympathy, and that we have a responsibility to provide the best possible care for them. Yet, there was significantly more fear of being in contact with people who have mental illness in 1994 than in 1993: more people thought mental illness was dangerous; more were afraid of living close to someone who had a mental illness; fewer people considered community care to be a good thing.

These findings were confirmed in a survey of key mental health service providers in the NHS and voluntary sectors (Repper et al 1997), which reported that over two-thirds had experienced 'NIMBY' (not in my back yard) campaigns. Most providers thought that opposition had increased

---

Box 14.2 Foci of concern about the development of local mental health facilities in order of importance

Fear of threat to local children
Fear that value of local houses will fall
Fear of threat to personal security
General dislike of people with mental health problems
Fear of violence
Fear of impact on local shops, traffic, parking and amenities
Fear that facility would 'lower the tone', 'not fit into this area'

From Repper et al 1997

Box 14.3 Factors affecting level of opposition

Less opposition		More opposition
	size	
small		large
	function	
day care/drop-in		residential
	users	
physically disabled		history of violence/drug abuse
diagnosis of dementia		diagnosis of schizophrenia
elderly		young
female		male
white		black
local/indigenous		from regional/national catchment area
	area	
early tenants on new site		established community
well resourced area		deprived/saturated area
familiarity with users		no previous contact with users
		family orientated community

From Repper et al 1997

during the 1990s. Most had had to delay opening at least one facility owing to community opposition, which ranged from protest letters and meetings to outright violence. The foci of protestors' concern are shown in Box 14.2.

This survey also clarified the nature of factors affecting the level of opposition towards people with mental health problems (see Box 14.3): most opposition could be expected towards young black men who were not local and had a diagnosis of schizophrenia, but discrimination occurs in all types of areas towards all types of people.

Racism

The additional fear expressed regarding black men is not surprising given the media's excessive use of black men in portrayals of the 'failure of community care'—most notably the photograph of Christopher Clunis on his way to court. All too often, articles on the failure of community care are illustrated with pictures of black men; a Panorama report on community care also explicitly stated that the public had more to fear from black men (Panorama, 13 October 1997)—however, this is not true since the Confidential inquiry into homicides and suicides by mentally ill people found that 80% of perpetrators of homicide were, in fact, white.

Discrimination in the criminal justice system

Anyone working in mental health services will know that service users—of whatever colour, sex or age, are more likely to be victims than offenders (Murphy 1993); how often do patients report jeering from local children, hostility from shopkeepers, lack of tolerance at the benefits office, delayed service in the pub—let alone more serious offences? (see also Read & Baker 1996, Repper et al 1997). Yet there is no record of the extent of such discrimination because people with mental illness are not seen to be credible witnesses by police and Crown Prosecution Service. This is yet another form of exclusion: access to justice is severely limited (Read & Baker 1996, Women Against Rape/Legal Action for Women 1996).

SUMMARY

People with mental health problems are likely to fit every given indicator of social exclusion: they are frequently impoverised, in poor housing or homeless, socially isolated and unemployed. But, in addition to all this, they are excluded from communities because of the widespread fear of mental illness. This fear is largely founded in saturation media reporting of tragedies. As Repper et al (1997, p. 39) summarize:

> Such is the ignorance of the nature and effect of mental health problems that the general public assume that violence and crime equate with mental illness; a view that is powerfully reinforced by sensationalised reports in local and national media ... None of the concern [in the survey] was based on personal experience of crime or violence by a person with mental health problems. ... In the majority of cases the cause was ill-informed fear and the outcome was delays to service development or abuse of service users.

Even when this is put into the context of the numbers of people with mental health problems who have never committed any crimes, the public appear to be unwilling to tolerate any possibility of risk. As Sayce (1995) has suggested, mental health service users appear to have been demonized, as part of a 'moral panic'. This would certainly appear to be true given Stanley Cohen's (1972, p. 9) description of this phenomenon:

> a condition, episode, person or group of persons [which] emerges to become defined as a threat to societal values and interests: its nature is presented in a stylised and stereotypical fashion by the mass media ... ways of coping are evolved or (more often) resorted to; the condition then disappears ... or deteriorates and becomes more visible.

Yet again, however, people with mental illness do differ from other groups with transitional 'outsider' status: their exclusion has been going on since the Middle Ages. Yet if moral panics 'bring boundaries into focus by accentuating the differences between the agitated guardians of mainstream values and excluded others' (Sibley 1995, p. 43), then the move from asylums to community care may have heightened consciousness of this boundary, and led to a tighter defence.

In addition to exclusion on the grounds of lack of material or practical qualifications and public attitudes, people with mental health problems may be isolated as a direct result of their mental health problems. They may experience symptoms that lead them to separate themselves from others—exclude themselves—as intense contact is difficult to tolerate, their symptoms may lead their friends and family to reduce contact with them, and their behaviour may overtly indicate the 'difference' that societies find so difficult to assimilate. Whatever the cause, and however social exclusion is defined, it is clear that people with mental health problems remain at least as excluded today as they were behind the asylum walls—no longer is even the dubious safety and relative tolerance of that institution available. The question for mental health workers lies in how to tackle this exclusion. As yet, there is little research to draw on; few innovative services have explicitly tackled social exclusion; fewer have evaluated their efforts in terms of impact on indicators of exclusion. The following section draws on work in related areas to make suggestions about the way forward.

TACKLING SOCIAL EXCLUSION

Policy initiatives

Whilst the principle of collaboration between health services, social services, voluntary agencies and private sector facilities in order to provide a comprehensive, flexible and complementary range of mental health services has been espoused since 1975 (in Better services for the mentally ill, DHSS), it is only in the past 5 years that the benefits of *interdepartmental* working have been recognized. Increasingly education, employment, leisure and housing initiatives for people with mental health problems or other disabilities have received joint funding from the Department of Health *and* other relevant departments (such as the Departments of Education, Employment and

Environment). The perceived benefits of such collaborative working have been confirmed in the new appointment of Minister of Public Health, a post working across departments to facilitate health gains through social changes, and the creation of the Social Exclusion Unit with the following goals (Social Exclusion Unit website home page—www.open.gov.uk/co/seu):

Improving understanding of the key characteristics of social exclusion and the impact on it of government policies; and promoting solutions by encouraging co-operation, disseminating best practice, and where necessary, making recommendations for changes in policies, machinery and delivery mechanisms.

Up to July 1998, the Unit's priorities included: reducing truancy and finding better ways of managing school exclusion, reducing street living to near zero and developing integrated and sustainable approaches to the problems of the worst estates. In addition, it was to improve mechanisms for integrating the work of different departments and draw up key indicators of social exclusion. In its first year of operation, the DOH has funded and jointly run three conferences on social exclusion and mental health with 'Focus' (a group of voluntary organisations), demonstrating some awareness of the relevance of the issue for people with mental health problems. However, this has not been received warmly by service user groups as it appears to run counter to the government's desire to reassure the public—restore confidence in community care—by introducing increasingly coercive measures (such as a review of the Mental Health Act with the introduction of community treatment orders and increasingly 'assertive' outreach teams). Since different stakeholders have different views, needs, goals and definitions of success, it is perhaps not surprising that a range of different—and sometimes contradictory—policies are developing. What is also not surprising is that the wishes of the general public take precedence over those of service users.

Campaigns to reduce discrimination

Outside the DOH, the issues of stigma, discrimination and community acceptance in relation to mental health have been recognized in a number of different initiatives. In October 1998, the Royal College of Psychiatrists (RCP) launched a 5-year campaign 'Changing minds: every family in the land' to combat the 'stigma' attached to mental health problems by increasing public understanding of mental illness. This has met with widespread disapproval among service user groups who do not want the public to receive a 'medical' understanding of mental health problems; the campaign runs alongside the RCP's support of proposals for compulsory community treatment and, even more contentiously, has not involved service users at all. As Steve Craine of the All Wales User and Survivor Network states:

> Psychiatrists hand out labels that stigmatise us for life and they systematically present us as dangerous nutters to justify coercive treatment
> Crane 1998, p. 5

A more welcome initiative has been set up by Mind. As part of their 'Respect: time to end discrimination on mental health grounds' campaign, they are holding an inquiry into 'Creating accepting communities'. An expert panel (chaired by Rabbi Julia Neuberger) will receive evidence from a variety sources concerning ways of increasing community tolerance and social inclusion.

Antidiscrimination law

The Disability Discrimination Act (DDA) makes it unlawful to discriminate against disabled people in employment, the provision of goods, services, transport and education. The Act is being implemented in stages. From December 1996 it has been unlawful for employers (of more than 20 people) to treat a disabled person less favourably than an able-bodied employee, unless they can establish a justified reason, and it requires them to make reasonable adjustments to the working conditions or workplace so that staff with disabilities are not at a disadvantage. Reasonable adjustments include: physical adjustments of the environment, altering responsibilities, transferring the employee to another job, altering working hours, allowing

time for treatment, providing a reader or interpreter and providing supervision. The Act covers people who have, or have had, a disability—defined as 'a physical or mental impairment which has a substantial or long term adverse effect on his ability to carry out normal day to day activities' (e.g. diabetes, epilepsy, heart disease, schizophrenia, progressive conditions such as cancer, multiple sclerosis, HIV, and previous conditions from which the individual has recovered—which makes discrimination on the grounds of previous mental health problems illegal). It is important for mental health workers to be aware of this Act so that they can help to advise service users if they encounter discrimination in their work and put them in touch with the appropriate expertise. Unison has published two booklets on the DDA (A fair deal for disabled members, and Unison and the Disability Discrimination Act—20 Grand Depot Road, London SE18 6SF) and further information is available from Mind (15–19 Broadway, London E15 4BQ).

The DDA has been strongly criticized by user groups and trade unions on the grounds that it is inadequate, and legitimizes discrimination in some ways (Cleary 1997). The Labour Government plans to strengthen it and set up the Disability Rights Task Force in 1997 to advise this process. The Task Force recommended a Disability Rights Commission to work proactively with employers and users to: develop good practice in employing disabled people, initiate investigations into discrimination and issue codes of practice. It is hoped that at least 50% of members would be disabled and would include users/survivors of mental health services (Sayce 1998b).

Strategies to enhance work opportunities

Work is not only integral to mental health, it is also a route out of poverty. Yet, since mental health problems vary in their nature, duration and impact, full-time work may not be possible for all those with mental health problems and a wide range of work options need to be made available: paid, voluntary, full time, part time, open, sheltered and supported.

The Labour Government has set up a welfare to work scheme with an emphasis on supporting the young, long term unemployed and disabled to achieve work; £50m a year (for 4 years) has been available for innovative schemes. However since project criteria include targeted numbers going on to full-time employment within relatively short periods of time, people with serious mental health problems find it difficult to fit into the schemes. Indeed, whereas employment projects for people with mental health problems have been successful in increasing quality of life and social functioning, they are less successful in achieving full-time employment for users. Funding for such initia-

tives has largely come from health, social services and charitable funds rather than employment agencies. Yet again, people with mental health problems are excluded from mainstream initiatives by placing responsibility for them in the 'caring' services, and by expecting them to fit criteria set for non-disabled people. There are some notable exceptions, for example the Pathfinder NHS Trust User Employment Project (which is summarised in Box 14.4). Although this initiative is funded by the local authority and health authority, of the first 18 volunteers taken on, 8 have gained paid employment within or outside the Trust.

Box 14.4 The Pathfinder Mental Health Services Trust User Employment Project

This programme is designed to increase employment opportunities within mental health services for people who have themselves experienced mental health problems (see also Perkins 1998). It comprises three parts:

Supported employment programme
This provides support for people who have experienced more serious mental health problems to gain and sustain employment in existing posts within the trust on the same terms and conditions as other employees. Users have been employed as mental health support workers, occupational therapy assistants and physiotherapy assistants. Applicants receive assistance at all stages of the recruitment process, training tailored to the needs of the post and ongoing individually tailored support. Most employees start on a part-time basis but half have moved on to full-time work as their confidence and abilities have increased. So far 16 user employees have been appointed and six more are being recruited. Most have a diagnosis of psychosis and all but one have been admitted in the past. They have been unemployed for a mean of 4.6 years and have now been employed for a mean of 14.3 months. Three are undertaking NVQ qualifications.

Volunteer programme
This enables people who have experienced mental health problems to gain the experience, confidence and references they will need to apply for open employment. All volunteers have a specific contract and receive training, ongoing support and assistance to look for and apply for posts when they are ready. Twenty-seven volunteers have been employed; of the first 18, 44% have gained paid employment within or outside the trust.

Decreasing discrimination in recruitment throughout the trust
In recognition of the discrimination that exists against employing people who have had mental health problems, the trust has introduced a charter for the employment of people who have experienced mental health problems. Within their charter the trust recognizes the detrimental effects that mental health problems can have on employment prospects, the deleterious effects of mental health problems on mental health, and the specific expertise that people who have experienced mental health problems can bring to the trust. 'Personal experience of mental health problems' has been specified as a desirable characteristic in advertisements for *all* posts within the trust. In the first 4 months of this initiative 13% of applicants, and 9% of those appointed, stated they had experienced mental health problems. The trust is aiming towards a target of 10% of the 1200 strong workforce being people who have experienced mental health problems.

Sayce (1998a) points out the need to reduce benefit disincentives as this clearly deters many people from trying work. In the UK, if individuals find themselves unemployed after gaining employment, there is a return to lower levels of benefits, which leaves them with a net loss of income as well as the experience of failed employment. Alternative models do exist; for example, in Germany employers are fined if they fail to employ sufficient numbers of disabled people and incentives are used to enhance job opportunities for disabled people.

Learning from other marginalized groups

The discrimination and exclusion that are experienced by people who have mental health problems is not unique, and it has been suggested that strength could be gained—and tactics learnt—by joining with other marginalized groups. Sayce (1998a, p. 337) summarizes the reasons for and against this:

> It may be objected to this that discrimination on mental health grounds is simply not comparable to discrimination on grounds of race, gender or sexual orientation: first because some users of mental health services cannot work or parent ....And secondly because other minorities do not perceive a necessary solidarity with users as a fellow minority group—they may rather want to distance themselves.

However, Sayce goes on to point out that disability rights activists have worked towards changing physical and social environments to make work possible. The same principles can be applied to mental health problems, with accommodations or adjustments—by making work or parenting accessible to people who are socially rather than physically disabled—people with mental health problems can work in the same way. She also suggests that:

> Discriminatory attitudes and behaviour cross-cut minority groups in complex ways. One of the greatest challenges facing anti-discrimination proponents is to build understandings of multiple discrimination ...

> Alliances between marginalised groups are vitally needed which effectively challenge one discrimination without compounding another.

Working with individuals: the social disability and access model

The principle of learning from other marginalized groups has been developed by Perkins & Repper (1996; 1998, pp. 22–23). They have drawn on the social disability model initially put forward by Wing & Morris (1981) to produce an overarching analysis of working *alongside* people who have mental health problems, to support them in gaining access to the communities, roles, responsibilities, facilities and opportunities of their choice. The main tenets of this model are as follows:

◆ Disabilities cannot be defined in a vacuum. A person is only disabled in relation to a particular social or physical context and the demands and expectations it comprises.

◆ A person who experiences the cognitive and emotional difficulties associated with serious mental health problems is socially disabled in much the same way that someone with mobility or sensory difficulties is physically disabled. A person with physical limitations is unable to negotiate the 'normal' (able-bodied) physical world without help, support and adaptation of that world. The handicap that someone with, for example, mobility problems experiences is far greater in the absence of adaptations such as ramps, mobility aids, wide doorways, transport and the like. These accommodations ensure access to roles, activities, facilities and relationships in an able-bodied community.

◆ A person who experiences the cognitive and emotional difficulties that characterize serious mental health problems is unable to negotiate the 'normal' (able-minded) social world without help, support and adaptation of that world. Accommodations and support that ensure access to work, housing and social/leisure activities facilitate access to roles, activities, facilities and relationships in an able-minded community.

◆ The support required by individuals to gain access to activities, facilities, roles and relationships might include specific interventions to reduce the cognitive and emotional difficulties associated with their mental health problems and enable them to maximize their role within the community. But it will also involve working within that community to reduce the social and economic disadvantages associated with social disability: facilitating access to housing, work, full benefits and other ordinary activities and supports to ensure that their needs are met in the same way as they are for the rest of the population.

Social disability is defined as the extent to which individuals with mental health problems are unable to perform socially at the level expected of them. This disability is a function of three interrelated processes. First, there are the primary symptoms of the individual's mental health problems. Secondly, there are the social disadvantages that either predate or succeed mental health problems (such as poverty, unemployment, isolation, poor housing, poor education and so on). Thirdly, there are individuals' responses to others' reaction to their mental health problems—the personal impact of discrimination (Perkins & Repper 1996, Shepherd 1984, Wing & Morris 1981). Such an understanding of mental health problems informs a far broader consideration of support than is conventionally the case in mental health services. It moves the focus of mental health work away from efforts to change individuals to fit their environment towards efforts to change the environment so that individuals can achieve their own goals. Rather than defining their role in terms of alleviation of symptoms, mental health workers need to focus on the specific barriers to individuals' lives within the community. No amount of help with voices is going to ensure that a person is tolerated by the next-door neighbour. Besides, what many people with long term mental health problems want is not so much to get rid of their symptoms but to gain a direction in their lives: a role which they—and others—value, access to the opportunities that most of us take for granted, opportunities that they are denied, rarely because of their symptoms per se, but because of the social consequences of their mental health problems. The support they require *might* therefore include

specific interventions to reduce their cognitive and emotional difficulties and enable them to maximize their role within the community, but it will also involve working within that community to set up the support structures needed and facilitate access to housing, work, full benefits, leisure activities and so on (for a full account of this approach see Perkins & Repper 1996).

Collaborative planning to promote social inclusion

In order for individual mental health workers to change their 'unit' of work from the individual to the local community, services need to work with the local community and all other local agencies. There are a number of different ways in which this can be achieved:

◆ Develop local community profiles to identify strengths, weaknesses, opportunities and threats for the integration and inclusion of people with mental health problems.

◆ Include members of the local community, local community groups, users and representatives of different services and agencies in strategic planning and management.

◆ Negotiate joint funding (e.g. from health authority, local authority, housing associations and education) to support housing projects; access to education initiatives; leisure schemes; employment projects and small business cooperatives.

Such developments would work towards 'mainstreaming' those with mental health problems: taking them out of an exclusively health (and frequently a perceived criminal justice) context, into the same communities as everyone else.

Increasing public understanding of mental illness

Alongside the essential work needed to combat structural inequalities, a huge challenge lies in dispelling fear and discrimination. Familiarization, getting to know people with mental health problems, is the one clearly useful strategy in reducing fear and prejudice—and this has been found to be most effective when combined with education

(Repper et al 1997). Thus local Mind associations have found that, where they have infiltrated local neighbourhoods by participating in church fund raising, local art exhibitions, etc., members encounter more support from neighbours and less hostility. This is something that mental health workers can capitalize on: identifying opportunities for service users to meet neighbours and, if the user wishes, accompanying them at first. This experience will be more valuable if users are able to meet others in a positive role—either as a mental health service user (for example, giving a talk on mental health issues to a local group) or not (for example, joining an aerobics class or entering a pub quiz night).

Once individual workers move beyond the problems of each individual to consider ways in which the community as a whole can contribute to their support, new areas of work are opened up. For example:

◆ educating the public through initiatives in schools and local groups; this is most effective when people who have themselves experienced mental health problems are involved

◆ changing the media representation of 'madness' by undertaking proactive work with local newspapers, radio and TV (see 'Challenge the media to get the facts right', a leaflet distributed as part of the Mediawatch campaign, which encourages the public to complain about media portrayals of mental health problems, available from The Mental Health Foundation, 37 Mortimer Street, London W1N 8JU)

◆ encouraging good relationships between local residents and mental health facilities by involving users, their families and local people in planning new facilities and encouraging joint purchasing/use of facilities (see Sayce & Willmot 1997)

◆ enabling users to make full use of community resources (e.g. banks, cafes, launderettes, job centres, education classes, religious events) by identifying specific named people in each institution and developing necessary structures and understanding. Also by supporting users in advocating for themselves

◆ identifying local employers and developing schemes to enable them to provide supported employment for people with mental health problems

◆ developing work opportunities for service users within the mental health service itself.

SUMMARY

Social exclusion is probably the biggest problem facing people who have mental health problems. The majority of those who have experienced more serious mental health problems are unemployed, in poor housing in areas ridden with social problems, socially isolated and facing personal discrimination on a regular basis. Inevitably this destroys self-confidence and engenders shame. Rather than face the prejudice and discrimination that follows disclosure of mental health problems, many people are forced to lie about their health. Others do not have this choice: they may not be able to hide their need for support; their behaviour may lead to others making assumptions about them; it may be apparent that they live, work or spend their days in a place for people with mental health problems. Few of these problems are a direct result of the primary symptoms that led to a label of mental illness. They are the consequences of the social exclusion that both predated these problems and occurred as a result of others perceiving them to be mad and therefore not to be trusted (see also Repper et al 1998).

There are many ways of working towards the inclusion of people with mental health problems. At a policy level, in national initiatives, at a service level, in local developments, and at the level of the individual mental health worker and service user, innovative projects are increasing. And this really is the time to grasp the nettle. There is a unique convergence of attention on social exclusion—from the government, professional groups, user groups, employment and housing agencies—with policies, campaigns, funding, partnerships, 'urban regeneration' and alliances between different groups. It is now time for mental health workers to consider carefully what this means for their work: Whom should they be working with?

DISCUSSION QUESTIONS

1. What is the relationship between social exclusion and mental health?

2. A social model of disability addresses both impairments (symptoms) and disadvantages (both preceding and subsequent to mental health problems). How would nursing care differ if a social disability model were adopted, rather than a medical model?

3. All nurses can promote social inclusion. Consider social inclusion strategies that might help:
   (a) a young woman admitted to an acute ward, leaving her husband and children at home
   (b) a man who lives in 24-hour supported accommodation in the community, but does little during the day
   (c) a woman in her late 30s, who wants to train to become a secretary, but continues to hear voices and has no previous qualifications
   (d) a man who has recently moved into a shared house in the community following a long admission?

Should their work continue to focus on making individuals 'fit' their community, or are there less stigmatizing ways of working that reduce the implied criticism of the person who does not 'fit' perfectly? What opportunities exist to promote social inclusion within their local 'patch'? What can they, as individuals, do to influence the media portrayal of mental illness? Who can they link up with to broaden the opportunities of service users? This chapter has only scratched the surface of these questions. No single approach will remedy the problems of social exclusion, but everyone can play a part by working with local users, community groups, agencies and establishments to develop local solutions.

REFERENCES

Allen D 1993 Mental illness for up to 50% of homeless people. Nursing Standard 19:42–43

FURTHER READING

Barham P, Hayward R 1995 Relocating madness. From the mental patient to the person. Free Association Books, London
This is an exceptionally readable book comprising an ethnographic study of the lives of ex-patients who have ongoing disabilities as a result of severe mental health problems. It graphically portrays their struggle to gain a toehold on community life, thwarted largely by negative attitudes, discrimination and disregard.

Perkins R, Repper J 1996 Working alongside people who have long term mental health problems. Chapman & Hall, London
This book describes the practical day to day work of mental health workers, both working with people's symptoms and facilitating access to the roles, relationships, activities and opportunities that they desire.

Read J, Baker S 1996 Not just sticks and stones. A survey of the stigma, taboos and discrimination experienced by people with mental health problems. Mind, London

Repper J, Sayce L, Strong S, Willmot J, Haines M 1997 Tall stories from the backyard. A survey of 'NIMBY' opposition to community mental health facilities experienced by key service providers in England and Wales. Mind, London
Both of the above reports, commissioned by Mind, illustrate the ongoing prejudice that people with mental health problems face. Whether applying for work, seeking parenting advice, embarking on education programmes or moving into specialist houses, the extent of discrimination is immense. Thus the struggle to recover from mental health problems is not only complicated by ongoing symptoms and impairments, but is also thwarted by social expectations and intolerance.

Barham P, Hayward R 1995 Relocating madness. From the mental patient to the person. Free Association Books, London

Chadwick P 1997 Schizophrenia: the positive perspective. Routledge, London

Cleary Y 1997 Disability discrimination. Mental Health Care 1(2):68

Cohen S 1972 Folk devils and moral panics. MacGibbon & Kee, London

Craig T, Timms P W 1992 Out of the wards and on to the streets? Journal of Mental Health 1:265–275

Craine S 1998 News digest. OpenMind Nov/Dec:5

Dahrendorf R 1985 The modern social conflict. Weidenfeld & Nicholson, London

Dayson D 1993 The TAPS project 12: crime, vagrancy, death and readmission of the long term mentally ill during their first year on local reprovision. British Medical Journal 162:40–44

Dear M, Taylor S M 1982 Not on our street: community attitudes to mental health care. Pion, London

DHSS (Department of Health and Social Security) 1975 Better services for the mentally ill. HMSO, London

Dobson J 1991 Sticking a plaster on the housing disaster. Health Services Journal 22 August:13

Foucault M 1965 Madness and civilisation. A history of insanity in the age of reason (transl of abridged version). Random House, New York

Fryer D M, Payne R L 1986 Being unemployed: A review of the literature on the psychological experience of unemployment. In: Cooper C L, Robertson I (eds) International review of industrial and organisational psychology. John Wiley, London

Glozier N 1998 (cited in) 'Survey reveals discrimination by employers' OpenMind, Sep/Oct, p. 5

Goodwin S 1996 Comparative mental health policy: from institutional to community care. Sage, London

Hall P, Brockington I F, Levings J, Murphy C 1993 A comparison of responses to the mentally ill in two communities. British Journal of Psychiatry 162(Jan):99–108

Helman C 1985 Culture, health and illness. John Wright, Bristol

Hitchcox M, Maurin J T, Russell L 1989 Obstacles to research analysis. Journal of Psychosocial Nursing 27:19–23

Leff J 1997 (ed) Care in the community. Illusion or reality? John Wiley, Chichester

Lewis D, Shadish W, Lurigio A 1989 Policies of inclusion and the mentally ill: long term care in a new environment. Journal of Social Issues 45(3):173–186

Lindsey A M 1989 Health care for the homeless. Nursing Outlook 37:78–81

Medical Campaign Project 1990 A paper outlining good practice on discharge of single homeless people with particular reference to mental health units. Policy Studies Institute, London

Murphy E 1993 Could do better. Care Weekly 18 November:6

Perkins R E 1998 An Act to follow? A Life in the Day 2(1):15–20

Perkins R, Repper J 1996 Working alongside people who have long term mental health problems. Chapman & Hall, London

Perkins R, Repper J 1998 Choice or control, dilemmas in mental health practice. Radcliffe Medical, Oxford

Philo G, Henderson L, McLaughlin G 1993 Mass media representation of mental health/illness: report for Health Education Board for Scotland. Glasgow University, Glasgow

Read J, Baker S 1996 Not just sticks and stones. A survey of the stigma, taboos and discrimination experienced by people with mental health problems. Mind, London

Reisdorf-Ostrow W 1989 Deinstitutionalisation: a public policy perspective. Journal of Psychosocial Nursing 27:4–7

Repper J, Brooker C 1996 Attitudes towards community facilities for people with serious mental health problems. Health and Social Care in the Community 4(5):290–399

Repper J, Sayce L, Strong S, Willmot J, Haines M 1997 Tall stories from the backyard. A survey of 'NIMBY' opposition to community mental health facilities experienced by key service providers in England and Wales. Mind, London

Repper J, Perkins R, Owen S, Robinson J 1998 'I wanted to be a nurse … but I didn't get that far': women with serious ongoing mental health problems talk about their lives. Journal of Psychiatric and Mental Health Nursing 6(5):505–509

Rogers A, Pilgrim D 1996 Mental health policy in Britain. Macmillan, London

Romme M, Escher S 1993 Accepting voices. Mind, London

Royal College of Physicians 1994 Homelessness and ill health. Royal College of Physicians, London

Royal College of Psychiatrists 1996 Report of the confidential inquiry into homicides and suicides by mentally ill people. Royal College of Psychiatrists, London

RSGB (Research Surveys of Great Britain for Department of Health) 1994 RSGB omnibus attitudes to mental illness, summary report. RSGB, London

Sayce L 1995 Violence: a framework for fair treatment. In: Crighton J (ed) Psychiatric patient violence. Duckworth, London, pp 127–150

Sayce L 1997 Motherhood: the final taboo in community care. Women and Mental Health Forum 2:4–7

Sayce L 1998a Stigma, discrimination and social exclusion. What's in a word? Journal of Mental Health 7(4):331–343

Sayce L 1998b Policy and campaigning update. OpenMind, May/June p. 4

Sayce L, Willmot J 1997 Gaining respect: preventing and tackling community opposition to mental health facilities. Mind, London

Shepherd G 1984 Institutional care and rehabilitation. Longman, New York

Sibley D 1995 Geographies of exclusion. Society and difference in the West. Routledge, London

Taylor C S, Warren B J 1993 What goals and interventions are important for nurses to use when working with homeless chronically mentally ill? Journal of Psychosocial Nursing 31:35–39

Tidmarsh D, Wood S 1972 Psychiatric aspects of destitutions: a study of the Camberwell reception centre. In: Wing J K, Hailey A H (eds) Evaluating a community service. Oxford University Press, London

Timms P W, Fry A H 1989 Homelessness and mental illness. Health Trends 21:71–72

Tomlinson B 1992 Report of the inquiry into London's health service medical education and research. HMSO, London

Tringo J L 1970 The hierarchy of preference toward disability groups. Journal of Special Education 4(3):293–306

Wadsworth R 1984 Turning point for the homeless. Nursing Times 80:48–49

Wing J K, Morris B 1981 Clinical basis of rehabilitation. In: Wing J K (ed) Handbook of psychiatric rehabilitation practice. Oxford University Press, Oxford

Women Against Rape/Legal Action for Women 1996 Dossier: the Crown Prosecution Service and the crime of rape. Women Against Rape, London

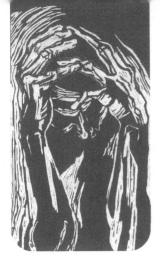

Chapter Fifteen

Antiracist practice: achieving competency and maintaining professional standards

Carol Baxter

AIMS

- ◆ To examine the implications of working in a multiracial society
- ◆ To provide an understanding of personal and institutional racism
- ◆ To lay the foundations of antiracist practice

KEY ISSUES

Origins of racism

Racism and rights

Poor health experiences

Stereotypical views

Personal racism

Institutional racism

Discrimination in hospitals

Double discrimination

Comparative stereotyping

INTRODUCTION

The message to all who choose to care for others is that, unless their actions are guided by a sense of importance of every human being, their competence and professionalism will remain questionable.
Nirza 1986

People who experience distress and illness come from all sections of society and from different racial and cultural backgrounds. If we are to maintain professional standards, then the appropriate attitude, knowledge and skills to meet the needs of all individuals regardless of their racial or cultural background is essential.

We need only take a look around us to appreciate that white people in Britain enjoy more privileges and have more opportunities and power than black people. Whiteness confers rights that are often denied to black people. Black people are more likely to live in run-down inner city areas and in substandard housing, to be found in semi- and unskilled jobs, to be disproportionately affected by unemployment and to be economically worse off than their white counterparts (Modood et al 1997, OPCS 1993). There is also evidence that black people have poorer health experiences and less access to appropriate health care (Balarajan & Raleigh 1993, HEA 1994). Even though the social security system applies the same rules to all, it can still create quite a wide range of inequalities in access to benefits for black and ethnic minority people.

These inequalities have their roots in racial discrimination. Racism is an ideology and an institution developed out of imperialism. Westerners needed to see African and Asian people as inferior and even subhuman in order to rationalize slavery, colonization and the furtherance of economic wealth and gain. Racism is thus based on the myth of the superiority of the white race. Stereotyping is one way in which racism is perpetuated.

Think back to your childhood and identify images you have about white and black people. These images come from family, school friends, literature, radio, television and newspapers. Spend a few minutes jotting down these images; it will become apparent to you that the words used to describe white images often reflect what you have learnt about the British Empire. They are generally positive images such as discoverers, powerful, inventors, scientific researchers, responsible, civilized and intelligent. Words that are used to describe black images are generally negative in contrast to those of white people—poor, needy, primitive, unreliable, helpless, incompetent, aggressive and subservient.

It may be comfortable to assume that all we have just said is merely of historical significance. These racist, stereotyped views are, however, still prevalent in our society. Black people who live in Britain today continue to be seen through this myth and continue to be discriminated against socially, politically and economically. There is evidence, from a recent survey (Modood et al 1997), of self-admission of racist attitudes in the UK. Indeed, the recent inquiry into the death of black teenager Stephen Lawrence revealed uncomfortable lessons for all public sectors including health and social welfare services (Macpherson 1999).

Racism is a complex phenomenon that operates at two different levels—personal and institutional. Although there will be incidents of personal racism, most people in the caring professions do not deliberately withhold care or treat people differently on the basis of their colour. Institutional racism is the more common and damning form of racism. This happens in a variety of ways—first, by default, where the way things are done within organizations do not take account of the needs of black people. For example, despite the fact that not all patients speak English as a first language, services are on the whole provided through the English medium only. Secondly, it happens where people in positions of power base their decisions on racist assumptions and stereotyping. An example of this is the popular view that black people do not need services because 'they prefer to look after their own'. Another very common form of racial discrimination within services is where the rules and regulations apply equally to all, but have the effect of excluding black and ethnic minority people while maintaining the privileged position of white people. McNaught (1985), from his analysis of a variety of reports, identified some practical ways in which racial discrimination against black patients in hospital has occurred:

1. *Patient's reception and handling*—ethnic minority patients kept waiting unnecessarily; staff making racist comments in earshot of the patients; addressing patients in a derogatory manner.

2. *Clinical consultation*—poor or no explanations offered to ethnic minority patients. Assumption that many are 'faking' or hypochondriacs. Inadequate or no examination before diagnosis and prescription of treatment. Delayed, inappropriate or even experimental treatment.

3. *Patient's consent to medical procedures*—inadequate explanations. Exceeding the procedures that the patient was advised were necessary without further consultation. Unnecessary procedures, said to be racially motivated.

4. *Nursing care*—offhand treatment. Racist slurs or comments to patients. Unnecessary medication, particularly of the mentally distressed.

5. *Health surveillance/diagnosis*—utilization of parameters and behavioural models that are culture-specific to white British people, for example, in mental health diagnosis, child health surveillance, social and medical assessment for special education.

DOUBLE DISCRIMINATION

Black people with mental health problems are particularly vulnerable in a racist society.

As is the case with mental illness, racism is also a form of devaluation and oppression. Parallels can be drawn between social role perceptions of people who are mentally ill and people who are black. Two of the most prevalent such role perceptions are that of being a *menace* and that of being *objects of dread*. Even today people with mental health problems are sometimes viewed as menacing or a threat. Attempts to establish community living are met with objections based on the *notions of danger* to local people, property and property values. Housing policies and practices aimed at keeping black people out of white neighbourhoods are commonplace. Black people are more likely to be locked away in mental institu-

tions and to receive custodial sentences and imprisonment (Cope & Ndequa 1991, NACRO 1989).

People with mental health problems are also largely still dreaded in society, often being avoided and denied social intercourse and conversation. Black people are also viewed as socially undesirable and unattractive. Many people will admit to fear and anxiety when there are large numbers of mentally ill people and (in the case of white people) black people around.

The relationship between black people and mental illness has increasingly been discussed in psychiatry. Classical psychiatry, having developed in the colonial era, reflects notions that emerged during the period of 'scientific racism'. Psychiatry prides itself in its scientific background based on anatomy and physiology and more recently in the social sciences. Within it can be found many of the simplistic assumptions of a racist society. Fernando (1988) states that:

> Historically speaking two important sets of ideas came into psychiatry from the basic sciences. First, the view that black people are born with inferior brains and limited capacity for growth; and secondly, that their personalities tend to be abnormal or deviant because of nature (genetic endowment) and/or nurture (upbringing). The influence of these themes ... was overt in the nineteenth century, but, although less obvious since the war, shows a tenacious persistence into the present.

The ongoing debates concerning the genetic background to mental illness have implications for the ways in which 'races' are perceived. This background, as well as the medical model within which much of psychiatric research is approached, can explain the concern with the prevalence of mental illness among black people. Although black people comprise less than one-fifth of the population, they make up a quarter of all inner city mentally ill patients. The widely debated study by Glyn Harrison in Nottingham (Harrison et al 1988), which is based on estimated populations of black people, reports a considerably higher incidence of schizophrenia among black people in Britain, especially among those born in the UK.

Traditional models of diagnosis are often inappropriate for black and ethnic minority people. Lack of recognition of the different experiences, pressures and lifestyles of black people within the method and process of diagnosis often leads to misdiagnosis. Consequently there is a failure of general practitioners to detect early signals of distress and minor forms of mental disorder such as depression and anxiety amongst black and minority people. This deficit may well be a contributory factor to the suicide rates well in excess of the national average amongst young Asian women (Balarajan & Raleigh 1993).

There is considerable concern that some black populations are being overdiagnosed with certain conditions (e.g. schizophrenia among Afro-Caribbean communities) (Burke 1984). Other ethnic minority populations appear to be under-represented in mental health services.

Black people are four times as likely as their white counterparts to reach a psychiatric hospital through the involvement of the police and to be compulsorily detained in hospital under the Mental Health Act legislation.

There are also measurable differences in the treatment that black patients receive compared with white patients. For black service users, there is greater reliance on physical treatment such as major tranquillizer and electroconvulsive therapy and they are less likely to be offered psychotherapy (Littlewood & Lipsedge 1982).

The commonly held view that all black people have self-supporting family networks and prefer to look after their own can have serious consequences for the aftercare of black people experiencing mental distress. Many patients are discharged into situations where the aftercare and support is not forthcoming. Carers usually do not have access to information about important issues such as the benefits and side-effects of medication, and about their rights as carers (Christie & Blunden 1991).

Racism is also considered as a contributory factor in the onset of illness among black people. Burke (1986) refers to the impact of racism on mental health as follows:

The evidence points to the conclusion that racism does lead to mental illness; firstly, by fermenting and maintaining social deprivation and so impairing chances of attaining mental health; secondly, by institutional factors which have the effect of withholding care; thirdly, by bully-boy/girl strategies of humiliating blacks into subordination and inflicting sado-masochistic attacks on them; and finally, when this fails, by implementing methods of social/medical control.

Fernando (1986) states: 'Racism causes depression by promoting blows to self-esteem, inducting experiences of loss, and placing individuals in a position of helplessness,' and he continues 'racism is not just an added stress to black and ethnic minorities, but a pathogen that generates depression in the individual'.

Even within the present climate of reform in services, it is still very questionable as to whether the very philosophies that underpin the changes will not in reality further work against black users of services.

One trend that has had a great impact on people who experience mental disorder is the move towards care in the community. Under the community care legislation voluntary organizations are playing an increasing role in providing services. This move could have severe effects on services for black people. Mainstream white voluntary organizations do not cater adequately for the needs of black people (Dungate 1984), being mainly based on the needs of the white majority population. However, the few black voluntary organizations that exist are too grossly underfunded and underresourced to take on this role. There will therefore be an increased burden on black families.

Criticism about other concepts and philosophies underpinning services are based on these very same principles. Services must recognize and address the effects of racism on the users and providers of services. Since service planners and managers are largely white it is possible that it is only those needs, wants and wishes of the mainstream society that will be considered as 'normal' or 'valued' experiences. An exercise carried out by a community mental handicap team in Harlesden, for example, demonstrated that what white staff would value for themselves would, in many cases, conflict with what black service users valued (Baxter et al 1990). The same can be expected in services for other client groups.

Refugees are amongst the most vulnerable section of the black and ethnic minority community. Compounding their similar experiences of racism, they also have less chance of learning the English language and thus communication barriers are often more acute. In addition their isolation from the wider community and lack of family support systems places additional stress on their lives and health. Adjusting to life in a new and strange country presents them with an enormous hurdle. Whatever their age, sex, family situation or cultural origin, coming to terms with the past, with the pain of separation and loss, as well as the uncertainties that lie ahead, can be a lifetime struggle. The acute dislocation that they experienced is intensified by the dearth of opportunities to improve their situation in Britain and the trauma of becoming and being a refugee can lead to particular mental health problems. Many refugees have the added problem of uncertainty about their position as immigrants: their status can be redefined as illegal at any time. Persons who have concerns about their relative legal status may be wary of any form of official intervention that might lead to investigation and many will be deterred from seeking treatment because it may involve questioning and disclosing important information to health staff.

What then, you may ask, about the response of black service providers? Should their presence in services not circumvent such negative interpretations? Black staff, especially those from backgrounds similar to service users, are indeed vital in providing services to a multiracial clientele. Experience shows that employing staff who can communicate with people in their own languages and who understand their cultures and share their experience of oppression can result in a dramatic increase in the take-up of services by potential clients who are from a similar background.

However, many black staff feel that their particular perspectives, experiences and skills are often not valued and that the initiatives and methods that they develop as more appropriate to the needs of black clients are seen as unprofessional by their colleagues and managers. Others feel that they are viewed as the 'expert' in caring for black service users and that black clients are 'dumped' on them to relieve white service providers of their professional responsibility. Furthermore, since service providers all undergo the same white-client-oriented training, not all black service providers therefore will have the necessary skills or feel confident and supported to work from an antiracist perspective. The majority of black staff tend to occupy low grade positions and their presence in services is not reflected at a managerial level. Very rarely, therefore, are black service providers in a position to become involved in informed decision making.

People with mental health difficulties often have to rely on others to plan their lives. Accordingly, the care programme approach enables service providers to recognize and meet individual needs. However, in many black communities the collectivity of the family and community may take precedence over the more self-centred individualism encouraged in majority white families. This difference in emphasis may be very important when working with users and carers from black communities.

Assessment of an individual's abilities is often based on white British norms, which bear little relationship to the everyday life of black people. Many standard assessment procedures involve approaches based on white, middle class lifestyle and experiences. A social worker of Afro-Caribbean background expressed these concerns as follows:

> The approach brought to assessment can be very Eurocentric. This can be very dangerous. A social worker I know was prepared to recommend that her Afro-Caribbean client was still very depressed and was not making progress. She based her decision on the fact that during a home visit the client offered her tea but had made her a cup of coffee instead. I had to explain to her that this was perfectly rational behaviour in many people of her generation, many of whom will use the term tea to refer to a warm drink.

The government required that clinical governance be established and in place by April 1999. This is the means by which health service organizations ensure the provision of quality clinical care by making individuals accountable for setting, maintaining and monitoring performance standards (DOH 1998).

At this time of great change when important decisions are being made and new systems and standards of support and care are being formulated, we should not miss this opportunity to design services to meet the needs of the whole community. The needs of black service users should not be considered as an afterthought or as additional or special, but should be enshrined within the concept of good professional practice. Connelly (1988) puts forward the following arguments in support of an antiracist perspective in services:

1. We all share a common humanity. To preserve this, all people should be given the opportunity to work for and enjoy all improvements in our society. Taking account of individual, racial and cultural diversity of needs is part of this process.

2. As tax and charge payers, black and ethnic minority people have a right as a matter of course to expect equal access to services which are appropriate and relevant to their needs. Planning and policies to enable this are crucial to social justice.

3. To maintain professional integrity, the competence of service providers hinges on their readiness, willingness and ability to apply existing and increasing knowledge to new situations.

4. Statutory and voluntary organizations have obligations under the Race Relations Act of 1976 to eliminate racial discrimination in employment and the provision of services.

5. Providing services which are appropriate to the needs of the population is making efficient and effective use of scarce resources. The multiracial community is indeed itself a resource and an opportunity to be utilized and cherished.

As we see what may be considered a return to organized care, particularly in a residential setting, it would follow that, because of the overrepresentation of black people in psychiatric services, there is likely to be a greater proportion entering residential care.

For inpatients, first and foremost, the issue of human rights should be addressed. It is now well recognized in services that all service users will need assistance in exercising their rights. As products of Western societies, we are all socialized into a racist culture and therefore have unwittingly accepted some of its attitudes, ideas and ways of doing things. We cannot change the past, but by recognizing its effects we can work towards developing higher professional standards in our practice.

For black users, therefore, attention should be focused on their right to be treated with dignity and respect as equal human beings. Those involved in providing services would find it helpful to address the following in relation to the design and maintenance of standards.

1. Is your relationship with black service users influenced by unhelpful racist stereotypes?

2. What measures have you taken to learn about and understand the nature of racism and how it affects your work practice?

3. Do you challenge racist jokes or slurs from other patients or colleagues?

4. What types of policies are there to ensure that where the client's rights are violated, the appropriate action takes place?

5. Black clients will need assistance to minimize destructive self-criticism and focus on their positive self worth.

FREEDOM OF CHOICE

Freedom of choice is an integral part of clients' rights. However, as professionals, we have the tendency to make assumptions about users' wants and wishes. This is particularly true for black users where white professionals are less likely to feel confident or take the time to get to know them as individuals. Even where there is some appreciation of the need to provide more individual and culturally specific forms of care, service providers often find it difficult to initiate dialogue in relation to a person's culture or racial origin. Further difficulties can arise when the service provider and service user do not speak the same language.

If choice is to become a reality for black service users, then it is important that the options and range of wants and needs are recognized. A priority must be to develop a closer working relationship with families. Included in this approach will be greater importance and confidence in working with and taking on board the views of a wider range of people, balancing the individuality, the position of the family and the long term relationships between them. Some ideas which will help to pave the way in developing a good partnership are listed below:

1. Black and ethnic minority people in the UK are most often British citizens by birth. To start off with questions about people's country of origin could give the impression that you feel that they do not belong in Britain.
2. Do not be blinded in your search for differences. Build up a rapport by acknowledging that you have things in common.
3. Build up a mutual trust and liking by reassuring patients and family members that you do not see their differences as a problem and that their differences will not detract from your ability to plan appropriately for their care.
4. Questions based on some existing knowledge indicate your interest and professional competence will increase as the client's and the family's confidence in you increases. For example, 'I know you are of the Muslim faith. Can you guide me on how I need to take account of this while caring for you?'
5. Do not rely too heavily on the cultural information in books that you have read because this could stereotype your clients. Use the information only as a guide to asking questions.

Unless they have a lot of experience in doing this, everyone has difficulty analysing what is second nature to them. Ask yourself the same question to make sure that you are not asking questions that are difficult to answer. There should be access to good interpreter services in those situations where there are language differences.

Personal hygiene, hair and skin care are very important to a person's feeling of well-being. It is important that staff are able to give the appropriate attention to these areas. The personal care and hygiene routines adopted at home should be followed:

1. Choice of either showers or baths should be available as not everyone would feel happy about sitting in a bath.
2. Support workers of the same sex may be preferred when carrying out intimate forms of care.
3. Differences in hair texture and skin colour have implications for routine physical assessment and care procedures. To use white hair and skin as the norm is dangerous.

Appropriate hair and skin care is still an area of gross neglect for black clients. Nurses and care assistants will need to appreciate that some people require their skin (and hair) to be moisturized, especially after procedures that deplete the body of moisture, such as a shampoo or a bath.

CULTURAL AND RELIGIOUS DIMENSIONS

Black service users in hospital will need assistance in maintaining their religious and cultural identity. Service providers should consistently work to the following criteria:

1. All clients should be addressed by their preferred name. Attempts should be made to pronounce accurately and record clients' names. These should not be changed to more English-sounding ones.
2. Clients should have the opportunity to have personal possessions which reflect their culture.
3. Appropriate and preferred dress is important in helping service users to maintain personal appearance. For example, nurses should be able to help an Asian woman to wrap her sari or a young Sikh man to wrap his turban.
4. Wall hangings, books, magazines, television programmes and other artefacts that portray positive images of a multiracial society should be utilized. Videos from most ethnic minority communities are now widely available and would be helpful.
5. The service user's religious beliefs (if any) should be established and respected. Assistance to make available places for those who may wish to practise their religion should be given. Mosques, Afro-Caribbean churches and Sikh gudwaras and

temples are welcoming to anyone who wishes to support members of their communities.

6. Catering arrangements should ensure the availability of a choice and range of foods to suit individual preferences. This should include those normally eaten at home. For example, vegetarian, halal and kosher meals should be available if required.

7. Service users should be encouraged to speak in their first language.

8. Daily routines should be of sufficient variety to promote positive identification with people's own racial and cultural background.

SUMMARY

The fact of disadvantage and discrimination as significant aspects of black and ethnic minority people's experience in Britain and the contribution of this to their mental health and welfare is now well established. The particular role of racism in contributing to the complexity of their experience of health care in terms of access to available care, equal quality of care and equal treatment is also widely acknowledged.

Within classical psychiatry can be found many of the markers of scientific racism, which have been in part responsible for poorer outcomes for this section of the population. To achieve competency and professionalism, services must therefore address the issue of racism.

Service providers will need to reflect consistently on their attitudes and values when delivering care and ensure that they develop the appropriate practical skills in relation to cultural and religious dimensions of the needs of people they serve. Without such efforts black and ethnic minority people will continue to have reduced access to services, experience unnecessary suffering and discomfort and probably death whilst the competence and professionalism of the service providers will remain suspect.

Antiracist practice therefore consistently:

◆ acknowledges the experience of racism and challenges this oppressive ideology within services

◆ values black and ethnic minority people, enhancing their self-esteem and identity, ensuring respect and dignity

◆ empowers black and ethnic minority users and carers, striving to ensure that services are strongly based on care and not control and facilitating them to exercise their rights

◆ involves users and carers in decisions about the planning and delivery of services

◆ renders itself accountable to local communities

◆ incorporates such perspectives in everything that it does

◆ develops policies and strategies to achieve these aims

◆ monitors performance against clear standards and goals.

DISCUSSION QUESTIONS

1. Is your relationship with black service users influenced by unhelpful stereotypes?
2. What measures have you taken to learn about and understand the nature of racism and how it affects your work practice?
3. Do you challenge racially discriminatory behaviour from patients or colleagues?
4. What is the policy on this in your workplace?
5. How do you measure up in terms of antiracist practice?
6. What skills and knowledge do you need to enhance your performance?
7. How can these be acquired?

RESOURCES

'Being white'—a video, 35 minutes. White people from different backgrounds talk about their understanding of the roots of racism and how they take account of it in their daily lives and work situations. Available from Albany Productions.

'Black'—a BBC film, 1983, 50 minutes. Examines the history of black and white relations and features young people talking about their experience of racism. Concord Films Council, 201 Felixstowe Road, Ipswich, Suffolk, IP3 9BJ. Tel. 01473 715 754.

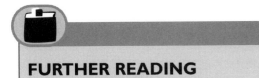

FURTHER READING

Baxter C 1985 Hair care of African, Afro-Caribbean and Asian hair types. National Extension College, Cambridge

Commission for Racial Equality 1976 Afro-Caribbean hair and skin care and recipes. Commission for Racial Equality, London

Fryer P 1984 Staying power. The history of black people in Britain. Pluto, London

Katz J 1978 White awareness. University of Oklahoma Press, Norman, Oklahoma

Mares P, Henley A, Baxter C 1985 Health care in multiracial Britain. National Extension College/Health Education Council, Cambridge

Shackman J 1985 The right to be understood—a handbook on working with, employment and training community interpreters. National Extension College, Cambridge

'The right to be understood'—a video about working interpreters. Available from the National Extension College, 18 Brooklands Avenue, Cambridge CB2 2HN.

'Black and in care'—in this video children talk about their experiences of being in care and how they have and are trying to overcome their difficulties. Available from Black and In Care Steering Group, c/o Children's Legal Centre, 20 Compton Terrace, London N1 2UN. Tel. 020 7359 6251.

REFERENCES

Balarajan R, Raleigh S V 1993 Ethnicity and health: a guide to the NHS. Department of Health, London

Baxter C, Poonia K, Ward L, Nadishaw Z 1990 Double discrimination—issues and services for people with learning difficulties from black and ethnic minority communities. King's Fund Centre/Commission for Racial Equality, London

Brown C 1984 Black and white Britain. The third PSI survey. Gower, London

Burke A 1984 Racism and mental illness. In: Cox J (ed) Transcultural psychiatry. Croom Helm, London, pp 135–157

Burke A 1986 Racism, prejudice and mental illness. In: Cox J (ed) Transcultural psychiatry. Croom Helm, London, pp 139–157

Christie Y, Blunden R 1991 Is race on your agenda? Improving mental health services for people from black and minority groups. King's Fund Centre, London

Connelly N 1988 Care in a multiracial community. Policy Studies Institute, London

Cope R, Ndequa D 1991 Ethnic difference in admission to regional secure units. Journal of Forensic Psychiatry 1:365–378

DOH (Department of Health) 1998 A first class service. Quality in the new NHS. Health Services Circular 198:113

Dungate M 1984 A multicultural society, the role of national voluntary organisations. Bedford Square Press, London

Fernando S 1986 Depression and ethnic minorities. In: Cox J (ed) Transcultural psychiatry. Croom Helm, London, pp 107–138

Fernando S 1988 Race, culture and psychiatry. Croom Helm, London

Harrison G, Owens D, Holton A, Neilson D, Boot D 1988 A prospective study of severe mental disorder in Afro-Caribbean patients. Psychological Medicine 18:643–657

HEA (Health Education Authority) 1994 Black and ethnic minority groups in England. Health and lifestyle. HEA, London

Littlewood R, Lipsedge M 1982 Aliens and alienists. Penguin, Harmondsworth

McNaught A 1985 Race and health care in the United Kingdom. Occasional paper 2. Health Education Council, London

Macpherson W 1999 The Stephen Lawrence Inquiry. Report of an inquiry by Sir William Macpherson of Cluny. Cmnd 4262–1. Stationery Office, London

Modood T, Berthoud R, Lattery T et al 1997 Ethnic minorities in Britain. Diversity and disadvantaged. PSI, London

NACRO (National Association for the Care and Resettlement of Offenders) 1989 Race and criminal justice. NACRO, London

Nirza V 1986 Race: the ingredient of good practice. In: Philpo T (ed) The residential opportunity? The Wagner report and after. Reed Business Publishing/Community Care, Wallington

OPCS (Office of Population Censuses and Surveys) 1993 Ethnic group of residents. OPCS, London

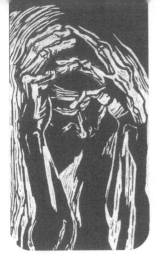

Chapter Sixteen

Women and mental health care provision

Clancy Borastero Karen Rea

AIMS

- ◆ To locate women's experience of mental health and distress within a historical, sociological, psychological and physiological framework
- ◆ To provide the opportunity for mental health practitioners to examine and explore their own professional practice and local, national and international policy and provision
- ◆ To utilize women's life experiences to understand the impact of gender insensitive services upon their lives and their experience of mental distress

KEY ISSUES

Historical perspectives of women's mental health and the impact on current service provision

The control of therapy and treatment in the health service

Women's experiences of power and power abuse

The impact of abuse on women's lives

Strategies for treatment and service provision and the importance of women's control over these

INTRODUCTION

The purpose of this chapter is not to tell mental health practitioners how to treat their clients who are women. The observations and concepts offered here can best be used to inform our practice. Theory is most useful when it affords us the opportunity to see what we otherwise might miss and then follow that up in our work and personal lives. Hopefully and ideally, what you read here will remain in the unconscious or preconscious until triggered by a real event. When it emerges it will be to serve its function—that of helping to explain and understand. What will be explored is how mental health care provision has evolved, from what basic premises, and how particular views about women have influenced the type of care and responses to mental distress that women as a gender often experience. All women are not the same, just as all men have individual traits, attitudes and behaviours. Different life experiences will affect both women's and men's opportunities and responses.

Underlying all discussion contained here is the fundamental belief that the experience of mental health is that of a continuum. At one end is optimal mental health and well-being whereby individuals' life is in relative harmony or they have the necessary skills and resources to maintain balance. At the opposite end is severe mental distress where individuals do not have the skills and resources to cope with all the stresses of life. The reality is that many people will experience movement up and down the continuum at least at some point during their lives. This model will be used to explore women's experiences of mental health and ill health, and their responses and differing abilities to deal with the factors that influence mental health.

Women's position and role in Western industrialized societies are of relevance to nurses and health care practitioners because it is women who have the major responsibility for their families' care (Doyal 1994, Glendinning & Millar 1993). If we take a purely functionalist view of the role of women as the care providers this means that we should therefore ensure that their health and well-being are of primary importance. Even in today's

society where women are increasingly becoming part of the workforce, the traditional role of carer still falls mainly to women (Miles 1991). The role of women as carers has been found to have profound effects on their health (Glendinning & Millar 1993, Miles 1991), both physical and mental. From an empirical perspective as formal carers, they comprise 90% of the nursing workforce and the majority of workers in the national health service as a whole (Clay 1987). Of informal (unpaid) carers two-thirds are estimated to be women. The role of the unpaid carer is of increasing importance in English society as the 1990 National Health Service and Community Care Act expressly identifies informal carers as a crucial element of community care. Service provision, according to the Act, should function to support carers and their dependants in order that the disabled, elderly and ill can remain within their community. If women as carers are therefore to be pivotal in the success of community care policies, it would seem to be common sense then that their physical, psychological and emotional welfare would also be of equal importance and high on the list of priorities, for service planners and providers alike. The importance of the family in modern society also means that women are responsible for the welfare of their family, from birth to death.

Yet is women's health and welfare the primary factor behind the design and provision of health care? Certainly there are many services identified for women; in health there are a number of services that would appear on first glance to provide health care facilities for women. Obstetrics, gynaecology, women's health clinics, reproductive technologies are all examples of this. Screening services for women's health problems such as breast and cervical cancer have been available for a number of years. However, what these services represent is a patriarchal and medical preoccupation with women's reproductive function, which serves to reinforce the patriarchal belief of women's role in society as being that of a mother and carer, and it could be argued this is more about maintaining the status quo in terms of roles and functions in society than about keeping women well (Ussher 1991). The stressful nature of being a mother and carer and its traditionally coercing nature has in the main been ignored by professionals (Barnes & Maple 1992). The work and influence of the women's health movement since the 1960s have emphasized the stressful nature of their patriarchally ascribed role (Graham 1992).

There is a recognition in today's society that stress can lead to mental distress. Feminists have pointed out that the stress women increasingly experience through what Doyal (1994) has identified as the dual burden of women, that of paid and unpaid work, needs to be recognized in any exploration of all aspects of their health.

In exploring women's mental health there is a need to examine historical, cultural, medical and patriarchal beliefs about women as human beings. Feminists have identified that misogyny and sexism, like racism, influences and informs social beliefs about what it is to be a woman. In the same way, however, the mental distress that women do experience needs to be recognized and woman-centred approaches to helping women identified and used.

To be a woman is to be 'the other'. Women live in a world controlled by men, for men. Accepted historical and present-day knowledge is dominated by men's thoughts and beliefs. This is what it means for a woman living in the world. In mental health, as in other aspects of health, man is the 'normal' and woman the 'abnormal'. Character traits that are admired and considered to be the more positive and superior are typically those ascribed to men. They include physical strength, emotional control, logical and rational thought, aggressiveness and ambition. 'Normal' women's characteristics are the opposite: passive, more in touch with their emotions, 'natural' nurturers and carers. As children, each gender learns which are the most appropriate for them. Hence the little boys learn to play with practical toys and not to cry, and the girl children learn to 'care' and ascribe to particular feminine appearances and behaviours through their toys. This is in fact 'learnt' and ascribed behaviour rather than 'natural' (Ussher 1991). Women and men who do not conform to these characteristics are 'different' and 'abnormal'. Conflict arises especially in women's lives in

the late twentieth century when choice, or economic necessity, either forces them to take on the dual role, or they choose to be 'different'.

HISTORICAL PERSPECTIVES OF WOMEN'S MENTAL HEALTH

To understand and explore both how much theoretical knowledge and discourse have been formulated about women and mental health care provision for them, we first need to look back in history. Although the Victorian era has perhaps been the most influential in producing medical theory, which has come to inform social life about women and mental illness, there is evidence from a much earlier period in history that women are treated differently from men in terms of their mental and physical health.

Elaine Showalter (1985) has identified how male-held beliefs about the role of women led to psychiatric practices in the nineteenth century that are still influential today. The role of middle class women in Victorian England was to be an asset to her husband. She was expected to look decorative, to be entertaining but not clever, and to ensure the smooth running of her husband's household. Medical beliefs of the time argued that too much education atrophied a woman's uterus and therefore affected her ability to bear children (Showalter 1985, Ussher 1991). Much of the psychiatric knowledge of the time was gained at the expense of women. They outnumbered men in the asylums by almost two to one. They were diagnosed as hysterics, a term which came from the Greek word '*hysterus*' meaning 'womb'. Much of the medical practice for mental distress at this time centred around curing the women by mutilating and removing parts of their sexual organs— including clitoridectomies and excising the labia (both of which were performed in order to prevent the woman experiencing sexual pleasure, either alone or with her male partner) (Ehrenreich & English 1979). The predominant view of psychiatrists and psychologists alike was that women's madness in this time stemmed from their sexual nature (Walsh 1978, Weinstein 1987). The Madonna/whore dichotomy was acted out during the Victorian times across the classes. Virtuous middle class women did not have sexual desires, whereas working class women were attributed with coarser and more base feelings, and promiscuous natures (Ehrenreich & English 1979). Women were seen as more vulnerable to mental disorder than men because of the instability of their reproductive organs. The link between uterus and brain was then used to remove the potential for women to attain success in the professions and in politics.

Much 'treatment' for 'madwomen' in the 1800s centred around the reinforcement and retrieval of women's 'natural' role in Victorian society. A class analysis also has to be included in any discussion of Victorian ideals about the 'normal' woman. Feminist discourses about historical perspectives on women and mental health has highlighted how the ideals of womanhood as identified in medical ideology and writings focused on women in the middle and upper social classes (Showalter 1985). The ideal of womanhood as a passive adornment to her husband's life applied only to the middle and upper social classes. Indeed, women in the lower social class were considered to be a completely separate group, who were much cruder, physically stronger and totally lacking in the feminine 'virtues' of their 'superiors'.

Charlotte Gilman Perkins, a woman married to a middle class man in the nineteenth century, wrote about her imposed removal from society by her physician husband (Showalter 1985, Ussher 1991). However, for some Victorian women (women who were married or related to men from the middle classes, that is), this was a voluntary choice, as they preferred to withdraw from a society where they felt they had no useful function. Many women ended up in 'asylums', often involuntarily, as they were committed by their husbands and/or male doctors.

The emergence of psychology allied to medicine and the ascent of psychiatry as a high status branch of medicine during this era also had a profound effect on women's lives. Much current psychological and psychiatric thought has evolved from the early work of men such as Freud. Past and present psychological studies are inadequate in their knowledge and understanding of the psy-

chology of women. There is a fundamental flaw in Freud's theory of penis envy in that he believed women to be essentially castrated males (Freud 1982). This implies that girls start life with a 'boyish outlook', which not only makes for a difficult reorientation at puberty but more importantly condemns them, as women, to lifelong envy of the male sex. Freud reached this conclusion without taking into consideration that many of the facts that led him to this belief were the product of cultural attitudes, and according to Schaef (1992), constitutes what she terms 'the white male system'. She states that this system controls almost every aspect of our Western culture. It makes our laws, runs our economy, sets our salaries and decides if we will go to war or remain at home.

Both Barnes & Maple (1992) and Ussher (1991) point out, though, that developments in the mental health arena in terms of treatment options during the twentieth century and those which are popular today are still dominated by very fixed patriarchal and sometimes downright misogynistic views of women. As Barnes & Maple (1992) comment, through all the 'innovations' and developments that the mental health field has both generated and experienced, medicine and medical ideology have remained dominant. At the start of the new millenium it is still the consultant psychiatrist who holds the purse strings in relation to mental health services and they still strongly control, influence and gatekeep over what is 'acceptable' and 'scientifically sound' practice.

Developments in mental health treatments, it would appear, have developed from what it could be argued are elaborate and at times highly complex theories to explain mental distress. The preoccupation with psychological reasons that dominated the nineteenth century gave way to even more highly elaborate psychological reasons and the birth of therapy. Just as physical treatments such as the use of ECT and psychosurgery dominated the latter part of the nineteenth century and first part of the twentieth century, so has the use of psychoanalysis and other 'talking' therapies dominated the middle and latter part of the twentieth century. Yet throughout all this what has remained dominant is medical control over what constitutes mental health care and provision. At times we have seen the use of several 'theories', a recent example being the attempt to discover the genetic marker for extreme violence, which it could be said to be a direct return to the beliefs of Lombroso in the nineteenth century (Ussher 1991).

To dismiss, therefore, the historical basis to the gendered nature of mental health service provision, and to argue that contemporary mental health services are based on gender neutral ideologies, would be extremely naive. Szasz (1977) argues that the principles and ideologies that formulated policy and practice are still prevalent today. A classic example of this is the diagnosis of hysteria. Women far outweigh men in the diagnosis of the hysterical and neurotic disorders. Where the diagnosis of hysteria is applied to men, it is often in situations where their 'masculinity' is being questioned. Hence, as Barnes & Maple (1992) report, gay men with AIDS may well end up being labelled as 'hysterics'.

CONTROL OF THERAPY AND TREATMENT IN THE HEALTH SERVICE

Allen (1992, p. 67) suggests that a: cursory examination of mental health statistics suggests that women are mentally sicker than men. We know that women outnumber men in inpatient hospital statistics, a situation which has descended from the Victorian era (Showalter 1985). It would appear then to be logical that, if women outnumber men in mental health statistics, then the services provided would be especially sensitive to their needs. Yet is this so? Many writers (e.g. Allen 1992, Showalter 1985) have argued that, far from being either gender sensitive or even gender neutral, psychiatry operates on a punitive framework for women, and that it has at times been justifiedly accused of being misogynistic (Ehrenreich & English 1979, Showalter 1985, Ussher 1991). Certainly historical and anecdotal evidence shows little understanding of the importance of women's lives in creating and maintaining illness, and also demonstrates a strong punitive element and

approach. Historically the removal and excision of women's sexual organs with the intention of denying them sexual pleasure and enforcing male ideas about women's normal sexuality have been excused on the grounds of curing their 'madness'.

These practices have their contemporaries in latter-day mental health and women's health services. The removal of women's uteruses during the menopause and the use of 'new' technologies such as hormone replacement therapy (HRT) have often been justified and medically diagnosed on the grounds of 'curing' middle-aged women's mental health problems. Yet, as feminist women's health activists have pointed out, the cause of women's mental distress during their 'middle' years may be more likely to be about their changing roles and functions (or perhaps their feelings of redundancy) during this time.

This is not the only example of the medicalization of sexuality and sexual life. Nurses working as family-planning advisors sometimes encourage women of colour in a inner city area to use a long-acting contraceptive (Depo-Provera), which once in place could not be removed (and which had been banned in their country of origin—the United States). The rationale for this is that the women who came to the family-planning clinic were often 'feckless' and 'could not be trusted' to use other forms of contraceptives correctly. Asked if the potential long term effects of this drug had been fully explained to the women opting for the treatment, the replies received were typically either 'no', because only a small number of women would suffer them anyway, or 'that was the responsibility of the doctor when he/she saw the woman'.

Chesler (1972) identified four premises that run through all the theories of psychiatry and apply to most clinical practices. These premises reflect how mental health professionals see women and how women have been taught to see themselves:

◆ everybody is crazy
◆ while everybody is crazy, women are crazier
◆ male homosexuality is sick and lesbians don't exist

◆ in order for a woman to be a real woman she has got to be a mother, and once you've become a mother everything that goes wrong with your family is your fault.

How then did these premises translate into service provision and what were the consequences for women with mental health problems?

◆ There is little or no understanding that women constitute an oppressed group in our culture and that oppression has negative psychological effects on women.

◆ Mental health professionals do little to reduce the professional distance and power imbalance between themselves and their clients, and even less to demystify the therapeutic process.

◆ Stereotypes of men and women, although limiting and unhealthy, are commonly held by health professionals and the lay person.

◆ There is little or no acknowledgment that the client is the expert on her own experience and

CASE STUDY: FLEUR'S STORY

Fleur, the younger of two daughters from an interracial marriage, began having problems with her body image during her final year at college. Although she was a beautiful, vibrant and intelligent young woman, she had a distorted image of herself. Her position became critical when she was having four or five showers in the morning as a result of perceiving herself as ugly and unpresentable when she looked in the mirror and, instead of correcting what she was unhappy about, she had to undo it (by having another shower) and start all over again. This went on for 6 months before her parents and sibling began to see the negative outcomes for her. By this time she had developed a fear of leaving the house and, when she did so, needed constant reassurance about how she looked. Her lack of concentration in relation to her studies resulted in her teacher advising that she withdraw from examinations rather than add to the stress levels she was already exhibiting just getting to college.

Fleur finally disclosed to her mother that she was finding life unbearable, was no longer able to control the anxieties she had through the rituals she was performing and had started to consider ending her life. Her mother immediately arranged an appointment with the GP. Having gotten to a point where she could acknowledge that something was wrong, and that she needed help, the GP, on hearing the reason for her visit, initially went into a lecture about the function of emergency appointments (that they could not last any longer than 5 minutes) and finally, under

pressure from the mother, agreed to refer Fleur to the psychiatric services at the local general hospital. Because the GP omitted to confer directly with the psychiatrist on call at the hospital, Fleur spent 4 hours waiting in the accident and emergency department to recount her distress to the doctor there who then referred her to the on-call psychiatrist, who undertook an hour-long interrogation (Fleur's perception).

At the end of the day, having seen three doctors, Fleur felt that she was wasting everyone's time as nobody had told her that she was not the only person who had these symptoms, and that there was help she could and would receive.

Within 6 months following this initial referral, Fleur had seen a psychiatrist three times, and was referred for counselling (this never got off the ground because the practice counsellor was on sick leave for 6 months). She was prescribed three different antidepressives, which were not effective, and a referral to the psychological services at the general hospital had not brought about an appointment.

Fleur's mother eventually located a counsellor, in private practice, who worked with adolescents and young adults with body image problems. She contracted to work with Fleur for 12 sessions. At the end of these sessions, Fleur has started to engage in a social life again, her ritualistic behaviours have reduced, but most of all she is not further hampered in her 'battle' by the members of the caring professions who appeared to require her to identify her 'fit' into *their* system.

is the best judge of what is right for her. (The nurse/therapist/psychiatrist/psychologist has a certain expertise related to knowledge and skills.)

◆ Women are socialized always to put others' needs first.

◆ Conforming to the adjustment model of mental health encourages women to conform to social expectations or norms.

In the past, and to a lesser extent at present, there was a lack of awareness and/or acknowledgment that women constitute an oppressed group in our culture. For some women, greater equity in both the personal and the political, or the private and public, spheres of their lives has led to positive experiences of mental health throughout their life. Yet to 'have it all'—that is, to obtain a good education, work and for many also run a home and have families, often brings its own stress. As Barnes & Maple (1992) comment, for many women the reality of employment both inside and outside the home means working in excess of 70 hours per week, and average of 11 hours a week more than male counterparts. It is not only culturally determined attitudes of men about women's sex role that have contributed to the lack of understanding of women, but much which even women themselves may attribute to the fact of their sex can be explained as a result of cultural pressure. This includes the acceptance by many women that women's inferiority is based on biological facts. Such a concept has obvious advantages for men, which make it more difficult for them to relinquish their beliefs, and, on the other hand, many women also have difficulties in freeing themselves from this idea, since their sex role socialization from childhood has supported this attitude. The con trick of society is that often the rules purport to suit everybody when in fact they usually serve the interest of one section in society. The oppressor needs to do little to control the oppressed because the oppressed will self-limit their own behaviour. Power of some sort is central to all relationships but, because people are accustomed to thinking of power as either manipulation or coercion, any discussion of power makes them feel uncomfortable. They try to pretend that it is not an issue.

WOMEN'S EXPERIENCES OF POWER AND POWER ABUSE

Before women can be empowered we need first to understand their experiences of powerlessness and oppression. For women, power and its use are complex: first, they experience power and power abuse through child and adulthood experiences, but in addition the coping mechanisms adopted by women to combat this oppression can take the form of the use of covert power.

The experiences of the abuse of power of women as adults and children have included:

◆ sexual assault or abuse in childhood
◆ rape or sexual assault as adult women
◆ violence or threat of violence
◆ inablity to speak through fear or rage
◆ racial abuse or exploitation
◆ lack of control over their bodies or lives.

These experiences need to be heard and understood, as they form the basis of each woman's experience of power and powerlessness. Within this context, though, there has to be a recognition that women do not constitute a 'homogeneous' group. Women of differing social classes and ethnic backgrounds experience different treatments at the hands of mental health professionals and indeed may, and often do, have differing reasons for their mental distress. Studies by Ussher (1991) and Barnes & Maple (1992) both highlight how women from lower social classes and women of colour are more likely to end up within the mental health care services, just as with the bias for men. An understanding of women's experiences of power and powerlessness informs us of the reasons for the strategies women use to survive. Their methods may in themselves appear to be destructive—for instance, in their strategies such as self-harm and in eating disorders (and are in fact often pathologized as further examples of the woman's 'madness'). Women report using strategies such as 'cutting up' (lacerations, incisions, gouging, etc. of their flesh) as a way of managing their pain and anger when it becomes intolerable. In this way an understanding of the covert use of power often employed by women can be gained. For women, the process of remembering and telling of their experience of power abuse may generate feelings of anger, pain and fear (Walker 1994).

Powerlessness

Sexual and social inequalities are created by imbalances of power; to understand the experiences of women's powerlessness, we need to explore the power dynamics. The 'naturalness' and 'other' experiences of women and their social roles can often lead to women expressing their feelings of distress in hidden, indirect and masked ways. In order to understand the 'problems' that women have we need to have an understanding of the power processes. For example, a woman who injures herself may be expressing internal rage and pain, or dieting disorders may be the woman's way of expressing her experiences of powerlessness in a society that values thinness as 'beauty'. For women, expressions of madness may provide them with the vehicle for speaking the unspeakable. Conveying pain and distress in indirect ways can alleviate or minimize the retaliation for not being a 'normal' woman. For women the social pressures that mould their very beings are often the processes that prevent their distress and pain being heard and acknowledged.

Women are expected to be 'good' mothers; their biological make-up informs their social role in a patriarchal society. They are 'natural' nurturers and carers, and their social identity is often dependent on this. The cause of the powerlessness they experience is directly related to this. Their experiences of sexual and physical abuse, assault and violence, rage and fear, and their silence, are attributal to their social roles and identities. In order to understand the processes that silence women we need to know about the causes of their oppression.

Empowerment

Understanding of women's experience of power and power abuses needs to be the starting point for empowering women. Feminists have highlighted how, in the sexual area of gender relations, rape is about power, not about sex. The social relations that exist between the genders need to be fully understood before there can be any meaningful discussion about empowering women. Denial of access to power and the use of it to women needs to be explored from the context of social processes. Making these social processes visible to and by women provides a way for making visible these power processes. The ways in which women use covert power, such as alcohol abuse, withdrawal and self-injury, can then be understood as just such a method of expressing power, given that access to the power attributed to men is denied them. This knowledge can be the beginning for women of understanding and valuing the other sources of personal power that they hold.

Empowering women should not be about asking them to give up their indirect power bases, but asking them to understand the costs of such actions, and why such methods have been used. This should provide the opportunity to explore and establish other sources of personal power they have. 'Feeling at home with our bodies' is about emotional empowerment. Emotional empowerment is about women finding their own voice, understanding why and not feeling shame about the indirect power they have used, lessening blame, feeling safe to speak, managing their rage in a way that both acknowledges their anger and allows it to be expressed in a safe way, feeling confirmed, being hurt, angry and sad about experiences of loss and abuse, and establishing rights and entitlements (Brown & Harris 1978).

To do this, though, one needs to relinquish one form of power (even if this has been damaging to the woman), which may too threatening to a woman if emotional empowerment has not fully taken place. It may be, therefore, that the woman continues to need to speak through her body until she feels fully confident and able to speak her voice. This change also requires the woman to acknowledge and understand the risks she is taking. Such risks of empowerment should not be underestimated; for women who wish to change the risks can be very real—that is, retaliation. The different forms that this can take (e.g. economic, physical, emotional) may vary for different women, but may have the same consequence: fear of change. Therefore it is important that practical and emotional preparations are made—for example, forming an 'escape plan', and that the woman identifies the sources of support that will be available to her. What should and must be of paramount importance is the acceptance of the woman's own knowledge of her safety and the need for change to be at the woman's own pace. Workers need to understand that women's caution and reluctance to move forward is based on their experience of being at risk. We need to listen carefully to the reasons for this caution.

Empowerment is also about helping women to gain access to more direct forms of personal power. This may include gaining access to housing, employment or employment training, and self-defence workshops. For women, often the major source of empowerment is through listening to each other in workshops and groups. The risks of moving towards the use of more explicit power may be too great for some women, even if the costs they experience in terms of mental health problems and self-harm are very high. To witness and accept this decision or choice can be very painful, and is a reminder that the costs of inequality for women can be very high.

DEPRESSION

A woman's description of her depression is as follows:

> I just wanted to sit and cry. I don't want to sleep or I'll sleep all the time. I don't want to be alive, but it would take too much effort to kill myself. Everything becomes completely out of control, it all goes too fast. It's like it is rushing on and dragging me kicking and screaming behind. It's like a dull empty ache inside; I can feel it physically. Then it can grow until it's an awful, awful pain and it takes over my whole self. It's like an enormous painful hole. And people say 'Well, do something to distract yourself'. If you're in really awful pain it won't go away, you can't ignore it, because it becomes you—it is you. And it can get beyond pain, to a point where everything disappears, and I have disappeared and it's like I'm in space, in total darkness, unattached to anything, wandering in circles in the dark.

(This account appears in Walker 1990, p. 101)

As a mood, depression is part of normal human living. The distinction between normal mood and abnormal depression is not always clear and psychiatrists do not always agree on the full range of emotional phenomena to be diagnosed as pathological. The fact that the depressions involve an accentuation in intensity and/or duration of otherwise normal emotions has mixed consequences for clinical judgement. On the one hand, this fact promotes the empathic understanding of mental health practitioners to the client's difficulties. Almost all human beings experience unhappy, sad, depressed and discouraged periods in their life, and therefore it is easy to acknowledge the client's emotional state and empathize with their distress. Conversely, this very familiarity sometimes interferes, making clinical assessment and differential diagnosis difficult in that there may be a lack of appreciation that the client has crossed the boundary area between the normal and abnormal. Very often the outcome is that mental health practitioners may tend to minimize the severity of affective disorders even when precipitating stressful events are apparent.

In severe forms, most depressed states are easily judged as pathological by criteria of intensity, pervasiveness, persistence and interference with usual social and bodily functioning. Considering that women have difficulty in having their views validated within the psychiatric system, that diagnosis includes an assessment of social functioning, that said social functioning is often defined by a patriarchal system that oppresses women and has expectations that women be subservient and dependent and any woman who cannot meet the 'ideal' and expresses her distress places herself at risk of being labelled depressed. Feely (1995) comes to the conclusion that depression is the medicalization of a normal response by women to their experiences in society. Taking a life cycle approach, women may (and often do) experience depression at times when their socially ascribed roles cause conflict within themselves. The classic example of this is the middle ages of a woman's life when her child-rearing 'function' ceases to exist and she (and society) questions her value. The role of mother and worker can and often does cause conflict, with an added stress of what Doyal

(1994) has termed the 'dual burden' that most women carry: that of worker and carer.

The most widely held theory about depression relates its onset and quality to the stress accompanying loss and separation. This theory is based upon the close similarities between the normal emotional reactions to loss and separation and the clinical state of depression. In recent years, the concept of loss has been extended to include not only separation and death, but also symbolic losses such as children leaving home and other forms of threats to self-esteem and impairment of interpersonal relations. Women who have experienced profound neglect, deprivation and abuse as children will be chronically depressed. This deep sorrow may not manifest itself with the classic symptomatology but may present itself as alcoholism, deviance, violence and aggression and women will find themselves at the hands of the criminal justice system, which is a whole other chapter, and their mental health needs will still be unmet.

> Depression in women almost always goes hand in hand with rage turned against self. The depressed woman suffers, and she has learned to use her depression as a weapon, making sure those around her suffer as well. Unfortunately she is often destroyed in the process.
> Schaef 1992

Research such as Brown & Harris's (1978) famous studies on depression among women found that precipitating factors were often related to experiences such as the loss of one's mother in childhood, having three or more children under 14 at home, no close confiding relationship and no paid job outside the home. From this we can deduce that 'women's work' is harmful to their health. Brown & Harris's study also needs to be viewed from a class perspective. Glendinning & Millar (1993) and Graham (1992) both identified that, for many women from working class backgrounds and women who live in poverty, opportunities to have time away from their family is extremely restricted, leading to both feelings and actual experience of social isolation and deprivation.

The statistics indicate that more women than men are diagnosed as suffering from depression. Sane (1993) reported that, in the United Kingdom, 3–4% of men and 7–8% of women suffer from moderate to severe depressive illness at any one time and Ussher (1991) asserts that women are more likely than men to be diagnosed as depressed. This would appear to be a significant mental health problem for women, but statistics that are based on the use of psychiatric services are not an accurate indicator of incidence (Feely 1995). He argues that women are predisposed to a diagnosis of depression because of the ongoing construction of the female and her role in society.

According to Johnstone (1993) certain life events may predispose some women to developing mental illness. Women without any adult companions who lack social supports or who are engaged in full-time motherhood appear to be more vulnerable to depression. One life event, and the ensuing emotional responses, that has been medicalized and pathologized is that of childbirth. Women who might be reacting to a number of stresses at that time, the shock and burden of responsibility, the loss of independence and earning power, and who may be reacting to these stresses by exhibiting emotional responses that range from general feelings of unhappiness or anger, can be pathologized and dismissed by being labelled as suffering from 'postnatal depression'. The term 'depression' neatly categorizes the woman, simultaneously denying her any right to her feelings, or any recourse to positive action that might alleviate them. Yet the other side of this double-edged sword, in which women are more likely to be pathologized for their complaints, is that women's concerns are invariably ignored, or dismissed as not being important (Ussher 1992).

An explanation of women's greater prospect of being diagnosed as depressed or suffering from a psychoneurotic disorder may be that the feminine gender role is more compatible with the sick role than is the masculine role. A woman's complaint of depression, insomnia or nervous breakdown has a higher degree of social acceptability than similar complaints on the part of a man.

SEXUAL ABUSE AND ADULT SURVIVORS

To understand how abused women react in adolescence and adulthood to childhood sexual abuse it is important to recognize the context of their abuse. In a society such as ours, in which men are well established in positions of power, misuse of this power over girls and women from early life onwards has long-lasting influence. Women's lack of power comes from the dominant position given to men in our society and from men's physical strength and greater propensity for violent response.

Women who have been abused in childhood may reach adulthood never having talked about their experiences. They may present themselves for help for all sorts of other problems: sexual dysfunction, eating disorders, depression, substance abuse or self-injury, or they may get into trouble with the law. Uncovering the fundamental trigger experience may be a lengthy process that will uncover fears, anxieties, neediness, hurt and rage. Working with women who have survived abuse is also about working with very hurt little girls who have been betrayed by those they thought they could trust. At that time they were unable to control what was happening to them. In many ways they had no power but they often had so much invested in them: the power to break up the family, if the abuser is within the family, the power to make the family fatherless if she broke her silence. Coming to terms with how much of their childhood they have lost and grieving for it can be a very painful process. The basic issues in therapy are disclosure, boundaries and working with the hurt child.

DOMESTIC VIOLENCE

One of the primary goals of therapy with women is centred around the empowerment of victims. The process of violence, be it sexual, psychological or physical, removes power and control from an individual. Feelings of powerlessness are closely associated with low self-esteem, anxiety, depression and somatic problems.

The following principles are basic to the empowerment of victims:

◆ a commitment to the belief that women and men are inherently equal
◆ an egalitarian approach to the practitioner–client relationship; the client is viewed as an equal partner rather than a helpless recipient of interventions
◆ focus during interventions on the enhancement of the victim's power
◆ focus during feedback and discussion on the victim's strengths and abilities
◆ respect for the victim's ability to understand her own experience
◆ family interventions that change destructive roles and expectations within the family system
◆ a willingness to state clear value positions about domestic violence and sexual abuse
◆ established social networks to decrease isolation and secrecy.

Success is measurable when the victims have:

◆ recognized that they are not to blame for the abuse and violence of others
◆ ended the denial and minimalization of psychological, physical and sexual violence against women and children
◆ demonstrated an awareness of strengths, skills and competencies
◆ re-established a sense of power over their own lives
◆ verbalized their right to express their own needs and to satisfy them.

TREATMENT OF CHOICE

If women's health problems are located in psychosocial stress and distress then the intervention of choice must be psychosocial. Unhappiness in respect of their relationship, domestic, social and political circumstances forms the bases of many women's problems. This unhappiness when medicalized and regarded as 'women's problems' only adds to the distress experienced. The use of feminist therapy and women's self-help groups, which seek to empower women to be active partners in their mental health care, are recommended. Such approaches involve listening not only to what women are saying about their distress, but also to what the themes in their communication and behaviour may be indicating with regard to their needs (Barnes & Maple 1992).

Mental health practitioners, like other professionals, have tended to be drawn from those groups in the population that have achieved sociopolitical power. These dominant groups often assume that their ways of behaving, aspirations and values are the only correct and intelligent ones (Showalter 1985, Ussher 1991). Even members of the dominant group who are less ethnocentric are apt to find it difficult to understand someone whose ways of communicating, thinking and living differ radically from their own. With the best will in the world, such a therapeutic situation is full of dangers and is apt to be more frustrating than helpful.

Although writing about counselling and psychotherapy, Walker (1990) attempts to identify whether practitioners really acknowledge the complexities of women's lives and incorporate this awareness into their work. She infers that the following groups may exist:

1. Those who are blissfully unaware that issues such as gender exist; whereas this situation may be acceptable to the practitioner, the same may not apply to the client.

2. Those who are aware but think themselves immune from falling into stereotypical traps. They intervene with clients with the belief that if they concentrate on the individual in a person-centred way they somehow become estranged from their gender. The problem is that gender as an issue is very often not confronted or acknowledged.

3. Those who have a theoretical knowledge gleaned during a training, which invariably did acknowledge the centrality of gender in the planning of courses but in the delivery of the course it was an 'add-on' rather than an awareness that should have been interwoven into the very fabric of the course material.

4. Those who acknowledge gender as a very significant issue. They have a political as well as a

psychological awareness and work within the context of both.

Tennov (1976) puts forward the view that a political and feminist stance clashes with a therapeutic approach, and that the former invalidates the latter. The argument has been mainly aimed at therapists who maintain that internal change is sufficient. Because of this perspective, traditional therapists are more likely to see pathology in normal behaviour. Yet psychotherapy has justifiably been criticized for expecting change to come from within, without recognizing the importance of the structural restrictions placed on an individual by any given society. A political and feminist stance would encourage empowerment of women that would recognize the need for change both at the macro and micro levels of women's lives, both external and internal.

Greenspan (1983) states that:

> As long as basic structural inequities of power exist in society, large numbers of women will manifest symptoms of this inequality. Working to correct social inequities is, in the long run, the only final cure for most forms of female emotional distress. Therapy can help people cope with certain intolerable social conditions, but it cannot improve those conditions unless it contributes to raising the consciousness of patients so that they will be less likely to tolerate them. On the one hand, this points to the necessity to demystify therapy so that people are no longer encouraged to believe that only individual psychological 'treatment' can cure what ails them. On the other hand, this points to the by-and-large unexplored potential of therapy to be an instrument of social change.

She argues that the ultimate goal of woman-oriented therapy is to help the female patient overcome the ways in which she colludes with her own oppression and thereby to help her more fully recognize her own power, both as an individual and as a member of a community of women. If this is not possible the therapist should at least recognize the commonality of women in particular contexts, be it social class, ethnic group, sexual orientation, age, etc. Nursing and social work are female dominated at a practice level and male dominated at a senior management and training level. This often has negative connotations for clients in that the worker assigned to them is not the one who can take decisions with regard to resources and policy making.

In the health service, men make up less than 10% of the nursing workforce, yet hold 50% of the management posts. The relative shortage of women in commissioning agencies may have affected the development of truly responsive services to meet the needs of women, despite the move towards more user involvement. Without a woman to represent and articulate the elicited views of women users in commissioning agencies, the likely outcome is provision of services that fit the male idea of what women need rather than what they really need. In a recent interview, Sayce (1997) asked Phyllis Chesler what had been the impact of the consumer/survivor movement for women. Her response was that, 'Feminists are allowed in to the consumer/survivor movement if they are prepared to put their feminism on the back burner. It's like going back to the 1950s—or the 1850s—if you keep quiet you're allowed to help.'

Traditional treatment for women has been based on helping them adapt to social circumstances and to view their identity in terms of success in predestined, socially decreed roles as wife, mother and sexual companion. Men and women working in the field of mental health are likely to share the cultural expectations of appropriate behaviour for men and women and this may influence the way in which they assess, diagnose, select therapeutic interventions and evaluate 'problem' behaviours. What can have detrimental effects is that there are mental health practitioners who see their work as reinforcing the current status quo, making their clients 'adjust' and suggesting to them that if they do not fit themselves into whatever model the therapist sees as appropriately feminine, they are failures as women and as human beings.

Being involved in a therapeutic relationship with a practitioner who sees women in stereotypical roles can be antitherapeutic as the practitioner's unexamined preconceptions and biases can seriously influence the processes in therapy.

Particular behaviours and characteristics may be viewed as indicative of pathology in women but not pathological in men. Broverman et al (1981) recommend that the causes of mental health problems would be better served if both men and women are encouraged toward maximum realization of individual potential, rather than an adjustment to existing restrictive sex roles.

Most often these unexamined preconceptions concern a woman's 'normal' role as a mother. Any indication that she is not willing to sacrifice herself and her interests to her children and husband is seen as a symptom that she is not a good woman. Women very often face a conflict between their own personal needs for autonomy and the stereotypes of society, which mental health practitioners often unquestioningly adopt, about how women, in order to be 'healthy', ought to 'adjust' to meet the needs and expectations of society as a whole—the opposite of autonomy.

Mental health practitioners need to understand women's relative powerlessness in the world, the psychological effects on women of this powerlessness and of devaluation and stereotyping. They need to be knowledgeable about the various problems experienced by women and with the strategies that they use to cope with them. Clients need to feel respected, to be treated with gentleness, to feel heard, seen and cared for without judgement.

Health professionals', including mental health professionals', concepts of health tend to exhibit similar gender biases (Broverman et al 1981). As a result of such stereotypes, women may internalize the belief that they are inferior and may feel disenfranchised by many of the circumstances of their lives and feel powerless to resist them. The onset of anorexia nervosa has been attributed to women's unhappiness with their social position (Orbach 1978). One of the most persistent stereotypes of women depicts them as passive and dependent. The fields of psychology and psychiatry have tended to foster and perpetuate this image, since the assumption that underlies much of the literature from these two disciplines concerning women implies that 'normal' women will find their identity and self-fulfilment completely in the role of wife and mother where they are dependent on and maintain their identity through others. Although, for some women, the roles of wife and mother as traditionally defined are sufficient for self-fulfilment, there is mounting evidence that for other women these roles, as historically defined, do not provide enough avenues for the realization of their true potential, nor do they reflect the present situation with regard to the functions which women are actually undertaking in society.

Prescribed drugs

Over several decades far more women than men have been prescribed psychotropic drugs, such as tranquillizers and benzodiazepines. This has kindled a dependence among women that is of almost epidemic proportions and, in some cases, women have used or abused tranquillizers at more than double the rate of men (Choiton, Spitzer & Roberts 1976). Many doctors have justified prescribing tranquillizers to older women to help them 'readjust' to domestic life. Because of this doctors have often been accused of being intent on maintaining the oppressed role of women. Some GPs too easily opt for pharmacotherapy as a treatment option because they work in oppressive conditions that do not allow them to spend more than a short period of time with their patients.

In her research Cooperstock (1978) concludes that women are more likely to request drugs and this is compounded by physicians being more likely to prescribe tranquillizers to women than to men presenting with the same complaints.

A Vancouver study of the prescribing of tranquillizers cites one woman's experience of the response she had when discussing her distress to her doctor. She said 'I feel that, essentially when a doctor prescribes a pill for me, it's to put him out of my misery'. Drug advertisements use images that favour traditional gender stereotypes. An analysis of the contents of drug advertisements over a 5-year period in the United States (Prather & Fidell 1975) showed the following:

1. There was a strong tendency to associate psychotropic drugs with female patients.
2. Non-psychoactive drug advertisements usu-

ally showed a male patient (this combination is particularly insidious because it indicates that real illnesses are experienced by men while mental problems are suffered by women).

3. The symptoms listed for male and female users of psychotropic drugs are significantly different. Men were usually depicted as presenting specific and work-related symptoms, whereas women were shown to complain of diffuse anxiety, tension and depression.

Joy Melville (1984) describes how, in 1 year alone, the British Medical Journal ran 115 advertisements for tranquillizers, antidepressants and hypnotics and that women were identified as the patient in 91 of them. One advertisement stated that the doctor could help an entire family by tranquillizing the mother so that she would be able to cook and serve their meals. The caption read, 'Treat one—six people benefit'.

Phyllis Chesler, author of Women and madness (1972), was quoted in a recent interview by Sayce (1997) as being aware of the positive role she now believes psychiatric drugs can play in the treatment of mentally ill women.

> I started talking to women about their experiences of using drugs for depression, and panic, and menopause; by the mid-1980's I realised that if women take responsibility and the drugs are properly monitored, then we have to use what works. Verbal therapy or feminist politicking doesn't always help; for some women, who do not sleep, or who hit other women, or who are suicidal, drugs work. But when we say we see a role for drugs, the difference is that we don't treat women with contempt.

ASSESSMENT

Mental health professionals have generally ignored the external factors that may have a major influence on a woman's state of mind. A recognition of these external factors would ensure the development of more appropriate care. A thorough assessment is the cornerstone to the effective delivery of appropriate care and this necessitates that the patient is viewed holistically. Solberg (1989) states that practitioners need to pay atten-

CASE STUDY: VANESSA'S STORY

Vanessa is a 45-year-old woman who has spent most of her adult life in various mental health units. In her mid twenties, after the birth of two children, she became extremely ill and was diagnosed as having schizophrenia. She was unable to cope with family life, her relationship broke down and she was left with the responsibility for two small children. Although her parents were very caring and supportive, Vanessa's behaviour became increasingly erratic and disturbed, causing many problems with her neighbours and extended family. Vanessa was eventually sectioned and detained in a local mental health unit. She would make small, temporary improvements in her health, would be discharged back to her parents' care and the whole cycle would begin again. Each time though, Vanessa's distress and anger would become more marked and difficult to manage. She was described as 'violent, aggressive, assaultive to staff and other patients, abusive, manic, prone to hysterical screaming fits of behaviour' in her various case sheets. She went from being admitted into the local psychiatric unit to being transferred to medium secure units and eventually a high security hospital because of her violent and unpredictable behaviour. Throughout this period Vanessa was prescribed various forms of antipsychotic medication and other therapies with limited success. During her time in a high security unit, Vanessa was eventually prescribed Clozaril, which effected an extremely positive change. Her mood swings stopped, her behaviour became much more stable and her ability to reason and interact with others improved beyond recognition. During this long period her parents had remained very loving, caring and interested in Vanessa's needs and she was discharged back to her local unit with the aim of returning to her local community. She appeared very committed to maintaining her health and had realized the improvements in her life that an effective antipsychotic medication had made.

tion to women's mental health as part of their overall health status and outlines the following specific areas for assessment.

1. *Self-esteem*—Does she value herself as a person? Does she perceive herself to be a valued member of her family, and society? How vulnerable does she feel? How confident is she in her life and in her work?

2. *Control*—Does she feel she has control over her own life and her career? Who or what does she see as barriers to living her life as she would like to live it? How uncertain is she about her life and what is happening to her? Does she feel she can make any changes in her life if she needs to change?

3. *Satisfaction*—How happy is she with her life and her accomplishments? Is she happy as a woman? How does her future seem to her? Does she have any unresolved conflicts in her life?

4. *Relationships*—Is she able to make and sustain meaningful relationships? How happy is she with her relationships? Are her emotional and affiliative needs being met? Is she socially isolated? How much interpersonal stress does she experience? Does she feel any social dissatisfaction and what are its sources?

5. *Stressors*—What changes have recently taken place in her life? How have such changes affected her? Does she have the resources to deal with any stressors present? What are her socioeconomic and employment statuses? What is present in her environment that may cause her stress?

SUMMARY

The future of services for women with mental health problems must develop on a different trajectory from those of the past and present. In the first instance it is necessary to understand the nature of women's distress and fully appreciate the various psychosocial factors that serve to impede all women from developing as mentally healthy adults. This requires all persons involved in mental health services for women to be educated about the ways in which, from birth, girls are exposed to a society where male definitions of what is and is not acceptable predominate. Girls are rewarded for dependency upon others and denying their needs for personal power and autonomy. They are punished for self-assertion and for presenting themselves in a manner that may not be satisfactory to men. This process of socially and psychologically shaping girls toward a traditional woman's role is ongoing and in many cases it is relentless. The result is that many women are unable to recognize their own needs; they have been processed to respond to the needs of others and to consider this proper. This, at least, must be understood and the relationship between it and the state of women's mental health admitted.

Barnes & Maple (1992) state that a working class woman is likely to accept full responsibility for child care, budgeting the family income, and ensuring everybody else's needs are met before her own. They state that 'Professional responses often imply that it is perfectly appropriate for adult women to be passive, dependent and unable to cope yet at the same time the myth of the all-providing wife and mother who should be able to meet all the family's needs in self-sacrificing way remains.'

This places women in a double bind, no-win situation in terms of personal and familial health and welfare. For women themselves the fact that they cannot cope produces feelings of guilt, low self-esteem and can perpetuate and exacerbate their mental distress. The inherent contradiction of a woman's 'natural' role can often lead to professionals feeling frustrated when it appears the woman 'won't help herself', and anger and dislike if the woman refuses to passively accept her 'lot'.

Claire provides a good example of this.

CASE STUDY: CLAIRE

As a young woman Claire belonged to a large local family. She had five siblings and was the youngest child. Periods of poor health, infrequent school attendance and small delicate stature led to her being sheltered and highly protected from much of social life by her mother.

At 19 Claire became pregnant, stayed in her family home and was very supported, in fact

CASE STUDY: CLAIRE (cont'd)

highly protected in her childcare of her son. At the age of 23, however, Claire's mum, who was the lynch-pin of the family, died and Claire was left with a father and child to care for.

Periods of depression followed until eventually Claire was considered to be neglecting her son to the extent that he was taken into foster care. Claire reacted extremely violently to this—both to professionals and her environment and ended up being detained under the 1983 Mental Health Act in two local secure provisions. Claire's depression was clinically treated but her requests to see her son were repeatedly denied. During a visit by her sister and young niece, Claire who had hidden a knife given to her by a male patient took her niece hostage, demanding to be released and to be reunited with her son. When the situation was resolved Claire was transferred to a high security environment, where she remains at present. The policy for Claire remains that it is not considered at present in the 'best interests' of the child that Claire sees her son.

What we can see here is a woman who, when she challenges stereotypes of passivity and compliance, albeit in two very dramatic ways, she meets with little sympathy from caring professionals. Another example is Mary's story:

'At a clinic visit to a consultant psychiatrist, to whom I had been referred by a locum GP when I felt I was at the end of my tether and had been considering driving into a wall at high speed in an attempt to "deal" with my unhappiness, I sat in silence while he reread the notes he made when he visited me in my home shortly after the referral. He did not look up from the notes until he had read all the way through them in front of me. This took 15 minutes and all the time I sat there in distress, looking to him for help, with him not looking at me but at his interpretation of me on paper. I began to feel frustrated and angry. I thought "Why am I letting myself be treated like this? I'm here in front of him and he hasn't even looked up from his notes. This is just making me feel *worse." When he finally did acknowledge me it was to inform me that he believed I was suffering from depression, to prescribe antidepressants and vitamin B injections and discharge me unless I instigated an approach to see him again. He was so cold that all I could do was cry, I wanted to bang the table and shout at him to look at me and talk to me. I was still crying when he concluded the consultation. All this without once interacting with me at a human level. I never went back and in fact felt I had been abused by a system which on the one hand (the locum GP) had tempted me to believe that help was possible, and on the other hand (the consultant psychiatrist) had reinforced the message that I was the helpless recipient of what he had to offer me.'*

Practitioners need to seek to understand the processes that make it difficult for women to articulate their distress directly. Rather than perpetuating the current misrepresentation of women throughout the process of service planning and delivery, policy needs to be reframed in relation to the nature of women and the mental health problems they experience. There needs to be a move away from the traditional biological and medical models that pathologize women's pain and distress primarily in terms of disease entities and chemical imbalance. These models, though generally ineffective in addressing the source of the issues, lead to expensive and dissatisfying interventions.

Traditional psychiatry encourages women to relate their misery to their own personal and internal deficiencies and to remedy these with 'treatment'. In reframing women's inner turmoil and confusion in terms of the human response to, at times, overwhelming helplessness, invisibility and confusion resulting from the socially constructed role definition of what it is to be female, we may achieve a more accurate starting point for intervention. In order to achieve this, however, it would be necessary for professionals to identify with these factors. As it is, there is a slim chance that high status professionals, especially men, who occupy the largest proportion of managerial and senior positions, would ever have been enabled to relate to the experience of vulnerability, disadvantage and stress that are likely to be central to the

life experience of the average woman user. It is also essential to reframe the patriarchal nature of facilities. This means that it ought not to be assumed that domestic pursuits, particularly those relating to serving others, are good therapy for women. Cooking, cleaning and other domestic activities are likely to reinforce the social influences that contributed to the women's mental health problems in the first place. It is far more appropriate to focus upon empowering, problem solving and creative behaviours.

In the Mind policy paper on women and mental health, titled Stress on Women (1992), details of service most likely to meet women's needs are identified as: 'crisis houses, information and advocacy, self help and support groups, housing with flexible support, employment projects, counselling and therapy in which women are involved in defining the help they are seeking, telephone crisis services and support for carers'.

In addition the Mind document (1992) emphasizes the importance of voluntary groups, women's groups and other self-help and support agencies being recognized and resources by statutory mental health service budgets.

There is ample evidence that life stress and physical and mental health are related, but not enough information about how they are related for women. Sources of stress for women need to be identified and life events lists broadened to include abortion, rape, physical assault, changes in childcare arrangements and incidents of sex discrimination. Greater specificity would yield a much more useful diagnostic tool. In addition, if data were gathered concerning the social supports and coping mechanisms available and useful to individual women or groups of women, we would be in a better position to help women deal with the outcomes of stress.

The threat to women's mental health will not be satisfactorily reduced until the reality of life for women is accepted throughout our society. No real change will be achieved until the disadvantage, oppression, injustice and abuse of women by men and by institutions are acknowledged and the balance redressed by policy and resultant attitude which is embedded in the very foundation of society.

DISCUSSION QUESTIONS

The following questions are intended to generate and provoke thought and discussion around the provision of services for women with mental health problems.

1. What is the purpose and validity of exploring women's experience of mental health services from a historical viewpoint?
2. Do we need to understand the past to identify future progress?
3. What changes (if any) in your clinical area do you consider, following the reading of this chapter, need to occur if women (and men) are to be provided with a mental health service that meets their needs and respects and values difference?
4. What political and policy changes need to occur to allow service provision to progress?

REFERENCES

Allen H 1992 Justice unbalanced. OU Press, Philadelphia

Barnes M, Maple N 1992 Women and mental health: challenging the stereotypes. Venture Press, Birmingham

Broverman I K, Broverman D M, Clarkson F E et al 1981 Sex role stereotypes and clinical judgements in mental health. In: Howell E, Bates M (eds) Women and mental health. Basic Books, New York

Brown G W, Harris T 1978 Social origins of depression: a study of psychiatric disorders in women. Tavistock, London

Chesler P 1972 Women and madness. Doubleday, New York

Choiton A, Spitzer W O, Roberts S R 1976 The patterns of medical drug use. Canadian Medical Association Journal 114:33

Clay T 1987 Nurses, power and politics. Heinemann, Oxford

Cooperstock R 1978 Sex differences in psychotropic drug use. Social Science and Medicine 12:179–186

Doyal L 1995 What makes women sick? Macmillan, London

Doyal L, Pennell I 1995 The political economy of health. Pluto Press, London

Ehrenreich B, English D 1979 For her own good. 100 years of the experts' advice to women. Pluto Press, London

Feely M 1995 Social constructionism and depression in women: psychiatry's role in maintaining the social order. Psychiatric Care 2(4):141–143

Freud S 1982 Female sexuality. In: Whittleff A et al (eds) The changing experience of women. Basil Blackwell, Oxford

Glendinning C, Millar J 1993 Women, health and poverty. The 1990's. Harvester, London

Graham H 1992 Women, health and the family. Harvester, London

Greenspan M 1983 A new approach to women and therapy. McGraw-Hill, New York

Johnstone L 1993 In the same boat. Nursing Times 89:27

Melville J 1984 The tranquillizer trap. Fontana, New York

Miles A 1991 Women, health and medicine. Open University Press, Milton Keynes

Mind 1992 Stress on women pack. Mind, London

Orbach S 1978 Fat is a feminist issue. Hamlyn, London

Prather J E, Fidell L S 1975 Sex differences in the content and style of medical advertisements. Social Science and Medicine 9:23–26

Sane 1993 Depression and manic depression. Sane, London

Sayce L 1997 Interview with Phyllis Chesler, 20th November 1996. Women and Mental Health Forum 2:20–24

Schaef A W 1992 Women's reality: an emerging female system in a white male society, 3rd edn. Harper/Collins, San Francisco

Showalter E 1985 The female malady. Virago, London

Solberg S 1989 Women and their mental health: a reflection of society's expectations and pressures. Recent Advances in Nursing 25:92–109

Szasz T S 1977 The manufacture of madness, 2nd edn. Paladin Granada, London

Tennov D 1976 Psychotherapy: the hazardous cure. Anchor, Garden City, New York

Ussher J 1991 Women's madness: misogyny or mental illness. Harvester, London

Ussher J 1992 Science sexing psychology: positive science and gender bias in clinical psychology. In: Ussher J, Nicholson P (eds) Gender issues in clinical psychology. Routledge, London

Walker L 1994 Abused women and survivor therapy: a practical guide for the psychotherapist. Walter, Denver CO

Walker M 1990 Women in therapy and counselling. Open University Press, Milton Keynes

FURTHER READING

Cogan J C 1998 The consumer as expert: women with serious mental illness and their relationship based needs. Psychiatric Rehabilitation Journal 22(2):142–154
This article explores how a gender blind paradigm overlooks important experiences that are central to women's lives. The findings of this study pose meaningful research questions worthy of further investigation in order to provide optimal community services to women with serious mental illness. The importance of researchers using the consumer as the expert approach to examine this issue further is emphasized.

Cook J S, Fontaine K L 1987 Essentials of mental health nursing. Addison Wesley, Menlo Park C A

Burr J A 1998 Some reflections on cultural and social considerations in mental health nursing. Journal of Pyschiatric and Mental Health Nursing 5(6):431–437
This article will provide the reader with valuable information on theoretical perspectives on mental health care and ethnicity, with particular reference to Asian women. The impact of poverty and racism on women's mental health in particular is emphasized, as is the problematic conceptual framework of Western mental health and the role it plays in perpetuating stereotypes.

De Beauvoir S 1988 The second sex. Picador, London

Roberts G L 1998 How does domestic violence affect women's mental health? Women and Health 28(1):117–129
This paper compares the mental health of women who reported domestic violence and women who reported no abuse in their lifetime. The aim was to explore the nature of symptoms and pattern of mental illness associated with domestic violence.

Hughes-Hammer C, Martsolf D S, Zeller R A 1998 Depression and codependency in women. Archives of Psychiatric Nursing 12(6):326–334
This paper reports on a study that aimed to identify the prevalence of codependency in women undergoing treatment for depression. The implications for this paper it is argued, are that the results of the study could be used to direct future research toward the relationship of codependency to power, alienation of self and personality disorders.

Steen M 1991 Historical perspectives on women and mental illness and prevention of depression in women using a feminist framework. Issues in Mental Health Nursing 12:359–374

Webb C 1992 Sexuality. In: Brooking J I, Ritter S A H, Thomas B L (eds) A textbook of psychiatric and mental health nursing. Churchill Livingstone, New York

Walsh M R 1987 (ed) The psychology of woman, ongoing debates. Yale University Press, New Haven, CT/London

Weinstein N 1987 Cited in Walsh M (ed) The psychology of woman, ongoing debates. Yale University Press, New Haven, CT/London

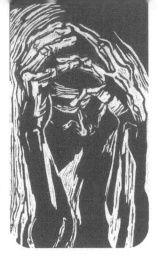

Chapter Seventeen

Suicide and deliberate self-harm

David Duffy

AIMS
◆ To introduce and analyse the concepts of suicide and self-harming behaviour
◆ To outline risk factors associated with suicide and self-harm
◆ To summarize approaches to the prevention of suicide and self-harm and the assessment and care of people at risk

KEY ISSUES
Definitions of suicide and deliberate self-harm
Social and historical background
Motivation for suicide and deliberate self-harm
Risk factors
Prevention
Risk assessment
Caring for people at risk
Suicide survivors

INTRODUCTION

Suicide, in which death is intentionally self-inflicted, must be carefully distinguished from a range of behaviours variously referred to as *parasuicide*, *deliberate self-harm* and *attempted suicide*. The term 'parasuicide' was introduced to denote 'any non-fatal act in which an individual deliberately causes self-injury or ingests a substance in excess of any prescribed or generally recognised therapeutic dosage' (Kreitman 1977). This definition includes acts that were intended to be fatal as well as those such as self-poisoning, for which the motives are often ambivalent, and self-injury such as cutting, which usually has no fatal intention and to which the notion of 'suicide' is not pertinent. Because any overall term needs to embrace self-injury, this chapter will use the term *deliberate self-harm (DSH)* to refer to the whole range of non-fatal self-harming behaviours.

Although suicidal and self-harming behaviours are extremely varied and individual, there are clear differences between people who complete suicide and people who engage in DSH. *Completed suicide* usually involves males. Men over 75 years are at greatest risk, although the rate has been rapidly increasing for younger men. *Deliberate self-harm* has, in the past, usually involved females, although the gender gap has been closing, and takes place mainly among younger people.

There are other differences: prevalence rates for mental illness are much greater in those who complete suicide and prevalence rates for personality disorder are much higher in those who engage in DSH, for whom living conditions, social circumstances and acute life upsets are more significant (Clark & Fawcett 1992).

However, the two groups do overlap to some extent. About 1% of people who engage in an episode of DSH go on to kill themselves in the year following—this is 100 times the risk in the general population—while many people who complete suicide have a previous history of DSH (Hawton & Catalan 1987).

THE EXTENT OF THE PROBLEM

Self-harming behaviour of all kinds is a major public health issue. Around 5000 people kill themselves in England and Wales each year (this figure includes both suicide verdicts and undetermined deaths). Each death represents both an individual tragedy and a loss to society, while the destructive ripples often spread out from the suicide to affect families and other 'survivors' economically, psychologically and spiritually.

A suicide kills two people, Maggie. That's what it's for.
Miller 1981

In recent years public concern has particularly been fuelled by the disturbing rise in the number of young people who kill themselves, especially young men in the 15–24-year age group, for whom suicide has become the second leading cause of death behind road traffic accidents. Along with these deaths there are very large numbers of people—perhaps as many as 142 000—who are admitted annually to accident and emergency departments because they have harmed themselves non-fatally (Hawton et al 1997). Even these numbers will be less than the actual total of people who harm themselves, since they may not attend hospital afterwards. Among admissions to accident and emergency departments for non-fatal self-harm, the majority involve self-poisoning; 10–15% tend to be cases of self-injury, with most of these involving cutting (Hawton & Catalan 1987). Many admissions are of people who have harmed themselves before and whose problem has therefore not been successfully addressed. Some of these people will go on to actually kill themselves (Hawton & Fagg 1988).

In response to the scale of the problem, the last Conservative Government made suicide prevention one of its key health policy priorities in setting the targets of reducing the overall suicide rate by at least 15% and reducing the suicide rate of severely mentally ill people by at least 33% by the year 2000 (DOH 1992). The present Labour Government has likewise identified a reduction in the rate of suicide as a measure by which it is prepared to be judged (DOH 1998).

Nurses and other health professionals encounter those who are at risk of self-harm or who have harmed themselves in many different settings and specialties—in general hospitals, in mental health services, in prisons, in primary care. They are therefore well placed to intervene effectively. Yet, disturbingly, there is evidence that not only do nurses and other health professionals sometimes have negative attitudes towards people who harm themselves (McKie 1994), but that they may even contribute to the suicidal mind-set of some patients by inducing 'malignant alienation' (Morgan & Priest 1991).

Suicidal people may well not wish to die or harm themselves, but may also find the idea of life going on as it is intolerable. It is possible to argue that suicide can be a rational response to such a situation. Physician-assisted suicides have made media headlines and a 'how to' manual for suicide has even been published (Humphrey 1991). However, the evidence is that most people who contemplate suicide or engage in DSH are influenced by depression and other mental health problems (Barraclough et al 1974). Significant numbers of people try to tell others about their intentions beforehand and many people are ambivalent in their motives. This very ambivalence provides an opportunity for others to step in, to listen and to offer help. This chapter will try to promote such a positive and empathic approach to self-harming behaviour by explaining some of the background to the phenomenon of self-harm and by setting out some ways in which health professionals can actively contribute to suicide prevention and to the care of those who harm themselves.

HISTORICAL BACKGROUND

Self-harming behaviour has been recorded throughout history. In the classical period, suicide was for some a matter of honour, but with the rise of Christianity it began to be seen as both a sin and a crime. The term 'suicide' itself is a legal, not a medical, concept and it is a coroner, a legal official, or the jury who decides whether someone has 'committed' suicide. In considering a verdict of suicide, coroners are required by law to try to determine beyond reasonable doubt not only whether a death has occurred from an act inflicted upon oneself, but also whether there is evidence of

intent to kill oneself (Todd 1992). If unable to determine actual intent the coroner will normally come to an 'open' verdict even if other evidence points to a suicide. In this context it is noteworthy that, historically, the goods of people found guilty of the 'crime' of suicide were forfeit to the Crown, often leaving survivors in poverty. If the person committed suicide while 'non compos mentis', that is, while the balance of the mind was disturbed, the survivors were not subjected to this draconian penalty. Even though the felony of self-murder was repealed in 1961, it is still the case that insurance companies may well not make payments to the relatives of suicides, adding economic pressures to their other problems. If we add the social stigma that is still associated with suicidal behaviour, possibly owing to its continuing status as a sin in some religions, it is unsurprising that coroners differ in their use of verdicts (Atkinson 1978, Renvoize & Clayden 1990). As a consequence of these factors it is generally assumed that the official statistics underrepresent the true incidence of suicide, and in England and Wales around 2000 deaths due to 'undetermined' causes are added each year to the total suicide figures.

WHY DO PEOPLE HARM THEMSELVES?

Individual motives

Interviews with overdose patients suggest that at least half did not want to die. Many of those who say they did want to die describe other reasons as well, the most common being that 'the situation was so unbearable that I had to do something and didn't know what else to do' (Williams 1997). It is often difficult for individuals to give a coherent explanation of their actions. This is unsurprising given the inner turmoil and ambivalence that is likely to precede and accompany self-harm.

And all at once she thought of the man crushed by a train the day she had first met Vronsky, and she knew what she had to do. With a light, rapid step she went down the steps that led from the tank to the rails and stopped quite near the approaching train …

'There,' she said to herself, looking into the shadow of the carriage, at the sand and the coal-dust which covered the sleepers—'there, in the very middle, and I will punish him and escape from everyone and myself …' And exactly at the moment when the space between the wheels came opposite her, she dropped the red bag, and drawing her head back into her shoulders, fell on her hands under the carriage … And at the same instant she was terror-stricken at what she was doing. 'Where am I? What am I doing? What for?' She tried to get up, to drop backwards; but something huge and merciless struck her on the head and rolled her on her back. 'Lord, forgive me all!' she said, feeling it impossible to struggle.
Tolstoy, 1901

Conscious of this complexity of motive, Freud (1917) suggested that suicidal people are acting out a fantasy and may experience their own body as a separate object that they can 'kill' while continuing in some way to survive. In self-injury such as cutting, the act is usually preceded by anger, self-hatred and, sometimes, depression, and the injury is often carried out in order to reduce feelings of unbearable tension (Hawton & Catalan 1987).

Fairbairn (1995) has proposed a classification of suicidal behaviour in terms of the individual's intentions. He argues that we can distinguish such forms as no hope, existential, dutiful, altruistic, revenge, political/ideological, judicial, other-driven and multiple/mass suicide.

Social processes

Emile Durkheim (1897/1952), the founder of sociology, believed that suicidal behaviour could be understood as a social phenomenon. By comparing the suicide rate in different countries with different social conditions, Durkheim arrived at a classification of suicide as egoistic, altruistic, anomic or fatalistic. This allowed him to propose, for example, that where 'anomie' was a feature of a society—that is, where social regulation through prevailing norms and values was reduced—individuals would tend to become less integrated with society and less protected from suicidal risk. Although derived from suspect data, this sociological explanation could help to explain, for exam-

ple, why the suicide rate tends to drop in wartime, when nations become united around a common purpose and anomie is therefore reduced.

RISK FACTORS

Although the motives of people who harm themselves are many and complex, research has provided us with a wealth of information about factors that are associated with an increased risk of this behaviour. This information does not *explain* the behaviour, but can deepen our understanding of when and by whom it is more likely to occur. Risk factors for suicidal behaviour can be divided into those associated with society as a whole and those associated with the 'clinical' profile of the individual person.

Sociodemographic factors

A range of population-based factors have been found to be associated with an increased prevalence of suicide and DSH.

Age

Suicide risk can be said to increase with age. However, the increase is far from constant. Suicide among young people under the age of 15 is very rare, yet among 15–24 year olds it is the third most common cause of death in England and Wales. Rates for men under 45 years are now higher than for those of older men, except for men over 75 years, who are at the greatest risk of any age group. However, over the last two decades the age-related pattern has been changing: the suicide rate in young men between 15 and 24 years has risen by 75% since 1982 (DOH 1993), whereas the rate for older people has been decreasing (Charlton et al 1994a).

For DSH, the evidence is that younger age groups, over the age of 12 and up to middle age, are at the greatest risk (Hawton & Catalan 1987).

Gender

Completed suicide is, and as far as we can tell always has been, more common in men than in women. The gap continues to widen. In England and Wales the rate for women has been falling in recent decades but has been steadily rising for men, for whom it is now four times as common as in women (Charlton et al 1994b). In general, males use more violent suicide means than females.

Reviewing their authoritative statistics, Charlton et al (1994b) confess: 'The main puzzle is why rates of suicide are increasing among young men but not among women. Further work is needed to explore this'.

The picture for DSH has until recently been very different. Women have for long been more likely to engage in DSH than men. However, the gender gap has recently been closing, with an increasing rate for both sexes but a steeper rise in men (Williams 1997).

Social class and employment

People of the highest social class (social class I, 'professional'), people of the lowest class (social class V, 'unskilled') and people who have no occupation are at greatest risk of suicide. Although the significance of unemployment for the suicide rate has been established (Platt 1984), Crombie (1989) has shown that the relationship between the suicide and unemployment rate is complex, depending, for example, on geographical location and the level of stigma attached to unemployment. Pritchard (1995) suggests that improvements in employment opportunities for women may be partly responsible for the decline in the female suicide rate.

DSH is more common among those who are unemployed and of the lower social classes (Hawton & Catalan 1987).

Family and relationship factors

The highest rates for both suicide and DSH are found in those who live alone and who are separated, divorced or widowed (DOH 1993). The increasing numbers of young men who are not married parallels the rise in the suicide rate in this group. Although motherhood is not in itself a protective factor, mothers of young children are less likely to kill themselves than other women. A fam-

ily history of suicide, alcoholism or depression is an indication of increased risk (NHS Health Advisory Service 1994).

For DSH, which is most prevalent among younger people, there is a strong association with ongoing family relationship problems (NHS Health Advisory Service 1994).

Social isolation

Isolation, often associated with loss of partners and older age, correlates with an increased risk of suicide (DOH 1993).

Religion

Members of religious groups—for example, Roman Catholics and Jews—that stigmatize suicidal behaviour and mitigate social isolation are less likely to engage in suicidal behaviour than those who are not affiliated (Williams 1997).

Ethnic group

There has been concern in recent years about an increasing risk of suicide in young Asian women, despite the fact that Asian people in general and women in particular tend to have lower suicide rates (Soni Raleigh, Bulusu & Balarajan 1990).

'Copy cat' effects

Studies have indicated that portrayals of suicide in the media can not only influence the means of suicide but also increase the suicide rate (Schmidtke & Hafner 1988). This is a major problem in devising large scale social prevention programmes that involve use of the media.

Imprisonment

People in prison, especially remand prisoners, have a high suicide rate, with one in six of such suicides occurring in the first week of imprisonment (Dooley 1990).

However, while the stress of imprisonment will undoubtedly play a part, Towl & Crighton (1998) observe that prisoners in general tend to have more suicide risk factors anyway—male, unemployed, history of substance abuse, etc.—than the general population.

Occupation

There are known to be certain occupational groups with heightened risk of suicide, although it is important to bear in mind that statistics about occupation are based on death certificates, which may record occupation when the person has in fact been retired for some time. Charlton et al (1994a) have identified veterinary surgeons, pharmacists, dentists, medical practitioners and farmers as high risk groups. Subsequently, Kelly, Charlton & Jenkins (1995) added farmers' wives to this list.

Geographical area

Rates of suicide and self-harm are high in economically and socially deprived areas such as inner cities. However, it must also be noted that in some rural areas the suicide rate may be even higher than in urban areas (Williams 1997). To a large extent this can be accounted for by the fact that farmers are a particularly high risk occupational group, but other factors such as high numbers of elderly and retired people and rural isolation should also be noted.

Access to means

The means used for self-harm is an important issue. There are clear gender differences in suicidal means, with males most commonly using car exhaust fumes and hanging and women most commonly using self-poisoning especially with paracetamol (NHS Health Advisory Service 1994). Access to suicidal means is a significant risk factor, with high risk groups such as health professionals having easy access to agents for self-poisoning and farmers having easy access to firearms and ropes (Hawton et al 1998). Different means are not necessarily interchangeable for those who intend to harm themselves, as is demonstrated by the fact that the change from toxic coal gas to non-toxic natural gas in this country in the 1960s and early 1970s was accompanied by a reduction not only in the use of gas as a means of suicide but in the overall suicide rate (Kreitman 1976).

Clinical factors

Physical

Investigations into the biology of depression in recent years have brought to light biological correlates for suicidal behaviour. The most consistent finding has been a link between self-harming behaviour and biochemical factors such as abnormalities in serotonin levels in the brain. Possible genetic markers for self-harming behaviours have also been noted (Motto 1992, Williams 1997). It is thought that these factors may be associated with increased impulsivity, aggression and anxiety but the research is still ongoing.

Physical illnesses such as cancer and AIDS carry an increased risk of suicide. A recent large scale study has identified a significantly increased suicide risk in stroke patients, especially in men under the age of 60 and in women. This appears to be related to depression consequent upon the stroke (Stenager et al 1998).

Psychiatric

Severe mental illness is one of the strongest risk factors for suicide, increasing risk by as much as 10 times (Allebeck & Allgulander 1990). A seminal study by Barraclough et al (1974) of a hundred cases of suicide indicated a diagnosis of major depression for 70% of the cases, alcoholism for 15% and schizophrenia for 4%. Other researchers have indicated that schizophrenia carries a greater suicide risk than this study suggests, and Miles (1977) and Dorpat & Ripley (1960) have estimated that 10–15% of people with schizophrenia ultimately die by suicide. Linehan (1993) has studied borderline personality disorder in detail and underlines the significance of suicidal behaviour in this group of people. In a recent meta-analysis, Harris & Barraclough (1997) have shown that virtually all mental disorders have an increased risk of suicide, with the exception of mental retardation and dementia.

Abuse of both drugs and alcohol is strongly associated with suicidal behaviour. Miles (1977) estimated that 15% of alcoholics ultimately killed themselves. In this context it should be noted that alcohol can act both as a depressant and as a disinhibitor, and can also be associated with suicidal means. Most of the rise in young male suicide has been related to higher levels of substance abuse (Needleman & Farrell 1997).

Psychological

Cognitive dysfunction, especially the mindset of 'hopelessness', and difficulties in interpersonal problem solving, are associated with suicidal behaviour. Indeed, hopelessness is more closely correlated to suicide intent than is depression per se and seems to be the key difference between depressed people with suicidal intent and those without (Weishaar & Beck 1990). One implication is that the suicidal person may not in fact desire to harm themselves, but can see no other option owing to the negative mindset in which they are trapped.

In terms of affective experience, suicide is associated with apathetic mood and DSH with anger (Farberow & MacKinnon 1974).

Psychodynamic

A number of clinicians have related suicide and DSH to the psychodynamic theory of mental conflicts. Freud himself (1917, 1957) proposed that suicidal behaviour involved turning aggression originally felt towards another towards oneself. This approach, postulating the origins of self-harm in inner fantasies and conflicts, has been elaborated by many psychodynamic theorists. Some of the relevant literature is lucidly summarized by Lovett & Maltsberger (1992).

Clearly, interpersonal issues, including relationships with health care workers, are of the utmost importance to the suicidal person. Henderson (1974), viewing suicidal behaviour as an example of animal 'care-eliciting' behaviour in humans, cautioned that an overtly caring response by the therapist could actually reinforce and intensify the suicidal, or care-eliciting, behaviour.

PREVENTION OF SELF-HARM

We have reviewed some of the ways in which we can try to understand suicidal behaviour and some of the factors that seem to increase its occurrence. The difficulties of preventing it loom large: the factors are many and varied, and arise from a whole range of social, economic and interpersonal problems that no one agency—certainly not the NHS—can control. These inherent challenges may lead some into a fatalistic attitude. It is easy to assume that prevention is not really possible or worth the effort (DOH 1993). The first step, therefore, in approaching prevention is to adopt an open-minded, problem-solving attitude. If we do so, we can distinguish two main approaches:

Population approaches to prevention

Population-based, or epidemiological, strategies target whole populations rather than individuals or high risk groups. Examples of this include the national 'Defeat Depression Campaign' organized by the Royal College of Psychiatrists in the early 1990s and the nationwide response to the rise in the use of paracetamol for self-poisoning (Gunnell 1994). This has led to a reduction in paracetamol pack size. Similarly, it is hoped that the increasing use of catalytic convertors in cars will influence the male suicide rate by reducing the amount of carbon monoxide self-poisoning (O'Brien & Tarbuck 1992). Such aspirations are based around the ambivalence and impulsivity of suicidal behaviour; if access to immediate means can be reduced then it is possible that the suicidal impulse will have time to pass.

Another population approach would be to address the economic deprivation that is strongly associated with suicidal behaviour. Most of these approaches require the development of 'healthy alliances' between different agencies (e.g. professional and voluntary bodies, national and local government, and the media).

Prevention by targeting high risk groups

The alternative preventative approach is to identify groups in the population who can be considered to be at high risk of suicidal behaviour through their statistical association with the risk factors we have already considered. People with mental health problems, for example, have been shown to be at high risk, so all admissions to mental health inpatient units could be systematically screened for self-harming ideation. Similarly, young substance misusers could be targeted for assessment and follow-up after DSH.

This approach has been argued to be appropriate and cost effective (Appleby 1997) but has also been criticized on the grounds that the risk assessment tools currently available for screening are insufficiently sensitive for us to effectively identify people at risk (Kapur & House 1988).

IDENTIFYING PEOPLE AT RISK

If we are to be of help to individual people with self-harming intent we first have to find out who they are. There are two main opportunities for detection: first, before the act of self-harm, for example with a person who is depressed, and secondly after someone has attempted suicide or engaged in DSH.

Before self-harm

Staff who work in primary care settings, for example health centres, and voluntary workers may be in a position to detect risk of self-harm. Barraclough et al (1974) noted that two-thirds of their sample of 100 suicides had visited a GP in the month prior to their death and 40% in the week before their suicide. These rates seem to have reduced nowadays (Elwood & De Silva 1998) but none the less Appleby et al (1996) found that as the time of suicide approached people still increasingly attended their GPs and in the final week before death 15% did so, although it was unusual for any impression of suicidal risk to be recorded. Mental health services are often involved in continuous observation and assessment of people who are at high risk of suicide, both to prevent self-harm and to prevent repetition.

After self-harm

People admitted to accident and emergency departments and medical wards for DSH must be assessed for risk of repetition. Assessment is still usually carried out by psychiatrists, but there is good reason for other health professionals such as nurses to be involved (Duffy 1993). In all settings, it is vital to bear in mind that suicidal intent may fluctuate rapidly and repeated or continuous assessment of the person may be necessary.

Approaches to assessing risk

Given what we know about the complexity of suicidal behaviour, risk assessment cannot be approached simplistically or on the basis of intuition and common sense alone (Duffy 1993). It must be based on an up to date appreciation of the risk factors and an empathic understanding of the person, facilitated by a positive and supportive approach to avoid further alienation of someone who may already feel isolated and hopeless. However, many of the skills and attributes essential for effective risk assessment are the skills and attributes of good nursing staff and other health professionals. It is no surprise that research has demonstrated that nurses can, if appropriately trained, assess suicidal behaviour as effectively as doctors (Catalan et al 1980).

For over a quarter of a century efforts have been made to devise ways of quantifying risk through the creation of assessment scales based on actuarial data (see, for example, Farberow & MacKinnon 1974, Motto, Heilbron & Juster 1985). Clearly, if it were possible to produce a workable scale, based on precise weightings allocated to particular risk factors, a major breakthrough would have been made in the prevention of suicide. However, all such tools have so far proved to be insufficiently sensitive, falsely indicating many people to be suicidal ('false positives'). Thus, on an acute inpatient ward, such an assessment is likely to predict suicide for the majority of the patients on the basis of mental health problems, unemployment and so on, even though many will turn out not to have self-harming intent.

The situation is further complicated in that risk

factors may themselves be offset by protective factors; for example, the fact that a depressed person has children may protect against an urge to self-harm.

The current limitations in suicide prediction are illustrated by the progress report of the national confidential inquiry into suicide and mental illness (Appleby 1997). The inquiry has found that the majority of suicides by people with mental illness occur in situations in which risk is perceived to be low, that few people who went on to kill themselves had been judged to be at high immediate risk at their last contact with services, that most were thought to be recovering and that most were under routine care. The report concludes that a key objective for mental health services should be improved recognition of those who are at risk—not just by training staff but by conducting research to improve the current state of risk assessment itself.

A risk assessment procedure

Given the limitations of our current predictive tools, health care workers are faced with the need to combine research-based knowledge of self-harming behaviour with interpersonal skills of empathic listening and relationship building if they are to effectively detect the risk of self-harm. Assessment schedules, if they cannot effectively predict, can provide valuable assistance in this process. For example, since hopelessness seems to be the linking factor between depression and suicide, the Hopelessness Scale (Beck et al 1974) can provide a robust measure of this state of mind.

The non-judgmental attitude promoted in counselling theory (Rogers 1967) is crucial from the very beginning of the risk assessment process. This is not only because it will help in eliciting information of which the person may feel ashamed. There is also the possibility that any personal opinions that the interviewer may hold *in favour of* the right to suicide may be inadvertently conveyed to the patient, thus encouraging them in their suicidal intent (Morgan 1990).

Information about the person's history and sociodemographic background should be collected in order to shape their profile in terms of longer term risk factors—for example, family history, occupation, economic circumstances, alcohol use, history of mental health problems. There will be a range of sources of this information—clinical records, relatives, neighbours and friends, and other staff. This profile should be refined by considering more short term risk factors. If the assessment follows DSH, there is clearly the risk of repetition, and the interview should explore the circumstances of the act, its apparent degree of lethal intent and the motivation behind it. Whether or not DSH has occurred, if the sociodemographic profile and general impression suggest that the person may be at risk, examples of relevant issues include: Has the person recently felt depressed? Have they recently experienced an adverse event? Have they become uncharacteristically religious? Have they recently made a will, or been untypically extravagant? Have they talked to others about harming themselves and, if so, how specific and practical have these plans been?

When interviewing individuals it is important first to try to establish a rapport with them. The approach used in a counselling situation, emphasizing warmth, genuineness and empathy in a comfortable, private environment, will help to overcome any resistance to disclosing information that may spoil suicidal plans. The person's mood (apathetic? angry?) and cognitive functioning (e.g. level of hopelessness) should be assessed during the interview.

The interviewer should lead gently and gradually from how individuals see the future and whether they feel life is worth living into more direct questions about suicidal intent. If the subject of self-harm is introduced too precipitately then rapport may be broken. However, at the right moment it is vital to be prepared to ask people directly if they have been considering harming themselves. It may well be the case that they are in fact relieved to unburden themselves of any feelings of fear or shame to someone who is prepared to listen non-judgmentally. If suicidal ideas are present, these should then be further explored with the person in order to evaluate how serious and imminent the risk is.

Careful written records should be made of the assessment and it should be shared with colleagues, including the responsible medical officer, as soon as possible.

CARING FOR PEOPLE AT RISK

Services

Care settings for people at risk of suicide and self-harm range from the person's own home, with a crisis intervention team providing intensive input, to other community services such as mental health resource centres, to mental health inpatient units. No one form of care environment will meet the needs of all who are at risk, and it is important for different agencies—primary and secondary health services, local authority social services and NHS trusts, housing departments and voluntary groups—to cooperate in ensuring such a 'continuum of care'. For many people, the general hospital accident and emergency department will inevitably be at least the first care setting, and the advent of liaison psychiatry with community psychiatric nurses and other specialist workers complementing the general team is an important development. It is known that young men, who are a particularly high risk group, are less likely to access services and more likely to discharge themselves (Hawton et al 1997). There is therefore a need for more targeted services for young men, for example open-house services and assertive outreach to keep patients involved in programmes of care.

Appleby (1992) concludes that the evidence is unclear as to whether the development of community care has negatively influenced the suicide rate. Certainly it has been clearly shown that at some stages of the care process people are at increased risk and that this is especially so in the period of transition from inpatient to community care (Goldacre, Seagroatt & Hawton 1993). It is also true that care settings themselves can be implicated in suicide. Crammer (1984) studied a series of inpatient suicides. Although 57% occurred outside of the hospital building, factors such as disruption of the patient's routine (e.g. by moving from ward to ward and changing staff) were significant. This is currently an important issue in view of the pressure for beds and staff in many acute mental health units.

Community care

If the person at risk is cared for in a community setting, careful consideration must be given to frequency of assessment and degree of contact with health professionals, including staff availability 'out of hours' either in person or by telephone. It is important to engage the assistance of the person's carers, relatives and friends in monitoring the level of risk, to ensure that any medication is prescribed in non-lethal amounts and to record and communicate the person's progress to all relevant agencies. The 'no-suicide contract' first described by Drye, Goulding & Goulding (1973) has had some success in community settings (Brimblecombe 1998). This is a combined assessment and management approach whereby the health professional and patient jointly create a contract stating that the patient will not engage in self-harm until an agreed date and time, before which the contract is reviewed. By agreeing a goal of staying alive until the next meeting, pressure on both health care worker and client is reduced.

Inpatient care

Although community care may well be preferred as a first choice so that problems can be worked through in the person's home, access to inpatient services is an important part of the range of care options. Even innovative community mental health treatment teams have found that around 16% of their clients need hospital admission at some stage in their care, with about half of these admissions due to increased concern about suicide risk (Brimblecombe 1998).

Inpatient units employ forms of increased observation for some patients to both provide ongoing monitoring of the level of risk and prevent self-harm. This activity, variously called special, constant or continuous observation is, although often carried out by unqualified staff, complex and demanding (Duffy 1995). Because it inevitably tends to be intrusive and often unwelcome to the patient, the intensity of the observation should be related to the level of risk and should be reduced when the clinical team agree that risk has reduced. Rotas of staff are usually involved in carrying out increased observation, and accurate records and communication are essential. The whole process should be monitored by the patient's primary or key nurse. Its purpose should be explained to patients and their visitors. Increased observation should be seen as a therapeutic intervention and integrated into the overall plan of care rather than viewed as a custodial practice. National standards have yet to be agreed but it is important that staff responsible for providing constant observation receive some form of training that covers such issues as responding to emergencies, risk assessment and development of therapeutic relationships.

THERAPEUTIC INTERVENTIONS

The therapeutic alliance

Effective care and treatment of suicidal people begins with the establishment of genuine therapeutic relationships. The Samaritans are a major voluntary service who specialize in assisting people who may be distressed and suicidal by using helping skills through telephone conversations. They place great emphasis on devoting listening skills, time and attention to the caller, trying thereby to convey the sense that the person is valued. Certainly, the 'neediness' of the suicidal person can require a patient and skilful response from the helper, volunteer or professional. Kullgren (1988) notes of patients with borderline personality disorder (a high risk group for suicidal behaviour) that they are 'particularly gifted at provoking rejecting and repressive behaviour in close interpersonal relationships, including their relationships with inpatient hospital staff'. Birtchnell (1983) suggests that latent suicidal tendencies exist in many people, including health professionals, and this may lead to a need on the part of staff to 'repress' and fail to respect suicidal behaviour in patients. Such people may be then be labelled by staff as 'difficult' and become examples of Stockwell's (1972) 'unpopular patient'. Morgan

& Priest (1991) have argued that this in turn may exacerbate existing alienation and turn potential into actual suicidal behaviour. The extent to which nursing staff do in fact adopt negative attitudes towards suicidal people is contentious. Platt & Salter (1987) found that nurses were more likely than psychiatrists to view DSH patients as 'attention seekers' and Patel (1975) argued that nurses had more positive attitudes towards patients with physical illnesses than they did towards people who demonstrated suicidal behaviour. However, Anderson (1997), comparing the attitudes of 80 CPNs and accident and emergency nurses towards suicidal behaviour, found generally positive attitudes in both groups.

We can be clear, however, that it is vital to maintain an empathetic and positive attitude. A balance must be struck between showing respect for the person and their wishes and at the same time avoiding reinforcement of suicidal behaviour by rewarding it with particular and overt attention (Birtchnell 1983, Henderson 1974).

Approaches to therapy

An individualized care plan, coordinated by a key-worker who can offer consistent contact and supervision of care, should be formulated to take account of the person's specific needs. A range of interventions should be selected with the person's involvement in the plan as far as possible. Examples include:

- appropriate and effectively monitored medication
- ECT
- problem-solving therapy
- cognitive behavioural therapy
- supportive counselling
- problem-solving family therapy
- assistance with practical issues such as finances, housing, etc.
- structured activities.

Cognitive behavioural therapy can help the person to become aware of and reframe negative states of mind. Problem-solving therapy is aimed at helping the person to identify specific problems, generate possible solutions and derive concrete and achievable goals. A study by Salkovskis, Atha & Storer (1990) showed a significant reduction in depression and hopelessness after problem-solving therapy in a group of people at high risk of repeating DSH. A more intensive version developed by Linehan (1993) has been similarly successful. People who injure themselves can be shown alternative ways of dealing with the build-up of tension that precedes their behaviour—for example, relaxation techniques and appropriate ventilation of feelings; cognitive approaches may also be of use.

During any form of care and treatment the level of risk will rarely be constant and may often fluctuate. It is essential to beware of false improvements: the person's apparent calmness may be due to a final decision for suicide having been made, while an increase in vitality as a profound depression lifts may provide the energy for a suicide attempt. Another danger is that the improvement has been dependent on the therapeutic setting, and the person relapses on discharge, leading to self-harm soon after.

DISCHARGE

People who have been effectively cared for while in a state of suicidal despair may be especially vulnerable when they return to their homes or when community staff withdraw, and there is significant clustering of suicide soon after discharge (Goldacre, Seagroatt & Hawton 1993). It is essential to plan the discharge process carefully beforehand and to ensure that withdrawal of care is as gradual as possible. The care programme approach (CPA) is intended to ensure that such needs are met, yet a study in Greater Manchester by Dennehy et al (1996) found that most of their sample of discharged psychiatric patient suicides had no identifiable keyworker—a crucial aspect of the CPA. Further, almost half of those who had committed suicide were not recorded as having been suicidal and in almost half of those who had expressed suicidal ideas the supervision or treatment was not changed. Clearly a follow-up plan must be agreed and coordinated by an identified, accountable clinician. Efforts must be made to

ensure adequate community support from friends and relatives and telephone contact with statutory and voluntary services made available.

SUICIDE SURVIVORS

It is only in recent years that the needs of people who are associated with the person who has completed suicide have begun to be systematically considered. These 'survivors' are, of course, the person's family and friends, but there are also people who can be traumatically affected by the suicide of those they were not conventionally 'close' to—for example, devoted fans of a celebrity suicide, or clinical staff who have cared for someone who has killed themselves.

Suicide survivors must not only undergo the normal processes of grief, they may also have to deal with trauma associated with discovering the victim; blame from others or from themselves; feelings of anger; real or imagined social stigma; or financial difficulties if the family breadwinner has died. Children may experience particular difficulties since adults may be unable to assist them in understanding the death (Dunne 1992). It is therefore unsurprising that suicide survivors may experience mental health problems and that they themselves are at increased risk of suicide (Roy 1986). The impact of a suicide may therefore be felt both widely and over generations. At present no coordinated service exists to meet the needs of survivors, although voluntary services offer support—for example Cruse, who provide bereavement counselling by volunteers, and the Compassionate Friends, who offer befriending to bereaved parents, including parents of suicides.

SUMMARY

Some have seen the prevalence of self-harming behaviour as an indicator of an unhealthy society (DOH 1998). Whether or not this is true, a healthy society would surely be characterized by a willingness to try to address states of mind in which so many people hang or gas themselves, need to have their stomachs pumped or inflict lacerations on their own bodies. This is not to lack respect for the wishes of people who self-harm, but to understand that very often such people are 'not themselves', that they have lost sight of other options in their lives. By being able to recognize such people and by understanding how to relate to them and how to provide guidance and support, health care workers can make a very real contribution to the health of society.

FURTHER READING

Atkinson J M 1978 Discovering suicide: studies in the social organisation of sudden death. Macmillan, London
Aspects of suicidal behaviour explored by a sociologist. A useful complement to psychiatric and psychological studies of the subject.

Bongar B (ed) 1992 Suicide: guidelines for assessment, management, and treatment. Oxford University Press, New York
A comprehensive collection of papers addressing the subject mainly from the perspective of psychiatry.

Hill K 1995 The long sleep: young people and suicide. Virago, London
A very readable and informative study of suicide among this high risk group.

NHS Health Advisory Service 1994 Suicide prevention: the challenge confronted. HMSO, London
A thorough and practical guide to the prevention of suicide.

Williams M 1997 Cry of pain: understanding suicide and self-harm. Penguin, Harmondsworth
A wide-ranging, up to date survey of the subject by a clinical psychologist.

REFERENCES

Allebeck P, Allgulander C 1990 Suicide among young men: psychiatric illness, deviant behaviour and substance abuse. Acta Psychiatrica Scandinavica 81: 565–570

Anderson M 1997 Nurses' attitudes towards suicidal behaviour—a comparative study of community mental health nurses and nurses working in an accident and emergency department. Journal of Advanced Nursing 25:1283–1291

Appleby L 1992 Suicide in psychatric patients: risk and prevention. British Journal of Psychiatry 161:749–758

Appleby L 1997 National confidential inquiry into suicide and homicide by people with mental illness: progress report 1997. Department of Health, London

Appleby L, Amos T, Doyle U et al 1996 General practitioners and young suicides: is there a preventive role for primary care? British Journal of Psychiatry 168:330–333

Atkinson J M 1978 Discovering suicide: studies in the social organisation of sudden death. Macmillan, London

Barraclough B, Bunch J, Nelson B, Sainsbury P 1974 A hundred cases of suicide: clinical aspects. British Journal of Psychiatry 125:355–373

Beck A T, Weissman A, Lester D, Trexler L 1974 The measurement of pessimism: the hopelessness scale. Journal of Consulting and Clinical Psychology 42:861–865

Birtchnell J 1983 Psychotherapeutic considerations in the management of the suicidal patient. American Journal of Psychiatry XXXVII:1

Brimblecombe N 1998 Supporting clients with suicidal impulses in the community. Nursing Times 94:49–51

Catalan J, Marsack P, Hawton K E, Whitwell D, Fagg J, Bancroft J H J 1980 Comparison of doctors and nurses in the assessment of deliberate self-poisoning patients. Psychological Medicine 10:483–491

Charlton J, Kelly S, Dunnell K, Evans B, Jenkins R, Wallis R 1994a Trends in suicide deaths in England and Wales. In: Jenkins R et al (eds) The prevention of suicide. HMSO, London, pp 5–12

Charlton J, Kelly S, Dunnell K, Evans B, Jenkins R 1994b Suicide deaths in England and Wales: trends in factors associated with suicide deaths. In: Jenkins R et al (eds) The prevention of suicide. HMSO, London, pp 13–21

Clark D C, Fawcett J 1992 Review of empirical risk factors for evaluation of the suicidal patient. In: Bongar, B (ed) 1992 Suicide: guidelines for assessment, management and treatment. Oxford University Press, Oxford, pp 16–48

Crammer J L 1984 The special characteristics of suicide in hospital inpatients. British Journal of Psychiatry 145:460–476

Crombie I K 1989 Trends in suicide and unemployment in Scotland, 1976–1986. British Medical Journal 298:782–784

Dennehy J A, Appleby L, Thomas C S, Faragher E B 1996 Case-control study of suicide by discharged psychiatric patients. British Medical Journal 312:1580

DOH (Department of Health) 1992 The health of the nation: a strategy for health in England. HMSO, London

DOH (Department of Health) 1993 Health of the nation key area handbook: mental illness. HMSO, London

DOH (Department of Health) 1994 The prevention of suicide. HMSO, London

DOH (Department of Health) 1998 Our healthier nation. HMSO, London

Dooley E 1990 Prison suicide in England and Wales, 1972–87. British Journal of Psychiatry 156:40–45

Dorpat T L, Ripley H S 1960 A study of suicide in the Seattle area. Comprehensive Psychiatry 1:349–359

Drye R C, Goulding R L, Goulding M E 1973 No-suicide decisions: patient monitoring of suicidal risk. American Journal of Psychiatry 130(2):171–174

Duffy D 1993 Preventing suicide. Nursing Times 89(31):28–31

Duffy D 1995 Out of the shadows: a study of the special observation of suicidal in-patients. Journal of Advanced Nursing 21:944–950

Dunne E J 1992 Following a suicide: postvention. In: Bongar B (ed) Suicide: guidelines for assessment, management, and treatment. Oxford University Press, New York, pp 221–234

Durkheim E 1897/1952 Suicide: a study in sociology. Routledge, London

Elwood P Y, De Silva P 1998 'The Health of the Nation', suicide and the general hospital doctor. Psychiatric Bulletin 22:150–152

Fairbairn G J 1995 Contemplating suicide: the language and ethics of self-harm. Routledge, London

Farberow N, MacKinnon D 1974 A suicide prediction schedule for neuro-psychiatric hospital patients. Journal of Nervous and Mental Disease 158:408–419

Freud 1917/1957 Mourning and melancholia. In: Strachey J (ed) The standard edition of the complete psychological works of Sigmund Freud, vol 14. Hogarth Press, London

Goldacre M, Seagroatt V, Hawton K 1993 Suicide after discharge from psychiatric inpatient care. The Lancet 342:283–286

Gunnell D 1994 The potential for preventing suicide. University of Bristol, Bristol

Harris E C, Barraclough B 1997 Suicide as an outcome for mental disorders: a meta-analysis. British Journal of Psychiatry 170:205–228

Hawton K, Catalan J 1987 Attempted suicide: a practical guide to its nature and management, 2nd edn. Oxford University Press, Oxford

Hawton K, Fagg J 1988 Suicide, and other causes of death following attempted suicide. British Journal of Psychiatry 152:359–366

Hawton K, Fagg J, Simkin S, Bale E, Bond A 1997 Trends in deliberate self-harm in Oxford, 1985–1995: implications for clinical services and the prevention of suicide. British Journal of Psychiatry 171:556–560

Hawton K, Fagg J, Simkin S, Harriss L, Malmberg A 1998 Methods used for suicide by farmers in England and Wales: the contribution of availability and its relevance to prevention. British Journal of Psychiatry 173:320–324

Henderson A S 1974 Care eliciting behaviour in man. Journal of Nervous and Mental Disease 159:172–181

Humphrey R 1991 Final exit. Dell, New York

Kapur N, House A 1988 Against a high risk strategy in the prevention of suicide. Psychiatric Bulletin 22:534–536

Kelly S, Charlton J, Jenkins R 1995 Suicide deaths in England and Wales, 1982–92: the contribution of occupation and geography. Population Trends 80:16–25

Kreitman N 1976 The coal gas story: UK suicide rates 1960–1971. British Journal of Preventive and Social Medicine 30:86–93

Kreitman N 1977 Parasuicide. John Wiley, Chichester

Kullgren C 1988 Factors associated with completed suicide in borderline personality disorder. Journal of Nervous and Mental Disease 176:40–44

Linehan M M 1993 Cognitive-behavioural treatment of borderline personality disorder. Guilford, New York

Lovett C G, Maltsberger J T 1992 Psychodynamic approaches to the assessment and management of suicide. In: Bongar B (ed) Suicide: guidelines for assessment, management, and treatment. Oxford University Press, New York, pp 160–175

McKie A 1994 Negative attitudes that lead to poor assessment: a survey of attitudes towards caring for suicidal patients. Psychiatric Care 1(5):186–190

Miles C P 1977 Conditions predisposing to suicide: a review. Journal of Nervous and Mental Disease 164:231–246

Miller A 1981 After the fall. In: Plays, vol II. Methuen, London

Morgan H G 1990 Suicide in psychiatric hospitals: to what extent is it preventable? In: Hawton K, Cowen P (eds) Dilemmas and difficulties in the management of psychiatric patients. Oxford University Press, Oxford, pp 77–89

Morgan H G, Priest P 1991 Suicide and unexpected deaths among psychiatric in-patients. The Bristol confidential inquiry. British Journal of Psychiatry 158:368–374

Motto J A 1992 Clinical applications of biological aspects of suicide. In: B Bongar (ed) Suicide: guidelines for assessment, management and treatment. Oxford University Press, Oxford, pp 49–66

Motto J A, Heilbron D C, Juster R P 1985 Development of a clinical instrument to estimate suicide risk. American Journal of Psychiatry 142(6):680–686

Needleman J, Farrell M 1997 Suicide and substance misuse. British Journal of Psychiatry 171:303–304

NHS Health Advisory Service. 1994 Suicide prevention: the challenge confronted. HMSO, London

O'Brien J T, Tarbuck A F 1992 Suicide and vehicle exhaust emissions. British Medical Journal 304:76

Patel A R 1975 Attitudes towards self-poisoning. British Medical Journal 2:426–430

Platt S 1984 Unemployment and suicidal behaviour: a review of the literature. Social Science and Medicine 19(2):93–115

Platt S, Salter D 1987 A comparison of health workers' attitudes towards parasuicide. Social Psychiatry 22:202–208

Pritchard C 1995 Unemployment, age, gender and regional suicide in England and Wales 1974–90: a harbinger of increased suicide for the 1990s? British Journal of Social Work 25(6):767–790

Renvoize E B, Clayden D 1990 Can the suicide rate be used as a performance indicator in mental illness? Health Trends 22:16–20

Rogers C R 1967 On becoming a person: a therapist's view of psychotherapy. Constable, London

Roy A 1986 Suicide. Williams & Wilkins, Baltimore, MD

Salkovskis P M, Atha C, Storer D 1990 Cognitive-behavioural problem solving in the treatment of patients who repeatedly attempt suicide. British Journal of Psychiatry 157:871–876

Schmidtke A, Hafner H 1988 The Werther effect after television films: new evidence of an old hypothesis. Psychological Medicine 18:665–676

Soni Raleigh V, Bulusu L, Balarajan R 1990 Suicides among immigrants from the Indian sub-continent. British Journal of Psychiatry 156:46–50

Stenager E N, Madsen C, Stenager E, Boldson J 1998 Suicide in patients with stroke: epidemiological study. British Medical Journal 316(7139):1206

Stockwell F 1972 The unpopular patient. Croom Helm, Beckenham

Todd C J 1992 Reduction in the incidence of suicide: a health gain objective for the NHS. Journal of Psychopharmacology 6(2)(suppl):318–324

Tolstoy L 1901/1972 Anna Karenin (trans. C. Garnett). Heinemann, London

Towl G J, Crighton D A 1998 Suicide in prisons in England and Wales from 1988 to 1995. Criminal Behaviour and Mental Health 8:184–192

Weishaar M E, Beck A T 1990 The suicidal patient: how should the therapist respond? In: Hawton K, Cowen P (eds) Dilemmas and difficulties in the management of psychiatric patients. Oxford University Press, Oxford, pp 65–76

Williams M 1997 Cry of pain: understanding suicide and self-harm. Penguin, Harmondsworth

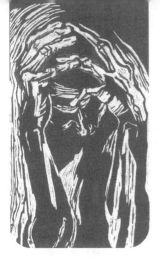

Chapter Eighteen

Developing a supportive service—a case example

Christine A Kirk

AIMS

- ◆ To understand the principles of providing an effective service for elderly mentally ill people and their carers
- ◆ To reflect on the successes, pitfalls and lessons learned in implementing a strategy for such a service

KEY ISSUES

Legislation

Values and policies

Style of service

Devising a strategy

Community mental health team for the elderly

Assessment services

Treatment and rehabilitation

Continuing care

Staffing innovations and community units for the elderly

Training issues

Evaluation

INTRODUCTION

For a long time it has been recognized that good practice for working with elderly mentally ill people and their carers requires the provision of comprehensive, flexible, caring, reliable, locally based services, to enable people to live independently in the community for as long as they are able. The guidelines relating to necessary components for comprehensive psychiatric services for elderly people have not been bettered since the Health Advisory Service (HAS) document, 'The rising tide' (1982).

The white paper 'Caring for people' (DoH 1989) and the National Health Service and Community Care Act (1990) set the then government's policy framework for community care. The policy guidance set out *what* was expected to meet the proposals on community care, but *how* it was done was left for innovation and flexibility at local level.

'The new NHS: modern, dependable' (DOH 1997) and subsequent guidance emphasizes evolutionary change, building on what has worked and reinforcing the need for partnership between all major stakeholders; and focusing on quality of care. Within the programmes, mental health and healthier older people are priorities in this social policy reform agenda.

The care programme approach (CPA) (DOH 1990) formalized previous good practice with people with mental health problems in emphasizing the need for an identified care manager (agreed between health and social services) to work with clients and their carers to plan, review and follow up a care programme.

In addition to the pressures from central government to provide a coordinated, comprehensive, integrated service for elderly mentally ill people and their carers, the increasing consumer voice of users of the service and voluntary organizations representing older people and their carers raise expectations of high standards of care and consumer choice. These are increasingly difficult to provide in a climate of cost conscious competition and at a time of reorganization of both health and local authority services.

In this chapter I will describe how one health

Box 18.1 Mental health partnership group statement of shared values

The partnership group for mental health recognizes the importance of sharing common values when planning mental health services between agencies. To foster collaboration and commitment, the agencies represented on the partnership group have agreed this statement of shared values, including the principles against which future plans and polices can be measured.

Aim

To provide a local, accessible and comprehensive mental health service, which is user centred and designed to promote the most acceptable quality of life geared to the individual's rights and needs.

Principles

Mental health services will be based on the following principles:

1. Services should be clearly defined in terms of rights. They should be local, accessible and non-stigmatizing.

2. Services should be supportive without encouraging unnecessary dependence. Information should be readily available and clearly presented so that meaningful choices can be made about the range of services available.

3. Services should be integrated to make the best use of existing resources, provide continuity and be sufficiently flexible to respond to changing need.

4. Services should cater for the needs and interests of families and carers.

5. Services must make clear statements to the community about priority and maintain effective services through regular reviews.

6. Services must take account of the ethnic, religious and cultural needs of service users.

7. Services should be participative by developing the involvement of service users.

---

trust implemented its plans to provide a good local service for elderly mentally ill people and their carers in collaboration with other agencies, and will highlight some of the pitfalls, lessons learned and the successes attained.

VALUES AND POLICY

The health authority adopted a statement of shared values via the planning partnership group for mental health (health, social services, voluntary sector, housing). This is detailed in Box 18.1.

The workers within the mental health service for elderly people work with all local statutory and voluntary agencies to plan the care with and for an individual and their carer. They involve the patient, the carer and significant others in producing the individual management plan, taking into account confidentiality issues.

STYLE OF SERVICE

At the time of planning (late 1980s), our health district served approximately 40 000 elderly people, resident in the four sectors of the mental health service. The population has now increased in line with national demographic changes. Providing a sectorized community service means that the specialist mental health workers can get to know and be known by the community workers, be more easily accessible, be more sensitive to the needs of the community and have earlier contact with patients than if they were all hospital based. Our system is similar to the hive system of psychiatric care described by Tyrer (1985), with the central hospital as a parallel to a honey bee hive and the workers coming to and from the hospital, to secondary 'units' close to the area of greater psychiatric morbidity. Psychiatric workers spend much of their time in the community, but like the bee have regular contact with the central hospital (hive), discussing the identified need and deploying resources within the community and statutory services' system to meet that need (Fig. 18.1).

DEVISING A STRATEGY

It is difficult to be sure of the exact prevalence of the commonest psychiatric disorders in elderly people (chronic organic brain syndromes—the dementias, affective disorders and paranoid disorders) because of difficulties in precise case identification, dependent on which instruments are used

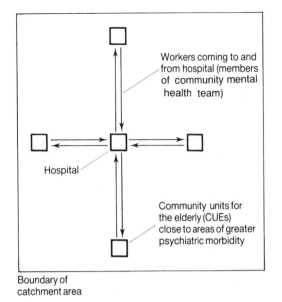

Fig. 18.1 The hive system of psychiatric care.

and whether appropriate cut-off scores are used (when does a case become 'a case'?). However, it is known that the prevalence increases with age, and with an ageing (particularly very old) population there will undoubtedly be more pressure on the statutory and voluntary services for this client group.

Very few places have the advantage of coterminosity between health and local authority boundaries, which increases the complexity for most planners in determining the expected need for specialist services. It is important, nevertheless, for some assessment to be made of the population need, by putting together expected changes in demography with the estimated prevalence of the commonest disorders. Our health district checked our prevalence of dementia (as identified by a validated instrument—the Clifton Assessment Procedures for the Elderly (CAPE)) in a local general practice sample of elderly people (Pattie & Moxon 1987) and we were relieved to discover that there was no more dementia there than elsewhere. The rule of thumb which I use in thinking of our likely local need is that, for the population over 65 years, 5% are likely to have a significant degree of dementia (with an increase with increasing age of the population—for example, for the over 80s about 20% will have dementia) and up to 20% depression. However, those with depression may not be so easily identified unless sought out, compared with those with dementia. In work with colleagues in social services it must be remembered that in 'special' places such as residential homes (compared with people in their own homes) there is likely to be a very much higher prevalence of psychiatric disorders (the client's mental state having determined the need for care in the residential home in the first place).

As well as knowing approximately how much psychiatric morbidity there is in the area, it is important to know who else is doing what in terms of dealing with this client group. No agency has resources to waste by duplicating what someone else is providing, and from the client's perspective a single access point to provide for a specific need is required. For example, in our area, social services have little specialist residential or day care for the elderly mentally infirm, but have developed an intensive domiciliary care scheme working alongside the community mental health team for the elderly. The private sector, similarly, has not developed much specialist residential or nursing home care for this client group and so it has fallen upon the health services to fill this particular gap, which historically, in our area, has been filled by the provision of continuing care beds in mental hospitals.

Our hypothesis was that, if we could be involved with patients and their carers early in the course of their illness, we would be able to provide a good, comprehensive, integrated, supportive community-based service with fewer long stay beds and still be able to cope with the demographic changes, with the increasing elderly (especially very elderly) population and the expected increased prevalence of psychiatric morbidity.

COMMUNITY MENTAL HEALTH TEAM FOR THE ELDERLY

Setting up a community mental health team for the elderly demands a great deal of time, effort and thought, with commitment to this style of working obtained from the multidisciplinary team of work-

ers, their professional line managers and the general manager of the mental health services. Issues relating to this and the continuing running of psychogeriatric teams are described in Lindesay (1991). The success of our team has been helped by the use of several 'time-out' sessions where, with an outside facilitator, we have clarified our operational policy, aims and objectives, and worked out roles and functions, both as individuals and as team managers. Having clear objectives and priorities for work has meant we can evaluate more easily what we are doing and tell other people who need to know (e.g. managers, other community workers) more readily what we are about. It is important for other workers with this client group to know how to gain access to our specialist skills, what they can and cannot expect from us and to spread the word of what is available via us to their clients and colleagues. If other workers do not know of our existence then our aim of early involvement with patients and their carers cannot be achieved; if they do not know the limits of capabilities then their expectations will be unrealistically raised, clients will be disappointed and our team will be swamped with inappropriate referrals with the resulting demoralization of all concerned.

The core community mental health team (for 20 000 elderly people) consisted of a secretary, four community psychiatric nurses (CPNs), a social worker, a clinical psychologist, a consultant psychiatrist and junior doctor, an occupational therapist, part-time physiotherapist, managers for the community unit for the elderly, and ward managers for the main assessment ward and day hospital. Special home care assistants and their home care manager (employed by social services) are also part of the team, but only come to the team meetings serving their particular geographical area. Team members follow the professional ethics and codes of practice of their own profession.

The weekly clinical team meetings act as an information exchange, an opportunity for report giving (assessment and progress), care plan changing, trouble shooting (seeking advice of team members at times of crisis) and the giving and receiving of support. The secretary notes significant information for the case records and data are collected for an audit of team activity. In addition, relevant (to the geographical area) members of the team meet in different areas on a monthly basis with other community workers (district nurse, social worker, voluntary sector workers, home care manager and special home care assistants) to exchange information about 'shared' clients in that particular area. Business meetings of the community mental health team are held every 2 months and there is a regular time-out meeting for team development every 6 months.

Referrals to our team can come from any source to any member, but we always ask the referrer to make sure that the general practitioner is aware of the referral. This gets around any difficulties produced by the reluctance of certain individuals to refer on for specialist psychiatric services, produced by the attitude of the 'non-referring' professional of 'what do you expect at her age?' and 'nothing can be done, so why bother busy people?' We hope that, by demonstrating what we can do to help, we will 'educate' that person, changing inappropriate, ageist views. The majority of referrals do in fact, come from GPs to the consultant, which is the traditional way of team working, but this ratio of consultant versus other team member referral is changing. Traditionally there is concern, if a person is referred to anyone in the team other than a doctor, that a potentially treatable medical condition will be missed, but statistically it is far more likely that a doctor to doctor referral will miss social or functional disabilities, which are better assessed by other members of the multidisciplinary team.

Team members use their professional skills to decide whether or not to bring each referral to them to the team meeting. The person to whom the referral is made is responsible for the initial assessment, including risk assessment, referring on to other team members for additional assessments if appropriate, and informing both the referrer and the client of what is happening. A care coordinator (CPA—see above) is identified who is responsible for devising, recording and reviewing the care plan.

The roles of team members are as follows:

CPN
◆ assessment of nursing needs, provision and evaluation of care plan

◆ advice to other professional workers in the community
◆ support for carers and relatives
◆ specific specialist treatment, e.g. giving injections, different therapies according to skill and expertise of individual CPN
◆ referring agent for different assessments and care
◆ education of others about mental disorders in elderly people

medical staff
◆ assessment of physical and psychiatric disorders by history taking, physical and psychiatric examination, and organization of appropriate investigations
◆ involvement in psychiatric treatments, e.g. medication, ECT, psychotherapy
◆ treatment and management of physical disorders, involving the appropriate specialists as necessary
◆ accepting medical responsibility for the patient referred by GP

occupational therapist
◆ assessment of daily living skills
◆ assessment of support systems, accommodation, social activities
◆ treatments including dressing practice, domestic work, relaxation, provision of appropriate aids and equipment to increase independence
◆ organization of activity/social groups

physiotherapist
◆ assessment of patient's physical condition, e.g. posture, coordination, mobility
◆ specific physiotherapy treatments
◆ advice on appropriate aids and appliances, e.g. seating, walking aids
◆ work with families, carers and other disciplines on physical aspects, e.g. mobility, lifting techniques
◆ group work particularly aimed at physical stimulation

psychologist
◆ assessment of cognitive, behavioural and emotional functioning
◆ specialist psychological treatments, e.g. anxiety management, cognitive therapy, behavioural therapy, hypnosis

- counselling and advice to carers and relatives on behavioural management
- advice and support to other disciplines, using psychological assessments and therapeutic approaches

secretary
- secretarial work for team
- liaising with relatives, carers and patients and putting them in touch with the right team member at the right time
- liaising with community-based organizations and other medical teams
- coordinating clinical information for relevant team members
- organizing trainee placements with different team members.

All team members are expected to 'educate' other team members about their specific specialist skills and experience.

ASSESSMENT SERVICES

Central to the provision of any specialist service is good quality assessment of need. The issue of needs-led assessment within the care management process cannot be dealt with here in detail. However, the specialist mental health assessment for elderly people and their carers and how this has been planned in our service will be described.

A multidisciplinary approach is employed to produce a comprehensive assessment of the physical, psychological and social needs and strengths of the individual. Each professional's individual assessment is integrated with information provided by other members of the extended team—that is, patient, family, home carers, district nurses, etc. It is most important to work out a sensible, realistic management plan with the patient and relatives (or other carers), involving all the key players in the community care 'package'. Often the interplay of physical, psychological, social and financial factors is so complex that if everyone is not 'signed up' to what is being attempted, and why, then the management plan is doomed to failure.

Information must be provided to the patient and carers about the illness, its possible treatment,

its likely course and the facilities and help that can be provided. It is sensible to provide this information in written form if possible, often in pamphlets, so that the individuals can take these away to ponder and discuss with, for example, other members of the family and come back and ask further questions if they do not understand it all, or some aspect of the care is not clear. We know from experience and research work in other areas that if relatives and other carers do not agree with, and cannot be persuaded about, a particular management scheme then it is unlikely to be successful for long. Information from carers about their views of things can be sought at formal case reviews or conferences, informally in the community by team members or at relative support groups. Sensitivity to the needs of carers is paramount in producing a long-lasting, effective supportive plan.

Individual carers (and individual patients) need individual opportunities to voice their opinions. Some people are quite happy meeting with a full multidisciplinary team to discuss their relative (client), whilst others prefer a quiet, informal discussion with one key member of the team, perhaps in the relative security of their own home, where they can display openly their feelings of, for example, grief at the illness of their relative. Helping them to be prepared for the future and what it may hold is a critical function of the team members. The aim is to avert potential crises before they occur. Even if this cannot be totally averted, at least the carer knows where to summon help and the team member knows the situation in considerable detail and can make a timely, appropriate response when the call for help comes.

It seems impossible to think of 'assessment' without thinking of management and treatment and the process of assessment is, of course, ongoing with review and evaluation of the management plan.

Up to a point, it does not matter where assessment takes place, but ideally it starts where patients are living, whether it be their own home, that of a relative, or a residential or a nursing home. If sufficient information is available from the patient and an independent informant, a physical and mental state examination and appropriate investigations have been carried out already and it seems after appropriate multidisciplinary discussion that no further assessment is needed, then a management plan can be devised immediately. However, further assessment may be necessary, for example by other professionals, which may take place in the patient's home, or different aspects may need to be assessed in different settings, for example the day hospital or hospital ward.

Such separate specialist assessments have different indications. For example, a patient with a chronic organic brain syndrome (dementia), with a fluctuating course, who lives at home with little support, can be assessed in the day hospital. The advantages of this are that the patient (who is already confused) is not uprooted totally, and attendance for 2 or 3 days a week gives the multidisciplinary team a chance to see different aspects of the same patient in different settings—at home and in a communal environment—and over a period of time. It then becomes possible to tease out which behaviours occur in which places and to look at possible influences of other people on the patients and their behaviour and illness.

After attendance for a reasonable period of time, for example, 2 days a week for 3 weeks, a review meeting is held with all concerned and a plan of action drawn up. Specific professionals of the community mental health team will be involved in this assessment process alongside day hospital staff, carers (formal and informal) and the patients themselves. Treatment and rehabilitation are provided as appropriate for patients with both organic brain syndromes and with functional illness. Other advantages of day hospital assessment are that it can test out the feasibility of day care as part of the care package, and relatives and the patient experience what it is like having support organized while the patient remains at home and is not removed to the unfamiliar, artificial surroundings of the hospital ward.

However, it may be necessary to arrange inpatient assessment if the situation has broken down at home; if it seems that alternative residential accommodation is needed and assessment is to include what type of accommodation is required, for example residential home or nursing home; or if 24-hour assessment is indicated because of problems, for example, during the night. Inpatient

facilities vary from place to place but generally are in either a psychiatric hospital or a general hospital. Obviously, for elderly people, who are likely to have both physical and psychiatric illness coincidentally, or interacting, it is ideal to have easy access to the investigative facilities and the specialist staff of a general hospital.

Our service has assessment beds for elderly mentally ill people in both the acute psychiatric hospital adjacent to the general hospital site and in a joint geriatric/psychogeriatric assessment ward in the district general hospital. Our facilities, shown below, seem to be a reasonable model for this type of service:

District general hospital	21 beds—joint geriatric/psychogeriatric assessment ward
Mental hospital	24 beds—organic and functional illness assessment
Community units for the elderly	variable—organic illness assessment

Approximately 1 bed per 1000 elderly people for organic assessment

Few places have successful joint geriatric/psychogeriatric inpatient units. However, geriatric/psychogeriatric liaison works increasingly well throughout the UK using different models of collaborative links, for example joint outpatient clinics and joint whole departments of medicine and psychiatry for elderly people. Our joint ward developed as a response to local GPs who felt that this would help fill a gap in the provision of services for elderly people with both psychiatric and physical illness. Factors influencing its success include having a multidisciplinary team dedicated to the ward; having all the beds designated as 'joint' beds and not a certain number of geriatric and separate psychogeriatric, which could lead to dispute; and the fact that the two consultants (one physician for the elderly and one psychiatrist for the elderly) involved in the ward get on well together and have a shared philosophy of how it should work.

Some places have opted to have psychiatric wards for elderly people where people with organic and functional illnesses are assessed alongside each other in the same ward. There are advantages in this for people who have mixed (organic and functional) disorders as they are correctly placed for the best specialist skills, as well as for all elderly people, as the staff have developed expertise in and interest in working with older people (compared with services where older people with functional illness are assessed with those of younger age and where frail, elderly depressed people may have to contend with, for example, young and difficult to manage schizophrenics on the same ward). Staff are geared to the slower treatment response and rehabilitation of older people, and some elderly functionally ill people in the rehabilitation phase of their inpatient stay seem to benefit from and enjoy helping other more disabled, demented people.

However, some people with functional illness are undoubtedly upset if they are nursed alongside severely demented people, possibly with deteriorated personal habits. So, if older people for assessment are in a common assessment ward there must be physical space and separate activities, as appropriate, for segregating those with dementia from those with functional illness, but with possibilities of integration for joint social activities.

Our service used to have beds for elderly people with functional illness in the wards serving the sector for general psychiatric practice. This has now evolved to having a separate elderly assessment unit, as above, which seems to be more efficient but does have slight disadvantages as outlined previously. In a service that is increasingly community orientated, it is helpful for the staff in the assessment ward to get to know the people involved in the community networks so that discharge planning and the care management process can be facilitated.

Why do we continue to do our assessments in a central hospital facility at all? It certainly is helpful in terms of communication with key staff, access to appropriate investigative facilities and the efficient economic use of highly trained specialist staff. However, we are assessing and treating patients increasingly in their own homes and in community day facilities, especially in the community units for the elderly (CUEs). This means

we and the patient are nearer to, or are part of, the informal community network; there is no stigma of being a psychiatric inpatient, which many patients and families prefer; and members of the primary care team can continue to be involved.

Different places have evolved different assessment procedures and documentation but, overall, the aim must be to produce a comprehensive assessment of the person's physical, psychological and social strengths and needs. This must be multidisciplinary, but not all cases will require involvement of all disciplines. The type of assessment, rehabilitation and treatment work that each discipline within the team carries out is shown in the list in the previous section. Devising the documentation to be used and defining operational details of the assessment process form part of the team-building process.

TREATMENT AND REHABILITATION

Treatment and rehabilitation are provided, as appropriate, for patients with both organic brain syndromes and functional illness. Any member of the community mental health team may be drawn in, as appropriate, to fulfil a specific specialist role and will work with the patient (and other formal and informal carers) wherever the patient is. These therapeutic endeavours will be continued as necessary when the patient moves from one setting to another, for example home to hospital and vice versa. Therefore it is very important that there is close liaison and coordination between hospital-based and community-based staff, which emphasizes the importance of a care manager being identified to guide the patient through the intricacies of the care system.

Specific therapies are dealt with elsewhere in this book. However, it is important to realize that elderly people, with the loss of adaptability that old age brings, often take longer to respond to specific treatments than do younger people. Developing an understanding of and expertise in this is yet another reason why specialist elderly care services have evolved to provide a high quality service for this client group.

CONTINUING CARE SERVICES

A decision had been taken to close one of the three mental hospitals in our area, with one remaining as the acute assessment hospital. One option would have been to pour money into the existing continuing care hospital to upgrade facilities and keep the Victorian buildings in a reasonable state of repair. However, the creative decision was made to involve local providers of specialist elderly mental illness (EMI) services in the planning of an innovative model of continuing care. The concept of Community Units for the Elderly (CUEs) gradually emerged, the objectives of which are:

◆ to provide a locally based unit with a comprehensive range of services
◆ to maintain people in their own homes through flexible use of resources as long as it is appropriate
◆ to be responsive to local needs and actively encourage local people to participate in the unit
◆ to encourage joint participation between health, social services and voluntary agencies
◆ to encourage cooperation between CUE staff, local GPs, primary care teams, community mental health teams, hospital services, social services and voluntary agencies
◆ the facilities to be available for use by the local community and others, e.g. Department of Social Security, citizens' advice bureaux, health education.

Each CUE services a population of 4500–5000 elderly people (with the health district eventually needing eight such units) to replace the continuing care beds, which would gradually reduce and eventually cease to exist with the closure of the Victorian mental hospital. Because of the lack of other specialist EMI residential accommodation in the area, it was important to reprovide continuing care beds for people with severe dementia requiring 24-hour specialist psychiatric care but to aim to provide them near to the patient's home (or that of the relatives) instead of in a central hospital, and make them of a more homely nature. A model for each CUE is as follows:

Community units for the elderly: model

For 4500–5000 elderly people:

◆ 14 residential beds
◆ 20 day places
◆ Resource centre
◆ Domiciliary outreach work
◆ Team members' base

With 14 residential beds in each unit we would eventually have continuing care bed numbers in line with the HAS (1982) suggested figures (2.5–3 per 1000 elderly people). Of the 14 beds, usually 10 are continuing care, with the remainder being used for organic illness assessment, flexible respite care—either regular holiday relief or night care, or respite admissions when required to give carers a break or in a social crisis. Obviously, there has to be very careful management of the usage of beds—a very precious and expensive resource. Priorities for bed usage must be established and clear, otherwise every elderly person in the vicinity may be signing on to such an attractive, free facility. Only the most disabled, psychiatrically disturbed people with dementia who cannot be coped with in any other settings can be offered a place in the CUEs for residential continuing care, following the health authority eligibility criteria.

In addition to the beds there are 20 day places, 5 days a week (with occasional flexible weekend use), for assessment and continuing care of people who live in the vicinity. These places and times are used flexibly to build up the appropriate care package for individuals and their carers. The advantage of having day places available in the same building as a residential facility is that times of the day service do not have to be rigid and if, for example, it suits a particular day visitor to come at midday for lunch and stay until after tea, or mid evening, there is no problem with this. Equally, if carers occasionally wish to leave a day visitor just for an evening, when they go to the theatre or a football match, it can easily be done and the patients are visiting somewhere that is familiar and has people they know. However, it is important to make sure that the design of the building is suitable for day visitors and residents to be separate from each other if they so wish (e.g. day visitors with some functional illness could be very disturbed if they had to remain all the time with a person with severe dementia with deteriorated personal habits). We have taken care in the design of our buildings to be sure that there are sufficient 'day' rooms available for several different activities to be going on at the same time, and for there still to be a place where someone can go just to relax and be quiet. The programme for each person is individually tailored and will include aspects of assessment and social and recreational activities, with appropriate members of staff and/or volunteers, and other clients of the service.

The design and function of the resource centre varies from CUE to CUE depending on what the local community requires of it. This is the interface between the NHS facility (definitely *not* a hospital) and the community. Voluntary organizations can use the resource centre for whatever they wish; information is available about elderly care services in the widest sense; trained volunteers are available to provide information and if they do not know the answer to the question they can seek help from the staff in the unit who will, we hope, be able to point the person in the right direction. The volunteers in the resource centre can work with day visitors or visit and befriend the residents, and in the first CUE the volunteers run a coffee shop in the resource centre, which attracts a large number of people from the local community, the nearby shops and health centre. Thus, the community is brought to the CUE!

A 'side-effect' of this is the raising of funds for the unit, and the 'Friends of ... CUE' have bought wonderful 'extras' for the CUE—for example, they provide weekly fresh flowers for the unit and pay for holiday activities for the residents and day visitors. The resource facilities are used on a regular basis by, for example, the Department of Social Security, to provide information and advice in the locality, and to supply hearing aid batteries for elderly people. Young people from local schools come into the unit on a regular basis, which not only stimulates the residents and day visitors but also 'educates' the young people about what we are doing, so reducing the stigma of psychiatric illness in old age and possibly the fear of the unknown for the young people.

Elderly people themselves, and their carers, frequently say that what they really want is help in their own homes to assist them in being as independent as possible. We have attempted to provide some of this care at home by the workers from the CUE going to people's homes to help with necessary tasks—for example, bathing, getting ready to go to the day centre, going to appointments elsewhere. There are advantages in the outreach worker from the CUE assisting the person with these tasks. The number of people who confused individuals have to deal with is reduced and they will often be more cooperative with someone they know and trust than with a relative stranger coming to the house. However, there rests a great deal of responsibility on the outreach worker working in a person's home and the type of work is different from that in a hospital with its readily available support from other staff members.

The detailed planning of each CUE was done by a task group, consisting of a local GP, a planning operational services manager from the hospital, a consultant psychiatrist for the elderly, a social services manager, a senior nurse (elderly), a voluntary sector person and/or carer, an administrator, the CUE manager (when appointed), and, as necessary, a housing department representative and the unit management accountant (with whom we worked on bed reduction targets for the base mental hospital). A separate planning group devised, with the architect, the detail of the actual building, but there was cross-over of individuals and ideas between the groups. We have learned a great deal as we have gone through the CUE strategy programme and we have always said that each CUE would be different because of different local requirements and that the first CUE, although good, will be the worst, because we will have learned so many lessons as we have developed.

Whilst we were planning the CUEs, various other developments were taking place:

1. A community, general practice random sample was undertaken, checking out the *prevalence of dementia* in our area.

2. *Interim day facilities* were established in already existing local venues. We based this on the concept of *travelling day hospitals* where the specialist psychiatric staff travel to local places, for example church halls, and run specialist day care in different localities on different days of the week, so that clients do not have to travel far from their homes and they go to places familiar to them with no stigma of mental illness attached to them. This is a relatively cheap way of providing local day care and can be of an extremely high quality with high satisfaction for staff, clients and carers alike. However, the ground work needing to be done to set this up is considerable—for example, it is time consuming and requires considerable diplomacy and expertise to find the right place with suitable facilities for caring for elderly people who are disabled; organize catering; negotiate the lease; and develop working relationships with, for example, the mother and toddler group who may use the facility on another day, and with the hosts who, in the case of church buildings, may also be able to facilitate care by organizing volunteers to work with us. The benefits of such a scheme, as a first phase of a CUE service, include giving the staff an opportunity to 'try out' working in that particular community, getting established in the existing networks of support, and emphasizing the CUE service and its philosophy, rather than just the building, which will eventually take its place in the community. Our experience has been that a great deal of enthusiasm for such schemes is generated amongst all concerned and an amazing amount of the highest quality work is able to be done in such limited facilities. Having to pack everything up at the end of the day is a chore, but one which people gladly do.

3. Planning and implementation took place for a *special home care scheme* (initially called the special home helps)—intensive domiciliary care, with our local social services department, which gave us some experience in what it would be like working in people's homes, the forerunner of the domiciliary outreach work for the CUE. For the pilot scheme, a self-selected group of home helps was interviewed and four selected to undergo a 2-week training programme, working alongside staff involved with elderly people with mental health problems in different parts of the health and social service provision, to understand the range of problems and how they can be dealt with. These special home helps are managed by their usual domiciliary care manager (social services) and work alongside the community mental health team, especially the CPNs, in the day to day management of clients. They also attend community mental health team meetings on rotation and their contribution at these meetings is highly valued as they are often the people most intimately in contact with our clients. They value attending the meetings as it provides them with helpful support.

The initial evaluation of this scheme showed it to be effective in supporting people in their own homes and helping to keep them out of institutional care. The amount of time spent with clients was not out of the range of care given previously to existing clients of the home care schemes. However, the special home helps were able to be more flexible in what they did with and for their clients and, within limits, could organize their time with people more flexibly than previously. Their roles included: befriending; accompanying clients to appointments; introducing them to luncheon clubs, day centres, etc; taking them to other social activities and staying with them if necessary; helping with personal care and finances; helping with looking after pets and almost anything else a family carer might do. Although it is difficult to prove, it is my impression that it is this sort of scheme that has made community care possible.

4. We held a *seminar with carers* to check out whether what we were planning was in line with what they felt was necessary. Conclusions from this day were that we should go ahead with what we were doing but that we should pay attention to how people access the service (carers felt that the service they got was good once they got into it, but some had experienced difficulty getting to the right place at the right time); we should not forget the needs of younger people with presenile dementia; and should make sure that continence help was available. To run such a seminar successfully, one needs to make sure that transport is available for carers to the seminar, that it is at a time when carers are likely to be able to come and that, if necessary, some form of 'sitting service' is avail-

able to care for their 'sufferer' reliably whilst carers are at the seminar.

Since the CUE service has been developing, we have taken the opportunity to ask carers how they see this working via the CUE evaluation process (see below).

5. We undertook a *community survey* to find out what services were already in the locality the CUE was to serve, and to find out how we would fit into the community and to develop local interest. This involved, for example, schools, churches, voluntary bodies and general practitioners. The name of the first CUE, Acomb Gables, was the result of a competition run in one of the local schools. Before Acomb Gables opened, we held two open days for anyone who wished to visit and we were very pleasantly surprised to have over 700 visitors, mostly from the local community. This local interest has continued and we feel we have established a place for ourselves in the community. At first, we were almost too successful in 'selling' ourselves in that people's expectations of what we were able to provide were unrealistic and it felt, at one time, as if everybody's granny wanted to come and live with us!

6. We were building up *links with the existing voluntary sector*, for example Age Concern and Alzheimer's Society, and helping establish new groups. The voluntary sector, as well as producing pressure on statutory services to close gaps in provision of services, can act in an advocacy role on behalf of a particular client group; can be in close touch with sufferers and carers to provide directly or indirectly for their needs; and can work in partnership with the statutory services to produce good, relatively cheap care—better than either the statutory or independent sector can provide separately. Through the voluntary sector and relative support groups, day care and sitting services have been established, which complement the health and social services provision. The local Alzheimer's Society branch, in which some of the local health and social services staff are involved, also provides an information and small counselling service. At times, it is difficult to know whether a particular community psychiatric nurse, for example, is wearing a CPN or a voluntary sector hat in their dealings with a particular client

and that is not a bad thing, contributing to a 'seamless' service.

7. *Utilizing existing community facilities* has become part of the development of the service—for example, pubs, clubs and a local cricket club providing a social facility for an afternoon session. Many carers, particularly of people with dementia, gradually lose their normal social lives and getting together with other carers in a social (not a formal support group) setting is important to them. They also like to continue a previous lifestyle that may have become impossible for them with their 'sufferer' whose personal habits may have deteriorated to an embarrassing point. By going out for a pub lunch on a regular basis with new friends who are in a similar position to themselves and supported by, for example, CPNs and special home carers, they have something to look forward to and a means of continuing something that they had previously enjoyed, and which is fun. This also acts, very often, as a starting point for someone with dementia to recommence social outings, which may eventually persuade them to accept some form of day care giving the carer some respite, but which inevitably depends on a separation from their carer, which previously they may have found difficult. The carer also learns that they can trust the people who will be looking after their loved one to care for them well and not to cause distress to them.

The cricket club group arose from the need for some form of low key, informal social 'club' for people in an early stage of dementia who may have lost confidence for joining in local 'normal' social activities, but who had fairly well-preserved social fronts and who would be distressed by day centres specifically for people with severe dementia. Their carers can go along with them and join in the activities, or just chat with others there, or can use the few hours of 'freedom' to get on with whatever they wish, or just put their feet up. Some carers find that this acts as an introduction to a relative support group and they suddenly find, unexpectedly, that they benefit from talking with another carer about the problems and solutions of caring for someone with dementia.

8. We were learning about *managing the closure of the continuing care mental hospital*. Issues

there included: keeping people informed of what was happening and when and whether we were on target; identifying with staff what the future held for them; organizing training programmes for the transition from hospital to community work; managing the reduction of beds in the hospital to coincide with the opening of the new CUE beds; keeping relatives up to date with what the future held for their loved ones; keeping up morale in the closing hospital; making sure that the financial resources were transferred from one budget to another as planned; and that the more distant managers who were involved in the eventual sale of the hospital site were aware that the priority for the site at that time was good quality patient care.

Staffing innovations relating to the CUEs

Even before the advent of health care assistants, we had decided to create *generic support workers* to assist the multidisciplinary staff in the CUEs. The idea was to make it less confusing for an (already) confused person by reducing the number of people relating to them in assisting them with their everyday care. Each person would have a key worker (one of the professional trained staff) and a few support workers who would work with them wherever they were—their own homes, in the day centre, or in the residential part of the unit. The tasks of these workers included physiotherapy and occupational therapy aide, nursing assistance, cleaning, and housekeeper and catering duties and they were recruited from existing staff in the hospital service—for example, porters, nursing assistants and domestic services staff.

Adjustment to working in a different way and different setting was aided by the training programme arranged and, as time has gone on and with new cohorts of support workers as the CUE strategy progresses, the training has evolved. Nevertheless the transition is stressful, undoubtedly, and considerable support is necessary. Details of the support worker role, training and conclusions about the concept are included in the Acomb Gables evaluation (Pattie & Moxon 1991).

From the idea of people living in their own local community despite needing long term continuing

psychiatric care as a result of their, for example, dementia, we developed the notion of asking the GPs if they would continue to look after their patients when they were involved with the CUE service. To implement this required considerable discussion with and 'education' of the GPs, often on an individual basis, about the CUE concept and philosophy and the fact that it was in line with their 'cradle to the grave' care. Obviously, some GPs were more enthusiastic about this than others, but the majority have remained involved with their patients. They have provided useful information to the staff of the CUE about patients and their relatives arising from the GPs' knowing them for many years, and give a good 'normal' general practice to people in the care of the unit. GPs 'use' the unit staff as a resource when they visit, including utilizing this resource with others amongst their patients who may not be in contact with the CUE. In the evaluation of the first CUE (Pattie & Moxon 1991), most of the responding GPs were pleased with the retention of general practice responsibility and the staff of the unit felt reasonably supported by the local GPs.

Training issues relating to the CUEs

Some of the training issues identified by the evaluation of the first CUE are:

1. Blocks of training are better than day release.
2. There needs to be ongoing training once the service is established—both formally and informally by knowledge sharing amongst individual staff.
3. Shared events for qualified and support staff help team building but cannot meet their differing needs, which require separate opportunities.
4. Clarification of roles, the extent of sharing tasks and role blurring need to be understood clearly to avoid unrealistic expectations of each other.
5. Specific training needs for transition from hospital (institutional) to community work must be addressed.
6. An understanding of the organization and procedures of other services for the elderly in the area facilitates integration into the local community and services.

7. Transition from temporary premises for day care to the permanent CUE building is stressful for staff. Preparation for, support of and recognition of their change of status are required.

8. Specific individual staff have specific training and development needs in providing a flexible, local service, e.g. dealing with bereavement, dealing with unexpected events in a self-supporting unit, career development specific to a new style of service.

9. The need for training and support should not be underestimated.

EVALUATION OF THE CUE

An evaluation of the first CUE, Acomb Gables, was completed by Pattie & Moxon (1991) and a summary of the report is also available. Topics covered in this are:

1. dependency/disability of elderly people in the care of mental health and other services
2. change in dependency, location and type of care over a 6-month period of study
3. transfer of elderly people from hospital care to Acomb Gables residential care and the perceptions of relatives and staff in relation to this move
4. use of residential places, length of stay, and mortality
5. the 'before and after' and transitional aspects of the old and new style services
6. client and carer perceptions
7. staff perceptions, training, expectations and morale
8. management issues, in relation to planning, setting up and running the service
9. impact on and contribution from a variety of professionals and services
10. architectural and use of the building issues
11. aspects of quality: the environment, care, atmosphere and subjective views
12. the resource centre
13. volunteer input.

A variety of qualitative and quantitative methods were used: dependency measures, interviews, questionnaires, rating scales and routine data collection involving staff, patients, carers and other service providers in the area.

The full details of the first evaluation cannot be included here but in summary they are:

1. The level of care reflected the dependency and was appropriate to the needs of the individual.

2. Very few very highly dependent people were able to remain in their own homes but some could if they had full-time carers and supportive services.

3. The service was enjoyed and appreciated by elderly people and their carers.

4. The generic support worker role seemed successful and the staff enjoyed working in the service.

5. There needed to be an adjustment in attitude and way of working for all staff in the transition to the new service.

6. The building and location were successful in use and function and the assessment of quality of service was very satisfactory.

7. It was difficult to get adequate data about the comparative costs but the service seemed no more expensive than the traditional service and waiting lists were no longer.

8. The strategy should continue.

THE STRATEGY HAS CONTINUED AND THERE ARE NOW SEVEN CUEs IN THE YORK TRUST AREA

CASE STUDY: MRS A

Mrs A was a 75-year-old married woman, living with her husband near to our CUE when she was first referred to the service by her GP as she had become unmanageable at home since they had come back from a recent holiday visiting a member of the family in the south. Their daughter and son who lived locally were very concerned for both of them and were demanding of the GP that 'something must be done'.

CASE STUDY: MRS A (cont'd)

The consultant psychiatrist for the elderly saw Mr and Mrs A at home and she and the GP confirmed by physical examination and routine blood and urine investigations that Mrs A was physically well apart from a urinary tract infection. However, detailed history taking revealed that she had become increasingly forgetful over the past 2 years and had been able to do less and less at home to deal with her personal hygiene and the day to day domestic tasks. Her husband had willingly taken these on but found it difficult to cope with her increasing confusion, constant packing and unpacking of clothes into a suitcase and wardrobe since they had returned home, and her deteriorating standards of personal hygiene and recent occasional urinary incontinence.

Her urinary tract infection was treated with appropriate antibiotics, which solved the urinary incontinence problem, and although the husband accepted the idea of day visitor assessment and respite at the CUE, Mrs A did not! She clung to him and was verbally aggressive to anyone suggesting she should go anywhere. The family were greatly relieved that a staff member from the CUE would visit the house on a regular basis to assist Mr A with his wife's care, to support him and gradually get him used to the idea of her dementia and what it meant. Eventually, Mrs A agreed to come to the CUE to some social activities with the support worker whom she had got to know in her home. At a later date she came as a regular day visitor and subsequently for respite residential care on a flexible basis when her husband wanted this and was able to persuade her to accept it. By this stage, she was requiring a great deal of assistance with personal care but was reluctant to accept it, was wandering aimlessly unless busy and supervised all the time, was irritable and could become aggressive if she were thwarted or anyone tried to persuade her to do something she did not wish to do.

Her family, for their own reasons, were unable to provide any further practical support but continued to be very concerned about their father's well-being. He found it very difficult to come to terms with his grief about her illness and loss of their previously happy relationship but derived some support from meeting with other carers at the carers' group at the CUE. He certainly enjoyed the social opportunities for activities at the CUE, which he took part in with his wife and with other people in similar situations.

Eventually he accepted that he could not manage with Mrs A at home much longer, and we, at a meeting with all the family, decided that no facility in the area other than the CUE would be able to cope with Mrs A with her present behaviour. Her name was placed on the waiting list for a continuing care bed and after a short time, when it became apparent that Mr A needed the bed to be available quickly, with a bit of juggling that bed was found. He was helped with dealing with his powerful emotions at that time by the staff of the CUE whom he had got to know well and trust.

A few months later, we were all saddened when Mr A was discovered to have cancer, deteriorated physically very rapidly and died. The family were not sure how to approach Mrs A during his illness and death and asked the staff at the CUE (her new family) to take decisions about whether and how she should be involved in the process of his final illness. Although she was severely demented and appeared to have little language function remaining by this time, she seemed to understand that something important and sad was happening and was helped by the staff in her grief. To the surprise of her family, she coped with going to the funeral and behaved appropriately there and afterwards.

We all felt that it would have been hard to have given her, her husband and her family the same quality support without the existence of the CUE service.

REFLECTIONS ON THE SERVICE AFTER THE COMPLETION OF THE STRATEGY

It may help to provide a SWOT analysis (strengths, weaknesses, opportunities, threats) to determine impressions of the service.

Strengths

1. A good service is given to people and carers—people want to come.
2. Most of the service is 'in the community' and part of it. It is respected and well liked.
3. There is good integration with other agencies.
4. The teams have credibility. They can achieve things both in terms of service changes and with individual patients and their carers.
5. The service has been able to evolve and cope with the need to increase assessment facilities and reduce continuing care beds. This has been possible because of the flexibility of acute, rehabilitation, respite and continuing care beds.
6. There is flexibility in providing support to the patients and carers and this is a high priority. This flexibility includes the hours the support is provided, the support itself, the tasks the staff are able to do, the availability of advice and other specialist input.
7. The service is a central point for elderly mentally ill people and their carers.
8. The central assessment facilities work well and are next to the facilities of the district general hospital.
9. All grades of staff have been 'empowered'.
10. Morale is good amongst staff despite the pressures.
11. It is cheaper to run this service in the new community buildings than in old Victorian asylum buildings.

Weaknesses

1. If a patient eventually needs residential or nursing home care there is an inevitable break with the CUE staff, which patients and especially their carers find difficult.

2. There are perverse incentives (e.g. financial), relating to continuing care and these will not be resolved until central guidance is clearer.
3. Agencies other than health in this area are doing less with this special client group than in other geographical areas.
4. Within our service there are some people who do not need quite as much of the specialist skills all the time, but other services have not been developed to provide them with alternatives. Carers would not get the same support elsewhere.
5. The service goes on 'coping' and attempting to 'expand' to deal with the need. This increases the pressures on staff without the commissioners of services really understanding it.
6. As there is considerable investment in buildings, as well as part of the overall service, this means there is less money available within the service to provide additional specialist staff.
7. Some carers have commented that the loss of the large grounds of the asylums is a slight disappointment to them.

Opportunities

1. This service is seen as a good model and therefore can influence others to provide high standards of care. Both national and international visitors spread good practice.
2. As we have good working relationships with other community groups, for example GPs, the voluntary sector and local authority workers, this is a good base from which to develop further partnerships and good practice.
3. There are excellent opportunities for multi-agency training.
4. We may be in a position to influence standards of practice and market forces in the development of specialist facilities elsewhere.

Threats

1. Demography (the number of people aged over 85 has nearly doubled since 1981 and will double again by the middle of the twenty-first century).
2. At present there has been little development of other specialist homes and day care, which,

combined with demographic change, could swamp our service.

3. There are pressures on all staff, as a result of 1 and 2.

4. There are many people being supported in the community by this service. The requirements of the care programme approach and the need to have multidisciplinary, multiagency reviews result in what has been called 'the review time-bomb'.

5. As staff within health services have been expected by some social services staff time to do most of the specialist work with this client group, there may be some 'deskilling' of, for example, social workers.

6. Because of pressures on local authority budgets the specialist intensive home care services may be under threat. Further evaluative work is going on to try to demonstrate the benefit of this service in terms of quality and cost effectiveness.

7. Ongoing training is most important for all staff. However, statutory training needs take priority, leaving little time and training budget for the more specialist aspects.

SUMMARY

Overall the strengths and opportunities far outweigh the weaknesses and threats. We continue to work with commissioning colleagues and those in other agencies to meet the original objectives in providing a quality service.

DISCUSSION QUESTIONS

1. What are the key elements of an effective review for elderly mentally ill people and their carers?
2. a) Who are the key members of a community mental health team working with older people?
   b) Who else needs to be involved in a comprehensive community service for older people?
3. Which criteria would you use to evaluate the success of the service?

FURTHER READING

Murphy E 1986 Dementia and mental illness in the old: a practical guide; understanding the problems—how to manage—surviving yourself. Paperman, London

Wattis J, Martin C 1994 Practical psychiatry of old age, 2nd edn. Chapman & Hall, London
These two books include straightforward descriptions of common mental health problems in old age, and some of the clinical issues and implications of these disorders.

Murphy E 1991 After the asylums. Community care for people with mental illness. Faber & Faber, London
This illustrates further points about community care for people with mental health problems.

REFERENCES

DOH (Department of Health) 1989 Caring for people. HMSO, London

DOH (Department of Health) 1990 The care programme approach. HMSO, London

DOH (Department of Health) 1997 The new NHS: modern; dependable, CM 3807. The Stationery Office, London

HAS (Health Advisory Service) 1982 The rising tide. Developing services for mental illness in old age. NHS Health Advisory Service, Sutton

Lindesay J 1991 Working out. Setting up and running community psychogeriatric teams. Research and Development for Psychiatry, London

Pattie A H, Moxon S 1987 Prevalence of dementia in York Health District. A report for Yorkshire Regional Health Authority. York Health Authority, York

Pattie A H, Moxon S 1991 Community units for the elderly in York Health District. An evaluation of the first CUE: Acomb Gables. York Health Authority, York

Tyrer P 1985 The hive system. A model for a psychiatric service. British Journal of Psychiatry 146:571

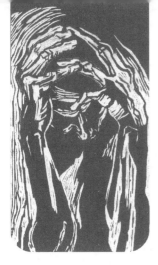

Chapter Nineteen

Drug abuse and mental illness: psychiatry's next challenge!

Colin P Vose

AIMS

- Define the terms of drug use, abuse, dependence, tolerance and addiction
- Explore underpinning theories of drug abuse
- Review the law in relation to illicit drug use and mental illness
- Examine the concepts of dual diagnosis
- Consider drug abuse, mental illness and dangerousness
- Identify treatment and management strategies
- Look at the need for training
- Review treatment and management strategies
- Investigate the relationship between cannabis use and psychosis

KEY ISSUES

Dual diagnosis
Law relating to drug use
Risk assessment
Care programme approach
Inter-disciplinary working
Training issues

INTRODUCTION

We see this [drug abuse] as the most serious peacetime threat to our national well being.
UK House of Commons 1985

At the end of the twentieth century and the start of the twenty-first, drug use would appear according to accounts in the media and supported to some extent by research (EC 1994), to have significantly increased, particularly amongst young people. The breadth and depth of drug use in modern society are issues of some debate, especially given the ever-changing nature of drug abuse. The reader may choose a variety of perspectives, but the recent experience of mental health services, be they community, acute or forensic, is that the rise in the number of clients presenting, in an extremely challenging way, with a potent mix of mental health problems and active drug use has been dramatic. This chapter seeks to examine the nature of such drug use and its interaction with mental illness.

DEFINITIONS OF DRUG DEPENDENCE

A number of different definitions of drug dependence and abuse exist, depending upon the theoretical perspective used to analyse the subject. Most definitions refer to certain physiological and psychological effects of repeated substance usage. The most widely accepted definition of drug dependence is that compiled by the World Health Organization (1969):

> *A state, psychic and sometimes also physical, resulting from the interaction between a living organism and a drug, characterised by behavioural and other responses that always include a compulsion to take the drug on a continuous periodic basis in order to experience its psychic effects and sometimes to avoid the discomfort of its absence. Tolerance may or may not be present.*

Within psychiatry two main systems of classification exist: those of the American Psychiatric Association (APA)—the Diagnostic and statistical manual of mental disorders (DSM)—and the World Health Organization—the International classification of diseases (ICD), both of which are consistently updated, the most recent being ICD-10 and DSM-IV (APA 1994). The two classifications identify similar categories of substance abuse disorders. In the ICD classification both alcoholism and drug dependence appear within the category 'neurosis, personality disorder, and non-psychotic mental illness', which specifically identifies 'alcohol dependence, drug dependence and non-dependent abuse of drugs'. Each system recognizes states of intoxication, abuse, dependence, withdrawal states, amnesic syndromes and drug-related psychotic disorders. In both classifications the criteria for diagnosing drug dependence are similar. They include: a strong desire to take the substance, progressive neglect of alternative sources of satisfaction, the development of tolerance and the presence of a physical withdrawal state. Tolerance is defined as a state in which, after repeated use, the effect of the drug is decreased, thus requiring increased dosages to produce the same effect.

In differentiating between substance use and substance abuse, DSM-IV criteria are helpful in identifying 'a maladaptive pattern of substance abuse leading to clinically significant impairment in the spheres of the individual's social, physical, psychological and legal well-being'. Substance abuse is the use of a substance in such a way or level that does cause such impairment.

UNDERPINNING THEORIES OF DRUG USE

Clear distinctions between experimental, recreational and dependent use are difficult to define. Experimental drug use is that undertaken by novices, usually adolescents, and may form part of the normal learning curve. This would include experimentation with cigarettes, alcohol, possibly solvents and illicit substances. This stage tends to be a short-lived phase. One of the difficulties with this form of drug use is that this is a process of learning that is based on ignorance. Ignorance of the substance, of the safe levels of dosage, methods of administration and the illicit nature of use drives that usage into environments that are inherently dangerous.

Recreational drug use is the regular, but controlled, use of drugs, in which the drug provides a focus for leisure activity without significantly impacting adversely on the individual's lifestyle. The problems associated with such usage will vary significantly among individuals and may be associated with unsafe methods of use or combinations of substances.

Dependent drug use is generally accepted to include physical, social, psychological and legal problems related to intoxication, excessive consumption or dependence resulting from use of a substance. The drug becomes central to the users' lives, dominating their very existence.

It is generally accepted that these three levels of drug use can be viewed as a ladder up which the individual may climb. For many drug users recreational use is the norm, an example of which is the social drinking in which large numbers of people indulge. The rate at which dependence occurs will be conditional upon the particular individuals—their mental state, the substance or combination of substances used and the sociological and emotional environment in which they function.

Table 19.1	Theoretical grid of drug use				
	Moral	**Disease**	**Symptomatic**	**Learning**	**Social**
Aetiology	Weak or bad character	Biological factors, possibly genetic	Another primary mental disorder	Learned behavioural disorder	Environmental factors
Focus of treatment	Control of behaviour through deterrent punishment	Abstinence to stop progression of disease	Improved mental health functioning	Learning behaviour alternative to or incompatible with substance misuse	Improved social functioning
Advantages	Responsibility for change lies with user	Not blaming or punitive	Not blaming or punitive; emphasis on importance of diagnosing and treating coexisting mental disorders	Not blaming or punitive; holds user responsible for new learning	Easily integrated into other models
Disadvantages	Punitive	Absolves user of responsibility to change Ignores cultural and environmental factors	Implies treatment of mental disorder is sufficient	Tends to ignore personality-disabling consequences of excessive substance misuse and irrationality of human beings	Implies change of social situation is sufficient

From Dr K. Checinski 1996 Department of Addictive Behaviour, St George's Hospital Medical School, London.

A number of theories exist that explain drug use; these include sociological, socioeconomic, psychological, behavioural, spiritual and medical models. Treatment models and philosophies on offer to drug users draw their impetus from such models. All theories and models have a validity when viewed in a narrow light, but by the very nature of human behaviour all models will inevitably have limitations. Ultimately it is the pragmatic mix of such theories identified in Checinski's (1996) theoretical grid of addictive behaviour (Table 19.1) that provides the basis for effective treatment pathways.

THE LAW RELATING TO DRUG USE

Box 19.1 details the legal changes relating to drug use.

Misuse of Drugs Act 1971

All drugs restricted by Home Office under the Misuse of Drugs Act have been given a class and a schedule. Classes determine criminal penalties. Schedules determine whether a restricted drug may be prescribed or not, and impose duties relating to record keeping, manufacturing, storage and distribution of drugs.

◆ *Class A*—heroin, Ecstasy, morphine, opium, cocaine, coca leaf, some hallucinogens, LSD, methadone, dicanol, mescaline, PCP, pethidine, psilocybin, active ingredients of cannabis, and any class B drug prepared for injection
◆ *Class B*—cannabis and cannabis resin, amphetamines, barbiturates, DF118, codeine in concentrations above 2.5%, and ritalin
◆ *Class C*—some stimulants, benzodiazepine tranquillizers, distalgesics and methaqualone.

Box 19.1 Historical development of drug legislation
1868 Pharmacy and Poisons Act Opium and later morphine sale restricted to pharmacists
1909 Shanghai Opium Commission Non-binding international agreement aimed at curbing UK opium trafficking and restricting opiates to medical use
1912 First Opium Convention (Hague Convention) International treaty committing signatories to pharmacy laws to restrict opiates and cocaine to medical use
1916 Defence of the Realm Act Regulation 408 Emergency regulation banning opium or cocaine possession or supply with prescription in response to cocaine epidemic among soldiers
1918 Treaty ending First World War Ratification of Hague Convention mandatory
1920 Dangerous Drugs Act and later regulations Implemented Hague Convention in UK making it a criminal offence to possess or supply opiates or cocaine without prescription
1925 Geneva Convention International treaty extending control to cannabis
1925 Dangerous Drugs Act Extended 1920 Act to cover cannabis and coca leaves
1926 Rolleston report Established that indefinite maintenance prescribing was a legitimate medical response to opiate addiction in Britain
1960s Youth culture Doctors lose control of spread of addiction; cannabis, stimulants and hallucinogens integrated into popular youth culture
1964 Drugs (Prevention of Misuse) Act Controlled amphetamines in UK, later used to control LSD
1967 Dangerous Drugs Act Implemented recommendations of second Brian report (1965) restricting the prescribing of heroin and cocaine to licensed doctors
1971 Misuse of Drugs Act Cornerstone UK legislation giving all Home Office-restricted drugs a classification that determines criminal penalties and schedules that determine level of restriction
1985 Intoxicating Substances Act Restricting the sale of solvents to adults
1986 Drug Trafficking Offences Act Outlaws sale of drug paraphernalia and allows confiscation of proceeds from drug trafficking

Schedules

There are five schedules:

◆ *Schedule 1*—these drugs are considered to have no legitimate therapeutic use and cannot be prescribed by a doctor or dispensed by a chemist. Possession is legitimate only with Home Office licence. These are issued only to doctors or scientists engaged in research. Schedule 1 drugs include cannabis and LSD.

◆ *Schedules 2 and 3*—these cover many controlled drugs considered to have medical therapeutic uses. These may be possessed by doctors, pharmacists, research establishments and medical staff working in hospitals, etc. A patient prescribed scheduled drugs by a doctor may legitimately be in possession, provided the drug is administered in accordance with the doctor's directions.

Schedule 2 includes heroin, morphine, pethidine, amphetamine and cocaine.

Schedule 3 includes diethylpropion, and other slimming aids, and temazepam.

◆ *Schedule 4*—this includes many benzodiazepines such as diazepam, etc. Persons listed under schedules 2 and 3 can possess these drugs. Supply for unauthorized use is illegal.

◆ *Schedule 5*—this covers compound preparations, e.g. cough medicines, antidiarrhoeal medicines that contain tiny amounts of controlled drugs. Some are sold over the counter.

Possession

Possession of many drugs is illegal. This may be direct possession or shared possession (e.g. two sharing a cannabis joint).

Control

If someone who, whilst not possessing a drug, is in control of that drug they can be deemed to be in possession and may be charged. This may be used by care staff wishing to control the actions and movements of known drug users in their care.

Defences to possession

Criminal law usually requires knowledge (i.e. some-one knowingly committed a criminal act). The burden of proof is on the defendant, however. Possession of clean needles etc. is not an offence.

Possession with intent to supply

This is a trafficking offence. Factors considered are the quantity of drugs involved and packaging along with other circumstances of the arrest.

Mental Health Act 1983

The Act states very clearly that people must not be deemed to have a form of mental disorder 'by reason of … dependence on alcohol or drugs'. The use of alcohol and other substances may precipitate a mental disorder to which the Act would therefore apply, but substance abuse without a mental disorder does not fall within the scope of the Act. Therefore the powers identified in Part 2 of the Mental Health Act cannot be used to detain or treat somebody who abuses substances but does not demonstrate a mental disorder.

DRUG USE AND MENTAL ILLNESS

The misuse of drugs and alcohol among those people who already have a diagnosed mental illness is now being recognized as an increasing problem (Smith & Hucker 1994). The term 'dual diagnosis' is now widely accepted as a suitable label by which to describe patients, or clients, who present with a mental illness and an allied substance abuse problem. The concept of dual diagnosis is one that Europe has inherited from North America, where there is a growing body of literature and research activity. It is only within the latter half of the 1990s that the experience of North America has been replicated in Europe. As in all areas of life the actual real life experiences are governed by the various actors on the ground at any one particular time. A consistent pattern is emerging from a number of different communities worldwide that identify common themes of clinical concern posing serious challenges to both the care and management of the mentally ill.

The actual level of substance abuse amongst the mentally ill is hard to substantiate reliably and will vary from area to area, and between social classes and genders, as will the actual substances of abuse. One reliable study, the Epidemiological Catchment Area Survey (Reiger, Farmer & Rae 1990) on the prevalence of substance abuse among the mentally ill, indicated that rates may be as high as 87% for individuals with antisocial personality disorders, 56% for bipolar mood disorders, 47% for schizophrenia and 32% for depressive disorders. Dixon, Weiden & Haas (1989), in a range of studies on clients diagnosed with schizophrenia, found a rate of substance abuse between 33–74%. Guebaly (1990) found that 10–15% of hospitalized schizophrenics and 80% of personality-disordered patients had serious drinking problems; the prevalence of alcoholism in clients suffering from panic attacks was between 10–15%. The multiplicity of the relationship between substance abuse and mental illness has been summarized by Crome (unpublished work, 1996) as follows:

◆ Substance use and withdrawal from substances may lead to psychiatric syndromes or symptoms.
◆ Intoxication and dependence may produce psychological symptoms.
◆ Substance use may exacerbate or alter the course of pre-existing mental disorder.
◆ Primary mental disorder may precipitate substance use which may lead to further psychiatric symptoms.

The abuse of substances by the mentally ill reflects the trends of substance abuse in the wider community. The 1992 British Crime Survey (Mott & Mirrlees-Black 1995) identified a number of trends in drug usage, namely: drug taking is most common between the ages of 16 and 29, and cannabis is by far the most commonly used illicit substance, with almost one in four 16 to 29 year olds reporting usage. This age group has seen a marked increase in the use of cannabis over previous studies, with the biggest increase amongst women. Offences concerning cannabis, a class B drug, accounted for over 80% of those found guilty or cautioned for breaches of the Misuse of Drugs Act in 1991 (Robson 1994).

Other illicit drugs most commonly used, again by the 16–29 year old group, are hallucinogenic and include Ecstasy, amphetamines and LSD, all of which are associated with the 'rave' dance culture. The multiple use of such drugs is becoming established reflecting a 'pick and mix' approach to recreational use of psychotrophic substances. In the survey of Leitner, Shapland & Wiles (1993) of people considered to be at high risk of drug taking, two factors were identified as significant: the combination of age (i.e. between 16 and 25 years) and living in a deprived location. In addition to this it is widely acknowledged that this period of late adolescence and early adulthood is a key period in the development of coping strategies, which include the refinement of adaptive and maladaptive behaviour patterns. This also is a period which, for some, sees the onset of psychotic episodes. Out of this cocktail emerges the person who may present to the mental health worker as disturbed, chaotic and confused. Is this state attributable to a pure psychotic illness or to the effects of a psychotrophic substance, or a combination of the two?

The effects of any interaction between an ongoing psychotic illness and associated substance abuse presents a range of possible and serious complications that may produce greater treatment resistance and severe clinical management problems. For some clients it is this presentation, and its associated risks of self harm and to public safety, that necessitates care in a more structured and secure environment.

The consequences of substance use and psychosis have increasingly become established. Thornicroft's (1990) review of studies relating to cannabis and psychosis found that heavy cannabis use produced brief acute organic reactions and psychotic episodes. When cannabis use is combined with that of neuroleptic medication, an antagonistic relationship is observed (Knudsen & Vilmar 1984), which is caused by the anticholinergic effect of cannabis reducing the effectiveness of the neuroleptic medication. Cannabis use also precipitates higher levels of awareness of the environment and reduces inhibitions. Franey (1996) identified a relationship between cannabis and persistent thought disorder, which can produce an increased risk of suicide, violent outbursts, treatment non-compliance and treatment resistance. The effect of cocaine when combined with schizophrenia is increased levels of paranoia and depression resulting in hospitalization (Brady, Anton & Ballenger 1990). The incidence of violence amongst the seriously mentally ill shows a dramatic increase if substance abuse is present. One study (Swanson 1990) identified the rate of violence amongst those with schizophrenia jumping from 8% to a staggering 30% where there was active substance abuse. This increased occurrence of high order psychiatric symptoms should precipitate a reassessment of the risk indicators of violence to either the self or others.

Dual diagnosis

Potential clinical complications include:

◆ increased rates of violence (Bartels, Drake & Wallace 1991, Franey 1996, Swanson 1990)
◆ increased rates of suicide (Allebeck, Varla & Kristiansson 1987, Franey 1996)
◆ non-compliance with treatment (Pristisch & Smith 1990)
◆ earlier psychotic breakdown (Breakley, Goodell & Lorenz 1974)
◆ exacerbation of symptoms (Alterman, Erdlin & McLellan 1980)
◆ relative neuroleptic refractoriness (Bowers 1977)
◆ increased hospitalization (Brady, Anton & Ballenger 1990)
◆ tardive dyskinesia (Dixon, Weiden & Haas 1989)
◆ homelessness (Gelberg, Linn & Leake 1988)
◆ poor prognosis (Drake & Wallach 1989).

It is now widely acknowledged that a considerable number of people experiencing psychotic illness utilize cannabis as a form of self-medication (Smith & Hucker 1994). Khantzian (1985) recognized that individuals were using a range of substances to alleviate the symptoms of mental disorder. The appeal of such self-medication should never be underestimated given the alternative of prescribed medication that for many clients offers only reduced psychiatric symptomatology and exposure to debilitating side-effects.

Risk assessment/assessment of dangerousness

The assessment and management of the risk of a psychiatric patient causing harm to another person is an integral part of psychiatric services (Royal College of Psychiatrists 1996). Risk assessment is concerned with carefully weighing up the likelihood of that particular risk occurring.

In a broad, diverse subject such as risk assessment/assessment of dangerousness the importance of a systematized approach is essential. It is important that precise and accurate recording and collection of relevant information in relation to a client's potential for dangerous behaviour are undertaken. It is widely believed that nothing predicts future behaviour better than the past (Gunn & Taylor 1993). In assessing the risk of violent behaviour, we attempt to forecast by referring back to previous behaviour.

Although there is no agreed definition of dangerousness, the Butler Committee (1975) said that 'dangerousness was a propensity to cause serious injury or lasting harm', whereas Scott (1977) defined dangerousness as 'unpredictable and untreatable tendency to inflict or risk irreversible injury or destruction'. The dangerousness of a person refers to dangerousness within a particular given situation or in a particular state of mind. There are a number of factors that should be considered in undertaking a risk assessment of dangerousness, Steadman et al (1993) identified five, which are:

1. the level and type of social support available to the person
2. how impulsive the individual is
3. reactions, such as anger, to provocation
4. the level and ability to empathize with others
5. nature of any delusions or hallucinations.

The University of Manchester/Department of Health ongoing study on risk assessment and violence (Alberg et al 1996) has identified the following factors that may increase the risk of violence in mentally ill people:

- history of violent behaviour
- high levels of anger/hostility
- clinical diagnosis
- medication—non-compliance and/or failing to attend appointments
- concurrent substance misuse
- homelessness
- presence of situational factors associated with past violence.

The importance of drug and/or alcohol misuse should not be underestimated. Such misuse is strongly linked to violence whether mental illness is present or not. Both drug and alcohol misuse present a greater risk factor for violence than any type of mental illness, but the combination of substance misuse with a mental illness puts the individual at particular risk for behaving violently. Alcohol and certain drugs disinhibit behaviour. In addition the crime associated with the need to obtain drugs increases the likelihood of violence (Alberg et al 1996). The relationship between substance abuse, mental illness and violence can be summarized as:

- alcohol/drug misuse and mental illness increases the risk of violence
- risk of violence amongst schizophrenics is 8%
- risk of violence in general population is 2%
- risk of violence by those with dual diagnosis is 30%
- the combination of substance abuse and mental illness leads to more diverse victims
- a level of violence that is more serious
- a greater likelihood of the use of weapons.

TREATMENT AND MANAGEMENT STRATEGIES

All treatment interventions with each client within the mental health services need to be the subject of a rational well thought-out intervention plan that is reflective of research findings and national and local policies. To take the latter first, all patients entering into the care of mental health services are subject to the care programme approach (CPA). This requires a systematic assessment of the client's health and social care needs, the development of a care plan, identification of a key worker and a regular review of that care plan. Good practice would indicate this CPA be managed by an effective multidisciplinary team.

In addition, the treatment of drug users within mental health services should be lodged within a clear local policy statement that identifies the criteria for treatment, clarifies issues of safety and security as well as issues of confidentiality, legal obligation and restriction—that is, the right to search, and the right to refuse treatment to problematic clients. Such a policy for the management of drug-related problems should be the subject of consultation with staff, managers, carers, service users and other professionals with clinical responsibility. It should include:

- the situation with regard to the law
- liaison with the police
- the procedures to be adopted when drugs are found on service provider premises or in the possession of service users
- informing carers
- the circumstances under which exclusion from service provision would apply
- access to specialist advice for service users with drug problems and referral procedures
- confidentiality
- clinical supervision of clinicians therapeutically engaging clients.

Individual therapeutic interventions should be located within a framework that does not view substance use as inherently wrong. Rather, they should focus on whether the use is problematic in nature and effect and most crucially identify the underlying drives that motivate the individual to use drugs. It is primarily within this area that treatment should ultimately be centred.

From this as the basepoint to develop treatment strategies the care worker should seek to clarify and reflect on the core spheres of health and in particular mental health. Health is defined by the World Health Organization as 'a state of complete physical, mental and social well-being and not merely the absence of disease or infirmity' (1981);

mental health may be better understood within the context of Maslow's (1954) hierarchy of needs and notion of self-actualization. Within these frameworks two core intervention strategies should underpin any care programme.

First, the concept of holism applies as much to the care of the drug user as to any other client with mental health problems. On this basis the drug, or drugs, of use should not be seen as the problem but as symptoms of a deeper problem. Whilst all drugs by their nature have an effect both physically and psychologically on the user, either positively or negatively, no drug has such an effect as to coax, bribe and force the non drug user into taking the drug in the first place. That motivation to use drugs lies within the complex web of psychological, social and emotional drives that are inherent within the individual or impinge on that individual. The focus of therapeutic intervention should have at its core the aim of untangling such a web and addressing factors leading to drug abuse or a pattern of abuse that is significantly harmful to individuals, their families and peers and to the wider society. Such intervention therefore accepts individuals as individuals and hence pays them due regard and respect. It is this principle that ultimately strengthens and enables the development of a meaningful and productive therapeutic relationship.

Secondly, given this fundamental tenet, therapists should recall the ethic that underpins their work: the promotion of health. Health promotion should be seen as the process by which we move the client from one level of health functioning to a higher level. If we accept health as operating in the spheres of physical, psychological and social dimensions then there is considerable scope for a range of interventions in any or all of the spheres. Health promotion activities in the field of drug abuse and psychiatry straddle paternalistic activities of supply control and humanistic activities of empowerment. Care workers should be conscious that their activities are located at some point on a continuum between these two points and seek to progress clients along the continuum towards that of therapeutic empowerment, whilst being conscious of the reality that for many clients the end goal may be a lifelong journey.

Clinical intervention continuum—dual diagnosis

Paternalistic therapeutic control———Humanistic therapeutic empowerment

The humanistic approach to health promotion is 'the process of enabling people to increase control over the determinants of health and thereby their health' (WHO 1981), whereas the paternalistic approach seeks to identify policy strategies that protect the individual from harm by restricting the activities of the individual.

An appropriate model of intervention is one that analyses the client's beliefs, values, attitudes and drives in relation to behavioural change. One such model providing a framework for change is that developed by Prochaska & DiClemente (1984). This is a 'directive client centred counselling style that is designed to assist the client in exploring and resolving ambivalence to increase motivation for change' (Miller & Rollnick 1991). This identifies five stages within the change process from which the individual will start and pass through. They are: precontemplation, contemplation, action, maintenance and relapse. The model accepts that clients will relapse in their substance abuse, but this relapse should be seen as a slip, or return to maladaptive coping techniques, rather than a failure. The vast majority of clients will relapse before achieving abstinence. Relapse is therefore a normal part of the process of change and is normally associated with high risk situations, in which the client would normally have used a substance. As part of the planning process the client should be encouraged to anticipate these situations and plan ways to cope.

It is important that the therapist recognizes that, for many clients, complete abstinence may be an unachievable goal. Many clients come into contact with services and present as chaotic, both in lifestyle and in patterns of drug use; for these individuals, stability in these two spheres would be significant milestones.

THE NEED FOR TRAINING

Substance abuse is posing significant clinical problems within the range of mental health services. For mental health workers across all sectors of the health and social care spectra there is an obvious but as yet largely unanswered need for extensive training. The first barrier for any effective training initiative to overcome is denial that a problem exists. Secondly, there is the belief that those with drug and alcohol problems are undeserving and unresponsive to clinical intervention. Indeed the extension of this view is that substance abuse problems should be tackled solely within a legal framework and therefore it denies the client any meaningful therapeutic input. These attitudes and feelings are significant barriers to non-judgmental care, allowing the process of labelling and stereotyping of clients to distract attention from individual clients' needs and focusing on the problem behaviour (i.e. on the drug use rather than the person who uses drugs). This, in part, reflects a lack of understanding of the issues surrounding substance abuse (Cranfield & Storeman 1996). A common coping mechanism of care workers struggling to cope is to deny their capacity to offer care and seek out expert opinion. Derricott & McKeown (1996) believe that this disempowerment of staff is facilitated through the construction of an edifice of mystery around the practice of staff who work exclusively with drug users, to the extent that this work is seen as expert and beyond the compass of ordinary practitioners.

The lack of training initiatives relating to substance abuse, and in particular dual diagnosis, leaves care workers with a knowledge base gained ever from the media, their client contacts or from their own varied drug-taking experiences. This thus significantly inhibits their own ability to act as health educators and reinforces the belief that such clients are not suitable for mental health services or require interventions that rely primarily on control rather than therapy (Vose 1998).

The statistics on drug use, particularly cannabis use, demonstrate that, whatever the legality of the act, cannabis use within the UK and throughout Europe is not only increasing but is here to stay. Mental health professionals in whatever sphere of work need now to rise to the challenge and act. They need, first, to enhance their own knowledge base about drugs by accessing appropriate train-ing and, secondly, to engage in programmes of health promotion that centre on the need to dispel the myths surrounding drugs and convince clients that their drugs use is harmful to their mental health and should be avoided. Failure to act will lead to a spiralling crisis of ever more disturbed clients entering a system whose inadequacies will become all the more exposed.

Training initiatives should be multifaceted in nature and multidisciplinary in delivery. Training on drug recognition, the legal rights to search, the 1983 Mental Health Act and physical and psychological first aid for the intoxicated patient should form the essential of any basic training package for mental health workers. The English National Board, in its guidelines for good practice in education and training of nurses (Cranfield & Storeman 1996), recommends the following areas for study:

◆ the social and cultural context of substance misuse
◆ personal and professional attitudes to substance misuse and substance misusers
◆ actions and effects of alcohol and other main drugs of misuse
◆ developing skills in assessment, brief interventions and information dissemination
◆ the professional and legal framework within which practice functions
◆ the range of specialist treatment services and referral routes.

Given the scale of client presentations throughout mental health and allied services such training should now become a priority for mental health workers to ensure effective care delivery.

DISCUSSION QUESTIONS

1. Is a key function of the mental health worker to minimize drug abuse amongst the mentally ill?
2. Is drug abuse contraindicated in psychosis?
3. What is drug abuse?
4. Can cannabis use be a form of self-medication?

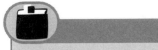

FURTHER READING

Alberg C, Bingley W, Bowers L et al 1996 Mental health risk assessment. University of Manchester, Manchester

Coyne P, Wright S 1997 Working with alcohol and drug users. Association of Nurses in Substance Abuse, London

Cranfield S, Storeman P 1996 Substance use misuse—guidelines for good practice in education and training of nurses, midwives and health visitors. English National Board for Nursing, Midwifery and Health Visiting, London

Gunn J, Taylor P 1993 Dangerousness in forensic psychiatry. Clinical, legal and ethical issues. Butterworth-Heinemann, London

Leitner M, Shapland J, Wiles P 1993 Drug use and drugs prevention. HMSO, London

Miller W, Rollnick S 1991 Motivational interviewing; preparing people to change their addictive behaviour. Guilford, New York

Prochaska J, DiClemente C 1984 The transtheoretical approach: crossing traditional foundations of change. Don Jones/Irwin, Harnewood

Robson P 1994 Forbidden drugs. Oxford University Press, Oxford

REFERENCES

Alberg C, Bingley W, Bowers L et al 1996 Mental health risk assessment. University of Manchester, Manchester

Allebeck P, Varla A, Kristiansson E 1987 Cannabis; a longitudinal study of Swedish conscripts. Lancet ii:1483–1485

Alterman A, Erdlin F, McLellan A 1980 Problem drinking in hospitalised schizophrenic patients. Addictive Behaviours 5:273–276

APA (American Psychiatric Association) 1994 Diagnostic and statistical manual, 4th edn. APA, Washington

Bartels S, Drake R, Wallace M 1991 Characteristic hostility in schizophrenic outpatients. Schizophrenic Bulletin 16:81–85

Bowers B 1977 Psychosis precipitating psychomimetic drugs. Archives of General Psychiatry 34:832–835

Brady K, Anton R, Ballenger J 1990 Cocaine abuse among schizophrenic patients. American Journal of Psychiatry 147:1164–1167

Breakley W, Goodell H, Lorenz P 1974 Hallucinogenic drugs as participants of schizophrenia. Psychological Medicine 4:255–261

Brian report 1965 Home Office

British Crime Survey 1992 Home Office

Butler Committee 1975 Report of the Committee on Mentally Abnormal Offenders. HMSO, London

Coyne P, Wright S 1997 Working with alcohol and drug users. Association of Nurses in Substance Abuse, London

Cranfield S, Storeman P 1996 Substance use misuse— guidelines for good practice in education and training of nurses, midwives and health visitors. English National Board for Nursing, Midwifery and Health Visiting, London

Derricott J, McKeown M 1996 Dual diagnosis. Psychiatric Care 3(suppl 1):34–37

Dixon L, Weiden P, Haas G 1989 Increased tardive dyskinesia in alcohol abusing schizophrenic patients. Comprehensive Psychiatry 33:121–122

Drake R, Wallach M 1989 Substance abuse among the chronically mentally ill. Hospital and Community Psychiatry 40:1041–1046

EC (European Commission) 1994 Community action in the field of drug dependence V/F/1 D(94), CEC/V/F/1/LUX/99/93, Rev 5,3–2, 16 June 1994

Franey C 1996 Dual diagnosis. Executive summary no 51, Centre for Research on Drugs and Health Behaviour, London

Gelberg L, Linn L, Leake B 1988 Mental health, alcohol and drug use, and criminal history among homeless adults. American Journal of Psychiatry 145:191–196

Guebaly M D 1990 Substance abuse and mental disorders; the dual diagnosis concept. Canadian Journal of Psychiatry 35:261–267

Gunn J, Taylor P 1993 Dangerousness in forensic psychiatry. Clinical, legal and ethical issues. Butterworth-Heinemann, London

Khantzian E J 1985 The self medication hypothesis of addictive disorders; focus on heroin and cocaine dependence. American Journal of Psychiatry 148:224–230

Knudsen P, Vilmar T 1984 Cannabis and neuroleptic agents in schizophrenia. Acta Psychiatrica Scandinavica 69:162–172

Leitner M, Shapland J, Wiles P 1993 Drug use and drugs prevention. HMSO, London

Maslow A H 1954 Motivation and personality. Harper & Row, New York

Miller W, Rollnick S 1991 Motivational interviewing; preparing people to change their addictive behaviour. Guilford, New York

Mott J, Mirrlees-Black 1995 Self-reported drug misuse in England and Wales: findings from the 1992 British Crime Survey Research and Planning Unit, paper 89

Pritisch C, Smith C 1990 Medication compliance and substance abuse among schizophrenic patients. Hospital and Community Psychiatry 41:1345–1348

Prochaska J, DiClemente C 1984 The transtheoretical approach: crossing traditional foundations of change. Don Jones/Irwin, Harnewood

Reiger D, Farmer M, Rae M 1990 Comorbidity of mental disorders with alcohol and other drugs of abuse: results from the epidemiologic catchment area study. Journal of the American Medical Association 264:2511–2518

Robson P 1994 Forbidden drugs. Oxford University Press, Oxford

Royal College of Psychiatrists 1996 ???

Scott P D 1977 Assessing dangerousness in criminals. British Journal of Psychiatry 131:127–142

Smith J, Hucker S 1994 Schizophrenia and substance abuse. British Journal of Psychiatry 1:13–21

Steadman et al 1993 From dangerousness to risk assessment—implications for appropriate research strategies. In: Hodgins S (ed) Mental disorder and crime. Sage, Newbury Park, CA

Swanson J 1990 Violence and psychiatric disorder in the community. Hospital and Community Psychiatry 41:761–770

Thornicroft G 1990 Cannabis and psychosis, is there epidemiological evidence for an association? British Journal of Psychiatry 157:25–33

UK House of Commons 1985 Fifth report of the Home Affairs Committee, misuse of hard drugs (interim report), Session 1984/5. The Stationery Office, London

Vose C 1998 Speaking out. Nursing Times 94(14) (April 8):21

WHO (World Health Organization) 1969 Constitution ???

WHO (World Health Organization) 1981 Constitution. Global strategy for health for all by the year 2000. WHO, Geneva

WHO (World Health Organization) 1992 International classification of diseases, 10th revision. WHO, Geneva

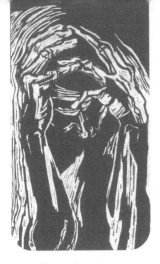

Chapter Twenty

Quality assurance in counselling and psychotherapy

Chahid E Fourali

AIMS

- ◆ Highlight the relevance of the concept of quality to mental health health institutions
- ◆ Highlight the relevance of the concept of quality to the work of counsellors and psychotherapists
- ◆ Introduce the main approaches to quality assurance
- ◆ Give a brief account on the development of the concept of quality assurance
- ◆ Address the issue of effectiveness and efficiency of treatment
- ◆ Offer the total quality management approach as a viable approach for comparing the quality of existing models of counselling and psychotherapy
- ◆ Test the total quality management approach in the context of a well-known cognitive behavioural therapy approach: rational emotive behaviour therapy.
- ◆ Highlight the current challenges to the quality of counselling and psychotherapy

KEY ISSUES

Promotion of concept and practice of total quality management in counselling and psychotherapy

Development of a general strategy for evaluating the relative effectiveness and efficiency of counselling and psychotherapy theory and practice

Evaluation of theory and practice of rational emotive behaviour therapy

Highlighting the need for culture sensitive counselling and psychotherapy services

This chapter has already appeared as an article in the International Journal of Psychotherapy 4(2):161–177, 1999 with the title: 'Quality assurance in psychotherapy and counselling'

INTRODUCTION

The quality of psychotherapy and counselling has always been at the centre of controversy, as has its therapeutic effectiveness. The controversy became more challenging after Eysenck launched his attacks on the utility of psychoanalysis and psychotherapy in general (Eysenck 1952, 1992). In his original attack, he claimed that whereas two-thirds of people with a neurotic disorder who undergo traditional (non-behavioural) therapy tend to recover, a similar proportion of neurotics who never benefited from any formal therapy tend to improve within an equivalent period. The study launched a wave of claims and counter-claims (e.g. Bergin & Lambert 1978, Eysenck 1992) from various corners with various orientations. Today the original claims have been tempered by results from researches with more refined methodologies such as meta-analysis (Smith, Glass & Miller, 1980). However, the initial challenge (which became known as the outcome problem) still remains. The challenge was that psychotherapists should demonstrate that treated patients recover significantly more and at a quicker rate than untreated patients. This issue became also associated with that of efficiency (Ellis 1989). Thus the challenge now for therapists is to show that their model effects quicker, more profound, longer-lasting recovery and changes at a cheaper price than any contending theoretical model (Pekarik 1993).

More recently, issues of efficiency and effectiveness are resurfacing under the guise of 'quality assurance'. This concept is quickly becoming a multifaceted criterion for assessing the adequacy of psychotherapy and counselling services (Steenbarger & Smith 1996). It is meant to address any aspect of products or services in order to assess their 'fitness for purpose' and points the way towards ways of improving them.

The aim of this chapter is to address the issue of quality assurance and illustrate its potential benefits in the field of counselling and psychotherapy. The chapter will first attempt to define the concept of quality assurance, trace the origins of the recent quality movement and look at what it may offer to the counselling and psychotherapy public service. It will draw on the debate that took place in an 'adjacent' area of service, the educational service, to give possible directions on how the quality movement can benefit psychotherapy and counselling institutions. It will also illustrate how the quality perspective can help mental health practitioners evaluate the validity and effectiveness of the theories of psychotherapy they use. The theoretical evaluation is illustrated by referring to a widely used brand of cognitive behavioural therapy known as rational emotive behaviour therapy. Finally, the chapter will draw conclusions and make recommendations that will point the way forward. (Note: this chapter does not focus on the differences between psychotherapy and counselling but rather assumes that there is a strong overlap in their functions and hence uses them interchangeably throughout.)

THE CONCEPT OF QUALITY AND ITS RECENT ORIGIN

Quality has many possible definitions. Here are some of them:

1. Quality is 'that which makes a thing what it is: nature: character: kind: property: attribute: … grade of goodness: excellence….' (Chambers English Dictionary 1988).

2. Quality is 'the totality of features and characteristics of a product or service that bear on its ability to satisfy stated or implied needs' (BSI 1987).

3. 'Quality is in its essence a way of managing the organisation' (Feigenbaum 1987).

4. 'The true criterion for judging quality is not conformance to tolerances but cost to society' (Bissell 1989, Macdonald & Piggott 1990).

Although the above definitions suggest that quality is about satisfying client needs, there remains considerable debate about what quality actually means and how to achieve it (Müller & Funnel 1991). In particular, different systems promote different constructs of quality (Elliot 1993) as well as different levels of implementation. Thus originally an industry-based concept of quality meant correcting mistakes; subsequently, it included the ability to prevent errors and finally the current view aims to delight the customer (Fourali 1994). According to some quality gurus there appears to be a small step toward a situation where clients become 'dictators' who imposes their view of what constitutes quality.

Since psychotherapy and counselling are a service and not a product made by a manufacturing industry, it is more relevant to our study to address the concept of quality from a 'service industry' perspective. Moreover, given that education is a service, it appears that the debate on quality in education can offer useful 'pointers' that may benefit a similar debate in the field of psychotherapy and counselling.

Elliot (1993) identified several systems of quality assurance currently being applied to further education, which reflect various 'ideological' concerns. These were:

1. *British Standards Institution (BSI) (e.g. the BS5750 or its international equivalent ISO9000)* —this model, which was initially developed for the manufacturing industries (BSI 1987), requires participating institutions to detail step by step procedures that contribute to the quality of the final product of an organisation.

2. *HMI (Her Majesty's Inspectorate) perspective*—this perspective can be understood by referring to 'Her Majesty's Inspectorate' publications about quality (e.g. DOE 1990, 1991). According to this view, quality rests chiefly on course monitoring and review and refers to the notion of internal and external stakeholders (e.g. course teams, academic boards, as well as validating bodies, training and enterprise councils, industries, etc.) (Elliot 1993).

3. *The stake holder model*—proponents of this model identify the main criteria as that which the various stake holders (i.e. those with a direct interest in the quality of a product/service such as parents, academic boards, validating bodies, training and enterprise councils etc.) view as clearly important in assessing quality and highlight them to those with the role of ensuring quality (Harvey, Burrows & Green 1992). This model promotes both credibility (by referring to the views of the professionals) and public accountability.

4. *The Training and Development Lead Body (TDLB) perspective*—these standards are based on the principles of the UK's National Council for Vocational Qualifications (which later on became part of the 'Qualifications and Curriculum Authority') whose primary aim was to develop vocational qualifications relevant to industry/business needs. Currently further education colleges as well as private companies involved in the running of National Vocational Qualifications (NVQs) are required to train their staff up to TDLB standards. Hence these standards have become a recognizable quality assurance feature.

5. *The self-managing model*—this model presents quality as a self-defined (as opposed to an externally imposed) core value adopted by an educational institution (e.g. school) to achieve its targeted goals of 'excellence' (Caldwell & Spinks 1992).

6. *The Strategic Quality Management perspective*—in this model managers refer to agreed quality characteristics/standards so that areas of concern are identified, measured and addressed with an overall drive to raise the quality of the learner's experience (Harvey, Burrows & Green 1992, Miller & Innis 1990).

The above quality systems show that there is a variety of purposes leading to a variety of procedures for implementing the systems.

Some of the criticism directed against quality assurance systems highlight their disregard of the influence of the environment, and levels of understanding, as well as the competing demands between staff, clients and business interests (Elliot 1993). In particular the social environment is known to affect significantly both meaning and implementation of quality initiatives (Lawn 1991). Moreover, quality assurance may be perceived as yet another tool that may reflect a particular ideology (involving market forces and academic freedom). If these issues are not addressed within the quality assurance initiatives, the outcome may be 'ritualism, retreatism or rebellion' (Merton 1970, p. 468).

Currently the buzzword for ensuring quality is 'total quality management' (or TQM). This concept comes under many guises. These include such expressions as 'continuous improvement' and, more recently in the UK, 'Business Excellence' (see British Quality Foundation, 1997). This is essentially a customer-focused framework where clients' needs are at the heart of the processes of improvements. The general strategy is to organize groupings of employees at various levels of the organization. These groupings adopt a problem-solving approach in that they watch for any (potential) problems, determine their root causes, generate solutions, select and implement them while monitoring the outcome. Total quality management is primarily known as a system that enables continuous learning to effect continuous improvement.

Many of the ideas of total quality management were developed in the 1930s. Their first applications took place in Japan after some American quality advisors developed the total quality management ideas and taught them to Japanese managers. It took a long time before the West realized the influence of such ideas in the Japanese economic success. However since the 1980s, as a result of fierce market competition, many American and British companies took notice of the philosophy.

A famous total quality management framework hailed as a model to follow is the Baldridge total quality management model (Marsh, unpublished work, 1991, Sallis 1993). This model (see Box 20.1) allows the integration of both routinized activities (such as BS5750) and the concept of continuous improvement.

This model has particularly been praised for its broader perspective, which includes vision, leadership and improvement processes (Marsh, unpublished work, 1991, Sallis 1993). More recently other models have come to the attention of the quality conscious public. For instance the European Quality Award (known also as the 'Business Excellence' model) set up to raise issues of total quality management in Europe and a UK equivalent, British Standard guide for total quality management, known as BS7850 (Sallis 1993). However it may be argued that the 'ingredients' making up the award are predictably similar except perhaps for a wider focus on 'organization's impact on society and environment' by the European award.

Box 20.1 Main components of the Baldridge model (Marsh, unpublished work, 1991, Sallis 1993)

Leadership
Values and management for quality
Information and analysis
Competitive comparisons, quality data and benchmarking
Strategic quality planning
Quality goals and plans
Human resource utilization
Employees' involvement, training and performance measurement
Quality assurance of product and services
Design, process control, assessment and continuous improvement
Measurement of outcome
Product and service, process and support, suppliers
Goals
Assessment and commitment to customer satisfaction

It appears that currently there is a move towards globalism and inclusiveness within quality initiatives. This is particularly true for global manufacturing companies who consider that any part of the world is a potential market.

The next section will look at the similarity between the psychotherapy and educational contexts to justify a possible mutual exchange between these two activities in terms of quality initiatives.

QUALITY IN EDUCATION VERSUS QUALITY IN PSYCHOTHERAPY AND COUNSELLING

The educational aspect of psychotherapy has been stressed by several authors in the field (e.g. Dryden 1991, 1994, Nelson-Jones 1982, Strupp 1983). Strupp (1983) reported Freud as characterizing psychoanalysis as a form of 're-education', whereas Prochaska & Norcross (1994) drew a parallel between psychotherapy and brain washing. Other psychotherapists (Dryden 1991, Nelson-Jones 1982) drew attention to the fact that psychotherapy can be used not only at the individual level but also at the group level in order to *educate* the public in psychological matters. Conversely, it can be argued that any debate, procedure or issue raised about improving the quality of education can have some direct bearing on 'psychological health'. Hence this section will attempt to extend the use of the quality assurance debate to psychotherapy. In particular it attempts to apply some approaches used to inform the quality assurance process in education to the problem of improving the quality of psychotherapy.

It may be useful to stress briefly at this stage that the expression 'quality assurance' needs to be considered in its larger meaning and not its usual 'industry-bound' meaning. Hence it may be noted that there is a difference between 'traditional' quality assurance outcome measurement based on 'tangible' assessment criteria, on the one hand, and 'measured' outcomes based primarily on clients' subjective values and uninformed models (as may be possible in a psychotherapy or educational setting), on the other. Accordingly, and as shown below, a robust quality assurance model needs to take into consideration such various dimensions as reflected in such a complex field as psychotherapy and counselling.

At the global level suggested in the previous section, some therapists propose that perhaps the most important aspects of a wider/total quality management perspective in a psychotherapy and counselling setting are three elements: leadership, system thinking and commitment to data collection and analysis (Steenbarger & Smith 1996). Indeed, it may be argued that leadership is necessary to act as the engine that establishes the mechanisms for inducing, recognizing and rewarding change. Systems thinking is also decisive in bringing together all the work roles within an organization and promoting a unified approach to the service. It also addresses issues of relations between staff within the organization on the one hand, and those between members of the organi-

zation and external clients and providers on the other. Finally the quality of data collection and analysis is essential to measuring the adequacy of the service as well as providing crucial pointers for improving it. Thus the selected quality goals can be systematically measured against the results of benchmark studies. As shown above, these three elements for ensuring quality of counselling and psychotherapy are also essential for ensuring the quality of education. Hence it is clear that the procedures highlighted by educational experts to improve the quality of education can easily be applied to and benefit a psychotherapy and counselling perspective. Thus Taylor & Hill (1993) adopted an open systems approach to the problem of analysing the process of educational delivery. Their approach highlights four critical points that characterize a higher education institution: input, process, output and outcome. Subsequently they built two models that enabled them to identify potential sources of problems at both the system and the delivery process levels. Given the similarity between psychotherapy and the educational perspective, both of their models can be easily adapted (with adequate changes) to the counselling and psychotherapy perspective, as shown below in Figures 20.1 and 20.2. (Note that Figure 20.2 expands the transformation process shown in Figure 20.1 by identifying the subcomponents of this process as predelivery, delivery and postdelivery.)

It is clear that the bird's eye perspective shown in Figures 20.1 and 20.2 helps to identify the various elements that contribute to the functionality of a counselling/psychotherapy institution. Such a broad analysis should enable the quality aware manager to identify more easily the possible areas for improvement. Such improvement in an institution's transparency not only enables its decision makers to improve its effectiveness and efficiency but also provides useful information to clients about both the quality of its organization and its orientation.

In addition, if a counselling/psychotherapy institution wants to heed the advice that the processes of delivery of a service can be as important to the customer as the 'formal' process of transformation (i.e. therapist–client interactions),

Input		Outputs	Outcomes
Capital			
Labour (managers, administrators, therapists)	**Transformation process**	Client (recovery, prevention, development)	Benefit to society
'Raw material' (self-referred clients, referred by others, e.g. doctors, court, etc.)			
Information (psychotherapy/counselling theory, background knowledge about client, background experience of therapist, rules, etc.)	Therapist/client interaction (including significant others)	Research New model of delivery Knowledge	

Fig. 20.1 Open system representation of a counselling/psychotherapy institution (adapted from Taylor & Hill's 1993 model, © MCB University Press, Bradford).

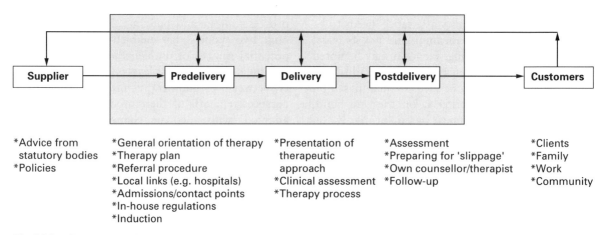

Fig. 20.2 Components of the delivery process from a psychotherapy/counselling perspective (adapted from Taylor & Hill 1993, © MCB University Press, Bradford).

there is a need to take into account all interactions at all levels between a client and a counselling/psychotherapy institution (i.e. from the very first contact by a client to the last one).

The next section will look at the reasons for the current drive for quality assurance in psychotherapy as well as the ways in which such a drive can be met. Subsequently an attempt will be made to analyse the adequacy of the rational emotive behaviour therapy model in the light of the previous debate about quality.

CURRENT CHALLENGES TO QUALITY IN PSYCHOTHERAPY

It is clear that recent moves in almost any area of activity are geared towards accountability. Such moves have been heavily influenced by at least four factors:

1. multiplication of the amount of therapies all claiming to be the best approach available (note that this proliferation was further

exacerbated by a similar proliferation of many 'professional' bodies that provide a stamp of approval upon their members)

2. adoption of a market perspective by clients who are keen to get some assurance that the service they are getting has been tested and offers value for money
3. anecdotal stories based on both facts and fictions that highlight the risks (health and financial) associated with using the 'wrong' therapy
4. higher awareness by clients of their legal rights regarding the quality of expected service (e.g. through the Citizens' charter).

Giles (1993) and Steenbarger & Smith (1996) add:

5. increasing budgetary pressures faced by counsellors/psychotherapists at a time of rising demand for services.

In the USA, such factors led to an increased pressure on mental health practitioners to demonstrate the quality of their service. This pressure culminated recently in the National Committee for Quality Assurance (NCQA 1996) accreditation of managed behavioural health care organizations. The accreditation requires providers of behavioural health care to be able to document the quality of their work. Such documentation should cover: client satisfaction, tangible clinical outcomes, adherence to verification and care guidelines. These areas had been the subject of several studies (Benson 1992, Hill & Corbett 1993, Steenbarger & Smith 1996, Zablocki 1995) and highlight a pressing need for standardization of measures of each of these areas as shown below. Note that these areas of focus fit easily within the delivery process model (Fig. 20.2).

Measures of satisfaction of clients

Steenbarger & Smith (1996) argue for the need to use more normed and standardized measures of client satisfaction instead of non validated self-made satisfaction questionnaires. They suggest the use of measures such as the Client Satisfaction Questionnaire (CSQ-8) and Service Satisfaction

Scale-30 (SSS-30). In particular they recommend the latter since it differentiates between satisfaction with the administrative compared with the professional aspects of service delivery. However, these measures of client satisfaction have been criticized for assessing the degree to which clients feel they have been helped by therapy and not the actual improvements in their life. This line of argument will be further developed below when discussing rational emotive behavioural therapy position vis à vis total quality management.

Measures of counselling/psychotherapy outcomes

Besides referring to clients' feedback about therapy, therapists often make use, at regular intervals during therapy, of a second type of measure that, irrespective of the views of the client, tries to address the question 'to what extent has the client benefited from therapy?' These measures, known as outcome measures, tend to focus on two areas (Steenbarger & Smith 1996): functional status and symptomatology of client. The first one addresses the level of functionality of clients given the problems they are presenting whereas symptomatology focuses on the frequency and degree of intensity of the presenting problems. These outcome measures have been criticized for focusing on psychopathology rather than on growth and development.

Measures of standard of care

Zablocki (1995) suggested the need to minimize the large variations between the practices among the mental health providers. Hence the need to create greater uniformity among practitioners through the establishment of standards of care. Barlow (1993) envisages the setting up of these standards in terms of clinical protocols that have demonstrated empirical efficacy. Subsequently, the achievement of such standards will be assessed in terms of performance indicators (Benson 1992).

In England the current move towards NVQs is believed to help standardize the counselling/psychotherapy process. This move, which was initiated in the mid 1980s by governmental agencies (e.g. the Department for Employment,

Training Agency, National Council for Vocational Qualifications), took on the challenge to rationalize the UK system of vocational qualifications. This rationalization, which was competence led as opposed to relying on 'time serving' (e.g. number of years spent studying or practising), encouraged subject experts to define as closely as possible the elements of the targeted competence. The level of competence of a candidate for an NVQ is subsequently determined mainly through 'tangible' evidence presented in a work-based environment (e.g. observable evidence offered in a psychotherapy practice). This NVQ system, which initially targeted industry-based occupational areas (e.g. motor mechanic, electronic engineering, etc.) progressively expanded to cover most existing occupational areas (including the counselling and psychotherapy area). According to this system, qualifications are developed by bringing together experts in an occupational area, who form the lead body (LB). Recently a lead body has been set up to develop national standards in counselling and psychotherapy. This lead body (which includes representatives from several recognizable professional bodies such as the United Kingdom Council for Psychotherapy, Alcohol Concern, British Association of Counselling, etc.) is known as the Counselling, Advice, Mediation, Psychotherapy, Advocacy and Guidance (CAMPAG). It is well on its way to developing the standards of competence covering the various facets of its occupational area. The standards being developed are meant to range from the most basic level of understanding and practice (represented in NVQs levels 1 and 2) to postgraduate/professional levels of achievement (represented in levels 3, 4 and 5). The implementation of these standards is backed by a multilayered quality assurance system involving both formal requirements (such as accreditation, training and assessment requirements) and desirable requirements (e.g. Investor in People and ISO9000). Although the NVQ approach is believed by many to bring more clarity and transparency in the assessment of competence process, as well as offering candidates nationally recognizable qualifications (i.e. recognizable by all main professional groups), the big test will be in the degree of acceptance shown by those who will pilot the new standards. Thus it has been argued that, although the system may offer clear advantages in certain occupational areas, it is not to be regarded as a panacea for all situations, and in some areas may lead to a more negative situation if applied indiscriminately (Fourali 1997).

Apart from budgetary difficulties, Steenbarger & Smith (1996) identified three reasons for non-compliance with outcome measurement procedures:

1. perceptions of administering the assessment material (outcome measures, etc.) as a non-essential task that is overlooked in budgeting for counselling/psychotherapy settings
2. difficulty in following up reasons for clients' drop-out of therapy (although it is always possible to assess changes on a regular basis (e.g. every three sessions) through set questionnaires)
3. resistance to data collection by some counsellors/psychotherapists who may believe that the information will be used to punish them or justify the introduction of new service demands.

It is clear that other reasons may contribute to the above stated non-compliant response. For instance, some psychotherapists and counsellors may argue that outcome measurement procedures may be suitable for behavioural orientations but may not reflect the 'ethos' of other non-behavioural orientations. Thus many psychotherapists of a non-behavioural persuasion many find them too mechanistic and detrimental to the process. Moreover a number of psychotherapists may question the practicality of such procedures, particularly in the private sector.

In addition to developing reliable measures for assessing the effectiveness of therapy there is also the need to develop a culture of continuous improvement, as suggested above in the total quality management and global approach to quality. It is clear that leadership commitment and support in the form of top management are crucial to determine and effect changes. It is also important that management shows genuine commitment to quality by applying the principles at all levels of the organization, thereby offering to the rest of the staff the new model to follow that crystallizes the newly adopted ethos.

Having provided a background to the issues surrounding quality assurance in general and how they may apply to a psychotherapy setting, the next part of the chapter will attempt to look at how the identified quality issues may be applied to evaluate both strengths and weaknesses of the model/theory adopted by psychotherapists/counsellors to guide their therapeutic interventions. The theory and method being used for illustrative purposes are that of the currently widely used approach known as rational emotive behaviour therapy. However, to start with, there is a need to introduce this model of therapy. This is done in the next section.

BRIEF INTRODUCTION TO RATIONAL EMOTIVE BEHAVIOUR THERAPY

Rational emotive behaviour therapy was developed in the 1950s by Albert Ellis who also had a decisive influence on today's cognitive behavioural therapies (Corey 1996). It is a multimodal, integrative approach which uses cognitive, affective and behavioural techniques (Corey 1996). This makes it a very potent type of therapy whose effectiveness is widely recognized (Kendall et al 1995, Lyons & Woods 1991, Smith & Glass 1977). Ellis argued that, although an emotional response 'C' may follow a critical activating event 'A', it is not A that causes C. The emotional reaction C is generally traced back to the individual's belief system B, which usually shows a dogmatic stance vis á vis the event. In particular, if C is undesirable it can be linked to the individual's irrational beliefs. To help reduce clients' disturbance, these beliefs are disputed through rational, empirical and pragmatic arguments (Dryden 1994, Ellis 1995). This form of therapy evolved from 'rational therapy' to 'rational emotive therapy' to its current name 'rational emotive behaviour therapy'. This progressive change of name results from the concern of its founder to highlight

the areas of focus of this form of therapy: mind, emotions and behaviour. Although the ABC idea was not new at the time of the creation of rational emotive behaviour therapy (e.g. Greek stoics and, more recently, Alfred Adler, quoted by Ellis (1995), had long before argued for the decisiveness of our 'inner response' to external stimuli in determining our emotional reaction) it was Ellis who developed it into a real system of psychotherapy. Among the specific aims of therapy that are encouraged by rational emotive behaviour therapy in order to promote in the clients a healthier approach to life are the following: scientific thinking, self-acceptance, self-interest, self-direction, social interest, tolerance, flexibility, acceptance of uncertainty, commitment, risk taking, high frustration tolerance, and own responsibility for disturbance (Corey 1996, Ellis & Bernard 1986, Ellis & Dryden, 1987). Dryden, quoted by Weinrach (1996), argues that rational emotive behaviour therapy can be defined as follows: 'Minimise your demandingness and awfulizing, raise your frustration tolerance and accept yourself and others as fallible human beings'.

Quality principles applied to rational emotive behaviour therapy

If the quality of a service is defined in terms of its efficiency and effectiveness, it may be argued that rational emotive behaviour therapy has always been aware of the need to deliver the best service with maximum efficiency. Ellis' main argument for discontinuing his use of both Rogerian therapy and psychoanalysis in favour of his new procedure, rational emotive behaviour therapy, was justified in terms of efficiency and effectiveness (Ellis 1989). Ellis (1989) and his followers are well aware of the need to protect the rights of consumers in terms of their purchase of products or services. However, he also gives strong warnings to protect these very consumers from their short range hedonism, which foolishly sabotages long range gains. This self-defeating or, at best, ineffective consumerism is argued to exist even when clients are presented with a selection of therapies to help them deal with their problems. Two types of factors appear to lead to an ineffective consumerism outcome: client-initiated ineffective consumerism and therapist-initiated ineffective consumerism.

According to Ellis (1989) the client-initiated ineffective consumerism results when clients opt for a type of therapy that may be unhelpful or even harmful to them. Some examples provided by Ellis (1989) include situations where clients select therapists who go easy on them, make them feel better (not get better), make them express their feelings and support them in their complaint about how the world has ill-treated them. Ellis argued that, in fact, these clients treat therapy and their therapists just as neurotically as they would deal with other involvements as their attitude towards therapy betrays a number of unhealthy irrational demands (i.e. 'musts' and 'absolute shoulds').

Therapist-initiated ineffective consumerism reflects a similar tendency to the latter in that it is induced by therapists who make demands regarding keeping clients, making a lot of money, making them 'feel better' (as opposed to making them 'get better') or adopt a dogmatic stance towards their theory, even if it is not helping the clients, to prevent a sense of shame and self-condemnation for 'failing' (Ellis 1989). Ellis argued that this type of ineffective consumerism is rife even among the most popular brands of cognitive behavioural therapies (e.g. Beck 1976, Goldfried & Davison 1976, Meichenbaum 1977, Raimy 1975). Among the examples given (Ellis 1989) are cases where these therapies:

1. are overly collaborative to the point where therapy is in danger of being derailed from decisive issues that may warrant an '*active-directive and persuasive*' stance from the therapist
2. do not target clients' dogmatic demands and address mainly the more superficial irrational inferences
3. adopt a mainly empirical, 'positive-thinking', problem-solving or skill-training approach and omit philosophical restructuring.

Such positions, Ellis (1989) argued, are at least unprofessional and at worst unethical and 'should' be avoided through setting up and enforc-ing clear and unequivocal ethical rules of psychotherapy practice.

The above argument shows how difficult it is to promote a total quality management view in therapy based on client satisfaction. This situation highlights the slippery concept of quality when it is applied to a service such as psychotherapy as opposed to a tangible manufactured product. However, detecting a difficulty in improving a psychotherapy service may not discourage therapists genuinely interested in the welfare of their clients from providing a better service. Ellis' above attack on ineffective consumerism can signal the need for more cautiousness from therapists in identifying the reasons behind their attitudes and strategies in helping their clients. In turn such cautiousness highlights the need for constant updating by therapists of their knowledge from research that will help them make sounder decisions about what is most helpful to their clients. Such an attitude of openness is not always present in therapists. However, the rational emotive behaviour therapy model appears to offer the 'ingredients' for such an attitude since it argues that one of its main tenets and aims in both therapy and training of its therapists is to challenge any absolute (Dryden 1991) and adopt a flexible view of the world that can be changed according to new evidence. It is clear that such a stance helps address effectively some of the discontents levelled against therapy (Dryden & Feltham 1992).

However, despite the above rational emotive behaviour therapy principles that demonstrate the view that this therapy supports the delivery of an effective 'quality psychotherapy', it appears that rational emotive behaviour therapy itself is in need of significant improvements.

Recently, a number of leading researchers in rational emotive behaviour therapy, including Ellis, identified a number of current issues within it that needed dealing with and resolving in order to help improve its effectiveness and efficiency (Kendall et al 1995). These issues, which were also raised by various other practising rational emotive behaviour therapists (e.g. Bond & Dryden 1996, Wessler 1996), fall into three categories—the scientific status of the theory, assessment and practice of therapy—as follows:

Scientific status of the theory

Rational emotive behaviour therapy does not have a strong reputation as a 'scientific' theory of psychopathology. This has been explained by a number of factors including ambiguities in the theory, flaws in the design of studies, scarcity of large scale clinical trials and lack of interest among rational emotive behaviour therapists to capitalize on clinical observations and translate them into testable hypotheses (Bond & Dryden 1996, Kendall et al 1995, Wessler 1996).

Assessment

Traditionally, it has been argued by rational emotive behaviour therapy practitioners that the best means of assessment consists in having several rational emotive behaviour therapy sessions with the clients (Dryden 1991, Ellis & Dryden 1987). This way they can be quickly helped while being assessed (Dryden 1991). However, it is becoming increasingly clear that unstructured clinical interviewing presents a number of serious difficulties that impede the adoption of a research perspective. These include difficulty in replicating results, and difficulty in isolating target variables (e.g. irrational beliefs) because of interference of other variables such as suggestion and reinforcement. In addition the majority of belief measures (e.g. irrational belief test, the idea inventory and the rational belief inventory) have been found to lack discriminant validity and may even be inappropriate for assessing irrationality (Kendal & Korgeski 1979, Kendall et al 1995).

Practice of therapy

Despite the well-reported effectiveness of rational emotive behaviour therapy as a method of therapy (Lyons & Woods 1991, Smith & Glass 1977), there has been a significant degree of criticism of the rigour of the studies that demonstrated this effectiveness (Kendall et al 1995). Hence there was a need to adhere to methodological protocols that facilitate a clear interpretation of research outcomes. Thus researchers are being encouraged to study at the micro level the therapy process including characteristics of the therapist, relation-ship factors, stages of application of rational emotive behaviour therapy and relative effectiveness towards different disorders.

Given the above presentation of rational emotive behaviour therapy principles and procedures, how does this therapy fare when seen in the light of a total quality management perspective?

Rational emotive behaviour therapy and total quality management

In order to evaluate the status of a psychotherapeutic approach in the light of the total quality management model, it is possible to apply any widely accepted total quality management model for its rigour and contrast its demands against the theoretical and practical characteristics of the psychotherapeutic approach. Hence, looking at the above description of the demands meeting the Baldridge quality model, it is possible to contrast them with the equivalent characteristics observed within a rational emotive behaviour therapy perspective as shown in Box 20.2.

The above description of rational emotive behaviour therapy and its evaluation in the light of a total quality management model showed a number of positive characteristics together with a number of issues of concern that need addressing by rational emotive behaviour therapy practitioners. Conversely, the Baldridge model showed good potential in helping evaluate the robustness of a particular psychotherapy orientation. Nevertheless it can be improved further by highlighting the social/environmental element (as done in the above stated European Award) particularly in an educational or therapeutic context. This point can easily be remedied by reminding users of the Baldridge model to address the social/environmental/global dimension at the levels of the 'quality assurance of product and services' and 'goals'.

Box 20.2 shows that rational emotive behaviour therapy appears to adhere to perhaps the most important total quality management feature: 'an on-going concern for continuous improvement'. Hence such an approach improves greatly its image compared with various other models that find it difficult to move away from earlier 'orthodoxies' despite clear evidence of inefficiencies.

Box 20.2   Applying the Baldridge requirements to the rational emotive behaviour therapy model

Leadership
As explained above, rational emotive behaviour therapy is led by a clear statement of the characteristics of a healthy approach to life. These characteristics reflect the attitudes and values, of clients and therapists alike, towards themselves, others and the world at large (e.g. self-acceptance, acceptance of others and a rational scientific attitude to life events). However, it appears that rational emotive behaviour therapy theorists have neglected the scientific status of their theory. Hence their current concern to rectify this situation by improving the rigour of rational emotive behaviour therapy research.

Originally the rational emotive behaviour therapy model was led by Ellis but, subsequently, this leadership became crystallized around a group of 'disciples' who encouraged the further development of the original ideas. However Ellis' views still remain decisive in the orientation of the model. For instance it is Ellis who recently decided to rename rational emotive therapy as rational emotive behaviour therapy.

Information and analysis
Rational emotive behaviour therapists were always aware of the need to gather information and carry out analyses that are essential for comparative analyses between the effectiveness of REBT method compared with others, despite criticisms about the rigour of these types of activities (Kendall et al 1995). Moreover rational emotive behaviour therapy showed great flexibility in integrating other 'proven' procedures (new and old) within its methodology as shown through its 'theoretically consistent eclecticism' (Dryden 1991).

Strategic quality planning
As mentioned above, rational emotive behaviour therapy, perhaps more than many other therapies, has a clear idea of what constitutes a healthy attitude to life and the need to design and plan therapy accordingly. However, it is also willing to compromise in cases where clients are not ready for 'radical' changes. Thus, although its ultimate goal is to induce a change in the client of the dysfunctional philosophical beliefs, rational emotive behaviour therapy practitioners are also known to revert to using other more moderate strategies generally associated with mainstream cognitive therapy (e.g. changing interpretations, changing inferences, changing triggering factors or relaxation, etc.) if the client is not ready for the deep changes.

Human resource utilization
Rational emotive behaviour therapy is keen to ensure a more consistent application of its 'proven' procedures by its followers. Hence the recent need to specify in more detail the rational emotive behaviour therapy steps (Dryden 1994) as well as ensuring that there are serious training courses and workshops available to those interested in using the procedure. If the method is adequately followed, it will be possible to measure more accurately its effectiveness compared with other methods. However, some recent research suggests that cognitive behaviour therapists in general need to increase their efficiency by considering possibilities for very brief treatments (e.g. three or four sessions) (see Pekarik 1993).

Quality assurance of product and services
Rational emotive behaviour therapy is goal orientated and has always aimed at effecting quality healthy changes in its clients. Consequently, the planning and process of therapy are designed to meet goals of therapy that reflect deep and long term changes. If these goals are not attained then there is a need either to reconsider the goals, or to reconsider the method or judiciously refer the client to another therapist or another therapy.

However, as will be argued below, rational emotive behaviour therapy could be perceived as being too individualistic since it always gives its main priority to the client—despite allowing 'a close second' to the rest of the world (Dryden 1994). This position could be challenged on either ethical or cultural grounds. At the ethical level, it may be argued that such a position could

Box 20.2 Applying the Baldridge requirements to the rational emotive behaviour therapy model *(cont'd)*

antagonize group or social (or even global) priorities. At the cultural level, it is clear that, in several non-Western cultures, individuals' well-being is very closely tied to their cultural/family group. It appears that a 'less confrontational' approach between individuals and the 'rest of the world' may prove more useful, as argued by the 'Beyond opposites' approach proposed by Fourali (in press 2000).

Measurement of outcome
Rational emotive behaviour therapy's *raison d'être* revolves around the idea of 'effectiveness'. This is particularly true since Ellis originally designed it as an effective alternative to other therapies such as psychoanalysis and Rogerian therapy. Hence it has always shown strong interests in comparative outcome studies. However, it appears that, initially, rational emotive behaviour therapists were more concerned with issues of practice to the point of neglecting issues of standardizations, objective assessment and large scale rigorous research (Dryden 1987, Kendall et al 1995). Recently, rational emotive behaviour therapy practitioners have become more and more aware of the need

for an adequate assessment of the outcome of their therapeutic treatments.

Goals
As shown above, rational emotive behaviour therapy's main concern is to effect real, deep and long term healthy changes in the clients. Consequently one of its targets at the early stages of therapy is to work with clients to achieve those goals that help them to 'get better and not simply to feel better' (Ellis 1995). Despite several studies demonstrating its comparatively higher therapeutic effectiveness, its practitioners are always keen to improve it by producing or adapting from other therapies effective therapeutic procedures. However, more recently there has been a debate as to what extent some of the 'values' identified by orthodox rational emotive behaviour therapy as healthy can stand to scrutiny. Thus Wessler (1996) recently challenged the validity of Ellis' position against religiosity and raised concern for rational emotive behaviour therapy's historical vulnerability to 'new fashions' or fads in psychotherapy.

However, it has also been argued that many psychotherapists, and in our case rational emotive behaviour therapists, may overlook the influence of their own cultural values and assumptions on psychotherapy/counselling theory and practice (Christopher 1996, Wessler 1996). This issue is particularly conspicuous by its absence in Kendall and colleagues' paper (1995), purporting to give rational emotive behaviour therapy theory a vision for the future, especially when, over two decades ago, Ellis (1973) stated: 'all psychology is, at bottom, a value system' (p. 28). Christopher (1996) argued that this view is promoted by many leading psychotherapists, who include Ellis, May, Wachtel and others. Despite this belief, he states: 'we seldom consider how cultural values and ideologies are enmeshed in the theory and practice of counselling [hence psychotherapy too]' (p.17). Christopher (1996) explains this tendency in

terms of Western culture's individualistic orientation, which induces therapists to think first and foremost of individual needs as opposed to the needs of the community/society. The view that we are brought into 'webs of significance' (Geertz 1973), which influence social practice, institutions and family life as well as the idea of 'good life', is also promoted by anthropologists (e.g. Geertz 1973) and hermeneutic thinkers (Gadamer 1975, Heidegger 1962). Hence it is clear that psychotherapy, including rational emotive behaviour therapy, should continuously challenge the values behind its methods and query their representation among the various cultural webs of significance. Such a perspective is particularly welcome at a time of postmodern relativity of values. In addition, any serious therapy should query whether it reflects only one version of the world cultures or whether it is truly 'global' in its perspective.

SUMMARY

This chapter addressed the issue of quality assurance within a mental health context. It looked at the approach to quality in an educational setting and showed the benefit that psychotherapy and counselling may derive by applying this approach. In addition it looked at the possibility of adopting a total quality management model in order to, systematically, identify problems and target them through research to determine adequate solutions. Such an approach should also highlight in a summary format the perceived strengths and weaknesses of a particular theoretical model.

The chapter has highlighted the current pressures on psychotherapists and counsellors to provide the best possible service in terms of both efficiency and effectiveness. In order to uphold such claims, the service will need to ensure quality at both theoretical and delivery level. In practice, the service needs to be satisfactory in at least three areas: client satisfaction, counselling/psychotherapy outcome and standards of care. The chapter has shown that all three of these measures can be problematic. In particular, rational emotive behaviour therapy argues that it is difficult to rely too much on clients' views as these views can be as self-defeatist as their problems that brought them to therapy in the first place. In addition, the issue of standard of care can be a 'red herring' too, in that different therapies may promote a different view of what is a standard of care because of their different orientations.

However, this does not mean that we cannot differentiate between a good and a bad counselling/psychotherapy service. Thus a clear and honest description of the philosophy and aims of therapy, as well as justification of its procedures (supported by rigorous research findings) can not only go a long way to stimulate debate among researchers but also provide a degree of confidence to the client to make responsible choices regarding what service they would like to get.

Eysenck (1992) had doubts about whether all therapies could be winners since they all claim to be different. However, it is still possible to establish, empirically, some generally agreed principles of practice that lead to long term successful out-

DISCUSSION QUESTIONS

1. How effective and efficient are the existing approaches to counselling and psychotherapy?
2. Is there a need for a quality assurance perspective in counselling and psychotherapy?
3. Why is the 'outcome problem' important?
4. Who benefits from adopting a quality assurance perspective to counselling and psychotherapy? Are there losers?
5. What are the difficulties in adopting a quality assurance approach to counselling and psychotherapy and how can they be avoided, if at all?
6. How does the concept of education relate to counselling and psychotherapy?
7. Compare and weigh up the pros and cons of two approaches to counselling and psychotherapy
8. Can you evaluate other models of counselling and psychotherapy using the total quality management approach suggested in the text?

comes. These, if demonstrated, should represent some general frame of reference for promoting mental health, which should help the researcher make sense out of the jungle of therapies that are currently available. For instance, it may be considered of paramount importance to involve clients actively in the aims, choice and process of treatment and not to make excessive demands/requests on them until they are ready, according to the principle of 'challenging but not overwhelming tasks' (Dryden 1991).

This chapter has illustrated the use of a total quality management model within a psychotherapy context by contrasting its principles with those identified in rational emotive behaviour therapy. The analysis showed that, despite some current problems facing rational emotive behaviour therapy, this type of therapy fits well within a total quality management perspective as its promoters are constantly aware of the need to improve its effectiveness and efficiency.

Finally, the author has argued that it is high time that therapies adopt a global approach towards quality—a perspective that does not sim-

FURTHER READING

Dryden W, Feltham C (eds) 1992 Psychotherapy and its discontents. Open University Press, Buckingham
This is an all-round very good reference about the many challenges facing counselling and psychotherapy ranging from those totally against any formal psychotherapeutic exercise to those favouring a cautious support for the work of psychotherapists.

Ellis A 1989 Ineffective consumerism in the cognitive-behavioural therapies and in general psychotherapy. In: Dryden W, Trower P (eds) Cognitive psychotherapy, stasis and change. Cassell Educational, London. pp 159–174
This article is very useful in raising awareness to serious weaknesses in the current practice of psychotherapy.

Fourali C in press 2000 Beyond opposites: extending the cultural boundaries of CBT methodology. Counselling Psychology Quarterly 13(2)
This article highlights the issue of improving effectiveness of the CBT model of psychotherapy as well as raising awareness of cultural effects on psychotherapeutic procedures.

Giles T R (ed) 1993 Handbook of effective psychotherapies. Plenum Press, New York
Provides useful information about trends towards effectiveness from several psychotherapeutic procedures as well as arguing for the need to make psychotherapy more respondent to current social needs.

Sallis E 1993 Total quality management in education. Kogan Page, London
A very useful introduction to the concept of total quality management, particularly in the educational context.

Steenbarger B N, Smith B H 1996 Assessing the quality of counselling services: developing accountable helping systems. Journal of Counselling and Development 75:145–150
A useful article highlighting a number of initiatives for improving the quality of counselling.

---

ply address some theoretical or practical issues within a particular culture (such as, say, that of a Western society) but attempts to question all aspects of both theory and practice from a variety of cultural perspectives. Indeed, the test of the robustness of a theory does not depend on whether it works in one particular place at one particular time of a society's history but to what degree can its precepts and practices be adopted everywhere, today and tomorrow.

ACKNOWLEDGEMENT

I would like to thank Tarik Enasr Fourali for his 'occasional' useful advice.

REFERENCES

Barlow D H (ed) 1993 Clinical handbook of psychological disorders, 2nd edn. Guilford Press, New York

Beck A T 1976 Cognitive therapy and emotional disorders. International Universities Press, New York

Benson D S 1992 Measuring outcomes in ambulatory care. American Hospital Publishing, Chicago

Bergin A E, Lambert M J 1978 The evaluation of therapeutic outcome. In: Garfield S L, Bergin A E (eds) Handbook of psychotherapy and behavioural change, 2nd edn. John Wiley, New York, pp 139–190

Bissell D 1989 Taguchi methods. Institute of Statisticians, London

Bond F W, Dryden W 1996 Why two central REBT hypotheses appear untestable. Journal of Rational Emotive and Cognitive Behaviour Therapy 14(1):29–40

British Quality Foundation 1997 Towards business excellence: a world in which organisations throughout the UK excel. British Quality Foundation, London

BSI 1987 British Standard 4778. Quality systems, parts 1 (same as ISO8402: 1986) and 2. BSI, London

Caldwell B, Spinks J 1992 Leading the self-managing school. Falmer Press, London

Chambers English dictionary 1988 edition W R Chambers, London

Christopher J C 1996 Counselling inescapable moral visions. Journal of Counselling and Development 75:17–24

Corey G 1996 Theory and practice of counselling and psychotherapy. Brooks-Cole, Pacific Grove CA

DOE (Department of Education and Science) 1990 Course monitoring and review in further education. HMSO, London

DOE (Department of Education and Science) 1991 Quality assurance in colleges of further education. HMSO, London

Dryden W 1987 Current issues in rational emotive therapy. Croom Helm, New York, Ch 10 Where is the evidence? Promoting quality RET research

Dryden W 1991 Reason and therapeutic change. Whurr, London

Dryden W 1994 Rational emotive counselling in action. Sage, London

Dryden W, Feltham C (eds) 1992 Psychotherapy and its discontents. Open University Press, Buckingham

Elliot G 1993 Whose quality is it, anyway? Quality Assurance in Education 1(1):34–40

Ellis A 1973 Humanistic psychotherapy. McGraw-Hill, New York

Ellis A 1989 Ineffective consumerism in the cognitive-behavioural therapies and in general psychotherapy. In: Dryden W, Trower P (eds) Cognitive psychotherapy, stasis and change. Cassell Educational, London, pp 159–174

Ellis A 1995 Rational emotive behaviour therapy. In: Corsini R J, Wedding D (eds) Current psychotherapies, 5th edn. F E Peacock, Itasca IL, pp 162–196

Ellis A, Bernard M E 1986 What is rational-emotive therapy (RET)? In: Ellis A, Grieger R (eds) Handbook of rational-emotive therapy, vol 2. Springer, New York, pp 3–30

Ellis A, Dryden W 1987 The practice of rational-emotive therapy. Springer, New York

Eysenck H J 1952 The effects of psychotherapy: an evaluation. Journal of Consulting Psychology 16: 319–324

Eysenck H J 1992 The outcome problem in psychotherapy. In: Dryden W, Feltham C (eds) Psychotherapy and its discontents. Open University Press, Buckingham, pp 100–124

Feigenbaum A V 1987 Total quality control. McGraw-Hill, New York

Fourali C 1994 Glossary of terms used in standards development, curriculum design, assessment and accreditation. City & Guilds, London

Fourali C 1997 Identifying and measuring knowledge in vocational awards: the NVQ experience. Research in Post-Compulsory Education 2(2):121–149

Fourali C in press 2000 Beyond opposites: extending the cultural boundaries of CBT methodology. Counselling Psychology Quarterly 13(2)

Gadamer H G 1975 Truth and method. Cross Road, New York

Geertz C 1973 The interpretation of cultures. Basic Books, New York

Giles T R 1993 Consumer advocacy and effective psychotherapy. In: Giles T R (ed) Handbook of effective psychotherapies. Plenum Press, New York, pp 481–488

Goldfried M R, Davison G C 1976 Clinical behaviour therapy. Holt, Rinehart & Winston, New York

Harvey L, Burrows A, Green D 1992 Criteria of quality: summary, quality in higher education project. University of Central England, Birmingham

Heidegger M 1962 Being and time (trans Macquarrie J, Robinson E). Harper & Row, New York

Hill C E, Corbett M M 1993 A perspective on the history of process and outcome research in counselling psychology. Journal of Counselling Psychology. 40(1):3–24

Kendall P C, Korgeski G P 1979 Assessment and cognitive behavioural interventions. Cognitive Therapy and Research 3:1–21

Kendall P C, Haaga D A F, Ellis A, Bernard M, DiGiuseppe R, Kassinove H 1995 Rational emotive therapy in the 1990s and beyond: current status, recent revisions and research questions. Pergamon, New York, pp 169–185

Lawn M 1991 Social constructions of quality in teaching. Evaluation and Research in Education. 5(1 & 2):67–77

Lyons L C, Woods P J 1991 The efficacy of rational-emotive therapy: a quantitative review of the outcome research. Clinical Psychology Review 11:357–369

Macdonald J, Piggott J 1990 Global quality. Mercury, London

Meichenbaum M 1977 Cognitive-behavior modification. Plenum, New York

Merton R 1970 Social structure and anomie, American Sociological Review 1938 3:672–680, reprinted in: Worsley P (ed) Modern sociology: introductory readings. Penguin, Harmondsworth

Miller J, Innis S 1990 Strategic quality management: the strategic management of a quality further education service—a working paper for LEA officers and college principles. Consultants at Work, Ware, Hertfordshire

Müller D, Funnel P 1991 Delivering quality in vocational education. Kogan Page, London

NCQA (National Committee for Quality Assurance) 1996 Draft accreditation standards for managed behavioural healthcare organisations. NCQA, Washington DC

Nelson-Jones R 1982 The theory and practice of counselling psychology. Holt, Rinehart & Winston, Eastbourne

Pekarik G 1993 Beyond effectiveness: uses of consumer-oriented criteria in defining treatment success. In: Thomas R G (ed) Handbook of effective psychotherapies. Plenum Press, New York, pp 409–436

Prochaska J, Norcross J 1994 Systems of psychotherapy: a transtheoretical analysis. Brooks-Cole, Pacific Grove, CA

Raimy V 1975 Misunderstandings of the self. Jossey-Bass, San Francisco

Sallis E 1993 Total quality management in education. Kogan Page, London

Smith M L, Glass G V 1977 Meta-analysis of psychotherapy outcome studies. American Psychologist 32:752–760

Smith M L, Glass G V, Miller T I 1980 The benefits of psychotherapy. John Hopkins University Press, Baltimore MD

Steenbarger B N, Smith B H 1996 Assessing the quality of counselling services: developing accountable helping systems. Journal of Counselling and Development. 75:145–150

Strupp H 1983 Psychoanalytic psychotherapy. In: Hersen M, Kazdin A, Bellack A (eds) The clinical psychology handbook. Pergamon Press, Oxford, pp 471–485

Taylor A, Hill F 1993 Quality management in education. Quality Assurance in Education 1(1):21–28

Weinrach S 1996 Nine experts describe the essence of rational emotive therapy while standing on one foot. Journal of Counselling and Development 74:326–331

Wessler R 1996 Idiosyncratic definitions and unsupported hypotheses: rational emotive behaviour therapy as pseudoscience. Journal of Rational Emotive and Cognitive Behaviour Therapy 14(1):41–61

Zablocki E 1995 Changing physician practice patterns: strategies for success in a capitated health care system. Aspen, Gaithersburg MD

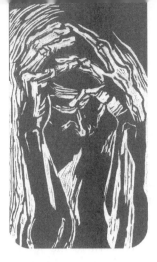

Chapter Twenty-one

Aggression management

Mike Musker

AIMS

◆ To introduce theories of aggression including psychoanalytical, ethological, psychosocial and biological perspectives

◆ To identify the difference between instrumental and affective aggression

◆ To discuss the issue of defining aggression

◆ To work through the phases of aggression management

◆ To outline approaches toward service users when they are agitated or in crisis

◆ To identify issues about aggression management in the context of the Code of Practice—Mental Health Act 1983

KEY ISSUES

Violence towards mental health professionals

Theories of aggression

Defining aggression

Managing a violent incident

Developing behavioural contracts

Drug dependency and aggression

INTRODUCTION

Managing aggression can prove to be the most difficult and frightening aspect of working in mental health. For nurses, fear of being attacked is based in statistical reality; evidence shows that nursing staff are 2.5 times more likely to be assaulted than other professional staff, and male nursing staff are 50% more likely to get injuries than female staff (Maier, Van Rybroek & Mays 1994). To help service users reduce their aggression we need to develop our own knowledge about what it is and to demonstrate less reliance on outmoded myths of traditional practice (Morrison 1993). Mental health professionals must endeavour to use evidence-based practice to further the scientific understanding of aggression and to determine effective outcomes of management interventions. In attempting to minimize acts of aggression we should listen to the subjective view of the service user who is experiencing the emotional difficulty, and combine this with objective evidence. The lay view of the service user can often be more enlightening than any theoretical knowledge of aggression. It is important that we take an holistic approach to aggression considering biological, psychological, social and cultural phenomena. Aggression management is a dynamic process and Deakin (1995) asks us to try to understand the feelings of agitation that can occur when living within a ward environment. Imagine life on a noisy ward full of disturbed people, 24 hours a day, 7 days a week, never being able to relax; only then can you begin to understand why someone might resort to an act of aggression. Additionally, people being admitted to hospital will invariably have to cope with serious mental health problems along with hallucinations, thought disorder and a variety of social problems. Their main desire is a place of safety and the help of supportive professionals.

THEORIES OF AGGRESSION

Aggression has developed during human evolution and can be considered to be a component part of our physiological prewiring (Moyer 1976).

History is littered with evidence of the ruthlessness of the human species, even the Bible describes allegorical stories of interpersonal conflict such as how Adam and Eve had problems with their children, when Cain slew his brother Abel out of jealousy (Genesis 4:1–16). When we consider some of the recent atrocities committed during international conflicts, it becomes difficult to understand the true nature of people. The human ability to be aggressive was a cause of concern to the seventeenth century philosopher Thomas Hobbes who advised that man is like a beast and argued that we need strong societal rules to protect us from our neighbours. Consequently, laws were developed to protect citizens from each other. In the mid nineteenth century mental health laws were introduced to remove all mentally ill into asylums regardless of their level of dangerousness. Today, the Mental Health Act 1983 continues to provide powers to remove from society those that are considered a danger to themselves or others.

Psychoanalytical explanations

Sigmund Freud, like Darwin with his theories on aggression in the previous century, created a controversy with his psychoanalytical theories about aggression in humans, which were publicized around 1920. He supported the idea of an innate drive or instinct for human aggression. Freud outlined how the 'Thanatos drive' or death instinct is in constant conflict with the 'Eros drive' or life instinct. He claimed that we have a natural drive to seek our greatest pleasurable experience, referred to as Nirvana, a feeling that we have only ever experienced in our mother's womb (Gross 1996).

Freud then proclaimed that the only way to achieve a similar mode of existence is through death. In order to prevent this urge for death we have to express anger outwardly, as suppression will lead to free floating anxiety and other problems emerging from the subconscious. Little credence was given to this theory until Dollard et al expounded the frustration–aggression hypothesis in 1939. They described a hydraulic type model of aggression, suggesting that when frustration builds up it must be released so that it does not accumulate to the point of explosive aggression. A simple analogy would be how a pressure cooker must let off steam.

Ethological explanations

Konrad Lorenz in his book 'On aggression', originally published in 1966, put forward the controversial view that aggression was part of an animal-like instinct in humans (Lorenz 1996). Lorenz used his observations of the patterns of aggression in animals to explain similar human behaviour. An example might be how animals and people try to make themselves appear bigger when they are trying to intimidate others. It has been identified that animals have 'innate releasing mechanisms', which are ritualistic demonstrations of strength or submission. The way a dog raises the hackles on its back is an obvious example. Animals are highly territorial, and rely on such non-verbal signals to prevent or limit serious episodes of aggression (Lorenz 1996). This is a survival tactic, which in nature reduces the likelihood of harm or even death. An analogous situation is how humans 'square up' to each other, and this is to give the opposition the opportunity to back down without an aggressive act.

Psychosocial explanations

Albert Bandura (1973) later refuted the inevitability of instinctive aggression, stating that it was a form of learnt behaviour, which could equally be unlearnt. He emphasized how humans, unlike animals, are capable of exerting executive control over their behaviour. Berkowitz (1993) has identified a major concern about the modelling and frequency of aggression in the media, describing how faulty role models have led to people imitating violent behaviours. Similar concerns have been expressed about violent films, which were believed to have contributed in the murder of James Bulger committed by two young boys in 1994 (Gross 1996). Serious acts of aggression like the Dunblane massacre are constantly being fed to us by the media, desensitizing people away from the horror of extreme violence. Here are some examples from the press to consider:

Slasher is given life ten times
'David Morgan 31 years old, went on a frenzied stabbing orgy at Rackmans store in Birmingham slashing 14 women aiming for their throats.'
Daily Express, 3/2/96

Care in the community killed off lunatic asylum
'John Rous 49 years old, telephoned police warning them before killing voluntary worker Jonathan Newby, stabbing him through the heart.'
The Independent, 21/2/96

Getting into the mind of a killer
'Jason Mitchell killed (strangled) retired stationmaster and his wife after reading about and watching "Silence of The Lambs". He later boasted to police that he'd planned to eat his victims. He also claimed he wanted to kill one person a day over the Christmas period.'
The Guardian, 28/3/96

No staff prosecution over predictable killing
'Andrew Robinson killed Georgina Robinson, an occupational therapist, stabbing her to death, after purchasing a knife during a shopping trip the day before.'
The Guardian, 28/6/96

Woman in knife attack sent to Broadmoor
'A woman, Perline Ayton aged 28 years, carried out a frenzied knife attack armed with four knives, five screwdrivers, which left one person with a knife embedded in their skull, whilst slashing at others.'
The Times, 19/9/96

The making of a machete maniac
'Horrett Campbell slashed at the faces of children with a two-foot machete in a school playground, St Lukes, in Wolverhampton. He idolised the murderer in the Dunblane massacre and his home contained news cuttings of such atrocities.'
Daily Mail, 10/12/96

Physiological explanations

Genetic

Advances in biological science have assisted in the scientific understanding of aggression. Some authors have identified that being young and male are factors that make you more aggression prone and that you are more likely to be homicidal (Archer 1994). However, other researchers have found that gender is not a clear predictor of aggression in mental health (Newhill, Mulvey & Lidz 1995). In the 1950s it was identified that people with phenotypic tallness (physical appearance) have a different genetic make-up, known as the XYY syndrome (genotype). The Y on the sex chromosome determines the male gender and it was thought that having an extra Y chromosome would cause the production of extra male hormones resulting in what has been referred to as the 'supermale' (Geen 1990). Falsely, the science community believed they had found a major cause of aggression and crime by providing some convincingly supportive statistics, but further epidemiological studies refuted this evidence (Archer 1994).

Neurological

The limbic system, also referred to as the 'emotional centre' of the brain, is known to exert physiological control over aggression. Its components are the amygdala, hippocampus and hypothalamus. These combine with the frontal and temporal lobes in processing thoughts and memories respectively (Stuart & Laraia 1998). Experiments on animals, and operations on people who have had cerebrovascular accidents or other brain pathology, have helped to investigate links between the limbic system and aggression. In one experiment a cat was observed to adopt an aggressive posture on direct stimulation of the perifornical nuclei (specialized cells) of the amygdala; arching of its back, hissing and piloerection were noted to occur (Tortora & Anagnostakos 1990). The limbic system can be affected by neocortical inhibition (executive or intellectual control). Neurotransmitters facilitate communication between these areas including seretonin, noradrenaline, dopamine, acetylcholine and the inhibitory transmitter GABA. Tranquillizers work by interfering with these transmitters, but are known to be very imprecise in their action (Mench & Shea-Moore 1995). Decortication of some animals has been used to confirm the inhibitory role of the cortex. Specific health problems such as epilepsy or brain

tumours are examples of how neuropathology can cause recurring aggression. As neuroimaging technology (such as PET scans) advances we will be able to determine specific physiological damage, creating a greater understanding of aggression (Garza-Trevino 1994).

Hormonal

Physiological control of aggression is mainly communicated to the body by the endocrine system. The hypothalamus, being part of the limbic system, controls the release of hormones via the pituitary gland (or master gland), which in turn sends hormones to the adrenal cortex and the gonads (Atkinson et al 1996). The adrenal cortex produces corticoids, and the gonads produce testosterone, which prepare the organs in readiness for aggression. The preparatory process is known as the 'fight or flight' response and is similar to the general adaptation syndrome in response to stress described by Selye (1979). The hypothalamus concurrently stimulates the adrenal medulla, via the sympathetic nervous system, which in turn stimulates the release of two other hormones adrenaline and noradrenaline (collectively known as catecholamines). Physiological studies show that noradrenaline is produced by the body during the act of aggression, whereas adrenaline prepares the body for imminent aggression (Tortora & Anagnostakos 1990).

DEFINING AGGRESSION

To understand and manage aggression we need to be able to define what it is. Aggression can be helpful in promoting human survival and can in some circumstances be viewed by society as positive in nature. Aggression during sport, when completing arduous tasks, or when it is part of our daily employment is referred to as 'instrumental aggression'. It is the alternative 'affective aggression' that can be problematic, which is when feelings are expressed with inappropriate behaviours. Violence, assault, dangerousness and threat are all synonyms that are used to describe this type of aggression. The term 'violence' is usually reserved

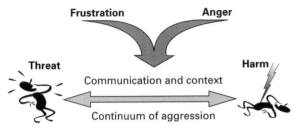

Fig. 21.1 Affective aggression.

for more serious acts of aggression such as physical assault or severe property damage (Siann 1985). You should not confuse aggression with assertion. Assertion is the ability to be direct and open about your feelings in defence of your personal rights, whilst at the same time respecting the rights of others. Any definition of aggression should attempt to capture the components of individuality and emotional feelings, whilst taking account of the contextual circumstances surrounding the aggressive behaviour (see Fig. 21.1).

A definition of 'Affective Aggression':

> *Any situation where behaviour is expressed to release emotional anger or frustration, with the intent of conveying these feelings to the self or others, reinforcing that communication with action on a continuum of threat to harm.*

PREDICTING AGGRESSION

Risk assessment is a rapidly growing science. We can sometimes predict aggression by observing the usual behaviours that occur before an assault— called prodromata (Guirguis 1978). Research has identified that people communicate their intention to assault up to 3 days prior to the actual incident by threatening gestures, verbal abuse, abnormal activity and threatening stances (Whittington & Patterson 1996). These are seen as 'normal' signs of potential aggression, and it is rare that a person will make an assault without some prior warning. Videotaped evidence of incidents have lead some researchers to state that we can predict up to 80% of aggression. This has been done by examining the behaviours immediately preceding an assault,

where assailants have been observed to: approach the victim rapidly, use intrusive gestures and to start yelling (Linaker & Busch-Iversen 1995). Other typical ways of communicating aggression non-verbally are through prolonged eye contact, speaking loudly, invading personal space, frowning and making threatening gestures.

These are usually supported by hostile verbal comments of a personal nature using statements like 'you never' or 'you always' (Stuart & Laraia 1998). Physical aggression has common outcomes, which include being choked, kicked, knocked out, thrown to the floor, punched, cut and stabbed (Sclafani 1986). People who have experienced such assaults suffer long term consequences to their disposition and behaviour, which is similar to post-traumatic stress disorder, usually in the form of anticipatory anxiety (Linaker & Busch-Iversen 1995). In order to obtain useful data on aggression we need a universally accepted tool, with consistent, accurate and objective recording.

CRITICAL FACTORS IN UNDERSTANDING AGGRESSION

Aggression within the community

It must be stressed that the majority of people with mental health problems are not aggressive. A variety of serious incidents, such as the killing of Jonathan Zito by Christopher Clunis, have emphasized the risk of dangerousness of the seriously mentally ill within the community, and such significant cases have given the impression that the cause of aggressive behaviour is mental illness. To compound this image, media influences have caused the public to fear the mentally ill, frequently portraying them within television programmes and films as the 'murderous hatchet-wielding psycho'. The reality is that community care has failed and the severely mentally ill are not receiving the care they need (Hodgins 1994). Criticisms have led to some new initiatives by the Labour Government, with the declaration of Frank Dobson's 'third way' for mental health. This bold development is supported by the Sainsbury Centre for Mental Health (1998) in their report 'Keys to engagement'. The Minister of Health declared that we need: 'a system in which both patients and public are safe and sound—a system which provides both security and support to all who need it'. New ideas proposed included more secure units, assertive outreach and changes in the mental health law to cope with the few mentally ill people who are dangerous. It will be the health care staff working at these secure units and within assertive outreach teams who are likely to be managing the aggressive minority.

Research and aggression

An epidemiological review of research on aggression has identified that there is no clear-cut evidence to show that the risk of assault from someone who is mentally ill is any greater than that from an individual in the average population (Arboleda-Florez, Holley & Chrisanti 1996). However, Monahan (1992), a well-known writer in the area of risk and dangerousness, has reversed his earlier beliefs on this matter, proposing that there *is* a greater risk of aggression from people who are mentally ill. Due to sampling errors and methodological limitations very few studies have been able to prove an unequivocal link between mental health and aggression (Link & Stueve 1995). What research has shown is that there are indicative behaviours that are displayed from service users who are more likely to become aggressive, allowing us to predict and manage individuals who are at greater risk of being dangerous. The most difficult time to predict aggression is upon admission when little is known about the person, but it is acknowledged that extra care should be taken when symptoms include paranoia, agitation and florid psychotic symptoms such as hallucinations and thought disorder (Kennedy 1993; Noble & Rodger 1989). If these symptoms are combined with some form of substance or alcohol abuse, the risk of aggression is much higher (Torrey 1994). In cases where there is aggression prior to admission to hospital, the person who is most likely to be attacked is a family member, but the majority of these assaults are usu-

ally minor in nature (Straznickas, McNeil & Binder 1993, Tardiff & Koenigsberg 1985).

Closer scrutiny of the statistics within hospitals has shown that the amount of aggressive episodes recorded can give a false impression about the frequency of violence. Aggressive episodes are generally underreported. The categorization of incidents makes it difficult to ascertain the severity of aggression, and it is difficult to make comparisons between hospitals because of the lack of standardized recording tools (Shah, Fineberg & James 1991). Davis (1991) indicated that hospital statistics on aggression are error prone owing to the obvious population bias; however, they have proved useful in identifying that a minority of people are responsible for the majority of aggressive incidents. In one typical study it was shown that 5% of the psychiatric inpatient population was responsible for 53% of all incidents over a 6-month period (Convit et al 1990). Statistics have also shown that the people who are most frequently attacked are nurses. The main reason is that the greater the contact with service users the more chance there is to be assaulted (Stuart & Laraia 1998). Two important factors compound the danger for nurses. First, once admitted to hospital individuals may feel safe to act out their aggressive feelings, assuming that nurses can help them bring their emotions under control. Secondly, in a study into antecedents of assaults, it was identified that 86% of incidents were caused by aversive stimuli such as setting limits on service users, forcing them to take medication, saying no, and asking them to perform behaviours that they do not want to do (Whittington & Wykes 1996). Aversive stimuli can be separated into three broad categories: *frustration* (refusal to meet a request, or preventing a behaviour), *activity demand* (a directive verbal statement) and *perceived attack* (comments, insults, or physical contact), all resulting in the possibility of an aggressive response (Whittington & Wykes 1996). Unfortunately, this incorporates the majority of nursing interventions and the custodial role of nurses does not ameliorate these aversive factors, particularly when those being detained under the Mental Health Act are often the people who pose the most danger to themselves or others.

MANAGING THE ENVIRONMENT

Goldstein (1994) proposed that, when trying to understand aggression, we must analyse it from the perspective of a 'person–environment duet'. In his book on the Ecology of aggression, he urged that we should consider the situational contexts of aggression, dividing these into micro (ward or home), meso (local community) and macro (city or country) environments. In considering some of the factors within the ward (microenvironment), it becomes apparent that there are many ways we can reduce the situational causes of aggression. An obvious example is, the more people crammed into a ward environment the greater the likelihood that there will be an increase in the amount of incidents (Haller & Deluty 1988). So we need to concentrate on creating a comfortable microenvironment with low occupancy levels. There is likely to be less aggression because of the reduction in noise stimulus, greater privacy, increased personal space and greater staff input for each service user (Palmstierna & Wistedt 1995). We all like to have a bit of personal territorial space and tend to feel quite protective of this area. People who are aggressive are known to require up to four times the normal interpersonal space (i.e. anywhere between 2 and 5 metres, or 6 and 16 feet). The way we manage the ward environment plays a major part in the management of aggression. It is important to have unambiguous ward policies, clear house rules and reasonable limit setting, which are consistently applied by all staff. This should prevent a hostile reaction when individuals are asked to adjust their behaviour in order to remain within these limits and also leaves less room for the dynamic process of splitting or transference. Conversely, wards that are too restrictive or oppressive and do not provide the individual with any positive hope for the future can also be a cause of aggression (Stuart & Laraia 1998). Evidence suggests that increased staffing, and high ratios of qualified to unqualified staff, will help to reduce episodes of aggression.

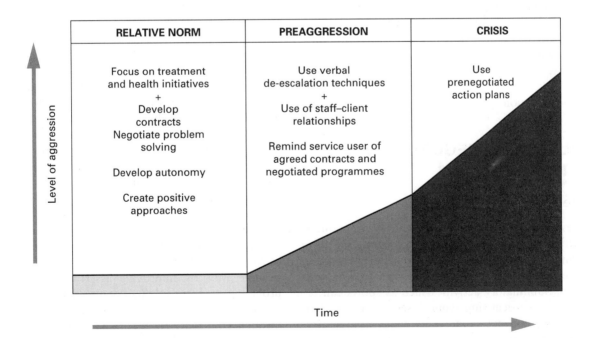

Fig. 21.2 The aggression cycle (adapted from Mason & Chandley 1999).

THREE PHASES OF AGGRESSION MANAGEMENT

Managing aggression should be a planned and systematic process. The care team needs to develop an action plan with the person involved through negotiation and partnership. We can divide the cycle of aggression up into three key phases (Fig. 21.2): the relative norm phase, the preaggressive phase and the crisis phase (Mason & Chandley 1999). Kaplan & Wheeler (1983) described two postaggression phases including the recovery and depression phase. The best way of managing aggression is to prevent it, and this can be achieved by knowing the early trigger factors of your client group, and by investing the majority of care in people when they are relatively healthy and calm.

For individuals who are frequently aggressive, much of the work must be done in the relative norm phase. This involves building a relationship with individuals when they are not aggressive. People who are prone to aggression should be encouraged to make positive use of their time by promoting healthy behaviours through a full rehabilitation programme. Plans and contracts should be formed to prepare for, and limit, future aggressive episodes. A common proclamation is that the best predictor of aggression is a past history of aggression. In working through the following case study, we can discuss the principles of managing changes in an individual's behaviour in relation to the aggression cycle.

PLANNING NEGOTIATED INTERVENTIONS

Relative norm phase

Develop a structured rehabilitation programme with John that takes up the main part of his day, which will channel some of the suppressed negative energy and frustration that can feed aggression. Sublimatory activities such as sports can be useful in occupying young service users, but beware that, for some individuals, competitive contact sports can also provoke aggression, leaving participants agitated long after the game has

CASE STUDY: JOHN

John is a 27-year-old man who is diagnosed as having schizophrenia, and was admitted because of an unprovoked attack on his neighbour. He currently suffers from paranoid ideation that others are going to restrain him and boil him in the ward cooker. He constantly looks warily about the ward, staring excessively at others. John often approaches nurses expressing his fears about the other people on the ward, stating that he must leave the ward because he is in fear of his life. At this point he has to be prevented from leaving by care staff owing to his being sectioned under the Mental Health Act. John then assumes everyone is against him and will panic, assaulting anyone who tries to prevent him leaving. He has even punched other service users without provocation when his paranoia overwhelms him. When John is not very anxious he is very pleasant and cooperative.

finished. A full and balanced timetable programme should aim to develop people's autonomy, with the objective of diverting them away from their anger by promoting positive behaviours. When John is settled enough to discuss his care, reflect on an aggressive incident and design some realistic interventions, which will be used during any subsequent episode of aggression. Planned interventions will include helping John to identify his angry feelings while he is still in control of them, at which time cognitive and positive behavioural strategies can be used to break the cycle. An example might be that John will request some time in his own room, utilizing the less stimulating environment to regain his confidence. Additionally, he could do some relaxation exercises on his bed or just listen to music. Attendance at a structured anger management group is helpful in learning to deal with feelings of aggression in a positive way, by improving assertiveness skills, providing problem-solving contingencies, and by learning face-saving alternatives. This is achieved through role play, psychodrama and education. Designing an intervention programme with John should include targeting each phase of the aggression cycle, so negotiation should take place about what happens when the aggression becomes uncontrolled and cannot be dealt with in the relative norm phase. Wherever possible you should involve and seek the support of family members in the management of aggression, as they are the people who will have to deal with John's aggression when he is discharged.

The preaggressive phase

In preparation for this phase some harsh negotiation may need to take place between John and his caseworker about dealing with his anger. This will involve some specific reality confrontation, which is a process of being direct, giving genuine and honest feedback about acceptable behaviour. Preparing for this phase in advance will promote cooperation between John and the staff. A plan should be written together that states, in clear bullet form, which actions will happen next in response to identified problematic behaviours. We know how John is likely to behave from his previous incidents, so we need to be very specific in describing his antecedent behaviour, the actual aggression and what consequences can be expected. John may be able to provide important data by explaining what he is usually feeling at these times. A behavioural analysis is useful here, which is an exact and objective description of what type of behaviours a person engages in throughout the day. This can be a very specific type of observation, for example, analogue assessment of the frequency of an identified behaviour per minute, which might be used to analyse the function of John's staring behaviour. Alternatively, there are time-sampling methods, which may be used to identify the function of other behaviours, such as the level of agitation at certain times of the day. This type of analysis is specialized and is usually performed with the supervision of a psychologist or behavioural nurse therapist. Other essential evidence that will help to shed light on aggressive behaviour is self-reporting, the clinical notes, reports from relatives and incident reports. One strategy that proved useful to break the aggression cycle in John's case was the negotiation about the use of the time-out facility on the ward. An agree-

ment is made with John that, when it is felt he may be in danger of assaulting others, he will be asked to take 5 minutes time-out where nurses can provide him with further support. This can take place in an interview room or a quiet area of the ward. When John does not demonstrate his cooperation at this point, the risk of assault is much higher and we are then approaching the crisis phase. It is useful to provide face-saving opportunities prior to his threats of physical assault and these should be discussed at the negotiation phase (Barash 1984). Once a plan has been developed prior to a serious incident, it is easier to manage people who are agitated, as they should be expecting the ensuing interventions. Gentle reminders about contracts and agreed consequences may be necessary. Here are some important factors to use in the approach of agitated individuals:

◆ Try to inform colleagues prior to your approach.
◆ Use confirming messages, expressing the person's worth.
◆ Model personal control, and the ability to stay calm during the expression of anger and resentment toward you.
◆ Use honesty, expressing your feelings congruently.
◆ Suggest the use of a quieter area of the ward environment.
◆ Set limits, and clear guidelines, which are consistently exerted.
◆ Use of structure to let people know in advance what is expected of them.
◆ Monitor and learn to recognize patterns of behaviour.
◆ Timely and calmly intervene (de-escalation) helping the person to work through their anger. Break the aggressive cycle.
◆ Facilitate expression—allow people to express anger and fear somewhere safely.
◆ Use non-verbal skills, avoiding threat, promoting calm and maintaining openness.
(Adapted from Lowe 1992)

Managing verbal aggression and intimidation

Verbal abuse, verbal threats, intimidation and

stalking are much more difficult to manage than overt aggression. You should attempt to find out why the person feels the need to be aggressive toward you. Talk to others about the possible functions of such behaviour. It may be a simple misunderstanding, or the basis of some form of thought disorder, and may be resolved through explanation and reassurance respectively. However, verbal threats are often a precursor to assault and they may be the way a person who has difficulty in communicating is attempting to warn you of their loss of control. In such situations, give the individuals concerned time and extra social distance and allow them to approach you later when they are calmer, or get another member of staff to arbitrate over the issue (Barash 1984). If the reason is thought disorder and hallucinations, clinical interventions such as dispensing prescribed medication may alleviate the verbal aggression. When people appear hostile, or have been reported to be disturbed earlier in the day, avoid isolating yourself with them.

It is imperative that wards avoid creating cultures where aggression toward other service users and staff becomes acceptable, as this can quickly become the relative norm. Aggression management should be seen as a care team problem and not just the responsibility of the people receiving the abuse. If you find you are suddenly being verbally abused, threatened or intimidated, enlist the support of colleagues, managers and other professionals. You may be surprised at the help you get, but you have to ask for it first. Make sure that every incident is recorded so others know what the atmosphere is like on the ward and the feelings you are experiencing. Do not shrug off this form of abuse, as this type of stress is unhealthy. Intimidation is sometimes very difficult to explain to your colleagues and an individual may target you at times when others are not observing. You have to be alert to such behaviour, and report it to the nurse in charge at the earliest opportunity. This facilitates more subtle observation of intimidating behaviours, allowing the care team to develop active strategies. Avoid becoming angry and confrontational, because you then become emotionally entwined in an interpersonal game of counter-transference.

The crisis phase

Section 19 of the Code of Practice (DOH & Welsh Office 1999) gives clear guidance on caring for 'Patients presenting particular management problems' with detailed reference to the use of restraint, medication, time-out and seclusion. Many hospitals are now taking up the initiative of training their staff to manage crisis situations. The emphasis of this training should be on verbal de-escalation and preventative methods. When approaching a disturbed person, you should do so as a member of a three-person team. When time permits, the person leading the team should be designated and an intervention strategy discussed. If possible, decide beforehand at which point you intend to use physical restraint and which signal the leading person will shout to coordinate the team's efforts. The lead person is the negotiator and must make the decisions for the team. This means that once your team has breached the safe distance of negotiation, the decision to restrain physically is with the leader. Essential points about the approach in a crisis situation are:

◆ Ensure all your staff are trained in crisis management—restraint is a last resort.
◆ Remain non-threatening and calm in manner—avoid counter-transference.
◆ Assess the person's position and possible mode of attack—adjust if necessary.
◆ Approach safely and gradually—do not be rushed.
◆ Keep talking and negotiating a non-physical alternative.
◆ Don't make promises or make offers you cannot keep.
◆ Provide at least one face-saving opportunity.
◆ The person leading the team should be aware of the safe threshold distance.
◆ As your team gets closer, move to a side-on position, reducing exposure to assault.
◆ If negotiation fails be decisive about reacting as a team.
◆ When an individual is secured, ask the person to move into a resting position on the floor.
◆ Allow the person time to relax; only one team member should do the talking and reassure.

◆ Use curtained screens to isolate the incident and protect the person's dignity.

◆ When the individual has calmed down, escort the person to a low-stimulating environment.

◆ Reintroduce the person back into the ward environment safely, in stages.

◆ Gradually reduce geographical limits around the ward and reduce observation.

◆ If the person is armed seek assistance from trained professionals (e.g. the police).

If the person has a history of assault, you should have negotiated an agreed action plan as described above, which is implemented as a consequence of such an event. This can include the amount of time that should be spent in a low-stimulating environment and the levels of observation required to ensure everyone's safety. A shared action plan should have explored the best way to approach the person and to use each new incident as a learning experience, altering the management plan accordingly. Part of the planning process should have strategies on how the trust in the staff–client relationship can be regained. If you work on an admission ward, your care team should have developed strategies and guidelines to support staff in managing assaults and aggressive behaviour (19.5 of Code of practice). Creating clear ward policies is important to prevent aggressors trying to play one team member off against another—splitting. These policies must be adhered to by all staff, and should be altered only with agreement by the care team. In units that use behavioural modification, agreed consequences should be applied as per individualized programmes. All staff must be consistent if behavioural change is to occur. Managing an aggressive person can be anxiety provoking, but the way carers behave during these episodes will determine the success of future carer–client relationships. Sometimes the expression of aggression is used to test staff to see if they will remain consistent, caring and professional. Assaultative people's crises do not end after the incident, because they will continue to feel guilty or angry toward the other people and their own behaviour. They will be hoping for supportive and caring messages from people around them. Restraint

should be used only as a last resort and never as a matter of course (19.11 of Code of practice).

POSTINCIDENT MANAGEMENT

The first priority is to enquire whether anybody has been hurt and to get additional support where required. Whenever physical restraint is used, it is important to inform as many members of the care team as possible. More specifically, ask the consultant psychiatrist or the registrar to examine the person involved after any hands-on intervention. Once you have informed all relevant areas, record the basic details of the aggression in the person's clinical notes along with the time, antecedent behaviours, what actions were taken afterward and when the interventions will be reviewed (19.23 of Code of practice). Most hospitals have their own printed incident forms that will help gather details about the circumstances of the aggression. The nurse in charge should make every effort to have a debriefing session with the staff involved in the incident, preferably when additional staff are still available from supporting areas. This is time spent with people to find out how the preparation went, how they felt during the incident, and whether they think the incident could have been managed differently. The debriefing process is helpful as an emotional release for staff and they should be encouraged to express their feelings openly and honestly, particularly anger and fears. Postincident discussion is also useful if it helps to manage and prevent future episodes of aggression, so notes should be made for this purpose. Nurses who have been assaulted may suffer shock and this may present as anger, anxiety, depression and self-blame (Stuart & Laraia 1998). Senior managers often facilitate the debriefing process, but what people value most is personal support from their colleagues.

Seclusion

Seclusion should be used only when a person is likely to cause harm to others, but every other avenue should be explored first. It should never be used because a unit does not have enough staff, or if people are likely to harm themselves (19.16 of Code of practice). There is increasing pressure to reduce seclusion, so staff need to identify a clear rationale when they intend to use it. Equally, managers should not put undue pressure on ward staff to reduce the use of seclusion as this then leads to dangerous management practices, more staff injuries and hence a reduction in the hospital's most valuable resource. A positive alternative in reducing seclusion would be to provide extra resources at the health promotion side of care, during the relative norm phase. When seclusion is necessary observation must be maintained, and a delegated nurse should be readily available at all times to make regular reviews (19.19 of Code of practice). Arrangements must be made for the person to be seen immediately by a doctor, and if seclusion continues for more than 12 hours over a 48-hour period an independent review by the care team must be organized (19.21 of Code of practice). When involved in aggression management, it is essential to work closely toward the guidelines of the Code of practice (DOH & Welsh Office 1999).

Records of seclusion will need to be available for scrutiny by visiting Mental Health Act Commissioners.

SUMMARY

Managing aggression requires mental health workers to take a detached view of their practice situation. You may be able to develop this skill by enhancing your personal knowledge of aggression and by viewing the extensive research available. It is sometimes difficult to maintain a positive outlook when overwhelmed by an aggressive situation. Developing self-awareness, seeking support and using personal stress-coping mechanisms can help when working with aggressive individuals. Aggression is not only frightening for those subjected to aggression, but is anxiety provoking for those displaying it. The loss of control can provoke feelings of guilt, which can complicate a person's seemingly hopeless situation, sometimes leading to greater interpersonal distancing and an intractable downward spiral of aggression. Service users will look to supportive professional carers for help in controlling their anger and frustration. Assaults on staff are far too frequent and organizations have an obligation to service users and staff in providing a safe working environment where aggression can be managed effectively (Chandley & Mason 1995). This can be achieved using proactive measures such as staff development, training in crisis management, verbal de-escalation skills, control and restraint methods and breakaway techniques. Research has shown that people with mental health problems and who also have a drug dependency are more likely to be violent. Providers of mental health services need to consider how this affects non-aggressive service users and the staff who have to care for them. An obvious alternative would be to provide separate facilities for those with drug dependency complicated with mental health problems.

DISCUSSION QUESTIONS

1. Why are nurses attacked more frequently than other professionals?
2. Can you create a care plan with someone to prevent his or her next episode of aggression?
3. How does the current Code of practice compare with your current practice?

ACKNOWLEDGEMENTS

Mark Chandley, clinical team leader—challenging behaviour; Pete Stoddart, behavioural nurse therapist; Matthew Byrne, clinical leader—challenging behaviour.

REFERENCES

Arboleda-Florez J, Holley L H, Crisanti A 1996 Mental illness and violence: proof or stereotype? Calgary World Health Organisation, Canada

Archer J 1994 Male violence. Routledge, London

Atkinson R L, Atkinson R C, Smith E E, Bem D J, Nolen-Hoeksema S 1996 Hilgard's introduction to psychology, 12th edn. Harcourt Brace College, Fort Worth

FURTHER READING

Berkowitz L 1993 Aggression, its causes, consequences and control. McGraw Hill, New York.
If you want a more in-depth look at the eclectic theories of aggression, this book provides a diverse overview by one of the leading writers in the research of aggression.

Breakwell G M 1989 Facing physical violence. British Psychological Society and Routlege, London
Examines some of the pragmatic issues of managing and facing violence.

DOH (Department of Health) & Welsh Office 1999 Code of practice: Mental Health Act 1983. HMSO, London
An essential knowledge of current practice issues and legitimate behavioural management can be obtained in the most recent code of practice.

Hamolia C C 1998 Preventing and managing aggressive behaviour. In: Stuart G W, Laraia M T (eds) Stuart and Sundeen's principles and practice of psychiatric nursing, 6th edn. Mosby, St Louis, ch 29
This chapter explores some realistic examples, and provides an excellent synopsis of aggression management.

Mason T, Chandley M 1999 Management of violence and aggression for nurses and healthcare workers. Churchill Livingstone, New York
This very recent text analyses the cycle of aggression, its causes and management. The authors have completed an extensive review of the literature on aggression, which is explored in detail.

Whittington R, Wykes T 1994 Violence and health care professionals. Chapman & Hall, London
An examination of the aggression process; some of the research examines possible precursors of aggression.

Bandura A 1973 Aggression: a social learning analysis. Prentice Hall, New Jersey

Barash D 1984 Defusing the violent-patient before he explodes. Registered Nurse March:35–37

Berkowitz L 1993 Aggression, its causes, consequences and control. McGraw Hill, New York

Chandley M, Mason T 1995 Nursing chronically dangerous patients. Psychiatric Care 2(1):20–26

Convit A, Isay D, Otis D, Volavka J 1990 Characteristics of repeatedly assaultative psychiatric inpatients. Hospital and Community Psychiatry 41(10):1112–1115

Davis S 1991 Violence by psychiatric inpatients: a review. Hospital and Community Psychiatry 42(6):585–590

Deakin M 1995 Using relaxation techniques to manage disruptive behaviour. Nursing Times 17(9):40–41

DOH (Department of Health) & Welsh Office 1999 Code of practice: Mental Health Act 1983. HMSO, London

Dollard J, Doob L W, Miller N E, Mowrer O H, Sears R R 1939 Frustration and aggression. Yale University Press, New Haven CT

Garza-Trevino E 1994 Neurobiological factors in aggressive behaviour. Hospital and Community Psychiatry 45(7):690–699

Geen R 1990 Human aggression. Open University Press, Milton Keynes

Goldstein A 1994 The ecology of aggression. Plenum Press, New York

Gross R 1996 The science of mind and behaviour, 3rd edn. Hodder & Stoughton, London

Guirguis E 1978 Management of disturbed patients: an alternative to the use of mechanical restraint. Journal of Clinical Psychiatry 20:295–299

Haller R M, Deluty R H 1988 Assaults on staff by psychiatric inpatients: a critical review. British Journal of Psychiatry 152:174–179

Hodgins S 1994 Schizophrenia and violence: are new mental health policies needed? (editorial) Journal of Forensic Psychiatry 5(3):473–477

Kaplan S G, Wheeler E G 1983 Survival skills for working with potentially violent clients. Social Casework 64:339–345

Kennedy M G 1993 Relationship between psychiatric diagnosis and patient aggression. Issues in Mental Health Nursing 14:263–273

Linaker O, Busch-Iversen H 1995 Predictors of imminent violence in psychiatric inpatients. Acta Pychiatrica Scandinavica 92:250–254

Link B G, Stueve A 1995 Evidence bearing on mental illness as a possible cause of violent behaviour. Epidemiological Reviews 17(1):172–181

Lorenz K 1996 On aggression. Routledge, London

Lowe T 1992 Characteristics of effective nursing interventions in the management of challenging behaviour. Journal of Advanced Nursing 17:1226–1232

Maier G, Van Rybroek G J, Mays D V 1994 A report on staff injuries and ambulatory restraint. Journal of Psychosocial Nursing 32(11):1–6

Mason T, Chandley M 1995 The chronically assaultative patient: benchmarking best practices. Psychiatric Care 2(1):20–26

Mason T, Chandley M 1999 Management of violence and aggression for nurses and healthcare workers. Churchill Livingstone, New York

Mench J, Shea-Moore M 1995 Moods, minds and molecules: the neurochemistry of social behaviour. Applied Animal Behaviour Science 44:99–118

Monahan J 1992 Mental disorder and violent behaviour: perceptions and evidence. American Psychologist 47(4):511–521

Morrison E F 1993 Toward a better understanding of violence in psychiatric settings: debunking the myths. Archives of Psychiatric Nursing 7(6):328–335

Moyer K 1976 The psychobiology of aggression. Harper & Row, New York

Newhill C E, Mulvey E P, Lidz C W 1995 Characteristics of violence in the community by female patients seen in psychiatric emergency service. Psychiatric Services 46(8):785–789

Noble P, Rodger S 1989 Violence by psychiatric inpatients. British Journal of Psychiatry 155:384–390

Palmstierna T, Wistedt B 1995 Changes in the pattern of aggressive behaviour among inpatients with changed ward organisation. Acta Psychiatrica Scandinavica 91:32–35

Sainsbury Centre For Mental Health 1998 Keys to engagement. SCMH, London

Sclafani M 1986 Violence and behaviour control. Journal of Psychosocial Nursing 24(11):8–13

Selye H 1979 The stress of life, revised edn. Van Nostrand Reinhold, New York

Shah A K, Fineberg N A, James D V 1991 Violence among psychiatric inpatients. Acta Psychiatrica Scandinavica 84:305–309

Siann G 1985 Accounting for aggression. Allen & Unwin, London

Straznickas K A, McNeil D E, Binder R L 1993 Violence toward family caregivers by mentally ill relatives. Hospital and Community Psychiatry 44(4):385–387

Stuart G W, Laraia M T 1998 Stuart and Sundeen's principles and practice of psychiatric nursing, 6th edn. Mosby, St Louis

Tardiff K, Koenigsberg H W 1985 Assaultive behaviour among psychiatric outpatients. American Journal of Psychiatry 142(8):960–963

Torrey E F 1994 Violent behaviour by individuals with serious mental illness. Hospital and Community Psychiatry 45:653–662

Tortora G, Anagnostakos N 1990 Principles of anatomy and physiology, 6th edn. HarperCollins, New York

Whittington R, Patterson P 1996 Verbal and non-verbal behaviour immediately prior to aggression by mentally disordered people: enhancing risk assessment. Journal of Psychiatric and Mental Health Nursing 3:47–54

Whittington R, Wykes T 1996 Aversive stimulation by staff and violence by psychiatric patients. British Journal of Clinical Psychology 35:11–20

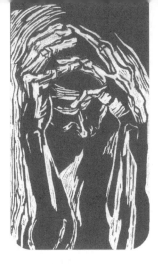

Chapter Twenty-two

Triumvirate nursing—a secure system for the delivery of nursing care

Pete Melia   Tony Moran

 AIMS

- ◆ To explore the relevance of personality disorder as a diagnosis of dysfunction
- ◆ To review the clinical patterns of presentation
- ◆ To explore the complex and intense interpersonal dynamics that occur between carer and the personality-disordered patient
- ◆ To suggest a more effective model for the organization and delivery of care to this patient group

KEY ISSUES

Poor understanding of health or functional deficit related to personality

Complex and intense interpersonal relationships

Therapy versus security

Question of treatability

Deliberate use of self as therapeutic tool

Talking therapies

INTRODUCTION

The notion of a health or functional deficit related to personality remains contentious with many mental health professionals who believe there is no such disorder, and many of those who acknowledge its existence believe there is nothing we can do about it anyway. Whilst such theoretical debates rage it is the nurse who provides continual care for these immensely damaged and damaging individuals and strives to make sense of these profound interpersonal problems. In this context our own health service model conspires against the nurse in interactions with clients whose very health deficit defines them as egocentric, self-centred and emotionally intense, in that the very canon of our profession dictates the therapeutic relationship as being one (nurse) to one (client).

We the authors, as experienced psychiatric nurses and health service managers, have attempted to deconstruct this canon in a care environment providing 102 beds for individuals with a primary (medical) diagnosis of personality disorder and a history of serious offending behaviours. Our clients have, therefore, been given into our custody by virtue of the Mental Health Act (1959) or the Mental Health Amendments Act (1983) and each carries the (legal) diagnostic label of psychopathic disorder. Our whole approach has been to redefine the nature of relationship being used as therapeutic tool, the emphasis being on bringing about change to those who are dysfunctional in their interpersonalness without bringing harm or change to the change agent—the nurse. We believe the primary nurse mechanism is not only damaging to the nurses faced with long term contact with personality-disordered clients for whom they provide care, but actually accentuates the egocentric components of the very disorder they seek to change. Such an approach as here suggested has proven highly effective with this client group.

THE NATURE OF THE CHALLENGE

Beck (1967), the pioneer of cognitive psychology,

defined personality disorder as 'a reflection of a specific faulty cognitive profile encompassing beliefs, attitudes, affects, and strategies relating to how the individual sees himself relative to others'. Whilst this goes some way towards identifying the human domain in which the nature of this disorder is rooted it gives no semblance of its aetiology, progress or maintenance. To date the notion of personality disorder as a health deficit remains equally as nebulous. It is recognized, however, that there is a psychosocial pattern demonstrable through the manner in which individuals perceive, interpret and relate to their environment and to others. In acknowledging this and trying to provide a treatment service for this challenging group of individuals it is crucial that 'relationship' is recognized as a key pathway towards providing appropriate clinical treatment.

The nature of a unit that provides a service to individuals whose health or functional deficit relates to personality and dysfunctional relationship must, therefore, have a sound and clear system for facilitating relationship in a safe and protective environment. Such a service is by definition somewhat different to many other services, especially those that are community based, particularly in the fact that it will deal with some of the most damaged and damaging individuals within the UK's health and criminal justice systems. The average length of stay for personality-disordered patients within special hospitals is something in the region of 9 years, with many of the more resistive personality-disordered patients staying for longer periods, in some cases as many as 30 or 40 years. The need then to ensure relationships are safe and developmental for both patients and staff is therefore imperative as the potential for practitioners to become damaged in such long term, intense relationships is so much greater. Concomitantly the risk of potentiating the more self-centred and egocentric components of the individual's personality disorder is so much greater when professional boundaries are deconstructed and surrogated by taut [pseudo] friendships masquerading as trust.

To explore this more fully then we must examine those aspects of the personality-disordered individual that will impact on the relationship and become manifest in the human environment. Most especially this must relate to dangerousness and the potential to commit serious offences against the person (self or others). As we, the authors, are employed in the Personality Disorder Unit at Ashworth Special Hospital we shall do this by examining this environment as a model in case.

The common characteristics of those developmental personality disorders that may underlie an individual's ability to commit serious offences, of a nature or to a degree that would warrant admission and detention within a high security hospital, are most succinctly described in 'Axis II of the DSM-IVR (APA 1994) and the ICD-10 (WHO 1992), Hare's psychopathy checklist (Hare 1980) and Blackburn's chart of interpersonal relationships in a closed living environment (CIRCLE) (1975).

In particular, such individuals demonstrate characteristics commensurate with a diagnosis of antisocial, narcissistic, borderline or histrionic personality disorder and frequently the diagnosis of more than one condition is necessary. In the human environment this translates into relationships being highly charged and often emotionally intense to the point where social interactions occur in a corrupted and exploitative manner. Such individuals demonstrate emotional extremes far beyond any continuum imagined in common social interactions, punctuated by a language embellished with superlatives and hyperbole. Levels of anger and hostility are particularly high and are most commonly focused towards those on whom individuals are most reliant, in effect the nursing staff.

In relating to others, such individuals demonstrate an expectation that they will be harmed, exploited and let down and they will relate to others with this expectation in mind, constantly looking for the signs that they are about to be rejected or abused. They will continually 'test' issues of loyalty and fidelity within relationships, demonstrating an intense concern for, and preoccupation with, the protection of self but showing little evidence of concern for others within their sphere of social interaction. They will often demonstrate seriously irresponsible and thrill-seeking behaviours with short term immediate gratification, but

with little or no concern for possible future consequences. They will often demonstrate an exaggerated moral outrage if they feel their own personal rights or wants have been violated, but will disregard the rights of others, demonstrating no remorse for having wronged another and showing no capacity to experience guilt or to profit from experience, often to the point where they will actually feel justified in having hurt or mistreated others. Such individuals are apt to be self-centred and egocentric, whose own sense of entitlement precludes the capacity to recognize or experience how their actions may affect others within the environment. In the living environment such individuals demonstrate no constancy in any value base or moral regulatory system but may feign a range of differing commitments depending on the circumstance at any given time. Such individuals are noted to develop a remarkable ability to rationalize their own actions to an exceptional degree, often shifting responsibility for their own actions and avoiding introspection through a process of blame and protest. They will constantly invite collusion from others via a range of linguistic and interpersonal techniques developed over very long periods of time. It is important to realize that some, or even many, of these characteristics may appear in any or all of us at given times within our lives. However, the diagnosis of personality disorder requires that such characteristics are a constant and pervasive feature of the individual's life.

Such processes are deeply ingrained within the mind set of patients suffering from the chronic and damaging disorders we consider here. The processes can relatively easily be explored through life history as individuals suffering these disorders can most commonly be seen as having come from home circumstances that may have been severely abusive and neglectful. It is likely that there will have been problems beyond the family in schooling and in the local environment indicative of conduct disorders in childhood; in adolescence they will have demonstrated excessively indulgent behaviours of an almost epicurean intensity in relation to alcohol/substance abuse, early sexual experience and thrill-seeking behaviours. There will be a pattern of seriously irresponsible behaviours, shifting into criminal offences (usually of increasing severity) through adolescence and into early adult life; such individuals will often have come to the attention of the criminal justice system at a relatively early age. Indeed many will have gone through care homes, special schools and young offender institutions before reaching the age of 18. Most will have experienced some period of incarceration within a penal institution.

In this environment, then, the issue of boundaries in interpersonal relationships is fundamental to the therapeutic process, both for the protection of the staff member and to aid the progress of the patient.

CHALLENGES IN THE CLINICAL ENVIRONMENT

Relationships

Clearly at the outset, the relationship between the patient and nurse is relatively neutral with relatively clear boundaries dictated by professional etiquette and cultural expectation. The process of assessment and treatment, however, can challenge the social construct of a neutral relationship as the discussion will often relate to the most intimate and intrusive components of the patient's life, experience and feelings. This can be particularly difficult for the nurse who will spend long periods of time with the patients in community settings and through a range of private and public experiences. Gutheil & Gabbard (1993) note three degrees or levels of challenge to relationship boundaries, namely 'boundary crossing, boundary violation and sexual misconduct'. They further note that the care environment can affect the integrity of normal professional boundaries: 'various group therapeutic approaches or therapeutic communities may involve inherent boundary violations'.

Moreover, the construct of the disorder is such that it will always tend towards a denial of responsibility for self and often complex rationalizations as to how the root of a particular problem was with some other party or group. Patients will essentially seek validation to the point of collusion from those staff who are significant to their cur-

rent circumstances. As in all relationships, they will be most strongly drawn towards those individuals who are less challenging and more accepting. This whole process is constructed around a tension in as much as, whilst the relationship is founded on an attempt to therapeutically challenge the way such patients perceive their [human] environment and relate to others, there is also a genuine need for carers to validate their individuality. This can have the effect of actually reinforcing the way the patients perceive their [human] environment and relate to others.

Splitting and secrets

The process of splitting in groups is well identified and recorded in the academic literature related to this field; put simply, it is a process of making individuals or groups feel different (normally better or worse) from their peers or those around them.

In practice the negative splitting behaviours are often quickly picked up—for example, some patients may claim specific members of staff (or staff groups) are victimizing them by not facilitating a request that they claim the staff should accept even if this is contrary to the ward/hospital policies. In this the patient is both exerting a pressure on any staff members directly concerned, who are attempting to maintain consistent practice, encouraging them to alter or 'bend' the rules *and* creating conflict between them and other staff members.

More destructive than this, however, are the seductive components of splitting, which are far more easily missed and can actually have a greater effect—for example, when patients invest an apparent trust and confidence in particular members of the care team and tell them 'you're the only one I can talk to, they [other member of the clinical or ward team] are not interested'. This is further complicated and distorted when patients invite therapists to maintain 'secrets' often in the name of confidentiality: 'Can I tell you something that I've never told anyone before?' or 'I need to talk to you about something that's really personal but you have to promise it won't go outside this room'. This is often used to compound the notion that the therapists concerned are 'different' from their peers, as it is explained 'they [other clinical team members] will use it against me or to wind me up!'. This can be particularly divisive when more than one discipline is involved and can lead to major conflicts within the clinical care team.

The level of conflict generated by such dynamics can be powerful and the ultimate effect is usually an avoidance or loss of sight of core matters in relation to the care of the patient and an overinvestment in day to day management issues and the 'power plays' that occur within groups. Moreover, such splitting amongst clinical team members frequently results in factions within the clinical team; these dynamics are quickly recognized and invested in further by the patient as per the overvalued ideation relating to loyalty and fidelity referred to above. The effect is in any case deleterious both to the care of the patient and to the functioning of the clinical team.

Rejection

Like many components of interpersonal relationships identifiable aspects or processes can be complex and multifaceted. Certainly the process of rejection by the patient can be a powerful yet highly complex relationship issue in as much as the nature of those disorders here cared for (as described above) is such that patients often expect to be exploited, harmed and let down. As a result they can be possessive and defensive in relationships, continually testing loyalties and ardently searching for signs that a 'let-down' is imminent.

At its most basic level, then, a rejection from the patient is merely a defence mechanism from one who fears being rejected by someone close (in this case the nurse) and who will negate the possibility by rejecting the nurse first. Such patients will reject you before you get the chance to reject them.

There is a far more profound effect of this in terms of a contributory factor in the deconstruction of professional boundaries or therapeutic relationships and in the shift towards personal friendships or more intimate relationships. The natural reaction in a social circumstance where rejection occurs is to assume some level of personal responsibility and a desire to rectify any wrongs done (or perceived to have been done). In this the nurse will often attempt to rectify the relationship with the patient by seeking the cause of the rejection rather than exploring the psychopathology of the feelings, thoughts and behaviour. Staff are, by necessity, constantly attentive to the demeanour of all patients and when such patients become hostile towards someone with whom they may previously have had a good relationship, it is common for the staff to attempt discourse to find out why the relationship has altered. In this, questions like 'are you annoyed with me?' or 'have I done something to upset you?' can unintentionally change the nature of the relationship, shifting it to a personal, rather than professional or therapeutic level, as the discourse focuses attention on staff members and their behaviour rather than the patients concerned and their thoughts, feelings and behaviours.

Following such a rejection experience these attempts to rectify the situation can be met with a highly intense level of anger and hostility as a result of the perceived wrongdoing, exemplified by phrases like 'I can't believe you of all people would do that to me' or 'I thought you were different, I thought I could trust you!'. The discomfort phase following such an incident can last for days before a gradual 'softening' occurs and the relationship resumes its previous status but, in consequence, is less professional and more personal.

Over prolonged periods of time such rejection experiences can have extremely undesirable, cumulative effects on even the most qualified and experienced of staff. Unchecked this can lead to prolonged duress stress disorders in some carers, but more importantly can lead to nurses losing sight of their own value base and conduct boundaries to the point where they may avoid challenging an issue or enforcing a policy, for fear of provoking the discomfort of a rejection experience and its inevitable aftermath. At worst such processes can also lead to a fragmenting of boundaries to the point where the staff may agree to bring in some small item, bordering on contraband, but more importantly establishing a level of intimacy based on 'shared secrets' and so beginning the slippery slope to professional ruin.

Whilst great efforts can be made to safeguard staff and patients by ensuring the maintenance of professional boundaries through clinical supervision, reflective practice groups, training and clear business planning strategies incorporating philosophy and policy statements, such relationships remain precarious and can be easily imbalanced. The range of national, professional and local standards relating to boundary and professional relationship issues are multiple but their enforcement has to remain focused in the clinical area and founded in current best practice. It is essential that, as a profession, nursing remains responsive to the needs of its users. The exceptional demands of this patient group in our setting has caused us to re-examine the system of delivering nursing care to personality-disordered patients.

THE CARE ARENA

Despite the enormously complex issues concerning the aetiology, progress and maintenance of disorders related to personality it remains apparent that the presentation or impact of such disorders is to be found in the way individuals perceive, interpret and relate to their environment, especially the human environment. The experience of the authors is that personality-disordered offenders who find themselves within the high security hospital often have disorganized and chaotic personal histories, which brings conflict with other patients—namely, there is no constancy, order, organization or routine to their life circumstances. Indeed there is a whole sense of disorganization in personal, social and relationship activities. Self-description and discourse related to personal circumstances and the circumstances which lead to referral to the care service (normally via the criminal justice rather than mental health system) are punctuated by evidence of non-teleological thought and motivational patterns that are not only chaotic but which also maintain a focus within the immediacy of the situation. The focus in the now and the frenzied lifestyle fails to engender development or maturity and tends to sustain a wholly chaotic existence.

In the care arena this issue particularly complicates the therapeutic relationship as personality-disordered offenders usually set out with the expectation that they will be harmed, abused or let down and will therefore continually 'test' the loyalty and trustworthiness of the nurse in ways referred to earlier. The cumulative effect of this is a gradual deconstruction of the therapeutic alliance and a shift in the relationship to a more personal and often intimate one, based on the need to sustain itself rather than to bring about personal and social growth in the patient.

A whole host of interpersonal dynamics, such as rejection, blaming, splitting, dependence and sharing secrets, contribute to this process and the effect is that professional interactions are excluded and replaced by 'friendship', validating the rationalizations and minimalizations of the individual and preventing purposeful talking therapy from taking place. Moreover this can have the effect of flattening or stultifying the professional impetus on the part of the nurse and in extreme cases can actually lead to psychological damage.

Tales of such horrors permeate the high secure psychiatric services and contribute actively to the way individuals working and living in the environment create their own realities through story telling (Said 1993) or anecdotal 'evidence'. The experience of the authors leaves us with little doubt that such factors are a major contributor to the polarized notion that high secure hospitals are either barbaric uncaring places where treatment is an alien concept or conversely that such patients are not disordered but simply evil and should be treated accordingly. We do not agree with either position.

The difficulty, then, is that, in recognizing the paramountcy of the need to use relationship as a therapeutic tool, we need to employ it in such a way as to protect the nurses who ply their trade in this difficult and challenging environment. To a large extent the development of clinical supervision encouraging reflection on practice by individuals and groups within supervision and ward environments has done much to help promote good clinical practice with this patient group, without further risking the psychological well-being of nurses. What remains, however, is the need to develop a service for individuals who maintain a poorly understood disorder in a financially overstretched health service with little evidence of conclusive research or evidence-based practice defining the efficacy of specific interventions or intended outcomes and clinical targets.

DELIVERING NURSING CARE

The challenge then is to enable the safe and effective delivery of nursing care to this group of individuals in such a way as to enhance the value of relationship as a therapeutic tool and promote human growth without compromising the integrity of the professional relationship or the quality of care. We argue that the most effective way of achieving this is through a pathways approach to problem solving within a social learning model of practice, the focus being on challenging the ways in which patients construct their perceptions of the environment and influence its continuance. In so doing it is equally as important that we should create a mechanism to enable and not stultify nursing practice.

The major problem in achieving this is the background of chaotic disorganized lifestyles with no notion of constancy, routine or order; this is an essentially insular and egocentric outlook that can actually be potentiated by exclusive one to one relationships (even with therapists) and perhaps most significantly a whole lifetime of abuse and neglect, which has taught such individuals to look on the human environment with an expectation that it will ultimately lead to their being harmed, let down, exploited and abused. In our work the delivery of nursing care was therefore shifted away from the one to oneness engendered by primary nursing to be replaced by a triumvirate model of nursing. This model was devised in order to promote human growth and social development within a community setting. The purpose was not only to create an acknowledgement that in a group or community environment the actions of the self affect those others in the group, but also that the individual actually has some responsibility for others within their own community or environment.

The mechanics of triumvirate nursing are quite simply that nurses work in a team of three, each with equal responsibility for the provision of care for their patients. Interventions are planned and outlined as part of the care programme assessment. Individual sessions are carried out by two nurses acting as cotherapists, following which a review takes place with the third nurse acting effectively as a clinical supervisor. The role of the third nurse is to challenge what went on in the session and to check out both colleagues in terms of their own emotional and professional state in relation to the care of that patient. The nurses are interchangeable so it is not necessary (and indeed is undesirable) that any one nurse should continually take on the role of supervisor or that any two nurses should continually take on the role of cotherapists, but each should fairly regularly shift and change roles within the triumvirate.

This method of working not only offers a developmental approach to relationship as therapeutic tool but also minimizes the risk of boundary violations occurring or undesirable interpersonal dynamics corrupting the therapeutic ethic. It also has the obvious advantage of having a supervision mechanism built into the operation of nursing in the environment. It is, however, a model that is fairly reliant on the organization of the ward or clinical area and is relatively specific to working with personality-disordered individuals. The environment or the organization of the environment has to sustain and support the notion of human growth and social learning, and at Ashworth we have developed a robust programme of therapeutic group work and a similar approach to structured activities centred very much around group and team activities. Namely, we discourage highly competitive individual pursuits such as playing squash, weight lifting or badminton and have developed more group and team activities, such as football, netball, water polo and hockey.

FOCUS OF CLINICAL IMPETUS

As earlier discussed, the notion of a health or functional deficit related to personality remains somewhat nebulous and ill defined. Further to this, the current debate about the measurement and classification of disorder related to personality further exemplifies the fact that traditional medical models and, to some extent, psychological ones have compounded this problem.

Hare's psychopathy checklist—revised (HPCL-R) (Hare 1990), designed for the diagnostic classification of such disorders, measures psychopathy or personality disorder on a categorical scale in terms of its severity. Whilst such measures are obviously of considerable value to those responsible for diagnosis and legal categorization, more helpful to those of us working in clinical practice is a multidimensional model of measurement as described by Costa & McCrae (1991) in their Neo five factor inventory: form S; this measures the so-called 'big five' personality dimensions of neuroticism, extroversion, openness to experience, agreeableness and conscientiousness. Similarly Blackburn (1975), in his typology cluster CIRCLE (chart of interpersonal relationships in a closed living environment), measures the extent of the disorder on the self and the environment (especially the human one) measuring dominance, coerciveness, hostility, submissiveness, compliance, nurturance and gregariousness. McGinn & Young (1996) describe 'domains' in which individuals function in relation to their core belief systems and around which expectations are built, these being dependence, subjugation/lack of individualism, fear of losing self-control, incompetence/failure, abandonment, defensiveness, unlovability, emotional deprivation, social desirability, unrelenting standards and guilt/punishment.

From this we can extract the process of thinking that defines the disorder and predicates the extremes of emotion, belief and interpersonal conflicts that punctuate the human environment of the personality-disordered client. Others have sought to define personality disorder in terms of intrinsically faulty fundamental beliefs about the self and the world and the resultant dysfunctional interpersonal styles of behaviour that they produce. Furthermore, the continuance of such maladaptive styles produces cycles of experience that reinforce this faulty interpersonalness and further validate it by the reaction elicited from others (Blackburn 1975). In challenging maladaptive or dysfunctional styles in clinical practice it is essential to identify precisely the process with which

you are dealing. McGinn & Young (1996) describe what they refer to as a 'schema'—that is, 'an extremely stable and enduring pattern of thinking which develops during childhood and is elaborated throughout an individual's life ... [encompassing] broad pervasive themes regarding oneself and one's relationship with others'. This notion of a schema being an implicit and unconditional template against which all experiences are processed is central to the nature of personality disorders and it is these processes that define the individual's behaviours, thoughts feelings and relationships with others.

Challenging faulty schemas in clinical practice demands considerable effort over a considerable period of time as by definition such schemas are self-perpetuating and very resistant to change. Moreover, there is evidence in clinical practice that the relationship between the schema and the domain in which it is operating is crucial and can be identified as having a specific purpose in either maintaining the schema, avoiding the schema or compensating for it.

This allows us to establish those dimensions of personality that can be isolated for particular therapeutic challenge. In this paradigm individuals may be seen to have components of the disorder that affect one or more of these personality dimensions or domains with differing degrees of severity, the degree of severity having a direct impact on such individuals and their relationship with their environment. In practice, therefore, it is the dynamic and interpersonal aspects of the relationship between carers and clients that may most effectively isolate those components of an individual's disorder in which the carers are trying to help bring about change. It is equally important that such practice also attempts to isolate areas of the individual's functioning which are not significant to the disorder, and indeed may be positive characteristics that should be maintained to as great a degree as is possible. Where these are healthy, functional components to an individual's personality these may be built upon as part of the treatment process to bring about adjustments or compensations for dysfunctional components of the individual's personality development. It is a particular feature of individuals who suffer from

Box 22.1   Components of personality disorder according to Cleckley (1976) and Hare (1984)

Psychopathic personality (Cleckley 1976)

Superficial charm and good intelligence
Abscence of delusions or irrational thinking
Absence of neurotic manifestations
Unreliable
Untruthful and insincere
Lacks remorse
Social behaviour inadequately motivated
Fails to learn by experience
Egocentric and incapable of love
Emotionally slow
Lacks insight
Socially unresponsive
Objectionable behaviour after drinking
Suicide threats and gestures without serious attempts
Impersonal sex life
No consistent goals

Psychopathy checklist (Hare 1980)

Glibness/superficial charm
Grandiose sense of self-worth
Need for stimulation/proneness to boredom
Pathological lying
Conning/manipulative
Lack of remorse or guilt
Shallow affect
Callous/lack of empathy
Parasitic lifestyle
Poor behavioural controls
Promiscuous sexual behaviour
Early behaviour problems
Lack of realistic long term plans
Impulsivity
Irresponsibility
Failure to accept responsibility for own actions
Many short term marital relationships
Juvenile delinquency
Revocation of conditional release
Criminal versatility

such damaging disorders that they will go to extreme lengths (particularly in focused therapy sessions) to avoid responsibility, deflect blame and sabotage the therapeutic process by introducing complex and often emotionally intense issues that are difficult to ignore but are of little or no significance to those functional components of the disorder that the therapist is attempting to challenge.

It is particularly important, therefore, that careful consideration is given to the assessment of the nature and extent of disorder within these dimensions as the planning of care is intrinsically based on maintaining the healthy or acceptable functional components of personality within the distal areas of activities. More focused therapeutic activity should target only those components of individuals' functioning which are significant to the impact of their disorder. It is, therefore, imperative that the therapist has a clear understanding based on careful assessment of the components of personality in which they are attempting to bring

about change (Box 22.1). Fundamental to this is the involvement of the client in planning and agreeing the care programme in advance of therapeutic sessions taking place. It is further important from the outset of the assessment process to attain a clear understanding and agreement of the relationship between the individual's cognitive processes and other behaviours, in particular offending behaviours.

This understanding of the relationship between cognition and behaviour is crucial for two fundamental reasons: first, part of the care process must be making the distinction between responsibility on the part of the individual for thought and behaviour. It is a core process in the therapeutic alliance that, whilst clients may not be responsible for their thinking processes and associated motivations, it must be a continual feature of the therapeutic relationship that they are reminded of their responsibility for any *behaviours* that result from these thought processes and motivations. This will enable the triumvirate team to engender a greater degree of self-management in the client (for example, we cannot blame paedophiles for the sexual attraction which they feel towards minors, but it is most certainly a deliberate choice on their part if they act on those fantasies). Secondly, there is an ever-increasing political demand for clear and careful risk assessment on the part of those responsible for the care of mentally disordered individuals (in particular offenders) and, although there is no clear model for risk assessment, there is a fundamental relationship between an individuals' history of offending behaviours and their attitude towards the object or objects of those behaviours at any given time. An absolutely essential component of risk management is, therefore, the ability of individuals to discriminate between their own thoughts, motivations and behaviours.

We emphasize therefore, that it is important for practitioners to recognize and understand that assessment criteria, particularly relating to risk, are not static but fluid. They are contextual in relation to patients' psychological state, situational (social) circumstances and the degree to which they are embedded in the social environment. The intelligence and interpersonal skills available to the individual at any given time are also variable and not static.

The focus of practice in the triumvirate nursing model is then to work on a problem-solving basis with the individual to isolate those aspects of the disorder in which change is desired. The care team must maintain an environment that supports therapeutic work and is fundamentally psychologically healthy, promoting personal and collective responsibilities through group activities, cooperation, reflectivity and shared learning in a manner that promotes individual dignity and respect for all involved. The planning of more focused therapeutic practice should be aggressively aimed at isolating functional and psychological attachments only to the components of those deficits in personality within the dimension and range of the disorder identified at assessment.

In relation to Figure 22.1, the normal social interactions would occur in the distal areas of functioning in relation to those parts of the individual's personality that are relatively well formed and culturally acceptable. The triumvirate would,

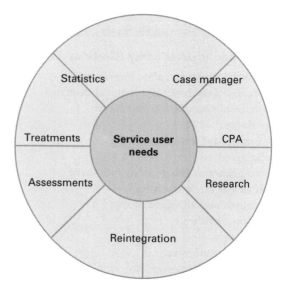

Fig. 22.1 Isolate only those domains in which disorder is prominent.

therefore, work with clients and their care team to agree on those areas of functioning that have failed to develop or have developed in an abnormal way. In such work, it is incumbent on the nurses within the triumvirate to isolate and challenge those traits of functioning that are ingrained within the individual to such an extent that they frame and define the individual's behaviours, thoughts, feelings and relationships with others. Within this problem-solving framework it is not entirely necessary that the origin or aetiology of the disorder or that domain or dimension within which the disorder is constructed be understood. It is far more important that its impact on the environment (especially human environment) be explored and some strategy for overcoming or compensating for such processes be constructed.

Traditionally it has been remarkably difficult for this to take place in one to one relationships with this client group as it is the relationship between client and therapist that becomes the focus of investment. The triumvirate process maintains impetus in relation to the client as the focus and the only pivotal point within therapeutic practice. The nurses within the triumvirate will continually shift in their position and therefore the relationship itself between the client and the carer is not a central component to the dynamics of the

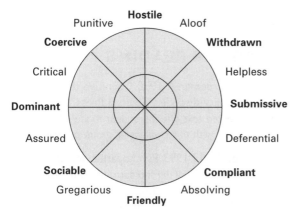

Fig. 22.2 A grid for analysis of the functional domains or dimensions of personality.

DISCUSSION QUESTIONS

1. Given that Blackburn's notion of the primary psychopath is someone who is genetically predisposed to psychopathy and the assertion that this is in fact simply a new metaphor for 'original sin', is the 'mad or bad' debate simply a reformation of the 'nurture v nature' debate?
2. With the knowledge that personality disorders are developmental with very early age indicators of aberrant behaviours should we be looking at changing social policy to promote collaborative working between health and education providers to ensure early detection and intervention?
3. Why is there a disproportionately low number of black and Asian individuals treated under the diagnostic category of personality disorder?
4. Given our assertion that the canonical model of nursing (Primary nursing) is inadequate for the delivery of care to personality disordered individuals, should we be looking at changing the organization of nursing care as is here asserted or should we be questioning whether nursing is the most appropriate professional model with which to provide care to this client group?
5. Given the poor understanding of intervention success and outcomes, is the notion of an 'untreatable psychopath' simply a reflection of the inadequaces of the psychiatric services?
6. Given the extent to which treatment receptivity and engagement vacillates should we have a system that allows movement between prisons and hospitals, to provide treatment when the individual is actively engaged in the care programme and containment when not?

therapeutic alliance (as it tends to becomes in one to one therapy with this client group). The only constancy, therefore, is the client and the focus of the disorder as has been agreed between client and carers at the assessment stage. The process by which we attempt to do this and to countermand the considerable and complex avoiders introduced by the client to distract from therapeutic focus we refer to as the 'critical referencing of self'. In this it is particularly important that the nurses within the triumvirate maintain a constant evaluation of the individuals, their sense of self and the position of that notion of self to the manner in which they apply corrupt interpretations on their [human] environment.

In this exchange, the focus of the alliance is on an analysis of clients by themselves, the critical reference being the responsibility of such individuals to reference or understand their thoughts, feelings and motivations in relation to their origins. It is the role of the nurses working with clients to ensure that they do not shift the focus on to issues outside of those that are central or those for which others in the environment may have been responsible. In this way nurses continually bring clients back to examining their own role in any given situation and what they were feeling, thinking and doing at the salient time. Concomitant to this process the cotherapists should be exploring with clients the more functional domains or dimensions of their personality (Fig. 22.2) which may be employed to compensate or adjust interpersonal

relationships and avoid the negative impact of the individual's disorder on the environment, especially the human one. In this it is the relationship that is used as the therapeutic tool to challenge and change the client's interpersonal processes. Significantly the relationship itself does not becomes a focus for examining itself, as in one to one relationships, and the entire focus of therapeutic interactions is on the individual and those maladaptive components of personality at issue.

SUMMARY

In working with the client the nurses working as part of the triumvirate identify and agree the domain in which their efforts will be focused and the strategy that will be employed. The assessment will inform the manner in which patients will formulate their own perspective of the environment and the way in which they see themselves in relation to others. Using a model of interpretation it is most essential for the nurses working within the triumvirate to identify the extent to which transference is a possibility/likelihood and to plan the strategy for intervention with this in mind. The therapeutic sessions are planned around the interpersonal focus of impact of the particular disorder and the interpersonal circumstances in which it becomes most profound.

REFERENCES

APA (American Psychiatric Association) 1994 Diagnostic and statistical manual of mental disorders, 4th edn (DSM-IV). APA, Washington DC

Beck A T 1967 Depression: clinical, experimental and theoretical aspects. Penguin, London

Blackburn R 1975 An empirical classification of psychopathic personality. British Journal of Psychiatry 127:456–460

Cleckley H 1976 The mask of sanity, 5th edn. CV Mosby, St Louis MO

Costa P T, McCrae R R 1991 Neo five factor inventory. Psychological Assessment Resources, Odessa FA

Gutheil T G, Gabbard G 1993 The concept of boundaries in clinical practice: theoretical and risk management dimensions. American Journal of Psychiatry 150:2

Hare R D 1980 A research scale for the assessment of psychopathy in criminal populations. Personality and Individual Differences 1:111–117

FURTHER READING

Beck A T, Freeman A 1990 Cognitive therapy of personality disorder. Guilford Press, New York
A well worked text offering a clear model of intervention with this challenging group of individuals.

Dolan B, Coid J 1993 Psychopathic and antisocial personality disorders: treatment and research issues. Gaskell, London
An excellent text which examines some highly pertinent issues around the aetiology, development, progress and maintenance of personality disorders.

Hare R D 1993 Without conscience: the disturbing world of the psychopath among us. Warner, London
The text offers an excellent insight into the impact of the personality disordered individual on his or her human environment.

McGinn L K, Young J E 1996 Schema focused therapy. In: Salkovskis P M (ed) Frontiers of cognitive therapy. Guilford Press, New York
Perhaps one of the best texts available in regard to its ability to deconstruct the multi-faceted components of the remarkably psychopathology of personality and thereafter, personality disorders.

Hare R D 1990 Manual for the revised psychopathy checklist. University of British Columbia, Vancouver, Canada

McGinn L K, Young J E 1996 Schema focused therapy. In: Salkovskis P M (ed) Frontiers of cognitive therapy. Guilford, New York, pp 278–301

Mental Health Act 1983. HMSO, London

Said E 1993 Culture and imperialism. Chatto & Windus, London

World Health Organisation 1992 ICD-10 Classification of mental and behavioural disorders: clinical descriptions and diagnostic guidelines. WHO, Geneva

Part IV
Issues for practitioners

This part considers more general issues affecting practitioners. It identifies recent developments in assessment, evidence-based practice, supervision and learning before turning to a description and analysis of the legal framework of provision and practice. Many of the ideas and insights are relevant across professions. They are also relevant to the challenges of providing a high standard of care. The chapters in this part hope to contribute to the development of high standards by supporting practitioners as they develop the ability to:

◆ identify, analyse and assess factors causing distress and illness
◆ make considered and effective interventions
◆ continue to develop their knowledge and skills and keep up to date with new ideas.

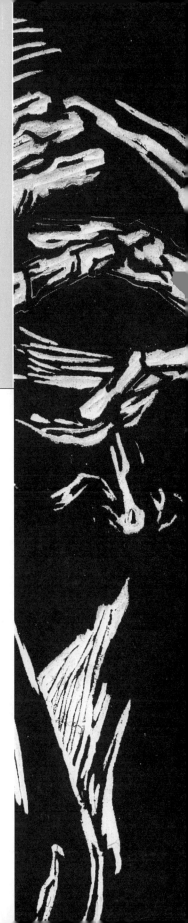

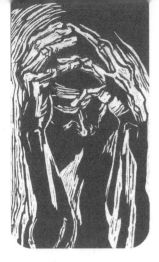

Chapter Twenty-three

Practitioner assessment skills

Robert Tunmore

AIMS

- ◆ To describe the therapeutic role and value of assessment
- ◆ Discuss the context of assessment in client care
- ◆ Promote involvement of clients and carers in the assessment process
- ◆ Critically appraise relevant assessment tools for practice
- ◆ Identify specific therapeutic skills for the assessment interview

KEY ISSUES

Assessment as part of a therapeutic relationship and as a means of gathering information

Client and carer involvement in assessment

Different approaches to assessment

Assessment tools

Assessment skills and the assessment interview

INTRODUCTION

Assessment is a systematic process that aims to:

1. provide a framework for the collection of information relevant to the client's health experience
2. engage the client in a therapeutic relationship
3. identify appropriate care, interventions and services.

Assessment is identified among the core skills and knowledge of the mental health nurse. The focus of mental health nursing is the human response to mental health problems for an individual and their family. Mental health nursing assessment is seen in terms of something that is done *with* people and not as something that is done *to* them. Assessment involves special skills and consists of far more than simply gathering information.

This chapter focuses on different approaches to assessment in mental health settings and the skills associated with practice in this field. These approaches range from broad frameworks for assessment to the use of specific assessment tools. The use of assessment tools for clinical practice is addressed and a means of critically describing and analysing these tools set out. Interpersonal therapeutic skills are a key component of the assessment interview. Preparation of both the client and the nurse for the assessment interview sets the context for the use of specific interviewing skills involved in assessment.

APPROACHES TO ASSESSMENT

Problems and needs

The assessment process involves assessment of *both* problems and needs. The assessment of health and social care needs may focus on the individual, a group, community or population. This main focus of this chapter is the assessment of individuals and the mental health problems that bring them into contact with mental health services. However, it is important to acknowledge the contribution nurses can make to the mental health of the population and public health.

The relationship between problems and needs may be put quite simply—for example, problems arise as a consequence of unmet need. Nursing care plans often have sections headed problem/ need suggesting, perhaps, that the terms are interchangeable. However, it is seldom so straightforward in mental health nursing. Problems may arise regardless of the needs of the individual, for example when the nature and severity of mental illness involves the risk of violence to others. Problems for the individual client may arise because of the health care system; for example, hospital admission may itself be distressing and disturbing. The needs of the individual client may be compromised by a range of factors including availability of social support, access to services, and treatment and care options.

THE NURSING PROCESS

The nursing process is a problem-solving approach to the care of the individual. In the UK it is described as a dynamic cycle consisting of four phases: assessment, planning, implementation and evaluation. Although assessment is described as a specific phase in this process it may be linked to each of the other phases in the process.

Assessment

Assessment involves activities associated with information gathering. The first phase of the nursing process may itself be identified as an ongoing process associated with the other stages in the nursing process. Assessment is ongoing and dynamic. It is the focus of assessment that varies through each phase of the nursing process. Assessment involves prioritizing, and goal setting.

Planning

Assessment identifies, describes and sets out the main areas of care that are to be included in the care plan. Assessment is used to define problems and needs from the client's perspective and set priorities in care. Goals are agreed and set and the interventions—possible and likely means of achieving the goals—identified.

Implementation

Assessment done *with* the client paves the way for implementation of the plan by providing opportunities to engage the client in the process of care. Assessment involves the initiation of a therapeutic relationship between nurse and client.

Evaluation

This may involve evaluation of the plan, of goals and achievement of goals, of interventions and outcomes, and of the original problem (i.e. a reassessment). Assessment sets out a baseline of comparative information—a measurement against which evaluative judgements about planning and implementation may be made.

Clearly, the relationship between assessment and other parts of this problem-solving approach is important. Sometimes this relationship is seen as a linear process with the interventions following on from the assessment. At other times assessment can be an ongoing process influencing intervention and outcome in a more dynamic interaction.

Although assessment is often seen solely as a process of gathering information it is important that it is not seen in isolation of other activities and processes but as an integral part of a comprehensive approach to care. Assessment must be purposeful, focused and of therapeutic benefit to the client. Indeed, used skillfully, the process of assessment should engage both clients and their carers in the development of a plan of care.

Client-centred assessment

A client-centred assessment will focus on the clients' perspective, experience and perception of their circumstances. It may include:

- history of current situation
- reasons for and understanding of hospital admission (if appropriate)
- previous health and illness history
- effect of illness on social roles and relationships
- worries and concerns
- stressors
- strengths, skills and resources

- coping styles and strategies
- work, employment and occupational activities
- recreational interests, enjoyable pastimes, play and leisure
- achievements, goals and aspirations
- self-care skills and abilities
- access to services
- satisfaction with services.

Relationships

The assessment of client needs and carer needs both involve a review of significant relationships. A client-centred approach will be based on the client's experience of those relationships and will acknowledge the perspective of others involved in the relationship. For example:

- clients' experience of self in relation to others—for example, how do clients see themselves in relation to others, how do they think others see them?
- the types of relationship they have—the identification of different types of relationship—for example, close, confiding relationships, or distant, continuous relationships
- who their friends are and how they describe their friendship relationships
- who they turn to in a crisis
- whether they ever feel socially isolated
- what support they have through other agencies and activities—for example, neighbours, colleagues, social support, financial support, religious groups, recreation, hobbies and pastimes.

User and carer involvement can be promoted through:

- providing summaries of assessments to users and carers in the form of a written care plan
- shared open communication between users and carers and professionals in needs assessment
- devising assessment tools in conjunction with users and professional carers
- having a key worker, advocate or other person present during assessment interviews.

Service users and carers are not a homogeneous group. Increasingly carers carry the burden of responsibility for supporting, monitoring and caring for users. The assessment of the needs of carers should be a component of routine practice. The needs of the users may be different to those of their carers. Clearly, tensions may arise in the assessment of individual need between users, carers and professionals.

The approach to assessment should take into account similarities and differences in the views of service users, carers and professional staff on issues including:

◆ assumptions about need and managing needs
◆ dependency on others and self-reliance
◆ safety, containment and promotion of personal autonomy.

The level and degree of involvement of service users and carers in assessment depends largely on the model of care and associated framework of assessment. Definitions of needs vary with different models of care. Medical models, institutional models and social models define need in different ways. For example, the medical model emphasizes individual pathology and disability, whereas social models will focus on relationships and systemic factors.

MENTAL STATE EXAMINATION

The mental state examination provides a structure for information gathered in the assessment interview. It provides a comprehensive overview of the client's current clinical presentation. Using the framework on different occasions over a period of time allows comparisons, and identification of changes—improvements and deterioration. Most of the mental state examination can be incorporated into a nursing assessment. Some parts of the examination may require specific types of question or testing—for example, cognitive functioning is usually assessed with specific questions for memory, concentration and comprehension.

During the interview nurses can identify any incongruity between what they observe and what the client states across the different components of the interview. For example, clients might report feeling distressed about a particular incident but make light of it with a joke or generalization. Alternatively they may say everything is fine and deny having any problems, but appear restless and agitated during the interview.

◆ *Appearance*—the physical characteristics of the client are noted as part of the interview—cleanliness, dress and clothing, personal hygiene, odour (body odour, alcohol, etc.), skin integrity, posture, facial expressions and pupil dilation.

◆ *Behaviour*—congruence with content of speech, mood and situation should be noted. Observation of behaviour includes levels of agitation, restlessness, relaxation, lethargy, any physical mannerisms, gestures and movement. Note changes in behaviour in relation to particular topics during the interview (e.g. change in eye contact and position). Possible signs of anxiety may relate to particular topics of discussion (e.g. wringing hands, playing with jewellery, reddening of neck or face, adjusting hair, etc.).

◆ *Speech*—note the speed (rapid or slow), tone, content, volume of speech, use of language (e.g. rhymes, neologisms, swearing and word associations). Other features include speech impediments (e.g. slurring and stuttering).

◆ *Mood*—this focuses on clients' self-report of their mood. They may say they are angry, irritable, frightened, anxious, worried, sad, excited, etc. Any incongruence with, for example, appearance, speech and behaviour, should be noted.

◆ *Affect*—observations focus on evidence of emotional expression, its intensity, duration and appropriateness to the situation. Clients may be expressive, demonstrable, labile, withdrawn, or blunted. The consistency and variation of expression should also be noted.

◆ *Perception*—note any beliefs about self and others, self-esteem, body image, personality, images, sounds, voices. Perceptual disorders include delusions and hallucinations. The nature and extent of these perceptual problems need a thorough assessment to identify potential risk of harm to self or others.

◆ *Thought content*—note current preoccupations, persistent worries and ruminations; expectations of self, others, the future; dreams and fantasies, recurring thoughts and ideas; unusual beliefs and belief systems.

◆ *Thought processes*—this section concerns the expression of thought through speech and behaviour rather than its overt content. For instance, is there a logical flow from one topic to the next; do particular patterns or themes emerge? Do they go over the same ground, returning to previous topics?

◆ *Judgement*—this concerns how choices and decisions are made and the extent to which they are based on a realistic appraisal and interpretation of current circumstances. There may be patterns or relationships between judgement and behaviour (e.g. impulsive behaviour, deliberate, planned behaviour). There may be errors in judgement; these errors may be consistent and repeated. Judgement patterns may involve, for example, an internal or external locus of control; they may be accusatory or accepting of self and others.

◆ *Intellect*—this involves assessment of levels of thinking and abstraction, clarity of thinking, literacy, formal education, level of knowledge and understanding, presence of learning difficulties and problem-solving ability.

◆ *Attention*—levels of concentration, consistency, and variability during the interview are assessed.

◆ *Comprehension*—note the response to and interaction with others, including verbal and non-verbal behaviours. Setting specific tasks may help the assessment of understanding of simple interactions and tasks.

◆ *Memory*—long term memory can be assessed as part of the client's history. This may need to be corroborated by other sources of information. Asking the client to recall the events of the last day or the 24 hours preceding the interview can assess memory of recent events.

◆ *Orientation*—the orientation with respect to time, place, person and self are used to assess levels of consciousness related to the current situation.

◆ *Insight*—note the client's understanding and awareness of the current situation, and the meaning of the inner experience to the client. Acceptance of mental health problems or denial of

them plays a critical role in the formulation and successful implementation of a plan of care and the establishment of a therapeutic relationship.

THE ABC MODEL OF ASSESSMENT

This approach considers human experience in terms of three interacting systems:

◆ Autonomic/physical system
◆ Behavioural system
◆ Cognitive system.

The autonomic/physical system refers to actual physical sensations experienced by clients. The behavioural system involves observation of what clients do—their actual behaviour under particular circumstances. The cognitive system involves clients' reports of their thoughts in relation to their problems.

The cognitive behavioural approach also addresses the relationship between individuals and their environment and the effect of this relationship on the problem. The approach focuses on the individual's part in initiating and maintaining the problem.

These actions are addressed in terms of their antecedents, behaviours and beliefs and consequences—a second ABC:

◆ Antecedents—things associated with the onset of the problem
◆ Behaviours and beliefs—the problem itself and the client's perspective of the problem
◆ Consequences—what happen as a result of the problem.

These two ABC sets may be used in the assessment process to define health problems from the client's perspective. This approach to assessment is systematic, specific and focused with precise specification of autonomic experience, behaviour and cognition. With the ABC assessment the main focus of the assessment is the presenting problem itself. A broader, more general assessment may complement the approach.

This model of assessment is derived from cognitive behavioural therapy. It may be used to make

Box 23.1 Evidence from mental health inquiries on risk assessment

Terms of reference	Inquiry

Examine all the circumstances surrounding the treatment and care, in particular:
 i) the quality and scope of health care, social care and risk assessments
 ii) the appropriateness of hospital treatment and inpatient care and subsequent support, supervision and after care in the community, in respect of:
   a) assessed health and social care needs
   b) assessed risk of potential harm to self and others
	Inquiry into the treatment and care of Raymond Sinclair (1996), West Kent Health Authority
	
	 Inquiry into the treatment and care of Francis Hampshire (1996), Redbridge and Waltham Forest Health Authority
	
	 Viner report (1996), Dorset Health Commission, Dorset Health Authority
	
	 Inquiry into the care and treatment of Nilesh Gadher (1996), Ealing, Hammersmith and Houndslow Health Authority

To establish the suitability of care in view of the patient's history and assessed health, social care needs, any previous psychiatric history or court convictions To establish the adequacy of the assessment of the patient's risk to self and others	Shaun Armstrong (1996), Tees Health Authority
Assessments from time to time of risk of harm to self and others	The case of Jason Mitchell (1996), Suffolk Health Authority
Recommendations for future assessment and care of people in similar circumstances to avoid possible harm to others	Grey report (1995), East London and the City Health Authority
To take due regard of all previous and ongoing assessment, treatment and care, both planned or received To assess the quality, range and delivery of the care and treatment, including assessments of risk, and whether it was suitable for the patient's needs	Woodley team report (1995), East London and the City Health Authority
The appropriateness of the care plan and care provided in the context of the patient's history and his assessed health and social care needs The suitability of the placement in view of the patient's history and assessed health and social care needs	Report of the inquiry into the death of Jonathan Newby (a volunteer worker) (1995), Oxfordshire Health Authority
To consider the implication of the state of the art of the assessment of risk and prediction of dangerousness posed by patients	The falling shadow (1995), South Devon Healthcare Trust

Box 23.1	Evidence from mental health inquiries on risk assessment
To inquire into the arrangements for the assessment, care, discharge and follow-up	Independent inquiry into the care and treatment of Kevin Rooney (1992), North Thames Regional Health Authority
An analysis of case records on the initial assessment and subsequent reviews, the decisions made, care and treatment plans and appropriateness of placement	Findings of the independent review of the case of Erieyune Inweh (1992), Kingston Health Authority

From Zito Trust 1997.

testable predictions about a client's behaviour and experience (Newell 1994). It is a client-centred approach to assessment that focuses on a specific issue or problem. It is this specific focus to assessment that helps the client and the nurse to identify appropriate interventions. Specific interventions should be employed to meet individual needs and address identified problems.

Using this approach to assessment it may be possible to predict:

◆ how a client will act in given situations
◆ the effects of these acts on the client's life
◆ the effect these actions may have on the client
◆ the effects of nursing interventions on the client's problems.

RISK ASSESSMENT

Risk assessment is a component of assessment identified among the key skills for mental health professionals (Sainsbury Centre 1997).

The importance of assessment skills relating to risk is highlighted by the reports of mental health inquiries. In Learning the lessons the Zito Trust (1997) summarizes events leading to the setting up of mental health inquiries and identifies their terms of reference. Assessment and risk assessment are a prominent feature of these inquiries. Box 23.1 identifies terms of reference relating to specific inquiries where matters relating to risk assessment have been addressed. The range of issues identified in these inquiries relating to risk assessment include:

◆ professional judgement
◆ training in the assessment of risk
◆ communication between professionals and agencies
◆ liaison and collaboration between agencies
◆ involvement of relatives and carers in the assessment and planning process
◆ the effectiveness of the assessment and care plan—delivery and compliance
◆ standards and quality of documentation and record keeping
◆ the likely influence of assumptions about race and background on social, housing, medical and psychiatric care
◆ assessment of the appropriateness of particular placement
◆ recommendations for future delivery of care.

Dimensions of risk assessment include concerns about safety related to severe mental illness. Building bridges (DOH 1996) identifies four components of safety in relation to severe mental illness:

◆ unintentional self-harm (e.g. self-neglect)
◆ intentional self-harm
◆ safety of others
◆ abuse by others (e.g. physical, sexual, emotional and financial).

Risk related to serious mental illness is considered in terms of:

◆ risk of self-harm
◆ risk of violence to others
◆ risk of self-neglect.

The aims of risk assessment are:

◆ to identify what must change to reduce the risk
◆ to propose means of reducing the risk and to identify interventions that might reduce the risk (DOH 1996).

Building bridges (DOH 1996) suggests that risk assessment involve the use of all available sources of information. These sources of information are identified in Box 23.2 along with key elements of risk assessment.

Box 23.2 Risk factors and sources of information in assessment

Risk factors

Patient's
◆ background
◆ history

Present
◆ mental state
◆ social functioning

Past
◆ behaviour
◆ previous court convictions

Patterns
◆ behaviours associated with the risk, e.g. people involved, circumstances—not taking medication, use of alcohol, or drugs
◆ frequency of these behaviours
◆ severity of the behaviours

Sources of information
◆ The client
◆ Relatives
◆ Friends
◆ Carers
◆ The treatment team
◆ Police
◆ Probation officers
◆ Housing departments
◆ Social workers
◆ Local press reports
◆ Neighbours

However, risk assessment is recognized as an inexact science (DOH 1996). The identification of 'risk factors' is based upon studies of populations at risk rather than on individual clients. Risk factors are correlates and not causes. Beware of statistical stereotypes. The presence or absence of risk factors must be considered in terms of individual history, responses, circumstances and relationships at any given time. This emphasizes both the need for a client-centred perspective to risk assessment and the importance of viewing assessment as an ongoing systematic process.

CASE MANAGEMENT AND THE CARE PROGRAMME APPROACH

A full risk assessment is an important component of the assessment process of the care programme approach (CPA). Risk assessment is a key element of good case management. The direct involvement of carers and users in assessment, care planning and review is one of the aims of the CPA. Key components of the CPA are:

◆ systematic *assessment* of health and social care needs
◆ an agreed *care plan*
◆ allocation of a *key worker*
◆ regular *review* of the client's progress.

A needs assessment under the CPA involves identification of the client's health and social care needs. Usually the professional to whom the client has been referred carries out this assessment. However, depending on the complexity of needs, it may involve multidisciplinary assessment meetings in conjunction with the client, carers and advocates to ensure that a broad range of appropriate and relevant health and social needs are assessed. Multidisciplinary perspectives on risk are likely to vary so it is important that risk assessment evolves around multidisciplinary teamwork. The key worker should have a clear understanding of the risk associated with individual clients in order to recognize warning signs both of self-harm and of harm to others (DOH 1996).

The following questions should be addressed when considering the roles and responsibilities of the colleagues in the multidisciplinary team in relation to an individual client.

- ◆ Who is responsible for the risk assessment?
- ◆ Who is responsible for conducting a social care assessment?
- ◆ Who is responsible for conducting a health care assessment?

Key workers should be aware of their own professional role in relation to risk assessment, and consider personal safety—for example, whether they interview alone or with another person present.

OTHER APPROACHES TO NURSING ASSESSMENT

The most commonly used approaches have been designed to identify a broad outline for the assessment process. They often organize a range of items relevant to a particular issue, problem area or concern. This approach helps to ensure that assessment identifies essential and relevant information as the basis for the development of a comprehensive and consistent care plan. It provides a standard format to the information that is gathered during the assessment process and should be tailored to the individual needs and problems of each individual by involving the client and carers in the assessment process. However, such broad approaches may need to be carried out in conjunction with a more focused approach (e.g. the ABC assessment or used with a specific assessment tool—see Box 23.4).

Examples of generic approaches to assessment include:

- ◆ Activities of daily living (Roper, Logan & Tierney 1980)
- ◆ Gordon's functional health patterns
- ◆ physical health—body systems
- ◆ specialist assessments.

Activities of daily living (Roper, Logan & Tierney 1980)

This has been used widely in nurse training and provides a broad overview of areas for assessment of individual health needs and problems. Roper et al's measures of activities of daily living include:

- ◆ maintaining a safe environment
- ◆ communicating
- ◆ breathing
- ◆ eating and drinking
- ◆ eliminating
- ◆ personal cleansing and dressing
- ◆ controlling body temperature
- ◆ expressing sexuality
- ◆ mobilizing
- ◆ sleeping
- ◆ dying
- ◆ worship.

Gordon's functional health patterns

This is a system of nursing classification that is a key component of the North American Nursing Diagnosis Association's (NANDA) approved categories of nursing diagnosis (Gordon 1997). The system identifies the following areas for assessment:

- ◆ health perception–health management pattern
- ◆ nutritional–metabolic pattern
- ◆ elimination pattern
- ◆ activity–exercise pattern
- ◆ sleep–rest pattern
- ◆ cognitive–perceptual pattern
- ◆ self-perception–self-concept pattern
- ◆ role–relationship pattern
- ◆ sexual–reproductive pattern
- ◆ coping–stress tolerance pattern
- ◆ value belief pattern.

Physical health—body systems

This approach to assessment addresses bodily systems and emphasizes the physical health of the individual. Although many people with mental health problems have concurrent physical health problems, their poor physical health is often a direct consequence of mental health problems and their treatment—for example, weight gain and sexual dysfunction associated with antipsychotic medication, neglect of physical self-care, including problems arising from poor diet, poor personal hygiene associated with enduring mental illness and somatic presentation of anxiety disorders.

Cardiovascular system	Cardiovascular disorders
Respiratory system	Pulmonary disorders
Gastrointestinal system	Gastrointestinal disorders
Genitourinary system	Genitourinary disorders
Musculoskeletal system	Musculoskeletal disorders
Neurological system	Neurological disorders
	Endocrine disorders
	Metabolic disorders

Clearly these broad approaches to assessment need to be adapted for particular client groups and specialist services and used in conjunction with more focused specialist assessments.

Specialist assessments

Many approaches to assessment are developed for clients with particular problems or to assess specific symptoms. For example, Brown (1998) has developed a framework for pre- and postadmission psychiatric assessment with a forensic focus to be used by professionals working with mentally disordered offenders and clients with challenging behaviours. Each part of the assessment identifies, through a range of subheadings, specific and focused areas for assessment for clients in forensic settings (Box 23.3). This type of assessment tool complements the more generic approach to assessment outlined above—for example, by incorporating them as 'basic care' issues.

Note the following general points with regard to the use of assessment tools:

◆ Ensure you are familiar with the assessment tool before you use it.

◆ Identify any training opportunities to practise using particular assessment tools.

◆ Incorporate the review of your skills in assessment as part of your ongoing learning needs and clinical supervision.

ASSESSMENT TOOLS

Approaches to assessment are often influenced by professional orientation, and service availability. Assessments may tend to be idiosyncratic, their

---

Box 23.3 Assessment for forensic psychiatric settings (Brown 1998)

◆ Basic care issues (see general approaches above)
◆ Medical history
◆ Incident history
◆ External network
◆ Behaviour at night
◆ Life experiences
◆ Security issues
◆ Previous placements and treatments
◆ Significant events
◆ Social behaviour
◆ Recreational activities
◆ Threat/fantasy issues
◆ Sexual issues
◆ Loss/bereavement
◆ Self-harming behaviours
◆ Hostage-taking history
◆ Eating issues
◆ Arson.

---

nature, form and content subject to and influenced by a range of factors. This may lead to the care plan and interventions being based on inconsistent and inadequate information.

Assessment tools are standardized assessment instruments designed to standardize the assessment process. A wide range of assessment tools are available to help guide or focus the assessment (Box 23.4). Different terms are used to describe assessment tools: terms such as 'scale', 'schedule', 'index', 'checklist' and 'test'. Sometimes the term used has a specific meaning or reflects some aspect of the development of the tool, its use or intended purpose. Some tools have been developed to aid clinical work; others may have been developed for research purposes. In general, assessment tools provide a focus for assessment (e.g. a particular symptom, its frequency, severity and occurrence) or they provide a measure of a particular attribute. You may come across a wide range of different assessment tools in different services and settings. It is important to use these tools appropriately and to ensure that the most relevant tools are used for particular circumstances.

Box 23.4   Examples of assessment tools

Name	Clinical focus or area	Approach	Reference
Camberwell Assessment of Need (CAN)	Direct identification of treatment needs	Observer rating	Phelan M et al 1995 The Camberwell assessment of need: the validity and reliability of an instrument to assess the needs of the seriously mentally ill. British Journal of Psychiatry 167:589–595
The Brief Psychiatric Rating Scale (BPRS)	General changes in psychopathology	Standard interview Observer rating scale Ideally requires two interviewers Completion time: 15–30 minutes Depends on good interview skills	Overall J, Gorham D 1962 The brief psychiatric rating scale. Psychological Reports 10:799–812 McGorry P D et al 1988 The development of the BPRS (nursing modification). Comprehensive Psychiatry 29:575–587
The Nurses' Observation Scale for Inpatient Evaluation (NOSIE)	Inpatient setting for people with chronic schizophrenia	Observer rating of behaviour Completion time: 5–10 minutes Helpful for withdrawn, mute, hostile and overactive clients	Honigfeld G, Klett C J 1965 The nurse's observation scale for inpatient evaluation: a new scale for measuring improvement in chronic schizophrenia. Journal of Clinical Psychology 21:65–71
Manchester Scale	Chronic psychosis positive and negative symptoms	Observer rating of behaviour Completion time: 10–15 minutes	Krawiecka M et al 1977 A standardised psychiatric assessment scale for rating chronic psychiatric patients. Acta Psychiatrica Scandinavica 55:299–308
Positive and Negative Syndrome Scale (PANNS)	Balance of positive and negative symptoms	Based on clinical interview Completion time: 30–40 minutes	Kay S et al 1987 The positive and negative syndrome scale (PANSS) for schizophrenia. Schizophrenia Bulletin 13:261–275
Characteristics of Delusions Rating Scale	Subjective experience of delusions	Visual analogue Self-rating Completion time: 20 minutes	Garety P, Hemsley D 1987 Characteristics of delusional experience. European Archives of Psychiatry and Neurological Science 266:294–298

Box 23.4 Examples of assessment tools *(cont'd)*

Name	Clinical focus or area	Approach	Reference
Dimensions of Delusional Experience Scale (DDES)	Subjective experience of delusions	Semistructured interview Completion time: 45 minutes	Kendler K et al 1983 Dimensions of delusional experience. American Journal of Psychiatry 140:59–65
Personal Questionnaire Rapid Scaling Technique (PQRST)	Auditory hallucinations	Completion time: 1 week	Mulhall (1978) Manual for personal questionnaire rapid scaling technique. NFER-Nelson, London
Liverpool University Neuroleptic Side-Effect Rating Scale (LUNSERS)	Medication side-effects	Self-report questionnaire 51 items 0–4 rating scale	Day J C, Wood G, Dewey M, Bentall R P 1995 A self-rating scale for measuring neuroleptic side-effects. British Journal of Psychiatry 166(5):650–653
Hopelessness Scale	Pessimism and negativity	Self-rating scale Completion time: 5–15 minutes	Beck A et al 1974 The measurement of pessimism: the Hopelessness Scale. Journal of Consulting and Clinical Psychology 42:861–865
Scale for Suicidal Ideation	Suicidal ideation among depressed and suicidal clients	Interviewer rating scale Completion time: 5–15 minutes	Beck A et al 1979 Assessment of suicidal intention: the scale for suicidal ideation. Journal of Consulting and Clinical Psychology 47:343–352
Suicide Intent Scale	Degree of suicide intent associated with suicide attempts	Interviewer-rated scale	Beck A et al 1974 Development of suicidal intent scales. In Beck A T, Lettieri D J (eds) The prediction of suicide. Charles Press, Maryland
Beck Depression Inventory (BDI)	Depression	Self-rating scale	Beck A et al 1961 An inventory for measuring depression. Comprehensive Psychiatry Journal 2:163–170
Hamilton Rating Scale for Depression	Depression	Self-rating scale	Hamilton M 1960 A rating scale for depression. Journal of Neurology, Neurosurgery and Psychiatry 23:56–62

Box 23.4	Examples of assessment tools *(cont'd)*		
Name	**Clinical focus or area**	**Approach**	**Reference**
Montgomery and Asberg Depression Rating scale (MADRS)	Depression	Clinical interview observer rating	Montgomery A, Asberg M 1979 A new depression scale designed to be sensitive to change. British Journal of Psychiatry 134:382–389
Zung Self-rating Depression Scale	Depression	Self-rating scale	Zung W 1965 A self-rating depression scale. Archives of General Psychiatry 12:63–70

There are a number of different reasons for using assessment tools. It is important to understand the reasons an assessment tool is being used. Assessment tools may be used:

◆ to gather clinical information as part of a client's care plan
◆ as a focus for therapeutic interaction (e.g. to facilitate discussion or to monitor changes over time)
◆ as part of a standardized risk assessment
◆ for data collection in a research programme
◆ to comply with organizational and service policy
◆ for purposes of clinical audit and quality monitoring
◆ to provide a valid comparison of data over time.

A single assessment tool may be used for a range of different reasons. It is important for both nurse and client to understand the purposes of using an assessment tool. Some tools require training before they can be used effectively; others will have been developed for specific client groups in particular settings and used under specific circumstances. Sometimes standardized assessment tools are adapted for use with particular clients. However, attempts to adapt or alter a standardized assessment tool may lead to problems associated with consistency, validity and reliability of information and the purpose and context of its use.

Other issues include:

◆ Different assessment tools may be used by health and social service staff and by different professional groups.
◆ The local development of tools inhibits broad comparison—for example, of outcomes of care.
◆ The use of assessment tools may lead to unrealistic expectations of services and practitioners.
◆ Assessments often identify unmet needs. Additional resources may be needed to address the outcomes of assessments.
◆ Different perspectives and approaches to assessment and the use of assessment tools may lead to conflict.
◆ Assessment may be seen as a one-off activity.

HoNOS: Health of the Nation Outcome Scales

The Health of the Nation Outcome Scales (Wing, Curtis & Beevor 1996) provide a numerical record of a routine clinical assessment that draws on a wide range of information from all sources. These scales have been developed to provide a national measure in response to the Department of Health's Health of the nation strategy. They aim to 'improve significantly the health and social functioning of mentally ill people' (DOH 1996).

There are 12 scales designed for use in secondary mental health care services. They address clinical and social areas relevant to adult mental illness and have been designed so that they can be completed in a short period of time by clinicians working in any setting. The scales provide a brief numerical record of the clinical assessment and this information has a variety of uses for clinicians, administrators and researchers. The scale also records the clinical setting and the client's primary diagnosis.

However, HoNOS do not take into account the cause of the problem, the duration of the problem, the effect on others, or future risk. Ratings are based solely on clinical judgements. HoNOS rating is *not* a structured interview. It does not set targets, nor specify interventions. Therefore it should be used routinely *in conjunction with* the clinical assessment, clinical notes, care plan and standard measures or tools.

Scoring

Comparison of any two HoNOS scores for a client will give a change score or outcome measure identifying trends and patterns—for example, on admission and at discharge from hospital.

They may be used to assess the most severe problems. Scales cover an agreed time period, for example the previous 2 weeks, the previous month, or since the last CPA review meeting. Wherever possible, the same person or team should complete successive HoNOS ratings. These must be qualified mental health professionals, and include the key worker or CPA team.

Severity of problems is rated on a five-point scale:

  0 = no problem
  1 = minor problem requiring no action
  2 = mild problem but definitely present
  3 = moderately severe problem
  4 = severe to very severe problem.

The 12 HoNOS scales are:

1. Overactive, aggressive, disruptive or agitated behaviour
2. Non-accidental self-injury
3. Problem drinking or drug taking
4. Cognitive problems

Box 23.5   A checklist for evaluating assessment tools

Items in the tool
Where did they come from:
◆ previous tools?
◆ clinical observation?
◆ expert opinion?
◆ service user reports?
◆ research findings?
◆ theory?
Has the tool been piloted and checked for:
◆ a clear scoring system?
◆ language and terminology?
◆ lack of ambiguity?
◆ lack of value-laden or offensive content?

Reliability
Has the scale been tested for reliability?
Has the scale been checked for internal consistency?
Does it have good test–retest reliability?
Does it have good interrater agreement?
Which client groups were used to test reliability?

Validity
Does the tool have face validity?
Is there evidence of content validity?
Has it been compared with other tools for criterion validity?
Is there evidence of construct validity?

Utility
Can the scale be completed in a reasonable time in the clinical setting?
What are the training requirements?
How easy is it to score?

Based on Streiner 1993

---

5. Physical illness or disability problems
6. Problems with hallucinations and delusions
7. Problems with depressed mood
8. Other mental and behavioural problems (specified)
9. Problems with relationships
10. Problems with activities of daily living
11. Problems with living conditions
12. Problems with occupation and activities.

Other scales

These include:

HoNOS–65+—Health of the Nation Outcome Scales for people with mental illness over 65 years old

HoNOSCA—Health of the Nation Outcome Scales for Children and Adolescents

HoNOS-LD—Health of the Nation Outcome Scales for People with Learning Disabilities

HoNOS-MDO—Health of the Nation Outcome Scales for Forensic Services.

Evaluation of scales and tools

HoNOS meet the following clinical requirements:

◆ they are short and simple for routine use
◆ they are acceptable to nurses and psychiatrists
◆ they cover a range of clinical and social functions
◆ they are sensitive to improvement, deterioration and lack of change over time
◆ they have been tested for reliability
◆ they are valid in relation to other established scales.

These attributes are important considerations for the usefulness of all rating scales and may be applied to the use of other scales. Streiner (1993) developed a checklist for evaluating the usefulness of rating scales, which can be adapted for a critical analysis of assessment tools and their use in particular circumstances (Box 23.5).

Development of assessment tools

Previous tools

Assessment tools may be developed from other assessment tools, combining different items to include a range of issues in the assessment. Sometimes assessment tools need to be updated— for example, if the language used is out of date or inappropriate for the client group it is to be used for.

Clinical observation

Assessment tools for clinical practice may be based on common clinical observations and presentations of particular problems, conditions, symptoms or disorders.

Expert opinion

A team of experts may develop assessment tools. The final tool represents the general consensus view of what is being assessed. It is important to know how this team has been put together and whether it is representative of particular stakeholders. For example, an assessment tool developed by a team of expert service users would probably look quite different from that developed by a team of professional experts.

Service user reports

Assessment tools based on the perspectives of mental health professionals are likely to focus on the behavioural or objective features of a disorder rather than the client's perspective of the problem and the personal context. As service users are increasingly involved in the planning of care, assessment tools need to take into account the subjective views of service users and their experience of mental health problems. Again, issues of representation are important considerations as individual experience varies from one person to the next.

Research findings

Assessment tools are increasingly based on research evidence but all research is open to critical analysis. Conflicting reports and counterevidence are not uncommon. Often it is difficult and inappropriate to apply research findings based on, for example, surveys of particular populations or groups to the assessment of particular individuals and their mental health.

Theory

Different theoretical perspectives on mental health incorporate a range of different concepts. For example, the medical model perspective focuses on mental disorders, symptoms and alleviation of symptoms though medical intervention. Sociological perspectives on mental illness will emphasize concepts of social support, social roles and relationships. The theoretical approach will influence the choice of items making up an assessment tool.

Scoring system

Some assessment tools include measures and scoring systems. These may, for example, be Likert-type scales—allowing for a range of responses on a five-point scale where respondents are asked to rate how strongly they agree or disagree with a statement or how much or little it affects them. The appropriate use of such scoring systems, if they are present, need to have been tested in a pilot study to ensure the system is clear, easily understandable and appropriate to the assessment. The simplest scoring system may provide a checklist of the presence or absence of particular items, but this may tell us little about the meaning to the client.

Language and terminology

Piloting an assessment tool helps to ensure appropriate language is used. Professional psychiatric jargon may include technical terms that are not understood or may be misinterpreted by the lay person. Terms such as 'mood', 'affect', 'depression' and 'anxiety' may have specific and shared meanings among professionals in mental health settings but may be seen differently by clients and their relatives. They may use terms such as 'stress' and 'nervous breakdown' more generally. The language and terminology of assessment tools can be tailored to the client group the tool is to assess. Similarly language and terminology should be free of ambiguity and value-laden or offensive content.

Reliability

A tool is said to be reliable if in tests it produces the same results from the same subject under the same circumstances at different times, or the same observation (or similar observations) from different observers of the same subject under the same conditions. Reliability may be measured in different ways, not all of which are appropriate for a specific assessment tool.

Internal consistency

This refers to congruency between responses to similar items in an assessment tool for a particular attribute. For example, in completing a self-assessment tool for anxiety people rating themselves as worried would also endorse items relating to nervous tension, preoccupation and feeling 'on edge'.

Test–retest reliability

Assessment tools should be consistent over a period of time and give similar results on successive trials, providing there are no changes in the external circumstances. For example, depressed individuals should give the same result on an assessment tool assessing depression from one week to the next, if there has been no change in their condition.

Interrater reliability

Those assessment tools that are completed by an observer rather than clients themselves are called observer-rating scales. Several observers assessing the same subject and achieving similar results test the reliability of these tools. Observer-rating scales often involve training in the use of the assessment tool; therefore, the quality of the training may influence the level of interrater reliability.

Choice of sample

Another factor influencing the reliability of an assessment tool relates to the client group for which it was developed (i.e. its intended purpose). This should be similar to that which it is being used to assess. If the group it is used to assess differs from that for which it was designed it may be necessary to retest its reliability with the current assessment group.

Validity

An assessment tool is valid if it actually measures what it purports to measure. There are different ways of addressing the validity of an assessment tool.

Face validity

Do the items appear to be relevant to the assessment topic? Face validity concerns the acceptance of the tool by the respondent as a measure of what it purports to measure.

Content validity

As with face validity, the items in the assessment tool should relate to key factors associated with the topic of the tool. For example, with an assessment tool addressing family functioning in severe mental illness key factors should be clearly identifiable by the respondent (e.g. communication issues, social support, family roles) and items related to these factors. The more items relating to a particular factor, the greater is the content validity.

Criterion validity

Assessment tools with criterion validity will compare well with other established, valid and reliable assessment tools addressing the same issue.

Construct validity

Assessment in mental health and mental illness often focuses on intangible concepts—for example, self-esteem, mood and anxiety. These are hypothetical constructs and so they cannot be directly measured or observed. We infer the presence or absence of these constructs from a range of variables that can be measured and observed. Construct validity increases with each study that investigates the relationships between these different variables.

Utility

This concerns practical considerations of using particular assessment tools.

Completion time

Assessment tools need be considered in terms of the time it takes to complete them in the clinical setting. Generally, the briefer they are the more likely they are to be completed and used. Their use needs to be considered in terms of their reliability and validity and in terms of benefits to client care and as a means of demonstrating effective clinical outcomes.

Training time

Training may be required to use assessment tools and to interpret their results. Some may require a mental health nurse or non-mental health professionals to complete them. Other non-mental-health professionals, for example practice nurses and district nurses, may use mental health professionals to assess the mental health of their clients.

The selective use of assessment tools may complement other approaches to assessment. They can be incorporated into clients' care plans where appropriate and used to engage clients and their carers in the process of care.

ASSESSMENT INTERVIEW SKILLS

Skills in assessment are among the core skills of a range of different professionals including mental health nurses, social workers, occupational therapists, psychiatrists, psychologists, GPs and primary health care teams who provide mental health care to adults with severe mental health problems. The Sainsbury Centre report (1997) 'Pulling together' on the future roles and training of mental health staff identifies a range of assessment skills as core competencies for these specialist staff. Box 23.6 identifies specific areas of assessment set out in the report as part of a template for core knowledge, skills and attitudes of professional staff.

Assessments should be objective and based on observation and collection of relevant information. Informal interviews may be more productive than question and answer sessions. It is important to communicate to your colleagues, and other

---

Box 23.6   Assessment skills

- Appropriate values and attitudes
- Listening and questioning skills required to make accurate assessments of individual need
- Skill in conducting a collaborative needs-based assessment
- Ability to develop a treatment and care plan based on a thorough and comprehensive assessment of the client, family and social system
- Apply knowledge of the issues and skill in the assessment and management of the combined problem of drug/alcohol abuse and mental illness
- Skills in the assessment of users' needs and requirements of housing, occupation and income
- Apply knowledge and skill in risk assessment and the management of violence and aggression
- Apply knowledge of factors related to the development of 'chronic crises' and skill in assessment and management strategies.

From Pulling together (Sainsbury Centre 1997)

Box 23.7   Guiding questions: preparation for the assessment interview

- Who initiates the interview?
- How do the parties involved perceive the interview?
- Has the respondent experienced this type of interview before—if so, how recently and with whom?
- What are the expected outcomes of the interview?
- How will the interview contribute to the client's therapeutic experience?
- What specific or new information is to be gathered?
- What skills does the interviewer possess?
- How motivated or able is the respondent?
- How long will the interview last?
- Where will it take place?

The assessment interview involves the exchange of information that is part of a therapeutic experience for the client. As part of a therapeutic process the interviewer needs to ensure that the respondent understands his or her role in the interview and that both parties share similar perceptions of the purpose of the interview.

Respondent preparedness

The level of preparation on the client's part for the interview will influence the appropriate use of open and closed questions. It is important for the respondents to have considered some of the topics to be covered in the assessment interview. Their response will be influenced by their opportunity to reflect on their experience. Reflection involves a process of recalling, organizing and evaluating experience. Open questions may be used in the interview to encourage this reflection and help respondents think through an issue so they can formulate opinions, perspectives and conclusions.

Interviewer preparedness

Interviewers may prepare themselves for the interview by addressing information from a range of

members of the multidisciplinary team, any information you have given to the client. Following your assessment, identify and record any recommendations for further assessment.

Preparation for the assessment interview

Preparation involves consideration of the purpose and expected outcomes of the interview as well as arrangement of the physical environment.

The physical environment should be comfortable and welcoming, and as free from disturbance and distraction as possible. The position of furniture and seating arrangement should be considered in relation to clients' needs—for example, is there somewhere for the client to hang their coat on arrival, is drinking water provided or are facilities for coffee or tea available? A box of paper tissues may be helpful in case clients should become distressed.

other sources prior to the assessment interview in addition to those areas identified in Box 23.7. They should be aware of what information has been collected to avoid unnecessary repetition of questions and duplication of information. Under these circumstance closed questions (see next section) can focus on, for example, clarifying specific details, matters of fact and interpretation. Open questions may be used to develop the interview with a client-centred focus, building on earlier work, for example, from a previous admission.

Guiding questions in Box 23.7 may be considered by those involved in the interview—both nurse and client—prior to the interview. They may be adapted by those involved—perhaps a working party on assessment with service users, carers, advocates and mental health worker representation—so that they reflect adequately the needs of your particular service setting.

The interview involves more than the interviewer collecting information. Clients may be motivated by an expectation that the interview will help relieve problems or lead to interventions that give relief from particular stresses or strains they have experienced. Alternatively, the client may be detained against their will and reluctant to take part in the interview. The interviewer may be seen as an important source of help or as an inquisitor conducting an interrogation.

INTERVIEW SKILLS

A range of interpersonal communication skills are involved in the assessment interview. The skills most frequently used for gathering information include open and closed questions. However, in order to engage the client in a therapeutic process, questioning skills need to be accompanied by and seen in terms of other interpersonal skills. The assessment interview involves skilled and sensitive use of interpersonal techniques—for example, those identified by Hays & Larson (1963) as characteristics of therapeutic interactions. Table 23.1 identifies these therapeutic techniques, which form the basis of skills used in the assessment interview.

Table 23.1 Interviewing skills: therapeutic interpersonal techniques

Skill	Rationale	Examples
Using silence	Provides an opportunity to reflect, collect thoughts, think and organize opinion	
Accepting	Conveys attitude of reception, permissiveness and regard	'I follow what you are saying', 'Go on', 'Yes', 'Uh hmm'
Giving recognition	Acknowledging, indicating awareness	'Hello Mrs Jones', 'You've had your hair done', 'I see you've updated your care plan'
Offering self	Unconditionally making one's *self* available	'I'll sit with you a while', 'I want to make sure you are comfortable'
Giving broad openings	Allowing the client to take the initiative in introducing the topic	'Is there something you would like to talk about?', 'What is on your mind?', 'Where would you like to begin?', 'Would you like to talk about yourself now?'
Offering general leads	Giving encouragement to continue	'Go on', 'And then?', 'Tell me about it'
Placing the event in time or in sequence	Clarifying the relationship of events in time	'What seemed to lead up to …?', 'Was this before or after …?', 'When did this happen?'

Table 23.1 Interviewing skills: therapeutic interpersonal techniques (cont'd)

Skill	Rationale	Examples
Making observations	Saying what is perceived, bringing your observations to the client's attention	'You seem tense', 'Are you uncomfortable when you …?', 'I notice that you are biting your lips', 'It makes me uncomfortable when you…'
Encouraging description of perceptions	Asking clients to talk about what they perceive	'What is going on now?', 'Tell me if you start to feel anxious', 'What does the voice seem to be saying?'
Encouraging comparison	Asking that similarities and differences be noted in relation to ideas, experiences and relationships	'Was this something like …?', 'Have you had similar experiences?'
Restating	Repeating the main idea expressed demonstrates effective communication and understanding, and encourages continuation	*Client:* 'I can't sleep. I stay awake all night' *Nurse:* 'You have difficulty sleeping' *Client:* 'I don't like the group. Who wants to know what I have to say anyway?' *Nurse:* 'You feel nobody is interested in your opinion'
Reflecting	Directing back to the client questions, feelings and ideas	*Client:* 'Do you think I should tell the doctor …?' *Nurse:* 'Do *you* think you should?' *Client:* 'My brother spends all my money and has the cheek to ask for more' *Nurse:* 'This makes you angry'
Focusing	Concentrating on a single point	'Shall we looking at this point more closely?'
Exploring	Delving further into a subject or idea	'Tell me more about that', 'Would you describe it more?'
Giving information	Making available the facts the client needs	'My name is …', 'I am here because …', 'I'm taking you to…'
Seeking clarification	Seeking to make clear that which is not meaningful or that which is vague	'I'm not sure that I follow', 'What would you say is the main point of what you said?'
Presenting reality	Offering for consideration that which is real	'I see no one else in the room', 'That sound was a car backfiring', 'Your mother is not here; I'm a nurse'
Voicing doubt	Expressing uncertainty as to the reality of the patient's perception	'Isn't that unusual?', 'Really?', 'I find that hard to believe'
Seeking consensual validation	Searching for mutual understanding, for accord in the meaning of words	'Tell me whether my understanding of it agrees with yours', 'Are you using this word to convey the idea…?'
Verbalizing the implied	Verbalizing what patients have hinted or suggested	*Client:* 'I can't talk to anyone. It's a waste of time' *Nurse:* 'Do you feel that no one understands?' *Client:* 'My wife pushes me around just like my mother and sister did'

Table 23.1 Interviewing skills: therapeutic interpersonal techniques *(cont'd)*

Skill	Rationale	Examples
		Nurse: 'Is it your impression that women are domineering?'
Encouraging evaluation	Asking clients to appraise the quality of their experiences	'What are your feelings in regard to …?', 'Does this make you feel uncomfortable?'
Attempting to translate into feelings	Seeking to verbalize the feelings that are being expressed only indirectly	*Client:* 'I'm dead' *Nurse:* 'Are you suggesting that you feel lifeless?', or 'Is it that life seems without meaning?'
		Client: 'I'm way out in the ocean' *Nurse:* 'It must be lonely', or 'You seem to feel deserted'
Suggesting collaboration	Offering to share, to strive, to work together with patients for their benefit	'Perhaps you and I can discuss this to discover what leads to your anxiety'
Summarizing	Organizing and summing up what has gone before	'Have I got this right …?', 'You said that …', 'During this interview you and I have discussed…'
Encouraging formulation of a plan of action	Asking the client to consider kinds of behaviour likely to be appropriate in future situations, using the assessment interview as the basis for a care plan	'What could you do to let your anger out harmlessly?', 'If this should happen again, what would you do to deal with it?', 'How would you like to proceed?', 'What do you think are the main things that should happen next?'

From Hays & Larson 1963.

Open questions

These free response or unrestricted questions invite the respondent to use their own words in their reply. These are most appropriately used to let respondents set the agenda on a particular topic and give an account from their own perspective. They allow the use of clients' own language and terminology.

Closed questions

Restricted or forced-choice questions direct the respondent towards particular alternative responses. The content, form and duration of the response are restricted. Closed questions are used most appropriately when the interviewer has advanced knowledge of the type and range of response and needs to minimize demands on the client

Interpersonal skills involving open questions are used most appropriately to learn about the client's perspective, attitudes, personal characteristics, attributes, opinions and feelings on different subjects. Closed questions are more likely to be used when the interview objectives focus on a specific topic or issue. Most interviews will involve a mix of open and closed questions—for example, open questions may encourage respondents to tell their story in their own words, while closed questions can be used to focus on particular areas of their experience, for clarification, understanding and detail.

Some interventions, for example, those involving closed questions, can be less demanding of clients. So if, for example, they find it difficult to focus or concentrate their thoughts and expression, a choice of response using a succession of closed questions may be appropriate. However, it may be the initial use of open questions that highlights these difficulties. Open questions may draw out whether respondents' ability to respond is associated with lack of information or uncertainty about a particular issue. For instance, they may be confused and unclear about their feelings.

Closed questions may be experienced as less demanding, less revealing and possibly less threatening. They may make extreme responses more amenable and more acceptable but they may also be restrictive, perhaps reinforcing any negative feelings respondents may have about their situation.

The assessment interview involves a balanced approach to the use of interpersonal skills in both the engagement of the client in a therapeutic relationship or therapeutic process and the collection of relevant, appropriate, accurate and detailed information.

GUIDELINES FOR DOCUMENTATION AND RECORDING ASSESSMENTS

Documentation of the assessment process provides a basis for the development of a plan of care. Record relevant information found during the assessment and interview under the appropriate heading in written reports. Ensure your report reflects the key findings of the assessment. Use the headings in the assessment tool to keep your assessment focused, clear and concise and relevant to the main areas of the assessment. Record any quotes from the client to illustrate your assessment. If scales are used, record appropriate ratings (e.g. severity on a scale of 1–10). Charting also includes the frequency of a particular behaviour over time (e.g. days of the week or months of the year).

If specific headings are used but no relevant information is found this should be stated in the report—for example, 'No relevant information identified during the assessment interview'. This reports clearly the findings of the assessment and may avoid giving the impression that an area of assessment was omitted or neglected. This may be important when the records are reviewed at a later

DISCUSSION QUESTIONS

1. Consider the approach to assessment in your clinical area. What are its main strengths and what are some of the drawback with its use in practice?
2. Identify an assessment tool that is in use on your clinical area. Apply the evaluation criteria for assessment tools set out in this chapter. What are your conclusions in relation to the use of the tool?
3. List the advantages of involving clients in the assessment process. Can you identify any obstacles and how might these be overcome?
4. Consider your approach to involving clients and carers in the assessment process? Are there some circumstances when they are always involved? How do the circumstances affect the level of involvement? What are the consequences of this?
5. Identify some of the skills you use in the assessment interview. Consider how you might improve your own interview skills. What resources do you need for this improvement and how might it be best achieved?

date. What is *not* identified during the assessment may also be important. There may be a lack of information or evidence on a particular issue. This does not necessarily mean that the issue is not important, but simply that no evidence was gathered.

Keep any of your own subjective opinions for a conclusion at the end of the report. If you record your subjective view then ensure it is clearly identified as such and distinct from the objective assessment information. Interpretations of and perspectives on factual information may vary.

SUMMARY

This chapter has identified a range of skills involved in the assessment of clients. A number of different but complementary approaches to assess-

FURTHER READING

Barker P J 1996 Assessment in psychiatric and mental health nursing: in search of the whole person. Stanley Thornes, Cheltenham
This textbook is essential reading for mental health nurses. It provides a detailed overview of assessment instruments and methods with an in-depth exploration of theoretical principles and their application to clinical practice. Moral and ethical issues are explored with specific chapters addressing holistic assessment relating to anxiety, mood, relationships, psychosis and the environment.

Howe G 1988 Mental health assessments. Jessica Kingsley, London
The second book in a series 'Living with serious mental illness' addresses assessment from the perspective of the sufferer or consumer of mental health services. It draws out key issues involved in the assessment process with recommendations for improvements. Drawing on a range of case studies the book identifies the role of different agencies—both health and social care—in the assessment process, emphasizing the significant role to be played by carers.

Newell R 1994 Interviewing skills for nurses and other health care professionals: a structured approach. Routledge, London
A very practical and helpful book for those learning about and developing practical skills in interviewing people with mental health problems. The chapters follow the interview process, opening the interview, developing a therapeutic alliance, the use of assessment tools, interpersonal skills used to explore, support and console, evaluation and learning from practice. The book is practice focused with numerous examples from clinical practice. Another essential read.

Robinson J, Elkan R 1996 Health needs assessment. Churchill Livingstone, New York
The focus of this chapter is assessment of individual clients and their individual needs and problems. It is important to take a broader perspective and to look at the health needs of the community at large. This book provides a useful introduction to the assessment of need from sociological and epidemiological perspectives and sets out the public health agenda. Topics including definition and measurement of health, inequalities in health, economics, screening and health profiling are addressed in terms of the implication for nurses.

ment have been identified in order to set the broad context for the use of these assessment skills in clinical practice. This context involves the client's perspective, assessment of risk and the appropriate use of assessment tools. The aim of assessment as a means of collecting data about the client's health status is acknowledged while the principle of using the assessment process as a means of engaging the client in a therapeutic relationship is emphasized.

REFERENCES

Brown V A 1998 Psychiatric assessment: pre and post admission assessment. Forensic Focus 8. Jessica Kingsley, London

DOH (Department of Health) 1996 Building bridges. A guide to arrangements for inter-agency working for the care and protection of severely mentally ill people. DOH, London

Gordon M 1997 Manual of nursing diagnosis; 1997–1998. Mosby-Year Book, St Louis

Hays J S, Larson K 1963 Interacting with Patients. Macmillan Co, New York

Newell R 1994 Interviewing skills for nurses and other health care professionals: a structured approach. Routledge London

Roper N, Logan W, Tierney A 1980 The elements of nursing. Churchill Livingstone, New York

Sainsbury Centre for Mental Health 1997 Pulling together: the future roles and training of mental health staff. Sainsbury Centre for Mental Health, London

Streiner D L 1993 Research methods in psychiatry: a

checklist for evaluating the usefulness of rating scales. Canadian Journal of Psychiatry 38(2):140–148

Wing J K, Curtis R H, Beevor A S 1996 HoNOS Health of the Nation Outcome Scales. Royal College of Psychiatrists, London

Zito Trust 1997 Learning the Lessons. Zito Trust, London

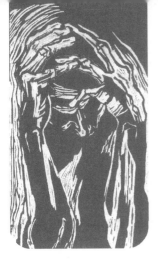

Chapter Twenty-four

Evidence-based practice and clinical effectiveness

Patrick Sullivan

AIMS

- ◆ To define evidence-based practice and clinical effectiveness, and to show why both are important in modern mental health nursing

- ◆ To demonstrate why experience and common sense must be supported by appropriate concepts, principles and theoretical models based on valid and reliable research evidence, if mental health nursing is to progress and develop as a profession

- ◆ To argue that mental health nurses should review their practice in light of relevant research and develop appropriate strategies to improve clinical effectiveness

- ◆ To describe how evidence can be applied to practice using a problem-solving process involving four key stages

- ◆ To explain how strategies to facilitate evidence-based practice and clinical effectiveness could be developed utilizing a management of change programme involving practitioners, managers, teachers and service users

KEY ISSUES

The idea that health care should be evidence based and clinically effective has caught the imagination of policy makers, professionals and service users. As a result mental health nurses must review their practice in light of the latest research evidence and develop appropriate strategies for improving clinical effectiveness

Strategies to facilitate evidence-based practice and clinical effectiveness will need to ensure that practitioners are informed about the best available evidence and use this information to change and monitor their clinical practice

Evidence-based practice can be conceptualized in terms of a problem-solving process that involves finding evidence, utilizing critical appraisal skills, practice development and evaluation of outcomes

Implementing evidence-based practice and clinical effectiveness is not easy, and will require changes in both culture and attitude. This will not occur automatically, and promoting change and innovation is a complex process that must involve practitioners, teachers, managers and service users

Evidence-based practice and clinical effectiveness offer both challenges and opportunities to mental health nurses; failure to meet the challenges and grasp the opportunities could have serious implications for the profession's future

It ought to be a matter of genuine concern—to patients, health professionals, politicians and taxpayers—that there is little, and often no scientific basis for most of the health care which is delivered under the name of the National Health Service.
Baker 1996

INTRODUCTION

This chapter will provide an introduction to evidence-based practice and clinical effectiveness in mental health nursing. Its aim will be to consider what this approach has to offer the practitioner and how it will benefit the service user. In adopting such an approach to their work mental health nurses will be emphasizing the importance of using empirical evidence in a rigorous way in order to demonstrate that the realities of their work has a sound conceptual base.

This is a complex area and it will not be possible to provide a model that can be applied to every practicality. The approach in fact reflects an attempt to provide an overview of the key issues, which means there will be a need to be selective. However, a balance will be maintained between theory and practice and wherever possible the points made will be illustrated by practical examples.

Underpinning the chapter will be four basic assumptions. First, mental health nursing is a specialized area of practice and the main focus of therapeutic activity is interpersonal processes used sensitively and in an antidiscriminatory way in order to bring about changes in behaviour. Secondly, different people perceive mental health nursing in different ways and from different theoretical perspectives. No single approach will satisfy everybody and the reality of clinical practice is a rather eclectic approach to intervention based on interprofessional and interagency working. Thirdly, despite this eclecticism and its very practical nature, mental health nursing is not just a matter of common sense and experience, although both are important; practice must also be linked to theory by the use of appropriate concepts, principles and theoretical models. Finally, a focus on evidence-based practice and clinical effectiveness can help bridge the gap between theory and practice and as such both are the business of practitioners, teachers, managers and service users.

EVIDENCE-BASED PRACTICE AND CLINICAL EFFECTIVENESS: A DEFINITION OF TERMINOLOGY

There is a growing literature on evidence-based practice and clinical effectiveness but, unfortunately, the variety of terms used to describe the process has resulted in some confusion (Kitson 1997). However, certain strands of activity can be identified.

First, there is a push to take research seriously, which follows the publication of a similarly titled report and led to the the launch of the NHS research and development (R&D) strategy in 1991 (DOH 1990, 1993). The strategy aims to create a research-based health service in which scientific evidence is used as a basis for decision making in policy development, service management and clinical practice. Research in this context has a very clear meaning. It is a systematic approach to inquiry that is designed to provide new knowledge needed to improve the performance of the NHS in improving the health of the nation. Such work must be based on a clear protocol, peer reviewed and generalizable (Task Force on R&D in the NHS 1994).

Secondly, there is a focus on evidence-based practice, which appears to derive largely from the concept of evidence-based medicine. This is a problem-focused process designed as a clinical learning tool in Canada at Macmaster University Medical School during the 1980s (Rosenberg & Donald 1995). It has been defined by Sackett et al (1996) as 'the conscientious, explicit and judicious use of current best evidence in making decisions about the care of individual patients'. Evidence-based medicine reflects a particular way of working based on a process of informed decision making. The adoption of this approach by a wide range of health care professionals suggests that evidence-based practice is a more appropriate term (Newman, Papadopoulos & Sigsworth 1998). It involves using a portfolio of skills to aid decision making and facilitate improved clinical practice. The essence is a problem-solving approach utilizing knowledge and understanding of the most recent research-based evidence.

Finally, the term 'clinical effectiveness' is related to the process of evidence-based practice, but rather than describing a way of working it is used in a broader sense to describe the process of utilizing research in order to improve patient outcomes. The NHS Executive publication Promoting clinical effectiveness described it as 'The extent to which specific clinical interventions, when deployed in the field for a particular patient or population, do what they are intended to do, that is, maintain and improve health and secure the greatest possible health gain from available resources' (NHS Executive 1996a).

WHY EVIDENCE-BASED PRACTICE AND CLINICAL EFFECTIVENESS ARE IMPORTANT IN MENTAL HEALTH NURSING

Mental health nursing is a practical activity and many nurses take the view that experience and the mere repetition of activity automatically lead to improved practice. The theory–practice gap in nursing is well documented and theory is often seen as remote, impractical and irrelevant. As a result clinical problems are often dealt with using an unsystematic approach to intervention based on a combination of common sense and routine ways of doing things. However, commonsense knowledge always reflects certain assumptions, and the practitioner inevitably utilizes some form of clinical-decision making model and associated knowledge base to guide interventions. Unfortunately, practitioners who function on the basis of unrecognized theory run the risk of using a very limited approach to intervention based on a very narrow perspective. The outcome is a wide variation in approaches and the use of out of date models which lack sophistication and whose only basis

is a combination of personal preference and institutional tradition. Interventions can then be ineffective or harmful and yet be incorporated into routine ways of delivering care.

The nursing profession generally and mental health nursing particularly, cannot allow such a situation to continue and, as Mason (1992) has quite rightly argued, it is inarguably better to base our practice on research evidence rather than tradition: on science rather than ritual. The rigour of the research process generates evidence that forms a more accurate basis for the delivery of care than tradition, and consistency in care giving is more likely to be achieved through research than through habit' (Mason 1992, p. 38). It should therefore come as no surprise that the idea that health care interventions should be based on valid and reliable research-based evidence has caught the imagination of policy makers, professionals and service users. Consequently the role of research and the concepts of evidence-based practice and clinical effectiveness have become the focus of attention from a variety of quarters, and during the 1990s there has been a concerted push to use research for the benefit of the service user and to take action to develop and implement a strategy for improving clinical effectiveness (NHS Executive 1996a).

EVIDENCE-BASED PRACTICE AND MENTAL HEALTH NURSING

These developments should come as no surprise as the nursing profession has long had an interest in identifying a clear theoretical basis for practice. In fact, considerable work has examined the relationship between theory, practice and research, and a broad professional consensus can be identified around the role research should play in clinical practice. In a mental health setting, Stuart & Sundeen (1983) have argued that theory must be generated on the basis of practical experience and validated through the research process. Such theory must then be utilized to direct clinical practice and effect clinical outcomes. If this is achieved then research is not merely an academic exercise.

A clear evidence base is increasingly important as psychiatric nurses focus their interventions on individuals with severe and enduring mental illness. When faced with clients who present with complex and challenging problems it is most important that interventions are based on valid and reliable evidence that is clinically effective. Variations in practice that cannot be explained are no longer acceptable and mechanisms must be found that can reduce uncertainty and encourage consistency in clinical practice. An increasing focus on evidence-based practice and clinical effectiveness is a means to this end. However, successful implementation of these approaches in mental health care depends on activity at three levels. These are to: (NHS Executive, 1996a, Nursing Times/NHS Executive 1998):

◆ *Inform*—ensuring that practitioners know what is clinically effective and that interventions are based on the best available evidence.
◆ *Change*—using this information to review, and where appropriate change routine clinical practice.
◆ *Monitor*—making certain that changes in practice result in measurable improvements in the quality of care provided.

These three main functions can be conceptualized in terms of a problem-solving process based on the following stages:

◆ finding evidence to help solve problems identified during nursing intervention
◆ evaluating the evidence and considering its applicability to practice
◆ implementing useful findings in the clinical situation by utilizing sustainable models of practice development in order to promote innovation and change
◆ evaluating the impact of implementation on clinical practice in order to ensure that interventions are more clinically effective.

FINDING THE EVIDENCE: THE PURSUIT OF QUALITY INFORMATION

The introduction of evidence-based practice is dependent on the successful integration of the realities of mental health nursing care with the critical analysis of the research literature. As a result, practitioners need to reflect on their practice and identify clinically important questions based on their experience. The next step is then to try to answer these questions based on the research evidence available. Success is dependent on obtaining good quality information and there are a number ways of achieving this. It is important to consider a number in some detail.

Some practitioners regularly access literature-searching facilities in order to facilitate this process and many nurses will be aware of the variety of information systems to support computerized literature searching. The most used are MEDLINE, CINAHL and EMBASE.

MEDLINE

This is the main database covering the international literature on medicine. However, it does include information from other health fields, as well as some broader information from the biological and social sciences. Information is included if it has a clear relationship with health care generally and medicine in particular.

CINAHL

This is the major database covering the nursing and allied health literature and covers the main journals that cover these topic areas. CINAHL is the database most used by nursing staff.

EMBASE

This covers medical literature and has a strong coverage of European work, particularly in areas such as pharmacology.

Other databases that may prove to be of value to mental health nurses are PSYCHLIT, which provides worldwide coverage of the literature relating to psychology, and SOCSCI, which contains information about educational, psychological and sociological research. Effective literature searching allows the practitioner to access research that is relevant to a clinical problem they may be facing in their day to day work and a number of detailed guides to this process are available.

However, not all practitioners have the time, skills or facilities to conduct their own literature searches and in recognition of this fact the Department of Health has been committed to increasing the body of available information. As a result there are a number of sources of information. Facilities such as the Cochrane Library, the NHS Centre for Reviews and Dissemination and the National Research Register may be useful.

Cochrane Library

This is a regularly updated electronic library incorporating four major databases that include information on systematic reviews, controlled trials and research methodology.

NHS Centre for Reviews and Dissemination

This centre is based at the University of York and aims to identify, review and disseminate the results of good quality research. For example, its Practice and Service Developments Initiatives (PDSI) is trying to provide a national focus for information on service and practice developments.

The National Research Register

This is a database of current research and development activity in the NHS.

The main difficulty with these three initiatives is that they are primarily designed to manage a large body of data about major R&D activity. As such they are of considerable value to psychiatric nurses engaged in such activity. However, as Ward & Reed (1997) have pointed out, these systems may not satisfy the needs of practitioners who want to use research to help deal with day to day clinical problems.

In response to this difficulty an increasing amount of published information is being made available that practising nurses may find more useful. For example, effective health care bulletins provide guidance on clinical practice based on a review of the available evidence. A number of reviews from the NHS Centre for Reviews and Dissemination have focused on topics of specific interest to mental health nurses. In addition publications like Effectiveness Matters and Bandolier also provide valuable information and journals like the Journal of Clinical Effectiveness and Evidence-based Medicine have published work on psychiatric issues. An example is the systematic review by Brooker, Repper & Booth (1996) of the effectiveness of community mental health nurses. The Journal of Clinical Effectiveness in Nursing and Evidence-Based Nursing are recent additions to the literature that focus on evidence-based practice from a nursing perspective.

There have also been a number of developments that relate specifically to the area of mental health. For instance, the report of the mental health nursing review team Working in partnership called for the establishment of a specific service for nurses in the specialty that would be run along the lines of MIDAS (Midwives Information Research Service), which provides the latest information on R&D in midwifery. Some progress towards developing such a service has been demonstrated through innovations like the Network for Psychiatric Nursing Research, which was formed in 1996. This is a project funded by the Department of Health and located in Oxford. Its aim is to provide a resource and contact for mental health nurses interested in research and practice development and possesses a database of information designed to support the implementation of evidence-based practice in the specialty. It publishes a regular newsletter called Network and regular updates are found in the Nursing Standard (Ward & Reed 1997). Another recent addition to published materials has been the newsletter from the Maudsley Hospital called The Evidence, which provides a means of communicating up to date research findings to those involved in planning and delivering psychiatric services.

Many practitioners also access the Internet on a regular basis. This is a means of gaining direct access to a vast array of information and allows participants the opportunity to communicate, obtain information, exchange ideas and network. There are an increasing number of sites on the Internet that contain useful information about health care issues and guides available to help clinicians find the information they require (Edwards 1995, Kiley 1996). There is in fact an evidence-based mental health website that includes a collection of tools to help practitioners develop skills relating to evidence-based practice, access to the journal Evidence-based Mental Health and the text of clinical guidelines produced by the Royal College of Psychiatrists. The main problem with the Internet is that it can be difficult to find appropriate information quickly and, given the volume of information available, there is no guarantee of quality.

Finally, no review of the information available would be complete without some consideration of the role of systematic reviews. These reviews provide a more rigorous approach to identifying evidence about a particular topic than can ever be achieved by an ordinary literature search. A systematic review constitutes a piece of research in its own right and involves examining all the available evidence about a particular clinical issue. Bannigan, Droogan & Entwhistle (1997) describe it as a process of 'finding, appraising and synthesising evidence from scientific studies to obtain a reliable overview of research in a specific area'. The aim of a review is to improve clinical decision making and as a result it is a valuable tool in supporting the drive towards evidence-based practice and clinical effectiveness. For example, Droogan & Bannigan (1997) have reported on a systematic review that found that family interventions with schizophrenia were effective in reducing relapse. The obvious clinical application of such information is that mental health nurses should consider using such interventions with this client group, either as an integral part of the treatment plan or in conjunction with other forms of treatment.

EVALUATING THE EVIDENCE: DEVELOPING CRITICAL APPRAISAL SKILLS

Evidence-based practice and clinical effectiveness involve using research findings and it is important that mental health nurses consider their approach to research not in terms of their ability to undertake original work, but rather in their ability to question practice and to make use of evidence. As Collins & Robinson (1996) put it, 'it is important to dispel the myth that all practitioners should carry out research, though they should use elements of the research process to develop a questioning and evaluative approach to care'. This means practitioners should be able to evaluate evidence in order to be sure it is of high quality, based on rigorous and systematic inquiry, and of potential value in the clinical situation.

Numerous guides to evaluating research are available and these describe how the application of skills in critical appraisal can help practitioners evaluate the evidence available to them. Key factors that need to be considered include:

◆ the relevance and importance of the work
◆ the appropriateness of the design and methodology used
◆ the representativeness of the sample
◆ the rigour of the data analysis
◆ the significance of the findings
◆ the quality of the conclusions
◆ the applicability of the findings to practice.

In considering the available literature, the practitioner is faced with a range of studies using a variety of research methods, including randomized control trials, non-randomized trials, observational methods, interviews, surveys and case studies, which are supplemented by their own clinical experience. Evaluating this evidence is complex and current policy initiatives are driven by a model informed by a 'hierarchy of evidence' (Long 1996). The different levels of evidence are as follows:

◆ *Level 1*—randomized controlled trials
◆ *Level 2*—controlled trials without randomization
◆ *Level 3*—cohort studies
◆ *Level 4*—time series designs
◆ *Level 5*—descriptive studies and informed professional opinion.

Clearly the scientific community has a preference for quantitative research techniques, which follow a natural science model. As a result the most appropriate methodologies are experimental or quasi-experimental designs, which emphasize empirical observations that lend themselves to mathematical analysis (Treece & Treece 1986). However, as Repper & Brooker (1998) have noted, there are few rigorous studies of this type that measure the impact of nursing interventions on health gain in a mental health setting. This reflects the very real difficulties experienced by researchers who attempt to achieve this objective. Although it should be possible to determine the value of any specific intervention by utilizing it in practice and observing the outcome, the reality is more complex. As Eddy (1984) has explained in relation to health care generally, 'uncertainty, biases, errors, and differences of opinions, motives, and values' weaken the links in the complex chain of clinical decision making. Nowhere is this process better illustrated than in mental health nursing.

The nature and origins of mental health problems remain controversial and the relationship between research, theory and mental health nursing skills has not been clearly articulated. As Chambers (1998) has argued, 'the primary functions of mental health nursing—the relationship building and therapeutic interactions—are couched in intangible language. There are problems in articulating and measuring them.' Consequently, there is considerable debate about appropriate modes of intervention and mental health nurses are faced with a 'conceptual pluralism' (Bolman & Deal 1984) when attempting to identify a clear body of evidence to underpin their clinical work. A range of approaches are described in the literature and the role of the psychiatric nurse is, in fact, difficult to define. Good practice seems to be an intuitive and experiential process that is difficult to analyse within a clear theoretical framework and this makes it difficult to examine in a scientific way. As a result, finding appropriate evidence can be problematic.

As there are few studies available that isolate and manipulate variables utilizing a clearly defined conceptual framework, we find a greater use of qualitative studies. These involve the non-numerical organization and interpretation of observations for the purpose of discovering important underlying dimensions and patterns of rela-

tionships (Polit & Hungler 1987). The findings from these studies need to be approached with some caution. Although there are qualitative studies that are rigorous and systematic, many are not. As a result, the practitioner must always be aware of the possibility of bias and subjectivity, which means the reliability and validity of such findings are then questionable. These difficulties mean that many existing studies relating to mental health nursing are potentially weak in both design and methodology. The danger of making use of research that is of dubious value is very real and this makes critical evaluation skills so important in mental health care. However, the body of available evidence is growing all the time and it is the application of evidence to practice that is often the most demanding aspect of any efforts to base interventions on evidence and improve clinical effectiveness.

MAKING USE OF THE EVIDENCE: PRACTICE DEVELOPMENT

The use of research evidence as the basis for nursing intervention requires the use of tools that enable practising nurses to utilize evidence in a practical way. It has been noted that bridging the gap between theory and practice 'requires both a means to translate research findings into the language and action of practice, and the opportunity to elicit sustained changes based on these findings' (Foundation of Nursing Studies 1996). A number of mechanisms exist that may help facilitate this process:

◆ the development of clinical guidelines based on sound evidence about best practice
◆ the setting of clinical standards on the basis of such guidance
◆ effective care planning to facilitate application of guidelines and the meeting of standards in practice
◆ the introduction of care pathways in order to help standardize best practice
◆ local research implementation and development projects.

Clinical guidelines are 'systematically developed statements which assist clinicians and patients in making decisions about appropriate treatment for specific conditions' (NHS Executive 1996b). The impact of clinical guidelines on medical practice has been evaluated systematically and it has been shown that they can be effective in changing practice and improving patient outcomes (Grimshaw & Russell 1993). Such guidance is applicable in a nursing context and offers a means of applying research evidence to practice, by providing precise and detailed guidance reflecting best practice for a specific client group (Antrobus & Brown 1996, Cheater & Closs 1997).

If used properly, such guidance can serve to provide the baseline for clinical standards that clearly state what is expected of nursing staff. This is achieved by specifying activity in relation to outcome and detailing the actual performance to be achieved in terms of a defined measure or indicator (Ovretveit 1992). Practical implementation is then dependent on the ability of nursing staff to incorporate the detail into the process of care planning. It is then possible to provide a clear rationale for each intervention and helps staff avoid ritual activity, which is merely a reflection of routine practice in the clinical area. A practical example of this sort of activity is provided by Robinson, Gajos & Whyte (1997). They describe how the development of a ward-based learning package was utilized in order to focus on the systematic process of care planning, which involved nurses finding and using research about therapeutic interaction in assessing, planning, implementing and evaluating nursing care.

This sort of process facilitates an evidence-based approach to everyday clinical problems and in the future is likely to be facilitated by the development of care pathways. These are essentially a map of the patient's planned care that specify anticipated interventions and are developed for individual patients based on their particular need (Walsh 1997). The rationale for care pathways is that individuals with a common problem will each receive a programme of care involving certain commonalities. As a result the predictable aspects of an individual's care programme can be pre-planned, whilst still focusing on specific individual needs as they occur.

According to Walsh (1997) care pathways provide a means to focus on outcomes, multidisciplinary collaboration and clear accountability. By planning each individual's pathway of care it is possible to identify critical points in the care programme with expected outcomes. The focus on a multidisciplinary approach means the professionals involved must agree their relevant contribution. Care pathways are a potential tool to support evidence-based practice and clinical effectiveness. By using multidisciplinary guidelines that incorporate local best practice, national guidance and research evidence it should be possible to develop pathways in mental health care that specify goals and proposed interventions based on clearly articulated standards of care across both disciplines and agencies. This provides the means both to facilitate and to evaluate the process and outcome of clinical intervention and to improve practice.

One mechanism that has been shown to be effective in promoting this type of innovation is the use of local research and practice development projects. A practical example of this sort of work is provided by the King's Fund programme Promoting Action on Clinical Effectiveness (PACE). PACE has been funded by the NHS Executive and has supported 16 local projects working on a clinical topic where there is known to be evidence about clinical effectiveness. An example from mental health is family support with patients suffering from schizophrenia. Projects have to be multidisciplinary and involve patients, clinicians and managers. What is becoming clear from this type of work is the need to focus on high priority issues and to have support from key senior personnel in all the local organizations involved.

The process is based on a systematic approach to assessing and managing a specific clinical problem and incorporates a number of key stages. First, there is assessment of current practice to identify the need to change. Secondly, a change programme is planned. Thirdly, there is put into place project management arrangements that focus on what is achievable using realistic timescales.

Finally, systems are developed to monitor the impact of the changes planned. This type of activity is best supported by practice development models that utilize action inquiry methods to identify real clinical problems and to derive strategies for change from observation of everyday practice (Kitson et al 1996).

The approaches described provide a means both to utilize research as a framework for nursing intervention and to translate the theoretical into the practical. They offer the practitioner a series of tools to help make sure that interventions are based on what is effective rather than merely thought to be effective. This is the essence of evidence-based approaches to nursing practice and the final part of the cycle involves demonstrating clinical effectiveness through regular evaluation.

EVALUATING THE OUTCOME: ENSURING IMPROVEMENTS IN THE QUALITY OF CARE

The application of evidence to practice should lead to improvements in clinical effectiveness. Consequently, any changes in clinical practice must incorporate appropriate feedback to ensure that the change has been implemented properly and that improvements in care can be demonstrated. In mental health care this involves considering improvements in areas such as symptom control, coping skills, social functioning and quality of life (Parry 1996, Thomas 1996). This requires systematic evaluation of processes and outcomes in the clinical situation, and this should always be built into the process of practice development. Kitson et al (1996) make this point very clearly when they state that, 'criteria for evaluating the impact of the intervention must be identified and agreed before implementing any change'. This has to be done scientifically and involves the rigorous collection of baseline information on current practice. This is followed by ongoing evaluation against clear outcomes after change has taken place.

Clinical audit provides a mechanism for this to be carried out by clinical staff. This is a 'systematic and critical analysis of the quality of clinical care', and offers a means by which judgements can be made against predetermined standards based on clinical guidelines. Ongoing practice development is then supported by continuous application of the audit cycle involving standard setting, observation of practice, evaluation against standards, action and constant review (Cheater & Closs 1997, Frost & Monteith 1996, NHS Executive 1996c).

Clinical audit involves a number of clear stages (National Centre for Clinical Audit 1997):

◆ deciding on a topic to audit, the reasons for doing the audit, how the quality of care is going to be measured in the audit, and the cases to be included
◆ collecting data on actual practice using the agreed measures of quality
◆ evaluating the findings of data collection to identify any shortcomings in care and their causes
◆ acting to make improvements in care
◆ repeating the data collection, evaluation and action steps as often as needed to achieve and sustain improvements.

Clinical audit is an essential part of any clinical effectiveness strategy. Unlike research it does not define evidence-based practice; rather it is a way of measuring the extent to which evidence-based approaches are utilized on a day to day basis. Unfortunately, in mental health care this process is not always straightforward, as outcomes are notoriously difficult to to measure. However, recent innovations like the Health of the Nation Outcomes Scales (HoNOS) may help in this respect. The Department of Health expects HoNOS to be incorporated into routine clinical practice and this may help nurses who are attempting to adopt evidence-based approaches to care. It is an assessment tool that incorporates 12 scales covering key areas of health and social functioning in individuals with mental health problems, and provides a means of recording progress on the basis of a series of outcome measures. By providing a numerical evaluation, it is easy to make comparisons across time and to assess the effects of interventions in a variety of areas (Wing, Curtis & Beevor 1996).

CHANGING CLINICAL PRACTICE: THE DEVELOPMENT OF AN EVIDENCE-BASED CULTURE

Unfortunately, as many practitioners will immediately recognize, the above remains a rather idealistic picture and does not reflect the realities of clinical practice in many areas of mental health nursing. As Lomas & Haynes (1987) stated of health care in general, 'in an ideal world, there would be no gap between what is known from sound research about the means to promote health and the means actually employed by health care practitioners in administering care to their patients. In fact, however, there is a distressing distance between care knowledge in general and the practices of individual clinicians for most validated health care procedures'. In reality, changing clinical behaviour is the biggest obstacle facing the development of evidence-based practice and those involved must understand the complex processes involved in implementing change.

There is a growing consensus regarding the factors known to impede the application of research in practice and these can be overcome only by addressing issues at a number of levels. This is a point made particularly well by MacGuire (1990) when she states that 'the integration of research and practice has to be addressed at all levels within an organisation; from policy statements to procedure manuals and from managers, educators and clinicians to support workers within the framework of the management of change'. This is a complex process that involves changing the culture and attitude pervading much of the professional practice in the NHS (Close & Cheater 1994). Such change will require moving away from what Griffiths & Luker (1997) have referred to as a 'non-challenging professional culture that sometimes stands in the way of optimal patient care'. In its place a more challenging and evaluative culture will need to develop. The basis of this must be formal structures that actively promote standard setting, clinical guidelines, care pathways, practice development models and regular audit in order to avoid widespread differences in

practice that cannot be explained in terms of variables like morbidity or social circumstances.

As Griffiths & Luker (1997) clearly demonstrate, evidence-based practice is not just about the critical review of research papers; it involves the critical analysis of practice followed by change when this is shown to be necessary. A sound knowledge of good practice and a working environment characterized by inquiry, initiative, innovation and learning are a means to this end. Such an environment would support the pursuit of excellence in practice and help mental health nurses to examine and improve the organisation and delivery of their work continually with the aim of constantly improving the care provided to the clients they work with. However, practice development of this type can be threatening and, as Robinson (1987) has argued, innovation and change 'can throw into question the meaning practitioners have given to their working lives for many years. We should not be surprised therefore if the validity of the proposals is denied and if practitioners maintain that because it is they who do the work, only they can be expected to know what is best.' For this reason practice development must always be based on the utilization of deliberate strategies to address the gap that often exists between scientific knowledge and its clinical application (Ketifan 1996). In practical terms there are, in fact, a number of key activities that must underpin any local framework for developing evidence-based practice and promoting clinical effectiveness.

First, health care management involves supporting staff in providing direct individualized care. The participation of service managers is, therefore, essential in the development of evidence-based approaches to care. For example, practitioners need to be supported by strategies that aim to improve the communication and dissemination of research findings. Practitioners can make use of evidence only if it is accessible, usable and properly communicated. This has resource implications as it requires investment in facilities such as libraries and information technology. For instance, every service should have access to some of the major sources of information considered earlier. In addition, every effort should be made to ensure that time is made available for staff to make use of this information and that local expertise and support are made available to ensure that time and facilities are utilized to maximum benefit. This has very real financial implications and it will be important for mental health services to pursue resources actively and make use of the opportunities offered by the funding arrangements for R&D.

Secondly, mental health services must create an environment that encourages professional development. This demands an organizational commitment to continuing professional education based on individualized training and development plans and a commitment to lifelong learning. This aims to bridge the gap between 'doing without knowledge' and 'knowledge without doing' (NHS Executive 1998), avoiding what Ashworth & Longmate (1993) call the 'unreflective day to day enactment of the work role'. This will be achieved only by training and development programmes that are designed to facilitate a questioning and evaluative approach to care. Such work-based learning programmes must be practice and client focused and avoid developing theoretical knowledge in isolation from experiential knowledge and clinical expertise. They must be clearly grounded in reality and facilitate the integration of theory and practice by emphasizing both knowledge and skills development in order to benefit the client.

In terms of content, educational programmes must provide practitioners with the critical reading and appraisal skills that are needed to understand, analyse and make judgements about the applicability of research findings to practice. However, in addition, practitioners must also be able to develop a fairly sophisticated awareness of the complex factors that contribute to the introduction of change and particularly the skills required in order to deal with resistance to innovation. This requires the utilization of a variety of teaching and learning methods that have the potential to integrate theory and practice. Examples from the literature include problem-based learning and practice write-ups. The former is based on work to improve problem-solving skills and relate theoretical principles to clinical

reality (Andrews & Reece-Jones 1996). The latter involves written analysis of routine experience and is a way of applying research by highlighting the evidence base being used in everyday practice (Gormley 1997).

Thirdly, evidence-based practice is about multi-disciplinary teamwork, and effective clinical leadership is essential in order to promote and support effective team performance. It is, therefore, imperative that suitably qualified staff are available in roles that provide the opportunity to develop the kind of working environment in which evidence-based practice can flourish. These individuals can act as role models who are able to demonstrate positive clinical attitudes and use their clinical expertise to develop models of good practice. Clinical nurse managers, ward managers, team leaders, lecturer practitioners, practice development nurses, clinical audit facilitators, nurse teachers and academics may all play their part in this process. They are able to provide the necessary expertise to utilize change management skills and apply change management theory to the development of nursing practice. This must incorporate the development of philosophies of care, approaches to care planning, systems of care delivery and processes of evaluation that are built around the needs of the client and reflect the application of evidence to practice. As part of this process, service providers should encourage the development of clinical guidelines and actively support the use of clinical audit and quality assurance programmes to change practice.

Finally, the most important part of the process is the activities of individual practitioners for, at this level, 'unless behaviour changes nothing changes' (Plant 1987). This means that learning and everyday clinical practice must be integrated. As a result all nursing staff must be encouraged to learn from both the problems and the successes of everyday clinical work. This requires each practitioner to be committed to their own continuous professional development and this needs to be reflected in a personal development plan. This provides a framework by which the individual practitioners' individual learning needs are clearly linked to the educational and managerial processes described previously. The major tools available to help practitioners learn from real experiences are systematic and structured clinical supervision and reflective practice. These enable nurses to consider their practice and to think about the interventions they use in terms of the theoretical knowledge base available. For this to occur it is important that supervisors have both the clinical and educational expertise to enable practitioners to undertake this process. It is only in this way that it is possible to facilitate evidence-based practice by grounding the application of evidence in the day to day clinical work of nurses and to improve the standard of nursing care through the systematic application of clinically effective interventions. As Fowler (1996) points out, theory can to some extent be 'taught' in the classroom, but it can only be 'mastered' through supervised practice.

SUMMARY

The move towards clinical effectiveness and the introduction of evidence-based approaches in mental health nursing involve making best practice routine and interventions outcome orientated. It presents a challenge to managers, teachers and practitioners that, if met, will have considerable benefits for those who use mental health services. Failure to meet the challenge will condemn mental health nursing to the dangers of complacency, stagnation and professional decline, leaving service users at the mercy of a series of interventions that at best cannot be shown to be clinically effective and at worst are potentially harmful, inequitable and even discriminatory. Mental health nurses must be able to demonstrate how their clinical practice is effective or their role is subject to challenge. Evidence-based practice and clinical effectiveness are two components of a health care agenda that poses both threats and opportunities. Failure to grasp the opportunities could have serious implications for mental health nursing roles in the future. A profession that fails to change its values and holds on to tradition and routine in the face of developing technologies, more knowledge, increased information and rising expectations is a profession that is unlikely to survive in any recognizable form in the future.

DISCUSSION QUESTIONS

1. Define evidence-based practice and clinical effectiveness and discuss their importance in modern mental health care.
2. Describe the facilities available to support evidence-based practice and clinical effectiveness in mental health nursing.
3. Describe an area of clinical practice and consider how the application of an evidence-based approach could encourage practice development and improve clinical effectiveness.
4. Consider the strategies required to develop a culture of evidence-based practice in mental health care.

REFERENCES

Andrews M, Reece-Jones P 1996 Problem based learning in an undergraduate programme: a case study. Journal of Advanced Nursing 23:357–365

Antrobus S, Brown S 1996 Guidelines and protocols: a chance to take the lead. Nursing Standard 92(23):38–39

Ashworth P D, Longmate M A 1993 Theory and practice: beyond the dichotomy. Nurse Education Today 13:321–327

Baker M 1996 Challenging ignorance. In: Baker M, Kirk S (eds) Research and development for the NHS. Evidence, evaluation and effectiveness. Radcliffe Medical Press, Oxford, ch 3, pp 19–26

Bannigan K, Droogan J, Entwhistle V 1997 Systematic reviews: what do they involve? Nursing Times 93:52–53

Bolman L G, Deal T E 1984 Modern approaches to understanding and managing organisations. Jossey Bass, San Francisco CA

Brooker C, Repper J M, Booth A 1996 The effectiveness of community mental health nursing: a review. Journal of Clinical Effectiveness 1(2):43–50

Chambers M 1998 Mental health nursing: the challenge of evidence based practice. Mental Health Practice 1(8):18–22

Cheater F M, Closs S J 1997 The effectiveness of methods of dissemination and implementation of clinical guidelines for nursing practice: a selective review. Clinical Effectiveness in Nursing, 1(1):4–15

Closs S J, Closs F M 1994 Utilisation of nursing research. Journal of Advanced Nursing 19:762–773

FURTHER READING

The range of information available on evidence-based practice and clinical effectiveness is already vast and is being added to all the time. Of particular value are a number of publications that are widely available and easy to read, and provide detailed summaries of the pertinent issues. These are listed below.

NHS Executive 1996 Promoting clinical effectiveness. Department of Health, Leeds

NHS Executive 1996 Clinical guidelines. Using clinical guidelines to improve patient care within the NHS. Department of Health, Leeds

NHS Executive 1996 Information on clinical effectiveness. Department of Health, Leeds

NHS Executive 1996 Clinical audit in the NHS. Using clinical audit in the NHS: a position statement. Department of Health, Leeds

NHS Executive 1997 Clinical effectiveness, resource pack. Department of Health, Leeds

Nursing Times/NHS Executive 1998 Clinical effectiveness for nurses, midwives and health visitors. Nursing Times, EMAP Healthcare, London

RCN 1996 Clinical effectiveness, a Royal College of Nursing guide. RCN, London

Walshe K, Ham C 1997 Acting on the evidence progress in the NHS. University of Birmingham HSMC, Birmingham

Collins M, Robinson D 1996 Bridging the research–practic gap: the role of the link nurse. Nursing Standard 10(25):44–46

DOH (Department of Health) 1990 Taking research seriously. HMSO, London

DOH (Department of Health) 1993 Research for health. A research and development strategy for the NHS. HMSO, London

DOH (Department of Health) 1994 Working in partnership: report of the Mental Health Nursing Review Working Group. DOH, London

Droogan J, Bannigan K 1997 A review of psychosocial family interventions for schizophrenia. Nursing Times 93(27):46–47

Eddy D 1984 Variations in physician practice: the role of uncertainty. In: Dowie J, Elstein A (eds) Professional judgement, a reader in clinical decision making. Cambridge University Press, Cambridge, ch 1, pp 45–59

Edwards M 1995 The internet for nurses and allied health professionals. Springer, Calgary

Foundation of Nursing Studies 1996 Reflection for action. FONS, London

Fowler J 1996 The organisation of clinical supervision within the nursing profession: a review of the literature. Journal of Advanced Nursing 23:471–478

Frost D, Monteith K 1996 About face. Health Service Journal February 29:30–32

Gormley K J 1997 Practice write ups. An assessment instrument that contributes to bridging differences between theory and practice for students through the development of skills. Nurse Education Today 17:53–57

Griffiths J M, Luker K A 1997 A barrier to clinical effectiveness: the etiquette of district nursing. Clinical Effectiveness in Nursing 1:121–130

Grimshaw J M, Russell I T 1993 Effect of clinical guidelines on medical practice. A systematic review of rigorous evaluations. The Lancet 342:1317–1322

Ketifan S 1996 Application of research to practice. In: Fulfilling the vision. Dissemination and application of nursing and midwifery research in practice and education. Post conference publication. University of Sheffield, Sheffield, pp 9–15

Kiley R 1996 Medical information on the Internet. A guide for health professionals. Churchill Livingstone, New York

Kitson A 1997 Using evidence to demonstrate the value of nursing. Nursing Standard 11(28):34–39

Kitson A, Ahmed L B, Harvey G, Seers K, Thompson D 1996 From research to practice: one organisational model for promoting research based practice. Journal of Advanced Nursing 23:430–440

Lomas J, Haynes R B 1987 Cited in: Department of Health 1995 Methods to promote the implementation of research findings in the NHS—priorities for evaluation. NHS Executive, Leeds, p. 6

Long A F 1996 Health services research—a radical approach to cross the research and development divide. In: Baker M, Kirks S (eds) Research and development for the NHS. Evidence, evaluation and effectiveness. Radcliffe Medical Press, Oxford, ch 6, pp 51–64

MacGuire J M 1990 Putting nursing research findings into practice: research utilization as an aspect of the management of change. Journal of Advanced Nursing 15:614–620

Mason C 1992 Research in practice: rhetoric or reality? Nursing Standard 25(27):36–39

National Centre for Clinical Audit 1997 Key points from the literature relating to criteria for clinical audit. National Centre for Clinical Audit, London

Newman M, Papadopoulos I, Sigsworth J 1998 Barriers to evidence based practice. Clinical Effectiveness in Nursing 2:11–20

NHS Executive 1996a Promoting clinical effectiveness. Department of Health, Leeds

NHS Executive 1996b Clinical guidelines. Using clinical guidelines to improve patient care within the NHS. Department of Health, Leeds

NHS Executive 1996c Clinical audit in the NHS. Using clinical audit in the NHS: a position statement. Department of Health, Leeds

NHS Executive 1998 Integrating theory and practice in nursing. NHS Executive, Leeds

Nursing Times/NHS Executive 1998 Clinical effectiveness for nurses, midwives and health visitors. Nursing Times, EMAP Healthcare, London

Ovretveit J 1992 Health service quality, an introduction to quality methods for health services. Blackwell, Oxford

Parry G 1996 Using research to change practice. In: Heller T, Reynolds J, Gomm R, Muston R, Pattison S (eds) Mental health matters. Macmillan, London, ch 34, pp 282–289

Plant R 1987 Managing change and making it stick Fontana, London

Polit D F, Hungler B P 1987 Nursing research: principles and practice. Lippincott, Philadelphia

Repper J M, Brooker C 1998 Difficulties in the measurement of outcome in people who have serious mental health problems. Journal of Advanced Nursing 27:75–82

Robinson J 1987 The relevance of research to the ward sister. Journal of Advanced Nursing 12:421–429

Robinson D, Gajos M, Whyte L 1997 Evidence based care through clinical practice. Nursing Standard 11(30):32–33

Rosenberg W, Donald A 1995 Evidence based medicine: an approach to clinical problem solving. British Medical Journal 310:1122–1126

Sackett D L, Rosenberg W M C, Gray J A M, Richardson W S 1996 Evidence based medicine. What it is and what it isn't. British Medical Journal 312:71–72

Stuart G W, Sundeen S S 1983 Principles and practice of psychiatric nursing. C V Mosby, St Louis

Task Force on R&D in the NHS 1994 Supporting research and development in the NHS. HMSO, London

Thomas B 1996 Principles of evaluation. In: Watkins M, Hervey N, Carson J, Ritter S (eds) Collaborative community mental health care. Arnold, London, ch 17, pp 330–349

Treece E W, Treece J W 1986 Elements of research in nursing. C V Mosby, St Louis

Walsh M 1997 Will critical pathways replace the nursing process? Nursing Standard 11(52):39–42

Ward M, Reed J 1997 Developing a research network for mental health nurses. Mental Health Practice 1(1):18–19

Wing J K, Curtis R H, Beevor A S 1996 HoNOS: Health of the Nation Outcome Scales report on research and development July 1993–December 1995. Royal College of Psychiatrists, London

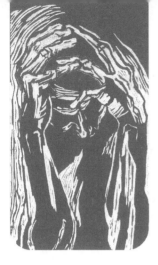

Chapter Twenty-five

Clinical supervision in mental health nursing

Karen Rea   Les Jennings

AIMS

- ◆ To encourage practitioners to reflect upon current professional practice and the role of clinical supervision in improving client care
- ◆ To provide a scheme for practitioners to examine their own current clinical supervision protocols by the exploration of a range of models and frameworks for clinical supervision
- ◆ To provide practitioners with the opportunity to examine difficult and contentious issues which may occur in the clinical arena and to identify management strategies for the resolution of these
- ◆ To encourage practitioners to explore the process of clinical supervision and their role in the facilitation and delivery of supervision

KEY ISSUES

Defining clinical supervision

The purpose of supervision

Benefits of supervision to the mental health nurse and to the service

Models of supervision

Key elements of supervision

Supervision as providing benchmarks for good practice

INTRODUCTION

The services for people with mental health problems have undergone significant and radical changes in recent times. Proposed governmental changes in mental health legislation, the work done by the NHS Confederation and Sainsbury Centre for Mental Health (1997) and the recent debates on mental health practitioner skills (Butterworth 1994, DOH 1994, Faulkner 1998), all indicate a 'shift' in consumer expectations and what constitutes best clinical practice.

What is evident is a growing realization that many practitioners in mental health will need to extend the parameters of their professional and vocational functions and become more autonomous and responsible for their practice. This autonomy, and related increase in the scope of practice for mental health workers, although welcomed, evidences a tacit acknowledgment of what Goldberg (1986) describes as a potential for 'increasing isolation and existential exhaustion'.

In addition, the work of Kennerley (1990) offers powerful indicators that many practitioners experience and report an increase in the level of anxiety and stress in their work. Contemporary management theory (Torrington & Weightman 1994), if translated into the world of mental health care, would suggest that there is a need for services that both support and facilitate practitioners whilst attending to the needs of the consumer. Supervision, if undertaken in a coherent, consistent and logical fashion, can offer the conduit or infrastructure required to help meet the needs of all parties within a service provision that is continually in a state of flux and change.

However, if you think for a moment about your current practice there will be occasions when, at least at some time, this change and complexity can leave you, the practitioner, in a state of 'stuckness' or disempowerment that, ultimately, will translate and parallel into 'real' working situations.

It is our intention here, therefore, to offer the theme of 'boundary violations' and 'stuckness' as the convenient, but complex, theme on which to hang the debate on supervision. This is based on our assumption that much of the contemporary debate concerning tensions within the therapeutic relationship hinges on the violation of acceptable professional boundaries and the resultant increased awareness of the need for supervision in all aspects of health care.

Evidence for our assumptions is based upon the work of commentators such as Briant (1997), Butler & Zelen (1977), Gemma (1989), Pennington et al (1993), Rushton, Ausberg & McEnhill (1996) and Totka (1996). Although writing from a variety of differing experiences, they all begin to explore and offer explanations about some of the 'unspoken and silent' tensions within the arena of professional relationships such as sexuality, what it means to care too much, what it means to care less in a way that might empower and the nature of the professional relationship and friendship. Although we acknowledge that supervision can, and does, extend beyond the apparent solitary issue of boundary violation, it is the above-mentioned accompanying tensions that provide the fertile ground required for the exploration of clinical issues that are pertinent and important in the world of your practice. Furthermore, the violations offer ready available source material within which to locate and explore the issues in a relevant and meaningful way. That said, further to the arguments expressed above, at a more pragmatic level Carroll (1997) argues that qualified practitioners all too easily become enmeshed in routine and forget to update their own learning, ensure that they are able to monitor and reflect on their own practice, and that they are working effectively to care for themselves and their clients and patients. These are reasons, we would argue, for clinical supervision.

In order to begin to address the issues described we shall structure the chapter and discussion under a range of subheadings as indicated below:

WHAT IS CLINICAL SUPERVISION?

Loganbill, Hardy & Delworth in 1982 defined clinical supervision as:

An intensive, interpersonally focused, one to one

relationship in which one person is designed to facilitate the development of therapeutic competencies in the other person.
Loganbill, Hardy & Delworth 1982, cited in Johns 1992

The UKCC's 1996 position paper on clinical supervision contends that:

Clinical supervision brings practitioner(s) and skilled supervisors together to reflect on practice. Supervision aims to identify solutions to problems, improve practice and increase understanding of professional issues.
UKCC 1996

For the British Association of Counselling (BAC 1992), however, the primary purpose of supervision is: 'To protect the best interests of the client'.

The Community Psychiatric Nurses Association document, Guidelines for supervision, describes supervision as 'the corner stone of clinical practice'. As Butterworth & Faugier (1992) comment, though, the implementation of clinical supervision in services has been very ad hoc, often developing from practitioners themselves as a desperate response to critical issues and events in their professional life. The lack, until recently, of any framework for clinical supervision has led to varying practices being identified as 'clinical supervision'. This has led to many practitioners being wary of accepting a practice that appears to have many definitions and interpretations. For nurses, the 1996 UKCC position statement on clinical supervision may go some way to establishing what it is.

Clinical supervision is a collaborative dynamic process extending beyond whilst incorporating a pastoral, nurturing role, which works positively towards 'enabling' the practitioner. In order to work effectively, it requires all parties involved in the relationship to participate actively towards ensuring that the needs of the client/patient are being addressed and monitored and that the supervisee is becoming a more competent practitioner.

Clinical supervision, as we will see in the following section, can and should have undoubted benefits for the practitioner working in the field of mental health. The benefits, however, are not restricted to the practitioner.

Of paramount importance is the potential beneficial effect the implementation of clinical supervision could have on service delivery, which in real terms for people with mental health problems should mean quality services that improve their lives.

WHY CLINICAL SUPERVISION NOW?

The provision of effective mental health care services is a constant challenge. The provision of services sits at times uneasily with economic constraints, ideological positions and the expectations of society and the general public. For practitioners working in this field this can (and often does) represent a mass of contradictions that render their role difficult and the provision of good quality care complex. The support of professionals undertaking such roles is crucial. In addition mental health practitioners have a duty to ensure that their practice is competent and the function of clinical supervision as educative as well as supportive and restorative (Hawkins & Shohet 1989) is critical.

The United Kingdom Central Council (UKCC) Code of professional conduct (1984) makes reference to the links between continuing professional education and the provision and improvement of the quality of patient care by stating that practitioners must:

◆ maintain and improve professional knowledge and competence
◆ acknowledge any limitations in knowledge and competence and decline any duties or responsibilities unless able to perform them in a safe and skilled manner
◆ assist professional colleagues, in the context of your own knowledge, experience and sphere of responsibility, to develop their professional competence, and assist others in the care team, including informal carers, to contribute safely and to a degree appropriate to their roles.

A principal medium for mental health nursing consists of the relationships that practitioners develop with individuals and groups. The initiation, maintenance, development and ending of those relationships can be problematic and stressful and require complicated and demanding skills. Reflection on practice and its effectiveness in meeting the changing health care needs of clients can lead to these skills being constantly redefined and sophisticated throughout professional life.

Clinical-based practitioners are at the heart of effective implementation of management strategies for improving quality of care. In this key position they need to feel valued as people, as professionals and as colleagues.

Feeling valued has two related aspects:

1. it involves nurses believing that what they are doing professionally is valuable, credible and worthwhile
2. and it involves feeling that what they are doing is valued by other whose views are respected and needed (employers, colleagues, clients and their 'significant others').

Within a broad framework of staff development the particular professional relationship within which the above can be systematically explored is clinical supervision. However, nurses working in the field of mental health face constant challenges, which often require them to reflect on the changing nature of their work and role.

Legislative and policy changes in the last two decades have led to an increasing number of practitioners facing major upheavals and differences in their working practices. The need to be constantly updating professional knowledge has never been more paramount and one method of updating knowledge is through the clinical supervision relationship. The 'specialization' process that has occurred in many health units and environments has also required practitioners to reflect upon their existing knowledge base and possibly adopt new strategies to meeting the needs of clients/patients with mental health problems. The supervises can be offered a unique and valuable opportunity to, as Power (1994, p. 105) suggests: 'Explore the often complicated dynamics of their professional, yet personal relationship with their clients, in a safe environment.' Supervisors can provide the supervises with new thoughts and insights into the problems or difficulties that are identified by the client/therapist or counsellor relationship.

It is often useful when reflecting upon therapeutic interventions and responses with a client to have the benefit of an 'outside' view. The gains of using clinical supervision in mental health practice can be identified as:

◆ self-growth
◆ increased job satisfaction
◆ support and sharing of feelings
◆ reduction in staff turnover
◆ reduced stress and burnout
◆ increased confidence and autonomy of practitioners.

For an increasing number of qualified and experienced nurses practising various forms of counselling and psychotherapy, supervision is an essential aspect of their clinical practice. The supervisory process in counselling and psychotherapy facilitates an objective overview and evaluation of the nurse–client relationship. Supervisors can provide the supervisee with new thoughts and insights into the problems or difficulties that are identified by the client/therapist or counsellor.

It is often useful when reflecting upon therapeutic interventions and responses with a client to have the benefit of an 'outside' view. For example, consider the case study outlined below.

CASE STUDY

A community nurse was visiting regularly a young woman with a history of attempted suicide by drug misuse. During one of their meetings the client revealed to the nurse that she was strongly attracted to him. On every occasion after this the young woman raised this attraction whenever they met, and made it clear that she felt their relationship had gone beyond that of the client/therapist.

In terms of clinical supervision there are several factors and issues that needed to be raised and explored. Although we do not provide an exhaustive list of issues, depending on the level of 'maturity' of the supervision relationship, the supervisor may examine with the supervisee:

◆ the client's transference
◆ community nurse's counter-transference
◆ ethical issues
◆ power relationships
◆ exploitation issues and other boundary issues
◆ previous management of the relationship
◆ future management of the relationship
◆ the client's feelings
◆ the community nurse's feelings
◆ attachment styles and responses.

WHY DO PROFESSIONALS WORKING WITH PEOPLE WHO HAVE A MENTAL HEALTH PROBLEM NEED CLINICAL SUPERVISION?

For the many practitioners working in the field of mental health the type of formal training they received was premised on hospital-based care. Policy, legislation and attitudes in the last two decades have led to large numbers of people with mental health problems living in the community. For nurses, this has meant substantial changes to the care and service they can provide. Furthermore, the form in which they can receive and provide support for one another has also changed. Within a hospital environment nurses could, and usually did, find that the level of supervision they received could be high, even if this only took the form of making sure that the daily routine was continued. The hierarchy of senior nurses (e.g. wards sisters) overseeing their members of staff's work at least provided nurses with the feeling that there was somebody who could help (or take over) if they got into professional difficulties.

The work of Carroll (1997) offers some insights and a reasonable account of how past changes have been 'played out' in the history of supervision. What is described is that the commencement of a social work model and developmental models of supervision created the first dent in the appren-

ticeship model. This history can be 'mapped' on to some of the changes that have taken place in the structure and delivery of mental health services. We would argue that in mental health services the first dent in the apprenticeship model described came with the deinstitutionalization of large numbers of those being cared for. As Carroll (1997) notes, the focus of supervision was now to be with the supervisee rather than the supervisor; a reversal of the master teaching the apprentice was noted. What became important was the learning of the supervisees and the management of such learning. We feel that an implicit growth and development model is a key feature of much of mental health training and service delivery today. It is, in the main, linked to the autonomous practitioner described by contemporary thinkers such as Johnson & Smith (1994).

The development of community services and the role of the practitioner in the provision of care to people with mental health problems has required the nurse to be a far more autonomous practitioner. It has also led, in many instances, to the nurse finding support and help from other professionals from different disciplines.

Furthermore, the nature of education provision for most students (but particularly those involved in mental health and learning disabilities) was somewhat different. Prior to the advent of the Project 2000 (UKCC 1986) initiative and the subsequent move into higher education many mental health training schools were small in nature with small numbers of students. A small group of students (usually 12) were 'managed' by a group tutor. One of the byproducts of this small enterprise was (in instances of good practice) an emergence of good relationships, built over time, which could offer a useful model for transportation and replication within nurse/patient relationships. This 'bonding' between the small group of students and the teacher could enable tensions within practice to be teased out. These historical changes, we would argue, are similar to the changes and refocusing of supervision practices described by Carroll (1997).

Similarly, the evaluation and appraisal of good management practice and service development redolent in initiatives such as interdisciplinary working and the needs led approach are testament to this significant change. Cooke (1992a) raises a pertinent point, felt by many nurses working in the field of mental health, when she highlights the fact that nurses working in the field of mental health are required (and have been for many years) to liaise with many professionals, and utilize a multidisciplinary approach to care provision. For many nurses working in this field, it has necessitated working in departments/offices other than nursing, and, for some, having line managers other than nurses. Geographical isolation from other nursing colleagues is yet another example of how nurses working in the community with people who have mental health problems have moved away from the traditional hierarchical structure of nursing management.

However, even with acknowledgement of the above, there does not appear to have been a uniform, standard model for the provision of care for people with mental health problems. Many of the key features of governmental legislation and advice have recognized this position. The 10 point plan (initiated by Virginia Bottomley of the then Conservative Government in 1993) paved the way for uniformity in approach. The care programme approach (CPA), supervision registers and supervised discharge, a main focus of the Mental Health (Patients in the Community) Act (1995), offer ready examples of the utilization of systems reasoning to bring equanimity into an unstructured and uncoordinated system. Debates at the time offered by Fisher (1996), Godin & Scanlon (1996), Prins (1996) and Rogers (1996) suggest some limitations in the thinking and service organization. However, what is a common theme is the need to develop services that are demand led as opposed to supply driven. Also, the key theme of an outcomes-driven service emerges. However, this potentiates a fundamental change in the nature of the therapeutic relationship. For example, recommendations by the National Development Team of Mentally Handicapped People (1982) have been widely interpreted. Reasons for the differences in care provision with this particular client group include:

◆ needs of the 'community' identified

◆ service provision identified as being 'priority' in terms of no existing service
◆ service provision being defined by groups of people—e.g. resettlement teams, challenging behaviour teams, children's teams
◆ availability of range of professionals
◆ financial constraints.

However for many nurses working mental health they will be in contact with a number of professionals involved in the care delivery to a individual.

All these factors require, therefore, the provision of some mechanism by which nurses can gain the support, education and facilitation that they need, in order to provide effective, competent, quality care. We would argue for a well-structured, coherent system of clinical supervision.

Clinical supervision can also ensure that the person receiving the care provided by the nurse is the best possible care. Nurses are encouraged to be 'empowerers', facilitating appropriate and optimal levels of independence for their clients. For many clients and their families, the nurse is a new experience. Often such care provision has been absent. It is, therefore, sometimes difficult for clients or their carers to 'know' fully whether the 'advice' and 'support' they are receiving is the best for them. To offer advice and support is a powerful element of the nurse's work, so the provision of an external person to that client–nurse relationship can, in the role of supervisor, provide the necessary balance.

Those working within the specialty of community nursing may argue that, for them, regular meetings with colleagues to discuss referrals provides the support they need. Where there is the provision of a truly multidisciplinary team, and there is the time available to discuss the clients' needs fully, this may be so. However, this is dependent on trusting relationships between the professionals represented in the team, and again adequate time. It may also be a very informal way of support, and lacking the structure that more 'formal' methods of supervision could provide. Very often the time when such discussions can occur is during case management, or individual programme-planning meetings. For support to be given fully to nurses, however, time between a designated person and themselves to discuss particular aspects of their professional life is essential.

Moreover, mental health nurses can and do play a pivotal role in the provision of care to people with mental health problems, yet they are still relatively small in number. For some this may mean that their supervisor is from a different professional background to their own. Whether this is successful or problematic may be down to several factors, including:

◆ trust between the supervisor and supervisee
◆ professional relationships within the team
◆ potential (and actual) interprofessional tensions
◆ perceived role and purpose of clinical supervision.

It is now accepted, however, that multidisciplinary teamwork and interagency collaboration are essential prerequisites for effective, high quality service provision to people who have mental health problems and their carers (Mathias, Prime & Thompson 1997). Changes in service delivery and service organization have meant that professionals working in this area have a responsibility to develop and maintain good working relationships with all their multidisciplinary colleagues. The advent of care management means that interagency and multidisciplinary practice are even more bound together. It would make sense, therefore, that, if a practitioner is used to working alongside another professional on a regular basis, clinical supervision across disciplines can be beneficial both for the practitioners, where there may well be an exchange of knowledge and information, and for the client whose care package may well be, in the main, organized, developed and maintained by several members of a multidisciplinary team.

However, Thomas & Reid (1995) highlight the causes of problems that can occur between the professionals working within a multidisciplinary team. These include: stereotyped views about each professional's role and function, lack of understanding about each team member's roles, working from different theoretical and knowledge bases, functional isolation and hierarchies. One of the ways to combat all of these problems, which

could begin with the understanding of each team member's roles, and which should lead to less professional jealousy and protectivism, is interdisciplinary clinical supervision.

Many practitioners working in the field of mental health have faced recent changes in their role from the perspective of provider to purchaser. For some nurses the introduction of case management has changed their relationships with their clients. They are now in the business of purchasing, contracting and arranging care, sometimes with the added responsibility of costing out that care. For the majority of nurses working in the direct provision of care to people with mental health problems this represents a fundamental shift in their working relationships with their clients. Changing existing working practices is often fraught with anxiety; nurses working in a field of care that has had many changes imposed upon it in the last two decades need support and supervision.

We would argue that, if the infrastructures of supervision are not put in place, the climate is ripe for the development of post-traumatic stress disorder (PTSD). This is usually discussed in relation to a single experience of great intensity but limited duration. However, it has been described by Ravin & Boal (1989) that a sequence of individual, less intense events can also lead to similar symptoms. Similarly, Scott & Stradling (1992) have stated that the predominant PTSD features of avoidance behaviour (absence/sickness) and intrusive imagery may also be found occurring in response to enduring circumstances involving prolonged duress and have coined the term prolonged duress stress disorder (PDSD). Work completed by Friis & Helldin (1994) identified the necessity of having a stable, experienced staff; clear leadership; and predictable, clearly structured staff functions in order to reduce the impact of both PTSD and PDSD.

A key feature of much of the work done by mental health professionals now relates to abuse issues. Lyon (1993) observed that staff members' reactions to patients' accounts of childhood abuse resemble some symptoms of PTSD. A detailed analysis of staff members' reactions reveals the themes of the 'toxic' or 'contaminating' quality of abuse description, feelings of isolation and alienation from other staff and friends and the questions of good and evil. If these observations are linked to the work of Silfin & Ben-David (1993), and issues surrounding work with violent and self-injurious clients, we can posit that the stresses of the transference/counter-transference relationship, and the resultant lowering of the practitioner tolerance threshold, make strong claims for a robust structure of clinical supervision

THE PURPOSE OF CLINICAL SUPERVISION

Supervision has many purposes, including the promotion of competent and accountable work that concerns both the client and the supervisee. Another purpose is the facilitation of professional and personal development.

Moreover, the process of supervision closely parallels that of the practitioner–client relationship. Both should be a learning process, a process that takes place within the context of a relationship that facilitates positive change, both at a professional and personal level. In this respect the supervisor may examine at what level (Stoltenberg & Delworth 1987) Chris is functioning at within the relationship with her client, Carol. For example, is Chris able to view the client in the wider context, present an overview that is cognizant of the client's personal history or life patterns? Is Chris able to remain fully present with the client despite the client's internal life circumstances, social context or ethnic background?

Respect must be the foundation stone for any supervisory relationship, not only for the process

---

CASE STUDY: CHRIS

Chris is a community nurse working with people who have mental health problems. One of Chris's more recent clients, Carol, has told Chris that she is pregnant. Chris is aware that Carol's first child was adopted as Carol was unable to look after the child. Carol is desperately keen to care for her second child when it is born, and is asking Chris for her support in order to do this. Chris has not met this situation before and is concerned that she will not be able to provide the level of support that Carol will need.

In clinical supervision, Chris raised this concern. The supervisor was able to provide practical advice in terms of giving Chris information about:

◆ support groups who might be able to help, and
◆ the name of another nurse in a nearby town who had had experience in providing this type of support.

The supervisor also emphasized that Chris was not to feel 'alone' in this, and that this issue should be raised whenever it was necessary, in supervision sessions.

CASE STUDY: MARK

Mark is a registered nurse (RMN) who has managed a small residential establishment for 10 people with enduring mental health problems for the past 8 years. In a move to further integrate this client group into the community, the unit is closing and Mark has been asked to manage this process, and has found that his role has radically changed from that of manager of a residential service to that of resettlement officer. He now shares an office with a social worker who has part-time input into resettlement and together they comprise the 'team'. Mark is now expected to liaise with hospital staff, statutory and voluntary agencies for the purpose of finding appropriate residential accommodation, occupational activities and episodic support for a significant number of people.

The isolation he feels at times and the pressure he was under to find suitable living arrangements for people working to a deadline have all led to high levels of stress. When Mark meets with his supervisor he is able to reflect on his practice, examine his working practices, identify his own development needs, establish priorities and identify possible solutions through the design, with his supervisor, of a 'care plan' for Mark.

of supervision, but also for the supervisor, the supervisee, the client and the organisation in which supervision occurs. Butterworth (1994) identifies that for nurses the development of their role as accountable, autonomous practitioners has evolved from the movement away from the medical model of health care by nurses. This development has left nurses with the need to develop strong 'protective' mechanisms, and to identify that with autonomous practice comes accountability. For nurses working in the mental health field, the power and protection by medics was never as strong as for other nursing professions, yet, by developing new roles, the need for support and supervision has never been more important.

For Booth (1992) the purpose of supervision is the provision of support to nurses, but it may also provide a vehicle for stress reduction reflection and the identification of problem-solving techniques.

If you think about the case study example of 'Mark' you will note that the approach described is consistent with the problem-solving approach described by Egan (1994). Implicit in the process of reflection is the establishment of the 'real' problem with guidance and advice for action, intervention and evaluation. Mental health nurses are familiar with the designing of care plans and individual programme plans for their clients, yet this can provide a useful tool for nurses to identify their own strengths and weaknesses, and priorities for care. The inclusion of a supervisor in this process can facilitate an objective viewpoint, provided the relationship between the supervisor and supervisee, is based on trust, non-judgmental attitudes and facilitation.

Clinical supervision should be addressing the clinical and practical aspects of nursing. Training and research needs can be identified through effective clinical supervision, and can provide a link between research and practice. It should help nurses appreciate clients as individuals, and should also examine the contribution of the nurse to the multidisciplinary team. Effective clinical supervision should identify and develop innovative practice. Cooke (1992a) identifies how, within traditional institutional settings, good practice could be seen even if it was not rewarded. Nurses working in the community are often isolated from colleagues and therefore examples of good practice may not be so readily identified. Finally, clinical supervision should support nurses with their feelings, thus leading to foster staff retention and morale.

There are many benefits to clinical supervision, not only for supervisees themselves, but also for the service for which they work.

Benefits to be gained by supervisees

These include the following:

◆ It provides regular space for the supervisee and supervisor to reflect upon the content and process of their work.

◆ It facilitates the development of understanding and skills within their work.

◆ It allows nurses space and time to receive information and another perspective concerning their practice.

◆ The nurse can be validated and supported both as a person and as a colleague.

◆ In a stressful occupation, or at stressful times, it helps to ensure that, as people and as practitioners, nurses are not left to carry, unnecessarily, difficulties, problems and projections on their own.

◆ It gives nurses the opportunity to explore and express personal distress, transference and counter-transference that have been brought about by their practice.

◆ It may facilitate interactions that help nurses to plan and utilize their personal and professional resources better.

◆ It encourages nurses to be proactive rather than reactive.

◆ It will allow nurses to use self-appraisal in respect to the quality of their work.

Benefits to the service

The service needs to be committed to the provision of clinical supervision, which requires time and energy to be effective. Planning, implementing, monitoring and evaluating a system of professional supervision in mental health service provision is justifiable if it brings the following benefits.

◆ Clinical supervision, as part of a staff development and support programme, could allow a sustained and detailed exploration of professional issues with a view to increasing job satisfaction, enhancing a sense of colleagueship and corporate purpose.

◆ The client's needs are being met through improvement in the quality of care provision.

◆ It would provide opportunities for valuing colleagues' strengths and identifying ways in which their professional needs could be met.

◆ It would encourage colleagues at all levels, across disciplines and agencies to become more confident in exploring their professional input at work in an open way, thus helping to build a climate of trust in which professional development could take place.

◆ It would involve practitioners working on a common problem or weakness or issue to create a greater sense of effective teamwork.

◆ It would provide a formal support system through periods of professional stress, crisis and confusion.

◆ Clinical supervision could be professionally empowering for nurses working within multidisciplinary teams.

MODELS OF SUPERVISION

Earlier on in the chapter we identified the mechanisms by which mental health nurses may be receiving some sort of supervision, other than identified sessions. It is fair to say that these opportunities may be more available to practitioners working within community support teams. For nurses working in residential or occupational/recreational settings, this type of supervision may not be available.

The most popular way of using supervision is for the supervisor and supervisee to meet regularly on a one to one basis, although supervision can be undertaken in many ways. Cooke (1992a) identifies four methods of undertaking clinical supervision, of which the most frequently used is the one to one method. Cooke argues that one to one supervision is often undertaken by the nurse manager. The potential problem with this is the

unequal relationship that exists between the supervisee and the supervisor. Most mental health community nurses now have to complete periodic records of their activities. These are usually submitted to their manager to provide information for future service planning. There exists, therefore, the potential danger that managers as supervisors may slip into their management role whilst being involved in supervision. The need for trust and mutual respect is therefore paramount in this type of supervision setting.

A method identified by Cooke (1992b) offers a most useful and potent example, that is perhaps exclusive to the role of the community nurse, as opposed to nurses working in residential settings; this is supervision of the home visit. Whilst this may allow the supervisor to see at first hand the relationship that the nurse has with the client and family, the stresses that this may put on that relationship may outweigh the benefits of this type of supervision. As a consequence, a level of trust, respect, aims and objectives and maturity in the relationship is paramount.

In some cases using role play to 'act out' situations that nurses may find themselves in—for example, dealing with uncooperative family members—either with the supervisor and supervisee meeting alone, or with the involvement of other staff, may help the nurse to develop the required skills.

Also, video playing these role play situations can provide the nurse with visual evidence of responses and methods of dealing with issues that are stressful or problematic. The supervisor and supervisee can examine together methods of developing the requisite skills. You will note, however, that the supervisor–supervisee relationship is crucial.

The model to which Cooke (1992b) refers is only one of several models or ways of working. We will now describe four main types.

One to one—the supervisor and the supervisee

This form of supervision has been discussed in the previous paragraph and is the most common form of supervision relationship but it is important to note that, within all supervision models, the UKCC Position statement on clinical supervision (1996) is quite definite in its stance as to what clinical supervision is. It argues that: 'Clinical supervision is not a managerial control system. It is not therefore: the exercise of overt managerial responsibility or managerial supervision; a system of formal individual performance review or hierarchical in nature.'

The role and function of supervision must, therefore, be very clearly identified by the practitioners involved in this relationship. For example, it would be of paramount importance that the contractual arrangements for the supervision were clear and understood by both parties. Issues such as the frequency and duration of the supervision must be explored, also what support will be offered to the supervisee, what constitutes clinical practice, developmental issues, confidentiality and personal issues. The caveat is that the supervisee is usually less experienced than the supervisor and that structures must be in place to manage the accompanying power relation tensions.

One to one cosupervision

This model involves two practitioners providing support for each other. The method used is to alternate the roles. This tends to presuppose equality of different levels of skill and expertise. Typically the supervision session is divided equally between the two.

Group supervision with an identified supervisor

There is a continuum of methods for providing this form of supervision. At one end of the continuum of supervision the identified supervisor will be responsible for appointing the times between the supervisees, and then concentrate on the work of the individuals in turn. At the other end of the continuum, it is the supervisees who organize their clinical supervision times, using the supervisor as a resource. Between these two alternatives, many different ways of working can operate.

Peer group supervision

This model of supervision takes the form of three or more supervisees providing supervision for each other within a group context. They are likely to be of equitable status, degree of training and experience. An example of this model could be that of three members of the multidisciplinary team providing support and help for each other.

Eclectic methods of supervision

This model is structured around combinations of the above models. Practitioners working in the field of mental health may need or choose to combine elements of the four models to suit their particular professional, working needs.

Within all these models of clinical supervision, Procter's (1986) ideas offer a useful representation or building block of the fundamental base on which supervision is premised. Procter perceives supervision as a working alliance between the supervisee and supervisor. This relationship focuses on casework being presented, with feedback and guidance then given. Procter sees the dimensions within this relationship as being educational, supportive and managerial. The model for supervision she has devised has normative, formative and restorative elements.

The normative element is concerned with professional and organizational standards of professional practice. They provide the quality in supervision. In this aspect the supervisor focuses on values, beliefs, evaluation of care, issues of caseload management and professional accountability.

The formative aspect of supervision is concerned with the identification and the development of skills, and with the integration of theory into practice. The training of many nurses was hospital based and nurses have had to adapt to changes in the care provision for people with learning disabilities with little or no training. The demands that such care provision often places on practitioners working in this field mean that they require both specific and generic skill development. The case study example of 'Mark', previously referred to, provides an example of this.

CASE STUDY: KIM

Kim is a registered nurse working in a residential facility for young people with mental health problems. Kim is concerned about some staff members' negative and punitive behaviour towards some of the young people who live in this particular house. Kim takes this concern to the supervision session, where it is suggested that staff development across the range of staff should be provided. Kim's response to speak out about unacceptable practices and attitudes is acknowledged, and Kim's decision to speak out is supported.

The third aspect or function of this model of clinical supervision, the restorative function, aims to provide supportive help for professionals. The practitioner will reflect on and seek to develop or improve personal coping strategies, and how to provide both high levels of support and challenge. This element of the model should also provide the opportunity to explore the stresses unique to their work environment, highs and lows of their work, and how to introduce, maintain and end (where necessary), supportive relationships.

ROLE OF THE SUPERVISOR

The role of the supervisor is characterized by two key features:

1. commitment on the part of the supervisor to the facilitation of growth, both educational and personal, of the supervisee
2. an acceptance of the voluntary nature of the contract.

These two features are fundamental to effective, safe, supportive clinical supervision, if the three elements or functions of supervision as described by Procter (1986) are to be met.

Procter (1986) describes supervision has having several key features, summarized below. Clinical supervision should be:

◆ enabling not dominating

◆ encouraging not judgmental
◆ valuing not belittling
◆ exploratory not dogmatic
◆ open not defensive
◆ developmental not restrictive
◆ accepting and yet challenging.

CASE STUDY: JIM

Jim is a gay nurse working with clients diagnosed as personality disordered in a therapeutic community setting. Jim has been the named nurse for Tony, a 24-year-old personality-disordered patient with behaviour frequently described as narcissistic and manipulative and, also, a series of convictions for sexual offences against young women.

Bob has been in a supervisory relationship with Jim for the past 9 months. Their relationship has moved through several developmental stages and functions, mainly at stage 3 as described by Stoltenberg & Delworth (1987). However, Bob has noticed that Jim's descriptions of his relationship with Tony and his therapeutic input evidences a qualitative difference. Jim refers to Tony as a close friend, often with a warm and seductive quality. In the supervision sessions Bob feels he is being drawn into the relationship between Jim and Tony. He feels a warmth towards Jim and postulates how he may explore those feelings.

We would argue that in order to explore a range of issues contained within the above case study Bob, as supervisor, would need to demonstrate a range of key skills linked to those described by Procter. For example, Bob may need to be open, accepting and challenging in respect of Jim's feeling but, more importantly, demonstrate those skills in respect of his own feelings. In terms of skill development, Hawkins & Shohet (1989) and their descriptions of the six-eyed supervisor offer potent guidance in the exploration of the relationship, internal processes, the here and now between the supervisee and the supervisor and the content of their session. Bob could readily utilize these ideas to explore the tensions at both a conscious and unconscious level within his relationship with Jim, and the dynamics of the relationship between Jim and his client and Bob's place within the dynamic.

SKILLS AND METHODS

Farkas-Cameron (1995) has identified some of the concerns nurses raise about clinical supervision. There may be a concern about the nature and purpose of clinical supervision—questions such as 'What is the purpose of clinical supervision?' may in fact be about feelings that their practices are being questioned in a negative manner. There may also be concern that supervision is about management and it is here, as has been mentioned previously, that the importance of the clinical supervision relationship being based on trust and being non-judgmental is paramount. Fowler (1996) suggests that the first question that needs to be asked when planning clinical supervision, whether at the individual or organizational level, is: What is the aim of the clinical supervision?

Davies (1993, p. 52) contends that: 'Supervision should be "for" the practitioner. It is not an audit of practice.' The aim of clinical supervision is to support, assist and facilitate the practitioner in the delivery of high quality care, but it is also about supporting and helping practitioners to manage the demands of their professional working life.

The introduction of clinical supervision into a service may meet with some initial resistance due to lack of understanding about the purpose of clinical supervision, fears about criticism of professional practice and a resentment that supervision will remove the autonomy of the practitioner. These fears and anxieties have to be allayed; it is in the methods and skills adopted in the introduction and implementation of clinical supervision that this can and should occur. For many people, the possibility that their professional practices may be criticized would be threatening. However, clinical supervision can assist practitioners to continue to develop existing good practice and learn new skills. Most practitioners informally discuss their clients' needs and ask for advice; clinical

supervision puts this into a framework that supports the practitioner and allows for the acknowledgment that in many instances the work that they are undertaking is difficult and that this difficulty needs to be recognized and shared.

To facilitate a supportive, trusting and therapeutic relationship within clinical supervision requires particular skills and a clear understanding of the purpose of the supervision.

Supervision allows for (Davies 1993):

◆ focusing directly on the practitioner case load
◆ focusing on the skills, interventions and evaluation of clinical/therapeutic interactions with clients and/or their carers
◆ self-evaluation and self-awareness
◆ guidance/advice on clinical practice and interventions
◆ validation of practitioners' positive clinical/interpersonal practice
◆ discussion of events and how the practitioner coped
◆ exploration of coping mechanisms and how harmful/beneficial these are.

If supervision is to be supportive, challenging, professional and effective the supervisor needs to have high levels of key skills that are used consciously in the supervision. The key skills are: clarification–exploration–progression–appraisal.

Butterworth (1994) has identified the need for supervisor training to ensure that supervisors have a knowledge of and sensitivity to the interpersonal processes that can occur between individuals and

CASE STUDY: HILARY

Hilary is a recently qualified nurse working in a local, acute services facility. She is allocated Colin, a newly admitted patient. Colin has a history of aggressive behaviour and sexual abuse within the family.

Hilary, during her assessment of Colin, experiences strong feelings of revulsion when discussing his history. She wonders whether she can continue to work with Colin. In clinical supervision she discloses these feelings.

groups and may impede the therapeutic nature of practitioner–client and supervisor–supervisee relationships. Key skills that facilitate effective communication are therefore vital.

Key skill—clarification

This skill involves identifying clearly a number of aspects of the style and methods that practitioners use in their everyday working life. Supervisees will be encouraged to explore their 'style of work', the effects that it has on clients, carers, colleagues and their understanding of the efficacy of this style. The skills that the supervisor will need to use include listening, questioning, summarizing, paraphrasing and checking out.

Being a good listener is not easy and supervisors should be aware of the difficulties that may arise. Supervisors also needs to be aware of any skill development they may need in listening to others.

Key skill—exploration

This phase of the supervision is a logical progression from clarification. It may involve the supervisor asking: 'now that your ideas about your practice have been clarified, can we explore one of your ideas that you currently manage the least effectively?'

A possible consequence of exploration is that it may seem threatening, and it is therefore vital that this skill is carried out in a supportive manner, which sets the supervisee at their ease and does not make the supervisee feel inadequate.

Exploration may well sound neutral—but it is in fact difficult and value laden. This skill involves coping with confusion—exploring options, considering different ways of working, examining the possibility of changing attitudes. This skill also requires the supervisor and supervisee to deal with conflict. The range of options suggested by the supervisee may not be options supervisors would themselves consider using. Whether this conflict is acknowledged and dealt with could affect the relationship.

Exploration involves challenging and this can result in the supervisee feeling inadequate. For the

CASE STUDY: LYNN

Lynn is a middle-aged woman in a medium secure unit for women diagnosed as suffering from a range of mental health problems. Her life as a parent has been somewhat complex, resulting in her only child being taken into care by the local authority. She has attempted suicide on a number of occasions and engages in self-injurious behaviour (regularly cutting herself with glass pieces and inserting sharp objects into the wounds). Most of the unit staff have labelled her behaviour 'attention seeking'.

Lorraine, an 18-year-old student with her own personal problems, has formed an attachment with Lynn. Some staff indicate that they feel the attachment is non-therapeutic. Lorraine discusses the issue with her clinical supervisor.

CASE STUDY: ALISON

Alison, a qualified nurse aged 28, is working in a unit for young persons diagnosed with severe, acute schizophrenic illnesses. She has been in a clinical supervision relationship with Ros for about 18 months. Ros feels that Alison remains overdependent on her for solutions to the problems she presents. Alison is anxious and insecure in her nursing role, lacks insight but is highly motivated. Ros wonders about progressing the supervision relationship.

act of challenging practice, beliefs, etc. to be positive it must therefore be perceived by the supervisee as supportive.

Exploration within the supervision session can provide information, identify goals and aspirations, and perceived and actual difficulties, and can improve skill awareness.

Key skill—progression

This is a generic skill that will be used throughout the supervision session. It is about avoiding going round in circles, becoming blocked down blind

CASE STUDY: MAUREEN

Maureen is a middle-aged woman who has been in mental health nursing for a considerable number of years. She is a highly skilled practitioner able to deal with a range of sensitive issues in supervision relationships. She is receiving clinical supervision from Clancy. However, during one supervision session Clancy observes that Maureen appears anxious when she suggests a review of her professional practice.

alleys and working only at the superficial level. This stage of the session involves identifying relevant action. It is necessary to identify and discuss problems; it is essential to discuss goals. This in turn should lead to greater clarity of actions, goals and aspirations. Part of identifying actions must include the exploration of resource availability. Learning to use colleagues as resources is important; seeing their skills and knowledge as useful and supportive can be the first break in the barriers that can often exist within multidisciplinary teams.

Key skill—appraisal

This skill is required in what is perhaps the most sensitive area involved in supervision. Assessment of professional practice can appear very threatening and produce high levels of anxiety. Appraisal is not only sensitive; it is also complicated. This skill involves and necessitates several subsidiary skills: the encouragement of self-assessment in which the supervisees analyse their own strengths and weaknesses, aims, criteria, strategies, etc. It involves being critical in a supportive way. Being critical involves making judgements, but the way in which those judgements are made will significantly affect how they are received.

The previously mentioned skills of clarifying and exploring are important—they will assist in the identification of future action, which assists motivation and continuation of good practice. This skill should be used to help the supervisee—to use reflective and evaluative practices and to identify the preferred styles of learning for continuous professional development.

SUMMARY AND RECOMMENDATIONS

What, then, is the benefit of clinical supervision? In this chapter we have identified the benefits to the service and to clients with mental health problems. The benefits to the practitioner can be numerous and include the following:

◆ It provides space for both supervisee and supervisor to reflect upon the content and process of their work.

◆ It facilitates the development of understanding and skills within their work.

◆ It allows practitioners space and time to receive information and another perspective concerning their clinical practice.

◆ The practitioner can be validated and supported both as a person and as a colleague.

◆ In a stressful occupation it helps to ensure that, as a person and as a practitioner, supervisees are not left to carry, unnecessarily, difficulties and problems on their own.

◆ It may facilitate interactions that help practitioners to plan and utilize their personal and professional resources better.

◆ It encourages practitioners to be proactive rather than reactive.

◆ It will allow practitioners to use self-appraisal in respect of the quality of their work.

It would appear therefore that the implementation of clinical supervision into services for people with mental health problems would be of benefit to all involved. For practitioners in particular, the implementation of clinical supervision may provide them with the essential support mechanism that they need to care for people with learning disabilities. It would be well to heed the words of Reg Pyne (1987): 'To care for and about our colleagues is to care for and about standards of patient care. Our consciences should not rest if we renege on that responsibility.'

In order to ensure quality supervision, certain criteria need to be met. The following section provides a list of actions that will assist in the facilitation of quality clinical supervision. Practitioners working in the field of mental health may find that this action list can provide a basic structure from which they can devise and implement their own systems of clinical supervision.

Actions to support benchmarks for good clinical practice

Organizational commitment would include:

- time and place for clinical supervision to take place
- clinical supervision as part of the organizational ethos
- the provision of formal arrangements, i.e. the use of contracts
- recognition of the importance of safety in the clinical supervision relationship
- respect and confidentiality
- opportunity to attend training sessions for clinical supervision
- clinical supervision arrangements forming part of an individual practitioner's regular review
- clinical supervision for managers
- maintainance of a record of clinical supervision.

REFERENCES

BAC (British Association of Counselling) 1992 Code of ethics and practice for counsellors. BAC, Rugby

Booth K 1992 Providing support and reducing stress—review of the literature. In: Butterworth T, Faugier J (eds) Clinical supervision and mentorship in nursing. Chapman & Hall, London

Briant S 1997 Too close for comfort. Nursing Times 93(6):22–24

Butler S, Zelen S L 1977 Sexual intimacies between therapists and patients. Psychotherapy: Theory, Research and Practice 14:139–145

Butterworth T 1994 Preparing to take on clinical supervision. Nursing Standard 8(52):32–34

Butterworth T, Faugier J 1992 (eds) Clinical supervision and mentorship in nursing. Chapman & Hall, London

Carroll M 1997 Clinical supervision: luxury or necessity? In: Horton I, Varma V (eds) The needs of counsellors and psychotherapists. Sage, London, pp 135–151

Cooke P 1992a Clinical supervision and mentorship in nursing. Chapman & Hall, London

Cooke P 1992b Mental handicap nursing. In: Butterworth T, Faugier J (eds) Clinical supervision and mentorship in nursing. Chapman & Hall, London

Davies P 1993 Value yourself. Nursing Times 89(4):52

DOH (Department of Health) 1994 Working in partnership: a collaborative approach to care. The Butterworth report. HMSO, London

Egan G 1994 The skilled helper: a problem management approach to helping, 5th edn. Brookes/Cole Publishing, California.

DISCUSSION QUESTIONS

1. 'Increasing isolation' and 'unspoken and silent tensions' may be accepted as given within mental health care work; how do you think they can be voiced within the apparent conflict between management and clinical supervision?

2. If you reflect on the contextual issues of your own practice, what issues emerge for you in terms of the relationship between the supervisor and supervisee if they form part of the same clinical/work network?

3. If selection of an appropriate supervision model is important, what tensions may exist between adopting an eclectic stance or adopting one particular model for your supervision practice?

4. In clinical supervision the voluntary nature of the contract is often stressed. How does it 'fit' within a health care system that is driven by economics, standards and contracts?

5. In the section of 'key skill—clarification', much is made of the unconscious process within supervision. In terms of the evidence base in what ways can you know, for certain, that such processes are 'real'?

6. If you think about the context of your own practice what would be the tension(s) evidenced in attempting to establish clinical supervision within a multidisciplinary or interagency structure/philosophy?

7. Most commentators describe clinical supervision as a 'good thing'. What is the evidential base for such a claim?

FURTHER READING

DOH (Department of Health) 1999 Making a difference. The New NHS. Department of Health, London
Although not a text specifically about clinical supervision, it focuses on improvement within the health service. Issues such as 'Improving working lives', 'Modernising professional self regulation', 'Strengthening education and training' and 'Working in new ways' offer a clear statement of the contextual reasons for a clinical supervision infrastructure within any caring environment.

Farrington A 1994 Defining and setting the parameters of clinical supervision. International Journal of Psychiatric Research 2:34–40
This article offers some research-based data relating to the establishment of clinical supervision processes. It is useful for those thinking of entering a supervision relationship as either supervisor or supervisee. The text clearly illustrates the limits and boundaries in supervision.

Jacobs M 1998 Psychodynamic counselling in action. Sage, London
This text offers a clear, easily accessed account of psychodynamic processes through the utilization of case studies. The link between past and present experience, the past influencing the way we deal with the present is evidenced. This is a useful text in exploring the ways in which we develop and manage relationship with others.

Playle J F, Mullarkey K 1998 Parallel process in clinical supervision: enhencing learning and providing support. Nurse Education Today 18:558–566
The writers firmly root the importance of the exploration of relationships, and in particular boundary issues, within the supervision relationship. A noteworthy aspect is the utilization of boundary negotiation as a legitimate focus for learning and support within the relationship.

Raffert M, Coleman M 1996 Educating nurses to undertake clinical supervision in practice. Nursing Standard 10(45): 38–41
A useful article for the nascent supervisor or teacher planning to teach or construct a module relating to clinical supervision. The article describes the design and structure of a module accredited by the Welsh National Board and the University of Swansea. The functions of supervision (adapted from Procter 1986) are described. Again, a useful text for those planning supervision.

Farkas-Cameron M M 1995 Clinical supervision in psychiatric nursing. Journal of Psychosocial Nursing 33(2):31–37

Faulkner J 1998 A head start. Nursing Times 94(43):39

Fisher N 1996 Managing the high risk psychiatrist. Psychiatric Bulletin 20:65–67

Fowler J 1996 Clinical supervision: what do you do after saying hello? British Journal of Nursing 5(6):382–385

Friis S, Helldin L 1994 The contribution made by the clinical setting to violence among psychiatric patients. Criminal Behavior and Mental Health 4(4):341–352

Gemma P B 1989 Can nurses care too much? American Journal of Nursing 89(5):743–744

Godin P, Scanlon C 1996 Community supervision. Nursing Management 3(5):12–13

Goldberg C 1986 On being a pyschiatric nurse. The journey of the healer. Gardner Press, New York

Hawkins P, Shohet R 1989 Supervision in the helping professions. Open University Press, Milton Keynes

Hughes R, Morcom C 1998 Clinical supervision in a mental health in-patient area. Nursing Times 3(3)

Johns H 1992 Professional supervision. Journal of Nursing Management 1:9–18

Johnson F C, Smith L D 1994 Personal and professional roles, skills and behaviours. In: Thompson T, Mathias P (eds) Lyttle's mental health and disorder, 2nd edn. Baillière Tindall, London, pp 12–40

Kennerley H 1990 Managing anxiety: a training manual. Open University Press, Milton Keynes

Lyon E 1993 Hospital staff reactions to accounts by survivors of childhood abuse. American Journal of Orthopsychiatry 63(3):410–416

Mathias P, Prime R, Thompson T 1997 Preparation for interprofessional work: holism, integration and the purpose of training and education. In: Ovretveit J, Mathias P, Thompson T (eds) Interprofessional working for health and social care. Macmillan, London, pp 116–130

Mental Health (Patients in the Community) Act 1995 HMSO, London

National Development Team of Mentally Handicapped People 1982 Third report. HMSO, London

NHS Confederation and the Sainsbury Centre for Mental Health 1997 Mental health care from problems to solutions. The Sainsbury Centre For Mental Health, London

Pennington S, Gafner G, Schilit R, Bechtel B 1993 Addressing ethical boundaries among nurses. Nursing Management 24(6):36–39

Power S 1994 A unique source of support and advice. The benefits of supervision in clinical practice. Psychiatric Care 1(3):105–108

Prins H 1996 Can the law serve as the solution to social ills? Case of the Mental Health (Patients in the Community) Act 1995. Medicine, Science and Law 36(3):217–220

Procter B 1986 Supervision: a co-operative exercise in accountability. In: Marken M, Payne M (eds) Enabling and ensuring: supervision in practice. National Youth Bureau, Leicester

Pyne R 1987 Confronting stress. Nursing Times 83(27):30–31

Ravin J, Boal C K 1989 Post-traumatic stress disorder in the work setting; psychic injury, medical diagnosis, treatment and litigation. American Journal of Forensic Psychiatry 10:5–23

Rogers B 1996 Supervised discharge: implications for practice. Mental Health Nursing 3(2):8–10

Rushton C H, Ausberg L, McEnhill M 1996 Establishing therapeutic boundaries as patient advocates. Pediatric Nursing 22(3):185–189

Scott M J, Stradling S G 1992 Post-traumatic stress disorder from prolonged duress. Counselling for post-traumatic stress disorder. Sage, London

Silfin P, Ben-David S 1993 The forensic psychiatric hospital. Analise Psicologica 11(1):37–47

Stoltenberg C D, Delworth U 1987 Supervising counsellors and therapists. Jossey-Bass, London

Thomas B, Reid J 1995 Multidisciplinary clinical supervision. British Journal of Nursing 4(15):883–885

Torrington D, Weightman J 1994 Effective management, 2nd edn. Prentice Hall, London

Totka J P 1996 Exploring the boundaries of pediatric practice: nurse stories related to relationships. Pediatric Nursing 22(3):191–196, 204–205

UKCC (United Kingdom Central Council for Nursing, Midwifery and Health Visiting) 1984 Code of professional conduct for the nurse, midwife and health visitor. UKCC, London

UKCC (United Kingdom Central Council for Nursing, Midwifery and Health Visiting) 1986 Project 2000: a new preparation for practice. UKCC, London

UKCC (United Kingdom Central Council for Nursing, Midwifery and Health Visiting) 1996 Position statement on clinical supervision for nursing and midwifery. UKCC, London

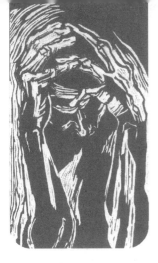

Chapter Twenty-six

Lifelong learning—a never-ending journey of development?

Fran Aiken

AIMS

- To consider the culture and systems that need to be in place to support professionals to develop
- To ascertain the skills and knowledge that are necessary for individuals in their professional development
- To critique the values of lifelong learning
- To outline some guidelines for organizations to promote lifelong learning
- To analyse strategies for the individual and the organization for lifelong learning

KEY ISSUES

Continuing professional development
Motivation
Guidelines for organisations
Personal development plans
PREP
Strategies for lifelong learning
Research agendas

INTRODUCTION

You may have recently successfully completed your preregistration diploma or degree and may be confident that you have the knowledge and skills to practise as a competent practitioner. However, can your previous learning keep up with changes in mental health care and new ways of working? Do you now find that other staff and disciplines' knowledge and attitudes are challenging yours? What is more important; do you want to develop, improve the standard of care you give and gain more job satisfaction rather than stand still? In this case, the process of continuing learning is relevant, not just as a newly qualified professional but throughout your career and life.

WHAT IS LIFELONG LEARNING?

The definitions of lifelong learning vary according to conceptual perspectives: Knapper & Cropley (1985) defined it as 'a set of organisational and procedural guidelines for educational practice aimed at fostering learning throughout life', which indicates learning as a policy statement rather than a personal belief. The government's consultation paper on the 'learning age' sees lifelong learning as 'the continuous development of the skills, knowledge and understanding that are essential for employability and fulfillment' (DEE 1998). It is also a key issue and cornerstone in the new NHS (Butterworth 1998): the recent paper from the Department of Health A first class service. Quality in the new NHS (DOH 1988) defines lifelong learning as: 'A process of continuing development for all individuals and teams which meets the needs of patients and delivers the healthcare outcomes and healthcare priorities of the NHS and which enables professionals to expand and fulfill their potential'. Hinchliff (1994) saw it as a process of continuing professional development (CPD) to enable the individual to keep up with change; this viewpoint emphasizes the autonomy of adult learners. Tensions, therefore, are evident between the individual's choice for self-growth and the policy of lifelong education. Certainly, the culture and systems need to be in place to support

professionals who have the necessary prerequisites, including the motivation to develop.

Some educationalists see lifelong learning as different from lifelong education, which Lawson (1982) described as a non-evaluative term encompassing the entirety of learning and education and therefore the term 'lifelong learning' may weaken the concept of education. Fundamental debates such as these need to be reconciled in discussions about lifelong learning: if the terms 'lifelong learning' and 'lifelong education' are used interchangeably (Maslin-Prothero 1997) the covert values of the language and terminology must be first made explicit. For the purposes of this chapter, 'lifelong education' is the *policy* for formal, informal and non-formal educational activities (Lawson 1982) while 'lifelong learning' is the *concept* of directed self-growth for continuing personal and professional development that should be enabled and supported by educational policy.

THE DRIVE FOR LIFELONG LEARNING

Lifelong learners have always existed and have been described by writers such as Matthew Arnold; however, it is now a favourite theme in institutional policy (Knapper & Cropley 1985), in political directives (DOH 1998, European Commission 1995) and professional standard setting (ENB 1995, UKCC 1991). These policy makers and institutions see lifelong learning as necessary for health practitioners in order to respond quickly to service needs and to enable purchasers and providers to achieve their objectives (ENB 1995). Communities and patients will benefit from professionals whose skills and knowledge are keeping pace with change—'A continuing process of updating and maintaining expertise will support the delivery of high quality, modern, effective healthcare in a fast changing world' (DOH 1998).

Policy makers and commentators have also identified the need to prepare for 'the dissolution of geographical boundaries and creation of trade blocks where goods, capital and services circulate easily and freely across borders in a climate of deregulation and decentralisation' (Affara 1997), and to update knowledge in order to overcome obsolescence of preregistration courses (UKCC 1991). Erosion of the applicability of knowledge has meant that professional obsolescence can start from between 2 and 5 years after registration (Grant 1992). However, there is also the drive to update and develop new skills in order to respond to the changing nature of employment where rapid and global change is a constant, and where technological progress and social change such as social dislocation, increased leisure hours and changing sex roles (Knapper & Cropley 1985) require workers to be more flexible. The deliberate strategy of career development through continuous learning (Hall & Mirvis 1995) is maybe as much a motivation for individuals as organizational or professional requirements.

For mental health professionals who use their personalities, communication skills and understanding of human emotions and behaviours to care for others, the need for self-development is critical (Johns 1997); we need to be accountable and reactive to criticisms, to protect clients from abuse and to protect ourselves from clients' manipulation by being aware of our own blind spots. We need to be aware, too, of our own limits. Proactively we can also continuously develop in order to learn about ourselves as social beings—'If lifelong learning is increasingly accepted as a central intellectual task in the field of continuing education, then we might fruitfully acknowledge and live out more consistently the need for lifelong emotional and social learning' (Johns 1997).

A study of registered nurses' reasons for participating in continuing education (DeSilets 1995) found that young, recently qualified nurses, in comparison with older nurses, were more concerned with professional commitment, reflecting on and improving their practice. The subjects were all interested in networking and interacting with colleagues and in improving personal benefits and job security. This study shows there may be a developmental aspect of motivation to continue learning that needs to be addressed by those who are planning and marketing formal programmes or providing any learning experience.

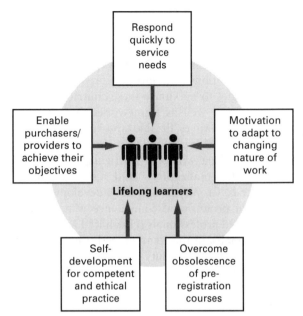

Fig. 26.1 Drives towards lifelong learning.

Whatever are the motivation and impetus for lifelong learning (see Fig. 26.1), there is a critical challenge for educationalists (for example, to provide the strategies), for employers (to support the learners) and for individuals (such as adapting study skills) to overcome. Organizational and educational responsibilities, flexibility of strategies and resources, integrating theory and practice and changing technologies are just some of the implications of lifelong learning that will be explored in this chapter.

THE VALUES OF LIFELONG LEARNING

The principles of adult continuing learning are rooted in the Western humanistic tradition. This ideology of andragogy offers a rationale for learning that is different from contemporary dictates (Gross 1982); the philosophy of adult-centred learning (Knowles 1984) recognizes that learning is ongoing, through formal and informal situations (Maggs 1996). Thus, in health profession, CPD provides the framework for individual accountability as enshrined in the UKCC Code of professional conduct (UKCC 1984). Following these beliefs, educational agencies and employers should recognize individuals' past experiences, value their contributions as adults and provide support and strategies to maximize these contributions to health care as well as frameworks that provide open, collaborative, flexible and available CPD programmes (Maggs 1996). For the adult learner, lifelong learning will offer particular chances to reach self-actualization and self-fulfillment (Knapper & Cropley 1985). Such development of a sense of professional competence is needed to retain skilled professionals (Hinchliff 1994).

Additionally, in the Kantian tradition of ethics, there is also the ideal, duty or obligation to develop and maintain our own autonomy through a knowledge of self and moral awareness and to assist others in educating themselves throughout life (Bailey 1988). Adhering to these beliefs, even defending them and developing them, then leads to a professional requirement to seek collectively, as well as individually, to advance and to nurture continuing education. Accountable practitioners then have the duty to disseminate knowledge to colleagues, to support reflectivity and development in others as well as continuing their own learning.

THE PREREQUISITES FOR LIFELONG LEARNING

There are certain factors that are necessary for lifelong learning to be meaningful: these can be clustered under three areas—psychological factors, competencies/skills and conditions.

Psychological factors

Individuals need intrinsic motivation to develop, to be self-directed and to learn. They may find they enjoy learning for its own sake and plan their learning in advance; this type of learner, the 'self-directed' or proactive learner, is often overlooked by educationalists (Jarvis 1987). Nevertheless, most adults learn because they want to use the knowledge or skills to cope with change in their lives (Aslanian & Brickell 1980) such as moving

to a new clinical area or working with a different client group. Other triggering events or transitional periods may be life events such as children leaving home. Whatever the trigger, the learning and development will occur unevenly, at different speeds or, as Gross (1977) put it, 'the rhythm of learning' will be uneven. Idealized lifelong learners (Knapper & Cropley 1985) will already be aware of the learning cycle (Kolb 1984)—in other words, that learning occurs all the time in real life and reflection in action will enhance knowledge and skills. They will also be highly motivated to lifelong learning, recognize their needs and have a self-concept that is helpful to lifelong learning. Houle (1980) believed there were three kinds of lifelong learners: those who used learning as a means to achieve a specific goal (for example, career progression), activity-orientated individuals who were interested in learning for the circumstances in which it took place (for example, in meeting colleagues outside of work), and those who sought learning for its own sake.

Lifelong learners need to be aware of their weaknesses and learning needs, need to be able to self-diagnose learning needs (Carpenito 1991) and need to be able to evaluate how learning has altered or affected these needs and deficits (Hinchliff 1994). Self-awareness and self-evaluation skills are therefore required. Learners also need a sense of control over what is learned and the pace of learning: if the locus of control is held by learners, rather than enforced from organizations or institutions, the learning achieved will be more significant and learners will become more autonomous and avoid learned helplessness, becoming more proactive and taking more responsibility for their own learning—for example, through using a learning log.

Competencies/skills

Lifelong learners must also set realistic learning goals commensurate with life circumstances and individual needs—for example, staff nurses with heavy family commitments, full-time employment and lack of knowledge of research methodology may not be able to achieve an MSc in a short time span. They must also have good study skills, awareness of the learning style best suited for them, and possess skills in using learning aids, such as open-learning material, and knowledge of resources and ability to access them. This may require additional resources and requirements beyond the individual. Self-managed learning is a requirement for lifelong learning but it requires personal commitment, devotion to goal setting and record keeping and openness to appraisal and support from others (Fair 1995).

Conditions

The individual cannot learn in a vacuum; there must be a culture of learning to support and augment the learning strategies and opportunities: 'for a culture of lifelong learning to develop the drive for enhancement and the sense of achievement is essential' (ENB 1998). A preregistration culture of emphasizing individuals' responsibility for learning strategies and development of inquiry skills, rather than only focusing on gaining knowledge and psychomotor skills, will encourage lifelong learning (Appel & Malcolm 1998).

Process-focused learning in the preregistration curriculum will develop the student's ability to question, challenge and learn independently (Carpenito 1991)—skills necessary for lifelong learning. Course content of postregistration programmes must be adapted to allow the learner to use and interpret materials and information from different fields; this is particularly effective in interdisciplinary shared learning—'the ability to integrate and maintain an overall perspective becomes critically important' (Knapper & Cropley 1985). The practitioner will then be more likely to be ready for decision making in the real world where resources have to be shared, team work is the norm and different viewpoints taken on board (Maslin-Prothero 1997). An active-learning approach in preregistration programmes has been suggested as an effective way of facilitating skills acquisition (McManus & Sieler 1998). Through utilizing resource-based learning such as skills laboratories the programme will be more likely to produce a competent, confident and reflective practitioner who is also self-directed and motivated to continue professional development.

Management support is essential not only to facilitate resources but also to value the active learner: through performance review and encouraging mentoring, the manager can give direction to the learner based on client and service needs in a framework of positive appraisal and support. The organization needs to value practice based on research that is relevant. The clinical learning environment will then allow practitioners to question practice and add to their own and colleagues' understanding (Maslin-Prothero 1997).

The process of CPD in a healthy, quality-driven organization has been identified by the DoH (1998). This document looks at the delivery of quality standards (Fig. 26.2) that describes assessment through training needs analysis and performance review, which take the form of organizational and personal development plans taking into account individuals' learning styles, identifying opportunities for shared and interdisciplinary learning and practice-based learning (DOH 1998). Further guidance for organizations is being developed.

Managers also have to develop strategies to support CPD as outlined in the requirements for clinical governance laid out by the Department of Health (DOH 1998). The organization is more likely to develop a learning culture through partnerships with educators basing formal programmes not on the interests or expertise of the education providers (Yuen 1991) but on the logically determined needs of the organization.

The environment needs to encourage analysis and change and time for these processes, along with individual performance review linked to personal plans for reaching two or three goals within a time-frame, and discussion groups (interdisciplinary) to discuss research findings. Care team meetings should encourage problem solving that is evidence based while acknowledging differences in styles of practice (Carpenito 1991). Organizational mentoring schemes (Annand 1997) can support and assist lifelong learners by harnessing peer-support groups and learning resource materials (Thompson & Mathias 1991) and providing a role model and advisor (Knapper & Cropley 1985).

Through encouraging a learning organization, managers will gain other benefits such as staff

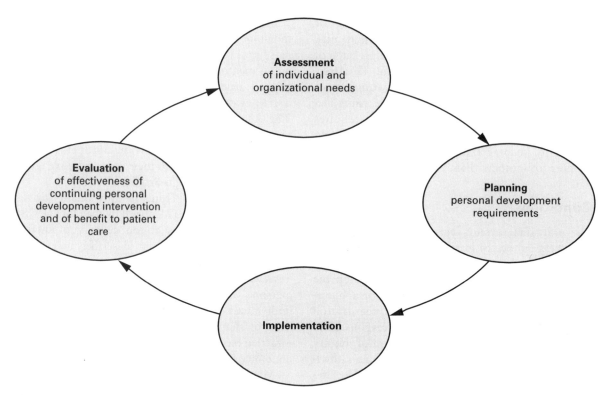

Fig. 26.2   A model of the continuing professional development cycle (from DOH 1998).

who can develop as expert practitioners with wider role boundaries; these staff will become valuable to organizations with transferable skills and new responsibilities (Fair 1995), particularly in the current NHS where there is a shortage of qualified nurses.

Some guidelines for promotion of lifelong learning are given in Box 26.1. Educationalists need to be aware that a preregistration education policy that will develop lifelong learners and promote lifelong learning should encourage (Carpenito 1991, Janhonen 1991, Jarvis 1987):

◆ learners to identify own needs and experiences required in clinical setting
◆ direction for learners to other learning experiences
◆ allowance for individual learning styles and personality differences
◆ more effective study skills
◆ self-evaluation
◆ peer review
◆ sharing between lecturers and learners of development of learning objectives
◆ responsibility of learners for their own learning.

Box 26.1   Guidelines for organizations to promote lifelong learning

◆ Training needs analysis
◆ Individual performance review
◆ Personal development plans
◆ Mentoring schemes
◆ Encouraging analysis and change
◆ Problem solving in care teams
◆ Discussion groups
◆ Shared learning
◆ Practice-based learning
◆ Reflective practice learning groups
◆ Valuing practice based on research

A strong continuing educational policy is a vital requirement for lifelong learning; when formal courses are planned they must be based on organizational needs by incorporating problem identification in the curriculum that focuses on health care (Jarvis 1987), using flexible strategies (see below) with facilitation and experiences that will meet learning objectives. Such clarity of purpose is essential in order to be helpful to the delivery of service and professional standards (Butterworth 1998).

STRATEGIES FOR LIFELONG LEARNING

An organizational training needs analysis is essential to formulate a robust training strategy that will provide professionals who are 'fit for purpose' at a cost that can be met within the available resources; however, individual learning needs assessment and action plans are also required for personal development plans that will meet the statutory body's needs for the minimum acceptable levels of continuous professional development—for example, the UKCC's requirements for reregistration for PREP (Pedder 1998). The personal development plan can form a key element of a personal professional profile that is required by the UKCC for reregistration every 3 years.

Through systematic and regular assessment and planning of learning experiences (see Box 26.2) professionals will develop a strategy for lifelong learning that is more meaningful to them, to the service and the client. The assessment can consist of objectives, assessment of time and resources, reflection of their own practice, analysis of current research, identification of other colleagues, research and development officers (Browne 1998) and educationalists as support or as a resource and an action plan with timescales and identification of costs (Pedder 1998). Reflection on learning can be enhanced through a learning diary in which the individuals record key points learned, how those might be applied to their practice, issues or areas that need further work, then assess how well they are using opportunities to learn in and outside of work, to review whether they are getting

Box 26.2 A personal development plan	
Stage 1: assessment	**Comments**
What do I need to do?	
What do I want to learn?	
Do I want to fulfil a personal training objective?	
Do I want to carry out practice at a higher standard?	
How much time have I got?	
What resources have I got already or are available?	
What aspects of my current practice do I need to change?	
What quality research is there already that might help me?	
Stage 2: planning	
What are my short term goals and the timescales for these?	
What are my long term goals and the timescales for these?	
What resources do I need to achieve these?	
Stage 3: reflection	
What are the key points I have learned?	
How might these be applied to my practice?	
Are there issues or areas that need further work?	
How well am I using opportunities to learn in and outside of work?	
Am I getting the most out of my learning?	
What feedback do my colleagues, mentor or supervisors give me on my development?	

the most out of their learning and then possibly involve other colleagues, mentors or supervisors on getting feedback on their development (Critten 1996). This model is similar to the approach suggested by Rath et al (1996) where individualized enhancement programmes were seen as the most appropriate way to impact significantly on competencies while using resources effectively. The process of the programme consisted of four phases from individual needs assessment, defining learning objectives written in the form of specific, measurable objectives, and assessment of available resources to evaluation of the learning experiences: 'This model encourages self-learning activities and recognises that individual learners have different learning styles and use unique learning strategies'.

Learning resources may be not just formally organized or academic courses but also self-directed work-based learning, or a combination of both. Jarvis recommends a balance of methods (Jarvis 1987). In reality, strategies will be somewhere along a continuum of learning, from informal student-directed methods to more formal approaches, which will probably be planned, facilitated and evaluated by educationalists (see Fig. 26.3).

Whatever the methods, accessing of information is vital for lifelong learning (Cheek & Doskatch 1998). Information-literate nurses can access the information superhighway and telecommunications systems to acquire knowledge and skills that relate to their roles and practice in order to enhance problem solving and decision making. It is not just the quantity of information, of which there is an abundance, that is needed. The nurse must also be discerning about the quality of information and needs critical thinking, analysis and evaluation skills to select material that is accurate, contemporary, reliable and relevant. However, Cheek & Doskatch (1998) found that students in preregistration programmes, despite being computer literate, had problems identifying, defining, analysing and articulating what exactly they needed from the information. To become an effective lifelong learner, the individual needs to realize that technology is just a tool, not the answer to knowledge.

As a developmental strategy, clinical supervision can assist with lifelong learning. The UKCC (1995) outlined six statements that would help in the development of a system of clinical supervision with ongoing evaluation of outcomes. These statements focus on support for practitioners to maintain standards, supervision being practice based, facilitated by a skilled supervisor, ground rules established and agreed, a realistic number of supervisees to each supervisor, preparation for supervisors and principles of supervision included in pre- and postregistration programmes and evaluation systems determined locally. However, clinical supervision can influence professional development only if it is made accessible regularly to all.

Mentoring has different interpretations although it has been recognized as a significant learning strategy (Jarvis 1995); one perspective sees mentoring as a structured and facilitated method for support, challenge and modelling, whereas others see mentorship as being possible only where the 'chemistry' is right (i.e. the individuals' choice is essential for the relationship to survive). Mentorship often occurs where mentees are newly qualified to help them reflect on practice and learn from their experiences. Whatever the context of the relationship and experience, a long term strategy is essential. Barlow (1991) reported that short

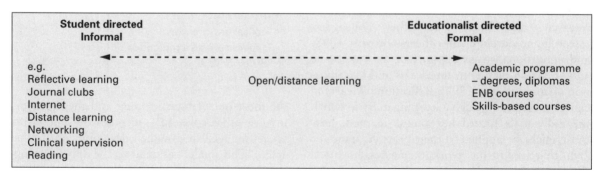

Fig. 26.3 A continuum of learning strategies.

term mentorship of students was not appropriate on clinical placements, particularly as mentors were often newly qualified nurses.

Reflection on and learning from practice is an essential component of CPD and critical to the growth of nursing as a profession: 'Reflecting—thinking purposefully about clinical practice to gain new insight, ideas and understanding—is becoming accepted as a vital element in the development of nursing' (Haddock & Bassett 1997). Reflection can take place informally by the individual, as in the personal development plan (see above), in clinical supervision, or in work groups. Carkhuff (1996) outlined reflective learning in work groups facilitated by staff development educators as groups could provide opportunities for nurses to become proactive learners. In the work groups by using the technique of reflection on action (including critical analysis, synthesis and evaluation), nurses identified what they had learned in the group by inquiry and also defined which aspects of learning that had occurred in the group were important to them. Reflection can also be used as a formal tool for assessment in academic programmes. Wallace (1996) described using reflective diaries to assess students formatively and proposed that adoption of learning diaries 'represents a move away from the concept of education as a product, towards emphasising nursing education as a lifelong process'. It was also recognized that this method had limitations as well as strengths—for example, keeping a diary depended on ability to express oneself and writing skills. There was also a risk that students might feel unprotected if disclosures were particularly deep. Mountford & Rogers (1996) described individual and group reflection in an ENB course focusing on summative course assessments and found that educational outcomes were positively influenced. Reflection as a learning strategy therefore seems advantageous, not only for the length of the academic programme or work group but as a tool for future individual development.

Reading some of the profusion of occupation-related books or journals also can provide an incentive to lifelong learning and will help the professional keep up to date with health care changes—'Reading is one the quickest, most accessible, most economical ways to accomplish this' (Armstrong & Gessner 1992). Yet a national study in the USA by Armstrong and Gessner found that, out of 721 staff nurses who were asked about their learning activities, only 15% preferred reading as a main learning activity and only 24% of the subjects used their medical/nursing library at least once a month. Factors that increased the subjects' reading were:

◆ belonging to nursing organizations
◆ subscribing to health-related journals
◆ purchasing one or more nursing books
◆ making one or more trips to the library
◆ reading at work.

The professionals in the study who did read, had received encouragement from managers or supervisors to read professional material; however, almost half reported little or no support. The study found that managers more frequently encouraged nurse managers and educators to read than supervisors encouraged staff nurses. Another study in the UK found that 45% of nurses read a journal on a weekly basis (Haig 1993). Certainly, reading is a cheaper option than study days and can be used at almost any time, in any place (Mathieson 1997).

While the commitment to reading is an individual one, encouragement and support from managers and clinical supervisors will provide a stimulus to lifelong learning, as will outreach schemes for journals, ward-based materials, journal clubs or flexibility of local professional library opening hours. Journal clubs in which group discussion and analysis can engender new ideas based on research and current literature are effective for professional development (Nolf 1996). A journal club should meet regularly and maintain direct focus on a particular topic at each meeting with a rotating group leader/moderator to organize, direct the discussion and conduct ongoing evaluation. Each member should present at least once a year. Through journals clubs nurses will be helped in learning and developing research-critical thinking skills; self-confidence will also be enhanced.

Networking has been viewed as a way of promoting individual growth and development (Gross 1977). Learning networks can be established informally in the work setting or internationally through e-mail with information exchange, support and dialogue, either around a particular interest or as a means of promoting coalition building for professional potency with powerful effects—for example, empowerment and political change. A study of learning networks in the USA (Bauer 1991) found that professional nurses learn important professional information informally, in a self-directed manner. Network members linked with one another because of experience and knowledge, recognized authority, rapport and accessibility. Listening, observing, asking helpful questions and offering alternative viewpoints and ideas are some of the skills of networking (Neubauer 1995). It is also a critical element in coping with change in health care and should not just be a skill solely used by executives and senior managers, as traditionally perceived, but the network must be used wisely (Gruber 1997).

Illich (1973) visualized learning networks as a web-like structure allowing learners to gain access to any educational resource they needed to achieve their learning objectives. Reference services, skills exchange and peer matching were the approaches he suggested but much of this requires organization and resourcing and would therefore be beyond the scope of the individual. These methods would, however, eliminate the dominance of institutionalized programmes.

A classic method of learning for those who cannot access formal courses is open and distance learning, particularly with the Open University. These methods fulfil needs for professional growth without the problem of being absent from family, occupational and social responsibilities (Joubert & du Plessis 1995). Learners often find that through open-learning courses their confidence improves and they are better equipped to give high quality care. However, students often feel isolated unless contact and peer support are built into courses. There are also resource implications as effective open-learning material is costly to produce. Evidence of effectiveness of open- or distance-learning material is therefore needed before utilizing such methods completely (Clark & Robinson 1994). Certainly it is an attractive option for professional development, not only for learners and education providers, but also for NHS employers who will be the customers (Ayer & Smith 1998), as such programmes allow for flexibility for study time to be planned around service needs.

Another means of providing flexibility for professional development programmes is the Credit Accumulation and Transfer Scheme (CATS). This is advantageous for professionals who change organizations and also promotes consistency of learning and specialization of postregistration practice while recognizing learning achieved in practice or from previous qualifications. Through Accreditation of Prior Learning (APL) and Accreditation of Prior Experiential Learning (APEL), which places academic credits on learning achieved by individuals in their practice, entry to academic programmes is widened. Learners then build up an individual programme of study using academic credits achieved through courses or modules of study at certificate, diploma or degree level to meet their personal and service needs. This programme will meet established academic and professional standards (Crooke & Marks-Maran 1993). The English National Board (ENB) framework is such a programme, but many individual higher education establishments provide other flexible routes towards academic awards. CATS has made higher education more accessible to nurses.

Many academic programmes for CPD recognize that the professional gains knowledge generated from experiential learning, which can be identified through reflection in practice. Work-based learning (WBL) recognizes the value of practice and offers a route to linking theoretical and clinical educational development (Hargreaves 1996). In WBL learners agree a contract outlining tasks and strategies to achieve learning in practice with educationalists and their manager. The learning achieved has to be supported by valid, current and reliable evidence before academic validation is given. This method of learning will benefit the organization, the learner and the academic institution.

Case studies

The following case studies are used to illustrate

CASE STUDIES

Bill is a 32-year-old nurse with a full-time job in mental health nursing and a young family; his wife does not work at present. He has had little time to study since qualifying but was interested in current developments in clinical work, especially in substance abuse, and read professional journals to keep himself updated. When the opportunity arose, he registered for a relevant ENB course. He gained confidence in his academic and clinical skills through this and, with managerial support, initiated and facilitated an inpatient substance abuse group. He continued his studies with a flexible degree pathway relevant to his clinical setting; taught modules were chosen based on his individual personal and professional needs in negotiation with his academic supervisor and in performance review with his line manager. There was also a work-based learning component in which he identified learning outcomes from his clinical groupwork.

He was motivated to continue his professional development as he was able to accrue academic credits at a pace that fitted in with his personal commitments, while basing his learning on professional interests and needs, thus maintaining a degree of control.

Sandy, an RMNH, aged 28 years, had attended various conferences and study days but felt they had little relevance to her clinical practice so wanted to update her knowledge and skills in a relevant area that would also meet the requirements for PREP. She heard of a skills-based course on working with the self-injurious client, which was an area that had not been addressed in her preregistration studies and in which she felt she needed more competence. The course carried academic credits but, at present, she was more interested in how the theory could be applied to practice.

Despite pregnancy and childbirth towards the end of the course, with support she completed the course. She also gained access to a network of resources that she would be able to use in the future to continue her learning. Her manager who had supported her throughout was prepared, on her return from maternity leave, to encourage her to develop related research projects and disseminate her knowledge to her care team.

Jean is a 38-year-old CPN who has been working in a very rural area for 10 years. Her only child has recently left home for university and she feels she needs an academic challenge herself but is unable to access university courses because of distance; she also wants something that will enable her to work more effectively with her clients whose problems range from anxiety and obsessive compulsive disorders to serious and enduring mental disorders. Her study skills are rusty so she first attends a short course in study skills at the nearest further education college. Then she rings the nearest university's library for information and is told about the Open University's newest course 'Mental health and distress: perspectives and practice' (K257S), which she enrols for and is able to work through at home. She finds the work stimulating, particularly when she is able to meet other students from a range of health and social care settings at study groups.

Jamilla, aged 30 years, an RMN, with managerial experience and NVQ level 4 in management, wanted to develop her clinical knowledge and skills in her area of nursing, specifically forensic nursing. She was able to gain credits under APL for her previous studies and commenced a degree pathway that incorporated the ENB 770 Nursing in controlled environments. For her 4-week placement for the course she negotiated with her manager and academic staff to visit and observe a range of forensic services in Canada. She established ongoing networking with these services through the Internet. On her return, she disseminated her findings to other students, as well as in her practice area. Further taught modules on research and assessment skills in forensic care were chosen through her own reflective practice to focus on skills she needed to respond to client and service needs.

John, aged 35 years, is a patients education teacher in a mental health residential setting. He had not done any further courses since his degree and felt stale and not focused on client needs. He identified a diploma course that would give him new knowledge and skills; however, after one module his manager said there were not enough resources to replace him while he attended the course. He had to withdraw but was encouraged by academic staff to continue updating himself with material from the course and he gained support and information from the students who worked in his area. He had also gained new information technology skills from the module so, through the Internet, found appropriate websites to gain access to ideas and contacts in his particular field.

He was able to identify a mentor in his own service who, although from a different discipline, was able to support him and guide him in specific areas of further reading.

the motivations and strategies used by individuals in the search for personal and professional development, some of the constraints they had to overcome and application of their learning to practice. Resources are also indicated, for example, peers and mentors, but the culture of learning at an organizational level, which is a crucial operational issue for CPD, has yet to be developed and researched adequately—in 5 years' time, hopefully, case studies or scenarios will include illustrations of good practice to illuminate the concept of lifelong learning.

Evaluation

Systems and organizational providers of strategies and resources for lifelong learning need to be evaluated for efficiency and flexibility. As Cowley (1995) points out, with increasing emphasis on managers playing a more active part in facilitating professional education, especially in the light of clinical governance, there is a need to look at how systems can enable or constrain learning for pro-

fessionals. In her analysis of a system that had deliberately abandoned its hierarchical provisions, there were still observable power patterns, inflexible communication lines, restricted interests, a narrow focus of learning, and managerial expectations of simplistic outcomes and, therefore, a likelihood of inhibition of CPD rather than valuing and encouraging skills and knowledge acquisition that will contribute to the whole organization.

Even in the USA, where continuous professional education has been evaluated, there are few data on the outcomes. A study in 1991 (Waddell) did find that 75% of those undertaking continuing education will deliver improved care and 90% of those learners had a positive perception of the impact. In the UK there is little empirical work on how CPD affects practice. Hughes (1990) claimed care planning was improved and others found that learners became more assertive, autonomous and competent (Lathlean, Smith & Bradley 1986, Turner 1991, Whitely 1992, Williams 1998).

Individual learner's needs and perceptions also need evaluated to understand and overcome constraints and barriers. Nolan, Owens & Nolan (1995) quote studies that have found that time, money, lack of information and availability of learning opportunities, workload and family pressures and lack of managerial encouragement all inhibited uptake of learning opportunities. Certain groups of staff are particularly disadvantaged (i.e. enrolled nurses, junior nurses, part-time nurses, night staff and private nursing home staff). Changes in practice have been even less evaluated. Whitely (1992) found that dissatisfaction and frustration after learning events could even be counter-productive. Nolan, Owens & Nolan (1995) found that perceived benefits were complex and included improvements to direct care.

Methods of evaluation can include self-report, record audit (independent review of patients' records) and direct observation by an independent professional (Grant 1992). Competency-based assessment by measuring outcomes, by subjective participant evaluation, and evaluation by an expert performance appraisal have also been suggested (Henwood, Edie & Flinton 1998). A wider perspective of evaluative methods is required, however, in order to capture the changes, through professional development, in attitude and values, the impact on the whole organization and the profession as well as a narrower focus on outcomes in a particular area of practice. Tripartite planning and evaluation of needs, function and outcomes may provide a more meaningful framework (Sunter 1993).

ACCREDITATION AND VALIDATION OF LIFELONG LEARNING

Whether CPD is a personal goal of the individual, a requirement for reregistration, an organizational responsibility or a quality standard set by government, there needs to be a consistent and recognizable method of accrediting the learning event or opportunity and validating the learning achieved. Where it is at an academic level the professional body and the Quality Assurance Agency (for higher education) will ensure quality but where, as in the case of profiles for PREP when reflective and experiential learning could be the major element, the cost of validators could be prohibitive, then the individual learners would have to self-validate their learning as the UKCC have proposed (Jasper 1995) with occasional auditing. However, as Jasper suggests, can nurses maintain, evaluate and ensure the quality of their learning? Can these methods ensure consistency?

The UKCC are about to produce and test guidelines on the types of appropriate learning and linkage to practice (Williams 1998). Then pilot studies will look at formats of profiles that can be audited, which will help them establish systems for auditing that are straightforward and equitable.

ISSUES AND DILEMMAS OF LIFELONG LEARNING

All of the above methods and strategies for learning can be either self-directed or voluntary, yet in the UK we now have mandatory continuing professional education in the form of PREP (UKCC 1995). This is described as a systematic framework for continuing professional education (Nolan, Owens & Nolan 1995) that must be tailored to the needs of the individual and relevant to the practice environment (Mitchell 1996). Surveys have shown that nurses have had difficulty with presenting evidence of the learning process and linking learning with practice needed to compile the required personal professional profile, although in reality the nurses did set goals and action plans (Williams 1998).

Indeed, the definition of CPD will cause tensions with a mandatory system as this limits the potential breadth of the continuing and developmental aspects of lifelong learning (Lindley 1997). There is a danger, however, that institutionalizing lifelong learning, as in mandatory CPD, will foster dependence in staff and, therefore, instead of empowering individuals to be autonomous, reflective and assertive learners, the individual could become passive, using learning opportunities not as personal achievements but as means to accommodate themselves to organizational or professional demands (Purdy 1997).

In a voluntary system, the individual decides whether and how to update or extend their competence and they do not have to record their learning. Australia's CPD is a voluntary activity that allows nurses to take advantage of learning opportunities as long as they are accessible and relevant. In obligatory CPD the professional body would require individuals to maintain their competence but would not enforce compliance and the responsibility to comply would rest with the individual. Oliveck (1998) claims that any compulsory aspect depresses motivation and professional enthusiasm, while Henwood, Edie & Flinton (1998) comment that the principle of adult learning is voluntarism; therefore mandatory CPD is a violation of this principle. However, mandatory education ensures nurses keep up with change and those who re-enter after an absence from employment will become competent (Yuen 1991).

Unless there is good evidence of the effectiveness of mandatory CPD in improving practice then there is a danger for reregistration. In reality, nurses may just give 'lip service' to CPD and passively resist learning opportunities: 'The desire of the learner to benefit from the learning experience is critical to the outcome of the process.' (Barriball,

While & Norman 1992). Not all nurses wish to progress, to develop, and may be actually threatened by mandatory CPD. In fact, Dill (1971) cautioned that some individuals may actually want their skills to decay and become obsolete as this may be more tolerable than any serious attempt to learn and develop!

There is also a tension between the traditional academic continuing education programme and experiential learning. Whereas the latter emphasizes reflection, is work based and allows self-direction, which is the cornerstone of lifelong learning, the former's rational and linear approach to curriculum planning increases educators' control over learning as they set the objectives; this decreases learners' autonomy and ability to be self-directing (Yuen 1991). However, formal continuing education aims to enhance practice through accumulation of a broad range of skills appropriate to varied settings (Sunter 1993), which is in opposition to many CPD issues. Educationalists themselves need to be more committed to self-directed learning: Janhonen (1991) found that nurse instructors failed to practise self-directed learning despite supporting it in principle. Yet, there is little research that proves the effectiveness of reflective learning (Grant 1992) and self-directed learning (Maslin-Prothero 1997) although these are central tenets in nurse education today as part of a humanistic and liberal ideology.

Responsibility for CPD, both financial and management, needs urgently to be addressed. If individuals are to fund their learning themselves then certain groups may be disadvantaged—for example, part-time staff, nursing home staff (Nazarko 1996). If funding comes from the employer then control is decentralized and CPD becomes more independent and rational in order to meet local needs (Yuen 1991). Local funding, though, carries the danger that meaningless and restrictive protocols may be built into service contracts in order to meet the minimum level specifications of provision, thus causing obstructions and constraints for individual learners (Cowley 1995). If employers are to invest at the outset of CPD systems and to continue to maintain programmes then they need to be convinced of the effectiveness of CPD in improving the service (Nolan, Owens & Nolan 1995). The fewer concrete benefits, such as individuals' improved critical skills, may then not be valued as much but, as mentioned previously, an organizational culture of learning that values such deeper level skills and attitudes is needed to change practice successfully.

Other constraints that need to be addressed by managers and educationalists are individuals' ability and willingness to undertake proactive and self-directed learning. There are certain boundaries that restrict nurses' ability to be self-directed (Candy 1991):

♦ perceived and disabling views about a lack of control over learning
♦ peer pressure leading to indifference or even antagonism to the learner from family or colleagues
♦ gatekeepers to learning placing obstacles in the way of learners, such as giving misleading information
♦ academic or professional language that differentiates an experienced learner from an inexperienced learner.

These issues need to be tackled to encourage lifelong learners not only at the individual and personal level, but also from a social and critical perspective.

FUTURE TRENDS AND NEEDS

Flexibility in provision of CPD programmes will be even more essential as local needs drive educational programmes. The long, developmental academic course will become a rarity as modular programmes become the norm; learners will demand strategies and resources that are accessible and equitable. Distance learning might be increasingly used in local training and education centres. Combination of video and TV programmes, mail systems and video-conferencing into a 'virtual university', where learners can participate in class discussions, communicate with peers and access tutorials or lectures, nationally and internationally (Davison & Rhodes 1996), is almost a reality. An example of a national project using an academic network is the Norwegian project, NITOL (Norwaynet with IT for Open Learning) where four universities and colleges joined forces in offering courses for credits, online on the academic network (Ask & Haugen 1995). Accessibility and flexibility are the obvious benefits. Issues such as a need for a shift from competition to common goals, rethinking to take full advantage of the potential of the new technology, copyright and ownership of knowledge, reliability of knowledge and problems related to openness of systems need addressed. The philosophical debate around how electronic communication in education separates the speaking body from the listening body also needs explored (Cheek & Doskatch 1998).

Flexible methods of registration and funding of vocational education and training have been outlined in the government's green paper The learning age (DEE 1998), which suggests career development loans offering people a deferred repayment loan. Technology will also help lifelong learning by using credit card-style individual learning credits, which would enable individuals to organize and pay for their own learning using employers' funds or their own earnings.

Ensuring standards of education provision, strategic direction of education and training and coordination of service needs with continuing education delivery, at a regional and national level, will be the role of the regional education and development groups proposed in the white paper The new NHS (DOH 1997). These groups will need to have real powers and resources as well as having a pragmatic perspective, or else there may be a danger they will just be more gatekeepers who can place obstacles or unrealistic specifications on continuing education delivery.

Learning in a multidisciplinary context will affect the lifelong learning of mental health professionals (Affara 1997) where constructive and effective team consolidation in the delivery of care must be taught and practised. Through more interprofessional education there will be more understanding and communication within teams (Skeil 1995). Other future directions for CPD include international links and exchanges possibly between institutions and between non-governmental organizations—for example, nursing exchanges

across professional organizations. Some of the educational activities for health professionals across international boundaries might be funded by multinational companies where scholarships or sponsorships could be utilized as long as these partnerships were in an ethical framework (Affara 1997). If international educational activities increased, there would be an accompanying need for accreditation to allow a mutual recognition of learning. The International Council of Nurses is currently looking at these issues.

Focused research agendas are needed in order to set future programmes, to satisfy purchasers' demands for proven, cost-effective CPD and to

Table 26.1

Learner focused	Assessing learners' perceptions of learning strategies, subjects, level and orientation to learning at different stages of the process; views of themselves as learners
Facilitator focused	Behaviours expected; commitment to personal autonomy as an educational goal; gatekeepers' strategies to meet learners' needs
Organization focused	Voluntary systems versus mandatory systems; hierarchical and academic systems versus local, employer-led systems; sources of financial support and resourcing; analysis of local needs
Process focused	What kind of educational perspective enables self-directed learning; facilitation skills needed to enhance lifelong learning; uptake and effectiveness of portfolio/profiles/personal development plans
Outcome focused	How continuing education improves quality of practice; how education overcomes professional obsolescence; contribution of CPD to career advancement and progression and staff retention; analysis of cost–benefits

satisfy the need for competent and self-directed professionals. The agendas may focus on different areas, as shown in Table 26.1.

SUMMARY

Uncertainty, lack of confidence and internal or external constraints may be the reason for evidence that the concept of CPD is maybe failing to become embedded in the nursing profession (Nolan, Owens & Nolan 1995, Whitely 1992). CPD is best encouraged as a cultural aspect of the profession (Oliveck 1998) and it must be the responsibility of not just the lifelong learner but also the educational advisers and providers, professional bodies and health care providers to promote and advance the culture of learning while removing the ideological and practical obstacles. The benefits for learners, as the green paper on lifelong learning states (DEE 1998), are that learning offers excitement and the opportunity for discovery as well as improving the chances of getting on; for employers, learning will make them more successful by keeping them up to date; for the nation, learning offers a way out of dependency and low expectation. For the health care profession there will be more fulfilled and competent practitioners: 'Through the acquisition of lifelong learning skills, nurses would be better able to meet the requirements of the profession and their clients and patients' (Maslin-Prothero 1997).

REFERENCES

Affara F 1997 Why lifelong learning? International Nursing Review 44(6):177–180

Annand F 1997 The mentor commitment. Insight 22(2):41–45

Appel A, Malcolm P 1998 Specialist education and practice in nursing: an Australian perspective. Nurse Education Today 18:144–152

Armstrong N L, Gessner B A 1992 Lifelong reading: putting reading first. Nursing Management June 24:61

Ask B, Haugen H 1995 The Norwegian JITOL experience and NITOL as a national extension. Journal of Computer Assisted Learning 11:203–209

Aslanian C B, Brickell H H 1980 Americans in transition: life changes and reasons for adult learning. In: Future directions for a learning society. College, New York

Ayer S, Smith C 1998 Planning flexible learning to match the needs of consumers: a national survey. Journal of Advanced Nursing 27(5):1034–1047

Bailey C 1988 Lifelong education and liberal education. Journal of Philosophy of Education 22(1):121–126

Barlow S 1991 The impossible dream. Nursing Times 87(1):53–54

Barribal K L, While A E, Norman I J 1992 Continuing professional education for qualified nurses: a review of the literature. Journal of Advanced Nursing 17:1129–1140

Bauer C 1991 Learning networks: a continuing education mechanism for nurses. Rutgers State University, New Brunswick

Browne A 1998 The role of the research and development officer. Nursing Standard 13(8):42–42

Butterworth T 1998 Speaking out. Nursing Times 94(42):21

Candy P 1991 Self-direction for lifelong learning. Jossey-Bass, San Fransisco

DISCUSSION QUESTIONS

1. Do you believe yourself to be continuously developing in order to learn about yourself as a social being, interacting with, and caring for, clients/patients and carers? If so, how can you support this process through professional development?
2. Which kind of lifelong learner are you:
   (a) one who uses learning as a means to achieve a specific goal (for example, career progression)?
   (b) an activity-orientated individual who is interested in learning for the circumstances in which it took place (for example, in meeting colleagues outside of work)?
   (c) one who seeks learning for its own sake?
3. What boundaries do you see restricting your ability to be self-directed? What strategies could you use to get over these?
4. How could you use the personal development plan (see Box 26.2) for your personal professional profile needed for PREP?

FURTHER READING

Carpenito L 1991 A lifetime commitment.
  Nursing Times 87(48):53–55
This article gives a succinct description of mandatory continuing education, from an American perspective, as well as a range of strategies for lifelong learning.

Cowley S 1995 Professional development and
  change in a learning organisation. Journal of
  Advanced Nursing 21:965–974
The article describes alternative approaches to organizational development with analysis on how the organization as a learning environment might be developed. An excellent source of information and debate for managers and educationalists.

Maslin-Prothero S 1997 A perspective on lifelong
  learning and its implications for nurses. Nurse
  Education Today 17:431–436
This article should be essential reading for all professionals, managers, trainers and educationalists interested in lifelong learning or CPD. The paper explores the literature on lifelong learning and relates how lifelong learning might contribute to the profession.

Nolan M, Owens R, Nolan J 1995 Continuing
  professional education: identifying the
  characteristics of an effective system. Journal
  of Advanced Nursing 21:551–560
The paper clearly outlines a functioning system of continuing professional education as well as benefits and barriers. A useful analysis for managers and educationalists.

Carkhuff M 1996 Reflective learning: work groups as learning groups. Journal of Continuing Education in Nursing 27(5):209–214

Carpenito L 1991 A lifetime commitment. Nursing Times 87(48):53–55

Cheek J, Doskatch I 1998 Information literacy: a resource for nurses as lifelong learners. Nurse Education Today 18:243–250

Clark E, Robinson K 1994 Open learning: the state of the art in nursing and midwifery. Nurse Education Today 14:257–263

Cowley S 1995 Professional development and change in a learning organisation. Journal of Advanced Nursing 21:965–974

Critten P 1996 Developing your professional portfolio. Churchill Livingstone, New York, ch 2

Crooke L, Marks-Maran D 1993 Learning that adds to your professional development. Professional Nurse Feb:284–287

Davison D, Rhodes D 1996 The virtual university. Nursing Standard 10(27):21–22

DEE (Department for Education & Employment) 1998 The learning age. A renaissance for a new Britain. The Stationery Office, London.

DeSilets L 1995 Assessing registered nurses' reasons for participating in continuing education. Journal of Continuing Education in Nursing 26(5):202–208

Dill W 1971 Obsolescence as a problem of personal initiative. In Dubin S (ed) Professional obsolescence. Lexington Books, Lexington MA

DOH (Department of Health) 1997 The New NHS. The Stationery Office, London

DOH (Department of Health) 1998 A first class service. Quality in the new NHS. The Stationery Office, London

ENB (English National Board) 1995 Creating lifelong learners: partnerships for care guidelines for the implementation of the UKCC's standards for education and practice following registration. ENB, London

ENB (English National Board) 1998

European Commission 1995 Year of lifelong learning. Guidelines. E.C. Brussels

Fair N 1995 Set up and grow. Nursing Management 2(2):24–26

Grant R 1992 Obsolescence or lifelong education: choices and challenges. Physiotherapy 78(3):167–171

Gross R 1977 The lifelong learner. Simon & Schuster, New York

Gross R (ed) 1982 Invitation to lifelong learning. Follett, Chicago

Gruber M 1997 Networking for nurses in today's turbulent times. Orthopaedic Nursing 16(2):25–30

Haddock J, Bassett C 1997 Nurses' perceptions of reflective practice. Nursing Standard 11(32):39–41

Haig P 1993 Nursing journals: are nurses reading them? Nursing Standard 8(1):22–25

Hall D, Mirvis P 1995 Careers as lifelong learning. In: Howard A (ed) The changing nature of work. Jossey-Bass, San Fransisco, pp 323–361

Hargreaves J 1996 Credit where credit's due—work-based learning in professional practice. Journal of Clinical Nursing 5(3):165–169

Henwood S, Edie J, Flinton D 1998 Continuing professional development—a re-examination of the facts. Radiography 4:5–8

Hinchliff S 1994 Learning for life. Nursing Standard 8(48):20–21

Houle C 1980 Continuing learning in the professions. Jossey-Bass, London.

Hughes R 1990 Evaluating the impact of continual professional education. Nurse Education Today 10:428–436

Illich I 1973 Deschooling society. Writers and Readers Publishing Co-operative, London

Janhonen S 1991 Andragogy as a didactic perspective in the attitudes of nurse instructors in Finland. Nurse Education Today 11:278–283

Jarvis P 1987 Lifelong education and its relevance to nursing. Nurse Education Today 7:49–55

Jarvis P 1995 Adult and continuing education: theory and practice, 2nd edn. Routledge, London

Jasper M 1995 The potential of the professional portfolio for nursing. Journal of Clinical Nursing 4:249–255

Johns H 1997 Self-development: lifelong learning? In: Horton I (ed) The needs of counsellors and psychotherapists. Sage, London, pp 54–67

Joubert A, du Plessis P 1995 Distance contact education bridging program: general nursing. South African Journal of Nursing 18(4):3–9

Knapper C, Cropley A 1985 Lifelong learning and higher education. Croom Helm, London

Knowles M 1984 The adult learner: a neglected species, 3rd edn. Gulf, Houston TX

Kolb D 1984 Experiential learning. Prentice Hall, New York

Lathlean J, Smith G, Bradley S 1986 Post-registration development schemes evaluation. NERU. Report no 4, King's Fund, London

Lawson K 1982 Lifelong education: concept or policy? International Journal of Lifelong Education 1(2):97–108

Lindley P 1997 Continuing professional development in the British Psychological Society: the differing needs of the profession and the professional body. European Psychologist 2(1):11–17

McManus E, Sieler P 1998 Freedom to enjoy learning in the 21st century: developing an active learning culture in nursing. Nurse Education Today 18:322–328

Maggs C 1996 Towards a philosophy of continuing professional education in nursing, midwifery and health visiting. Nurse Education Today 16:98–102

Maslin-Prothero S 1997 A perspective on lifelong learning and its implications for nurses. Nurse Education Today 17:431–436

Mathieson A 1997 Using journals and books for professional development. Nursing Times Learning Curve 1(4):2–3

Mitchell M 1996 The continuing professional education needs of midwives. Nurse Education Today 16:394–401

Mountford B, Rogers L 1996 Reflection in and on assessment. Journal of Advanced Nursing 24:1127–1134

Nazarko L 1996 Nursing home nurses need support to update skills. Nursing Times 92(42):38–40

Neubauer J 1995 The learning network: leadership development in the next millennium. Journal of Nursing Administration 25(2):23–32

Nolan M, Owens R, Nolan J 1995 Continuing professional education: identifying the characteristics of an effective system. Journal of Advanced Nursing 21:551–560

Nolf B 1996 Journal club: a tool for continuing education. Journal of Continuing Education in Nursing 26(5):238–239

Oliveck M 1998 So what is CPD? Therapy Weekly March 26:8

Pedder L 1998 Training-needs analysis. Nursing Standard 11(6):50–53

Purdy M 1997 Humanist ideology and nurse education. 2. Limitations of humanist theory in nurse education. Nurse Education Today 17:196–202

Rath D, Boblin-Cummings S, Bauman A et al 1996 Individualised enhancement programs for nurses that promote competency. Journal of Continuing Education in Nursing. 27(1):12–15

Skeil D 1995 Individual and staff professional development in a multidisciplinary team: some needs and solutions. Clinical Rehabilitation 9:28–33

Sunter S 1993 The effectiveness of continuing education. Nursing Standard 8(6):37–39

Thompson T, Mathias P 1991 Standards and mental handicap: key to competence. Ballière Tindall, London

Turner P 1991 Benefits and certificates of continuing education: an analytical survey. Journal of Continuing Education in Nursing 22(3):104–108

UKCC (United Kingdom Central Council for Nursing, Midwifery and Health Visiting) 1984 Code of professional conduct for the nurse, midwife and health visitor. UKCC, London

UKCC (United Kingdom Central Council for Nursing, Midwifery and Health Visiting) 1991 The report of the post registration education and practice project. UKCC, London

UKCC (United Kingdom Central Council for Nursing, Midwifery and Health Visiting) 1995 PREP and you—your professional development UKCC, London

Waddell D 1991 The effects of continuing education on nursing practice: a meta-analysis. Journal of Continuing Education in Nursing 22(3):113–118

Wallace D 1996 Using reflective diaries to assess students. Nursing Standard 10(36):44–47

Whitely S 1992 Evaluation of nursing education programmes: theory and practice. International Journal of Nursing Studies 29(3):315–323

Williams M 1998 Surveys reveal nurses getting the message about PREP. Nursing Times Learning Curve 2(10):2–3

Yuen F 1991 Continuing nurse education: some issues. Journal of Advanced Nursing 16:1233–1237

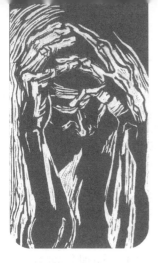

Chapter Twenty-seven

The law relating to mental health and disorder

Written by Enid E Wright and updated by Colin P Vose

AIMS

- ◆ To provide a review of the legislation that applies to people experiencing mental disorder
- ◆ To provide a reference to relevant sections within the legislation

KEY ISSUES

Mental Health Acts 1959 and 1983

Care in the Community Act 1995

Actors within the Act

Exclusions from definitions of mental disorder

Legislative duties and powers of health service personnel

Other statutory services (legislative base)

Children and young people

Other legislation

INTRODUCTION

Many people suffer from mental disorder during some stage of their lives, either personally or through their families or friends. The relevant law varies according to the mentally disordered person's condition at different times.

There is a continuum of relevant legislative provision ranging from that which promotes good mental health, through preventative/enabling/ rehabilitative measures, to statutory powers and duties relating to acute mental disorder. The application of preventative/enabling/rehabilitation legislation by social workers, nurses and others can help move the focus of their work with mentally disordered people along this continuum towards the mental health end.

Legislation can also be used to support the families of mentally disordered people and others who feel overwhelmed by traumas and personal problems. Professional support, with timely application of enabling legislation, can often prevent them also becoming mentally ill.

It is important, however, to know the difference between statutory duties and enabling powers. While all local authorities, for example, must fulfil their statutory duties, the extent to which enabling powers are used depends on the policy and resources of the particular authority. In this respect, social workers can bring pressure to bear on their employers in the interests of their clients and families.

Some legislative provisions are specific to mental health or disorder whereas others apply to mentally disordered people as they do to other vulnerable citizens. This chapter will consider both types.

CURRENT LEGISLATION

Current legislation includes the following:

Children and Young Persons Act 1933
Disabled Persons (Employment) Act 1944
National Assistance Act 1948
National Assistance (Amendment) Act 1951
Disabled Persons (Employment) Act 1958
Mental Health Act 1959

Criminal Procedure (Insanity) Act 1964
Health Services and Public Health Act 1968
Chronically Sick and Disabled Persons Act 1970
Local Authority Social Services Act 1970
Matrimonial Causes Act 1973
Juries Act 1974
Social Security Act 1975
National Health Service Act 1977
Nurses, Midwives and Health Visitors Act 1979
Education Act 1981
Health and Social Services and Social Security Adjudications Act 1983
Marriage Act 1983
Mental Health Act 1983
Representation of the People Act 1983
Police and Criminal Evidence Act 1984
Registered Homes Act 1984
Enduring Powers of Attorney Act 1985
Housing Act 1985
Disabled Persons (Services, Consultation and Representation) Act 1986
Social Security Act 1986
Access to Personal Files Act 1987
Children Act 1989
National Health Service and Community Care Act 1990
Social Security Act 1990
Criminal Justice Act 1991
Criminal Procedure (Insanity and Unfitness to Plead) Act 1991
Registered Homes (Amendment) Act 1991
Community Care (Residential Accommodation) Act 1992
Mental Health (Patients in the Community) Act 1995
Sex Offenders Act 1997

Rules of the Supreme Court 1965
County Court Rules 1981
Mental Health Act Commission (Establishment and Constitution) Order 1983
Mental Health Act Commission Regulations 1983
Mental Health (Hospital, Guardianship and Consent to Treatment) Regulations 1983
Mental Health (Nurses) Order 1983
Mental Health Review Tribunal Rules 1983
Court of Protection Rules 1984

Nursing Homes and Mental Nursing Homes
Regulations 1984

Court of Protection (Enduring Powers of
Attorney) Rules 1986

Local Authority Social Services (Designation of
Functions) Order 1989

Children (Secure Accommodation) Regulations
1991

Representations Procedure (Children)
Regulations 1991

Owing to space limitations, it has been necessary to restrict the section on children and young people. However, much of the rest of the chapter applies to them and there are suggestions for further reading.

CURRENT LEGISLATION SPECIFICALLY RELATING TO MENTAL HEALTH DISORDER

Mental Health Act 1959

Although the Mental Health Act 1983 consolidated much of the law of England and Wales specifically relating to mentally disordered persons, certain provisions of the Mental Health Act 1959 have not been repealed, including the following.

s.8 Function of welfare authorities. This section enables local authorities to provide residential accommodation for the care or aftercare of mentally disordered people under the National Health Service Act 1977 even though they are required or authorized to provide such accommodation under s.21 of the National Assistance Act 1948.

s.128 Sexual intercourse with patients. This section makes it an offence (i) for a man on the staff of, or employed by a hospital or mental nursing home to have extramarital sexual intercourse with a woman who is receiving treatment for mental disorder in that hospital or home either as an outpatient or an inpatient, and (ii) for a man to have extramarital sexual intercourse with a woman who is subject to his guardianship or is otherwise in his custody or care. No offence is committed

under s.128 if the man did not know. and had no reason to suspect, that the woman was a mentally disordered patient.

Mental Health Act 1983

This Act consolidated much of the law of England and Wales specifically relating to mentally disordered persons. It applies to Scotland and Northern Ireland only to the extent provided for in sections 146 and 147 respectively, which mainly relate to the removal of patients between the different countries of the United Kingdom.

The DHSS memorandum (DHSS 1983a) on Parts I-VI, VIII and X of the Mental Health Act 1983 provides guidance on the Act. The revised Code of practice (DOH & Welsh Office 1993) required under s.118 of the Act was prepared by the Mental Health Act Commission and published by the Secretaries of State for Health and for Wales in August 1993. It came into force on 1 November 1993 (DOH 1993a, DOH & Welsh Office 1993).

The Code is not mandatory in that professionals carrying out functions under the Act are not legally obliged to follow the advice contained in the Code. However, a failure to have regard to the Code could be used in legal proceedings as *prima facie* evidence of bad practice although the effect of non-compliance will largely depend upon the nature of the provision in the Code that has not been followed. Section 118 of the Act requires the Secretary of State to revise the Code from time to time.

The Act is divided into 10 Parts and six Schedules. This chapter gives a guide to key aspects of the application of the Act and the main definitions relating to patients, nurses and approved social workers under the Act. There is no space, however, to consider the other provisions in the same detail. In any case, this would duplicate what is more authoritatively stated in the legislation itself, the DHSS memorandum and the Code of practice, and more comprehensively dealt with in legal manuals and law books. The Mental Health Act manual (Jones 1991) is especially useful as it both updates the legislation and comments on it, with references to government circulars, cases and other documents. The chapter refers to relevant delegated legislation and other Acts where appropriate. It also considers the key themes reflected throughout the legislation, DHSS memorandum and Code of practice.

Part I (s.1) sets out the application and extent of the Act and defines 'mental disorder'

s.1(1) says 'The provisions of this Act shall have effect with respect to the reception, care and treatment of mentally disordered patients, the management of their property and other related matters'.

s.1(2) defines 'mental disorder' and three of the four specific categories of mental disorder as follows:

> In this Act—
>
> 'mental disorder' means mental illness, arrested or incomplete development of mind, psychopathic disorder and any other disorder or disability of mind and 'mentally disordered' shall be construed accordingly;
>
> 'severe mental impairment' means a state of arrested or incomplete development of mind which includes severe impairment of intelligence and social functioning and is associated with abnormally aggressive or seriously irresponsible conduct on the part of the person concerned and 'severely mentally impaired' shall be construed accordingly;
>
> 'mental impairment' means a state of arrested or incomplete development of mind (not amounting to severe mental impairment) which includes significant impairment of intelligence and social functioning and is associated with abnormally aggressive or seriously irresponsible conduct on the part of the person concerned and 'mentally impaired' shall be construed accordingly;
>
> 'psychopathic disorder' means a persistent disorder or disability of mind (whether or not including significant impairment of intelligence) which results in abnormally aggressive or seriously irresponsible conduct on the part of the person concerned.

The DHSS memorandum (DHSS 1983a) points out at para. 10 that the term 'mental illness' is undefined in the Act and says 'its operational definition and usage is a matter for clinical judgement in each case'.

The actors within the Act

The patient. s.145(1) defines the 'patient' as 'a person suffering or appearing to be suffering from mental disorder', except in Part VII, which relates to the management of patients' property and affairs, and unless the context otherwise requires.

However, the applicability of the condition of 'mental disorder' and of the specific conditions varies between different sections of the Act. Who is 'the patient', therefore, also depends on the particular section of the Act under consideration. More than one of the conditions may, of course, affect the patient at any one time (CCETSW 1992).

For many purposes of the Act a general diagnosis of 'mental disorder' is not sufficient and a diagnosis of one of the four specific categories of mental disorder—mental illness, mental impairment, severe mental impairment or psychopathic disorder—is required. A specific diagnosis must be made for an admission for treatment (s.3), a reception into guardianship (s.7), a hospital or guardianship order made by the court (s.37), an interim hospital order (s.38) and a transfer from prison to hospital (s.47). On the other hand, a specific diagnosis is not required in relation to admission for assessment (s.2), admission for assessment in cases of emergency (s.4), application in respect of a patient already in hospital (s.5), warrant to search for and remove patients (s.135) and mentally disordered persons found in public places (s.136).

See Chapter 29 of the Code of practice (DOH & Welsh Office 1993) for definitions and discussion relating to mental handicap/learning disabilities. See also the DHSS memorandum (DHSS 1983a) and Jones' Mental Health Act manual (Jones 1991).

A 'patient' for the purposes of Part VII—management and administration of property—is defined in s.94(2). Most patients are informal patients (see s.131 below).

Exclusions from the definitions of mental disorder. s.1(3) of the Act says:

Nothing in subsection (2) above shall be construed as implying that a person may be dealt with under this Act as suffering from mental disorder, or from any form of mental disorder described in this section, by reason only of promiscuity or other immoral conduct, sexual deviancy or dependence on alcohol or drugs.

Paragraph 16 of the memorandum (DHSS 1983a) advises:

This means that there are no grounds for detaining a person in hospital because of alcohol or drug abuse alone, but it is recognized that alcohol or drug abuse may be accompanined by or associated with mental disorder. It is therefore possible to detain a person who is dependent on alcohol or drugs if they are suffering from a mental disorder arising from or suspected to arise from alcohol or drug dependence or from the withdrawal of alcohol or a drug, if all the other relevant conditions are met. Similarly sexual deviancy is not of itself a mental disorder, for the purposes of the Act, which can provide grounds for compulsory detention.

Relatives. The terms 'relative' and 'nearest relative' are defined in s.26 of the Act. See also para. 68 of the memorandum (DHSS 1983a). Section 26, which defines 'relative' and 'nearest relative' for the purposes of Part II of the Act, also applies to patients who have been placed under hospital or guardianship orders by a court under s.37.

A person who has been identified as the patient's nearest relative can authorize any person, other than the patient or a person disqualified under subsection (5), to perform the functions of the nearest relative. The authority can be revoked at any time. Both the authority and the revocation must be in writing (see Regulation 14 of the Mental Health (Hospital, Guardianship and Consent to Treatment) Regulations 1983).

Section 27 as substituted by the Children Act 1989 defines the nearest relative of a child or young person in care. Under this section, if an unmarried child under the age of 18 years is in the care of a local authority by virtue of a care order

in England or Wales, that local authority becomes the child's nearest relative.

Section 28 as amended provides for a person who has been appointed as a child's guardian (other than under the Mental Health Act) or a person who is named in a residence order (as defined by s.8 of the Children Act 1989) to be that child's nearest relative.

Sections 27 and 28 also apply to children who have been placed under hospital or guardianship orders by a court under s.37.

Section 29 relates to the appointment by a court of an acting nearest relative. The section gives the county court power to make an order directing that the functions of the nearest relative shall be exercised by another person, or by a local social services authority.

Section 30 provides for the discharge or variation of an order made by a county court under s.29 for the appointment of an acting nearest relative. It also specifies the duration of an order which has not been discharged.

National Health Service personnel. A wide range of health service personnel are involved with mentally disordered patients in hospitals, residential and day services and the community generally. These include consultants, psychiatrists, psychologists, psychotherapists, hospital managers, doctors, nurses, occupational therapists, ambulance personnel, porters and receptionists. The legislative duties and powers of nurses include the following.

Nurse of the prescribed class. This term is defined in s.5(7) of the Mental Health Act 1983 which says 'In subsection (4) above "prescribed" means prescribed by an order made by the Secretary of State'. The Mental Health (Nurses) Order 1983 prescribes the class of nurse for the purposes of subsection (4) of this section as 'a nurse registered in Part 3 (first level nurses trained in the nursing of persons suffering from mental illness) or Part 5 (first level nurses trained in the nursing of persons suffering from mental handicap) of the register prepared and maintained under s.10 of the Nurses, Midwives and Health Visitors Act 1979 (the professional register)'.

Section 5(4) provides for nurses of the prescribed

class to invoke a 'holding power' in respect of a patient for a period of not more than 6 hours. Guidance on this is contained in Chapter 9 of the Code of practice (DOH & Welsh Office 1993). Jones (1991) submits that, as this Part of the Act applies only to mental nursing homes that are registered to receive detained patients, a nurse of the prescribed class who works in a mental nursing home could exercise the power provided for in this subsection only if the home in question is so registered.

Nurses generally. Nurses nurse mentally disordered patients in hospitals, mental and other nursing homes and in the community. They also have particular roles under ss.57 and 58 of the Act, which deal respectively with treatment requiring consent *and* a second opinion and treatment requiring consent *or* a second opinion. Section 57 provides that certain of the most serious forms of medical treatment for mental disorder can be given only if the patient consents to the treatment and three independent people, one being a doctor, have certified that the patient understands the treatment and has consented to it. The doctor must also certify that the treatment should be given because it will have a beneficial effect. Section 58 provides that certain forms of treatment shall not be given to a patient unless the patient consents or an independent medical practitioner has certified that either the patient is incapable of giving his consent or that the patient should receive the treatment even though he has not consented to it. Under both sections, before issuing the certificate the doctor must consult two other persons who have been professionally concerned with the patient's medical treatment and one of these shall be a nurse. See Chapter 16 of the Code of practice (DOH & Welsh Office 1993) and DHSS Circular no. DDL (84)4 'Mental Health Act Commission: guidance for responsible, medical officers—consent to treatment (DHSS 1984a). Chapters 14–26 of the Code, which relate to treatment and care in hospital, are also especially relevant.

The Act also defines the responsibilites of the responsible medical officers, managers, doctor and health authorities and considers approved social workers as follows.

LOCAL AUTHORITY SOCIAL SERVICES PERSONNEL

Approved social workers. An 'approved social worker' (ASW) means an officer of a local social services authority appointed to act as an approved social worker for the purposes of the Mental Health Act 1983.

Section 114 provides for the appointment of approved social workers by a local social services authority for the purpose of discharging the functions conferred on them by this Act. No person shall be appointed by a local social services authority as an approved social worker unless approved by the authority as having appropriate competence in dealing with persons who are suffering from mental disorder. In approving a person for appointment as an approved social worker a local social services authority shall have regard to such matters as the Secretary of State may direct.

In respect of approved social workers' functions the relevant sections are:

s.4	Admission for assessment in cases of emergency
s.10	Transfer of guardianship in case of death, incapacity, etc. of guardian
s.11	General provisions as to applications
s.13	Duty of approved social workers to make applications for admission or guardianship
s.14	Social reports
s.18	Return and readmission of patients absent without leave
s.29	Appointment by court of acting nearest relative
s.30	Discharge and variation of orders under s.29
s.40	Effect of hospital orders, guardianship orders and interim hospital orders
s.87	Patients absent from hospitals in Northern Ireland
s.89	Patients absent from hospitals in the Channel Islands or Isle of Man
s.115	Powers of entry and inspection
s.135	Warrant to search for and remove patients
s.136	Mentally disordered persons found in public places

s.138 Retaking of patients escaping from custody.

Other sections of the Act also involve approved social workers. Indeed, the whole Act is relevant to their role to some extent.

DHSS Circular no. LAC(86)15/WO circular no 51(86) (DHSS 1986) contains revised directions from the Secretary of State, made under s.114 of the Mental Health Act 1983, on the appointment of approved social workers. Paragraph 4 says:

The new arrangements provided for in this Circular are designed to ensure that all approved social workers receive appropriate and adequate training for the statutory duties they are required to perform. CCETSW will be responsible for approving training courses and for monitoring the standard of training provided by authorities—whether singly or in consortia: no costs will arise to authorities for this. Authorities themselves will be responsible for ensuring that only staff who have been properly trained and who are competent to perform statutory duties are appointed.

CCETSW's revised training requirements are in CCETSW Paper 19.19 (CCETSW 1993).

Paragraph 8 of the above Circular says, in judging the number needed, full allowance should be made for the time that these trained and experienced mental health social workers need to spend on preventive work which avoids the need for compulsion.

Paragraph 14 says:

Approved social workers should have a wider role than reacting to requests for admission to hospital, making the necessary arrangements and ensuring compliance with the law. They should have the specialist knowledge and skills to make appropriate decisions in respect of both clients and their relatives and to gain the confidence of colleagues in the health services with whom they are required to collaborate. ... Their role is to prevent the necessity for compulsory admission to hospital as well as to make application where they decide this is appropriate.

Paragraph 15 of the Circular stresses cooperation with other services.

The Code of practice (DOH & Welsh Office 1993) spells out in Chapter 2 the role of approved social workers in assessment and paras 2.10–2.17 stress the individual professional responsibility of the ASW. Paragraph 2.10 says:

It is important to emphasise that where an ASW is assessing a person for possible admission under the Act he has overall responsibility for co-ordinating the process of assessment and, where he decides to make an application, for implementing that decision. See also paras 2.28–2.29 of the Code on disagreements between different professionals and paras 2.30–2.31 on the choice of applicant for admission.

Other chapters of the Code are also especially relevant to ASWs including Chapter 3 'Part III of the Mental Helath Act—patients concerned with criminal proceedings', especially para. 3.12 on the role of the ASW, Chapter 6 'Admission for assessment in an emergency', Chapter 11 'Conveying to hospital' and Chapter 13 'Guardianship'.

Social workers, residential workers and other staff in local authority social services. Paragraph 8 of the above DHSS/WO Circulars (DHSS 1986) says that 'social workers to be approved should be selected from amongst those engaged in the wide range of mental health work in their departments'. Many sections of the Mental Health Act set out the other powers and duties of local authority social services. These include s.14, which places a duty on social services authorities to arrange for a 'social worker of their social services department' to interview the patient and provide hospital managers with a social report on a patient's social circumstances if the patient has been admitted to hospital pursuant to an application made by his nearest relative under either ss.2 or 3. Local authorities also have a duty to provide social circumstances reports to Mental Health Review Tribunals (MHRTs). Other local authority responsibilities under the Act include those relating to guardianship (ss.7 and 37, and Chapter 13 of the Code of practice) and aftercare (s.117, and Chapter 27 of the Code). Local authorities also have a responsibility to provide social work support to the health service, including psychiatric hospitals. HO Circular no. 66/90, annex F (HO 1990) sets out the responsibilities of local authority social services departments in relation to mentally disordered offenders. In addition to social workers, a wide range of staff in the personal social services, including residential workers, day-care workers, home help organizers and home helps, provide services to mentally disordered people of all ages.

Probation officers. Probation officers are particularly involved under Part III of the Mental Health Act 1983 with patients concerned in criminal proceedings or under sentence. Chapters 3, 7, 17 and 28 of the Code (DOH & Welsh Office 1993) are especially relevant as are HO Circular no. 66/90 (HO 1990) and the Police and Criminal Evidence Act 1984 and its Codes of practice (HO PACE 1991).

Voluntary and private sector staff. Many social workers, residential and other staff work in the voluntary and private sectors.

Police. The police have powers and duties under the Act, including s.135 relating to warrants to search for and remove patients to places of safety, s.136 relating to removal to places of safety of mentally disordered persons found in public places and s.137 relating to provisions as to custody, conveyance and detention. Chapters 3, 7, 10, 17 and 28 of the Code (DOH & Welsh Office 1993) are especially relevant as are HO Circular no. 66/90 (HO 1990) and the Police and Criminal Evidence Act 1984 and its Code of practice (HO PACE 1991).

Lawyers. Lawyers have responsibilities under the Act including those relating to MHRTs, both as tribunal members and as solicitors with experience of tribunal work, as well as in relation to the management of property and affairs, for example, as Lord Chancellor's Visitors.

The prison service, prison medical service and forensic psychiatric service. These services also have responsibilities under the Mental Health Act 1983 and are dealt with in HO Circular no. 66/90 (HO 1990). The chapters in the Code (DOH & Welsh Office 1993) relating to criminal proceed-

ings and medical treatment are also especially relevant.

The courts. Courts, including Magistrates Courts, and the Crown Prosecution Service, have responsibilities under mental health legislation including those set out in the Act, Code (DOH & Welsh Office 1993) and HO Circular no. 66/90 (HO 1990) relating to criminal proceedings.

Generally speaking, all the main 'actors' are involved to a lesser or a greater extent in most parts of the Act. In any case, each needs to know the roles played by the others.

Medical treatment. It is worth noting that the term 'medical treatment' includes nursing, and also care, habilitation and rehabilitation under medical supervision' (s.145).

The community. The term 'community' is not defined in the Mental Health Act, but it is where most mentally disordered people live.

The law should not be applied in isolation, but needs to be seen in the context of social work, nursing, medical and other professional practice.

Part II of the Act (Sections 2–34) relates to compulsory admission to hospital and guardianship

Documentation must be in the form set out in the Mental Health (Hospital, Guardianship and Consent to Treatment) Regulations 1983. Many chapters of the Code of practice (DOH & Welsh Office 1993) are also relevant. Part II contains the following provisions:

s.2 admission for assessment

(2) An application for admission for assessment may be made in respect of a patient on the grounds that

(a) he is suffering from mental disorder of a nature or degree which warrants the detention of the patient in a hospital for assessment (or for assessment followed by medical treatment) for at least a limited period; and

(b) he ought to be so detained in the interests of his own health or safety or with a view to the protection of other persons.

(3) An application for admission for assessment shall be founded on the written recommendations in the prescribed form of two registered medical practitioners, including in each case a statement that in the opinion of the practitioner the conditions set out in subsection (2) above are complied with.

This section authorizes compulsory admission to hospital for assessment (or for assessment followed by treatment) and for detention for this purpose for up to 28 days. If applicants are approved social workers they must inform the nearest relative about the application, although the nearest relative cannot prevent an approved social worker making an application. The approved social worker is required to have regard to any wishes expressed by relatives of the patient, but is not required to consult with them.

DOH/WO Circular letter of 18 February 1992 (DOH & Welsh Office 1992) removed an obscurity from the former Code of practice on the Act, which seemed to suggest that people would be admitted compulsorily only if they were a danger to themselves or others. It has now been made clear that people can be compulsorily admitted for the sake of their health alone. The amended Code could help reduce the number of mentally ill people sleeping rough.

Paragraph 23 of the memorandum (DHSS 1983a) points out that the conditions for s.2 admissions are not quite so stringent as those for s.3 admissions because assessment may well be used for the purpose of determining whether the more stringent conditions for admission for treatment are met.

s.3 admission for treatment

(2) An application for admission for treatment may be made in respect of a patient on the grounds that:

(a) he is suffering from mental illness, severe mental impairment, psychopathic disorder or mental impairment and his mental disorder is of a nature or degree which makes it appropriate for him to receive medical treatment in a hospital; and

(b) in the case of psychopathic disorder or mental impairment, such treatment is likely to alleviate or prevent a deterioration of his condition; and

(c) it is necessary for the health or safety of the patient or for the protection of other persons that he should receive such treatment and it cannot be provided unless he is detained under this section.

(3) An application for admission for treatment shall be founded on the written recommendations in the prescribed form of two registered medical practitioners, including in each case a statement that in the opinion of the practitioner the conditions set out in subsection (2) above are complied with; ...

Compulsory admission to hospital for treatment and subsequent detention can last for an initial period of up to 6 months. Under s.3 if approved social workers make the application they must consult with the patient's nearest relative if practicable and cannot proceed with the application if the nearest relative objects. The applicant must have seen the patient within the previous 14 days and an approved social worker applicant must interview the patient before making an application.

Applications under ss.2 and 3 can be made by either the patient's nearest relative or an approved social worker and should be addressed to the managers of the hospital to which admission is sought.

Whether it is appropriate to detain a patient under ss.2 or 3 is considered by the Code of practice (DOH & Welsh Office 1993) and Chapter 5 of the consultation documents relating to revision of the Code (DOH 1992a, 1993a).

s.4. s.4 provides for **admission for assessment in cases of emergency** for a period of up to 72 hours. Applications may be made either by an approved social worker or the nearest relative and shall be sufficient in the first instance if founded on one of the medical recommendations required by s.2 (see Code of practice at para. 6.1 *et seq.* (DOH & Welsh Office 1993)).

s.5 Applications in respect of patients already in hospital. This section provides for applications for compulsory detention under ss.2 or 3 to be made by a registered medical practitioner for up to 72 hours in respect of mentally disordered patients who are already receiving treatment in hospital as informal patients. It also sets out the procedures that can be used if it is considered that a patient might leave the hospital before there is time to complete an application under ss.2 or 3.

Subsection (4) provides for nurses of a pre-scribed class to invoke a 'holding power' for up to 6 hours:

If, in the case of a patient who is receiving treatment for mental disorder as an in-patient in a hospital, it appears to a nurse of the prescribed class:

(a) that the patient is suffering from mental disorder to such a degree that it is necessary for his health or safety or for the protection of others for him to be immediately restrained from leaving the hospital; and

(b) that it is not practicable to secure the immediate attendance of a practitioner for the purpose of furnishing a report under subsection (2) above,

the nurse may record that fact in writing; and in that event the patient may be detained in the hospital for a period of six hours from the time when that fact is so recorded or until the earlier arrival at the place where the patient is detained of a practitioner having power to furnish a report under that subsection.

See also the Code of practice (DOH & Welsh Office 1993).

s.6 The effect of an application for admission. This section authorizes applicants or anyone authorized by them to take and convey the patient to hospital within specified periods and the hospi-tal managers to detain the patient once admitted. See Chapter 11 of Code of practice (DOH & Welsh Office 1993).

s.7 An application for guardianship. This section specifies the circumstances whereby a patient aged 16 years or over may be received into the guardianship of a local social services authority or a person who is acceptable to the authority. Neither the authority nor individual is obliged to accept the duties of guardian. The grounds for a guardianship application in respect of a patient are that:

(a) he is suffering from mental disorder, being mental illness, severe mental impairment, psychopathic

disorder or mental impairment and his mental disorder is of a nature or degree which warrants his reception into guardianship under this section; and

(b) it is necessary in the interests of the welfare of the patient or for the protection of other persons that the patient should be so received.

A guardianship application must be founded on the written recommendations of two registered medical practitioners and may be made by either the patient's nearest relative or an approved social worker. The latter cannot make an application if the nearest relative objects, which can cause difficulty if the relative seems to be acting irre-sponsibly towards the patient (Jones 1991). It is not possible for a mentally handicapped person whose impairment is not associated with abnor-mally aggressive or seriously irresponsible conduct to be placed on a guardianship order.

A patient may also be compulsorily admitted to a hospital or residential care facility under s.47 of the National Assistance Act 1948 or in an emer-gency under s.1 of the National Assistance (Amendment) Act 1951. In practice, the use of these provisions tends to be confined to elderly people, living alone and unable to care for them-selves. Under s.47 a local authority may make an application to a Magistrates Court to remove a person from home on the grounds (i) that the person is suffering from grave chronic disease or, being aged, infirm or physically incapacitated, is living in insanitary conditions; (ii) that the person is unable to devote to himself or herself, and is not receiving from others, proper care and attention; and (iii) that removal from home is necessary, either in the person's own interests or for prevent-ing injury to the health of, or serious nuisance to, other persons.

s.8 Effect of a guardianship application etc. This section confers specific powers limited to restrict-ing the liberty of the person under guardianship only to the extent necessary to ensure that various forms of treatment, social support, training, edu-cation, occupation or residence are undertaken. The guardian does not have the power to detain the patient, use or dispose of the patient's proper-ty, or carry out any financial transactions on the patient's behalf. The guardian is subject to the duties laid down in Part III of the Mental Health (Hospital, Guardianship and Consent to Treatment) Regulations 1983. See also para. 13.7 of the Code of practice (DOH & Welsh Office 1993).

s.9. s.9 empowers the Secretary of State to make **regulations as to guardianship.**

s.10. s.10 provides for the **transfer of guardianship** where the guardian dies, becomes incapacitated, wishes to relinquish the function or is found to be performing his functions negligently.

s.11. s.11 contains **general provisions as to applications for admission for assessment or treatment or guardianship.**

s.12. s.12 contains **general provisions as to medical recommendations.**

s.13. s.13 sets out the **duty of approved social workers to make applications for admission or guardianship** if they consider that applications ought to be made and are of the opinion, having regard to any wishes expressed by relatives or any other relevant circumstances, that it is necessary or proper for them to make the applications. Before making an application for admission to hospital, the approved social worker must 'interview the patient in a suitable manner and satisfy himself that detention in a hospital is in all the circumstances of the case the most appropriate way of providing the care and medical treatment of which the patient stands in need'. If so required by the nearest relative, the local social services authority has a duty to direct an approved social worker to consider making an application for admission to hospital. See Chapter 2 of the Code (DOH & Welsh Office 1993).

s.14. s.14 provides for **social reports** and places a duty on social services authorities to provide hospital managers with a report on a patient's social circumstances if the patient has been admitted to hospital pursuant to an application by his or her nearest relative under s.2 or s.3.

s.15. s.15 relates to **rectification of applications and recommendations.**

s.16. s.16 provides for **reclassification of patients.**

s.17. s.17 provides for **leave of absence from hospital.** This section applies to the granting of leave for all patients detained under Part II of the Act. Leave of absence can be granted only by the responsible medical officer. This section should be applied to cover all leave from the shortest period of absence to extended absence. The period of leave can be extended in the patient's absence.

Conditions may be imposed on the patient whilst on leave for the protection of the patient's interest or that of the general public. These conditions may include a place of residence, attendance at day care services or visits by a key worker. The granting of leave and conditions attached to it should be recorded in the patient's notes. The patient, the key worker and the patient's GP should be made explicitly aware of the granting of leave and relevant conditions. Section 17 is the appropriate section for detained patients to participate in escorted leave whilst in the custody of a designated staff member of the hospital.

s.18. s.18 provides for the **return and readmission of patients absent without leave.** In such condition where a patient absconds or disregards the conditions of leave as stipulated in Section 17 the patient may be taken into custody by:

◆ an approved social worker
◆ any police constable
◆ any officer on the staff of the hospital.

s.19. s.19 provides for **regulations to be made by the Secretary of State as to transfer of patients.** See Mental Health (Hospital, Guardianship and Consent to Treatment) Regulations 1983.

s.20 Duration of authority for detention or guardianship. This section provides for patients who have been detained for treatment or placed under guardianship to be detained or kept under guardianship for an initial period of up to 6 months. It also sets out the renewal criteria to be satisfied which can be for one further period of 6 months and subsequently for 1 year at a time.

These renewal provisions can be used to renew the authority to detain a patient only if the patient's mental condition requires his detention as a hospital inpatient (*R. v. Hallstrom, ex p. W.; R. v. Gardner, ex p. L. (1986) 2 All E.R. 306*). The decision in the *Hallstrom* case has generated a debate on whether there should be legislation to introduce a new 'community treatment order', which would permit the compulsory administration of drugs to patients living in the community (see below).

s.21. s.21 makes **special provisions as to patients absent without leave** and s.22 **special provisions as to patients sentenced to imprisonment, etc.**

s.23. s.23 relates to **discharge of patients**. For discussion, see Hoggett (1990) and Jones (1991).

s.24. s.24 provides for **visiting and examination of patients** and the production of documents relating to discharge (see Reg. 10 Nursing Homes and Mental Nursing Homes Regulations 1984). See also Chapter 26 of the Code of practice (DOH & Welsh Office 1993).

s.25. s.25 relates to **restrictions on discharge by nearest relative.**

ss.26–30. ss.26–30 relate to **functions of relatives of patients** (see above).

s.31. s.31 relates to **procedure on applications to county court.** See County Court Rules 1981.

s.32. s.32 relates to the Secretary of State's power to make **Regulations for purposes of Part II.** See Mental Health (Hospital, Guardianship and Consent to Treatment) Regulations 1983.

s.33. s.33 makes **special provisions as to wards of court.**

s.34. s.34 relates to **interpretation of Part II.**

Part III (Sections 35–55) relates to patients concerned in criminal proceedings or under sentence

This Part deals with the circumstances in which patients may be admitted to and detained in hospital or received into guardianship on the order of a court or transferred to hospital or guardianship from penal institutions on the direction of the Home Secretary. Guidance is contained in the Code of practice (DOH & Welsh Office 1993) and Home Office Circular no. 66/90 'Provision for mentally disordered offenders' (HO 1990), which contains sections on the police, Crown Prosecution Service, Magistrates Courts, probation service, prison medical service, psychiatric services, health services and local authority social services.

The Police and Criminal Evidence Act 1984 and its Codes on detention and questioning (HO PACE 1991) are relevant both to the role of the police and to the social worker's role as 'appropriate adult' for mentally disordered people and juveniles.

Section 4 of the Criminal Justice Act 1991 requires that, where an offender is or appears to be mentally disordered, the court shall normally obtain a medical report before passing a custodial sentence. It also requires the court to consider the likely effect of such a sentence on that condition and on any treatment that may be available for it.

Under common law, a person is considered unfit to plead or 'under disability' if unable to instruct a legal representative, understand a charge against them, follow evidence, or challenge a juror. These aspects of the common law are not affected by the Criminal Procedure (Insanity and Unfitness to Plead) Act 1991. The 1991 Act was a response to civil liberties campaigns that complained that under the Criminal Procedure (Insanity) Act 1964 the only option available to the court was a hospital order without restriction of time—that is, potentially indefinite detention without trial. Moreover, the evidence relating to the alleged offence used not to be heard by the court, so there was a presumption of guilt. Now, where an accused person has been found unfit to be tried, the Criminal Procedure (Insanity and Unfitness to Plead) Act 1991 provides for a 'trial of the facts' by a jury.

s.35 Remand to hospital by the courts for the purpose of assessment and preparation of report. This applies to persons charged with offences that could lead to imprisonment. Duration of this section is for an initial 28 days with an option to extend to a maximum of 12 weeks.

s.36 Remand to hospital by courts for treatment. If a person is charged with an offence before a

Crown Court, with a offence which could lead to imprisonment, that person can be remanded to hospital to receive treatment. This section cannot be used in the case of a person with a previous conviction of murder or stands accused of murder.

s.37 Interim orders. These provide a temporary alternative to allow the court to decide if the best course of action is Section 37 or imprisonment, fine or probation.

s.41 Restriction orders. Where a Crown Court makes a Section 37 hospital order, it also has the powers to impose restrictions on the patient's discharge. These restrictions are such that leave may only be granted with the agreement of the Secretary of State (Home Office), transfers require Home Office approval, discharge can only occur with Home Office agreement. In order to impose a restriction order the Court must be satisfied that it is necessary for the protection of the public from serious harm being mindful of the nature of the offence, the person's criminal history and the risk of reoffending if allowed to go free. The duration of the restriction order is determined by the Court and is often indefinite. The Home Office has the powers to end the restriction order, leaving the original hospital order intact, to discharge the patient absolutely or allow conditional discharge. The MHRT has similar powers on appeal.

ss.47 and 49. These cater for the **transfer from prison to hospital** of a convicted prisoner to hospital for treatment of a mental disorder. s.48 makes provision for the **transfer of a remanded prisoner to hospital.**

Part IV (Sections 56–64) relates to consent to treatment

This Part, which overrides the common law, applies only to treatment relating to the patient's mental disorder. It clarifies the extent to which treatment for mental disorder can be imposed on detained patients in hospitals and mental nursing homes. It provides for two categories of treatment which have different legal consequences. These are, first, the most serious treatments, which require the patient's consent *and* a second opinion (s.57) and, secondly, other serious treatments, which require the patient's consent *or* a second opinion (s.58). Treatments that do not come within either category can be imposed on a detained patient who understands the nature and purpose of the treatment, but expressly withholds consent (s.63). The safeguards provided for by ss.57 and 58 can be overridden if the treatment is required urgently (s.62). See the Code of practice (DOH & Welsh Office 1993) especially Chapters 15 and 16, the Mental Health Act Commission's guidance in DHSS Circular no. DDL (84)4 (DHSS 1984a) and the Mental Health (Hospital, Guardianship and Consent to Treatment) Regulations 1983. For further advice on capacity and consent, see also the Law Commission documents 'Mentally incapacitated adults and decision-making: a new jurisdiction' and 'Mentally incapacitated and other vulnerable adults: public law protection' (Law Commission 1992, 1993).

For a discussion of supervision and treatment in the community, see 'Future developments' below.

Patients presenting particular management problems

For guidance, see Chapter 18 of the Code (DOH & Welsh Office 1993).

Part V (Sections 65–79) relates to mental health review tribunals

These tribunals are empowered under the Act to review the cases of many detained patients and can also hear applications in relation to patients who are subject to guardianship orders. They have no jurisdiction over informal patients. Provisions relating to the constitution of MHRTs are in Schedule 2. Tribunals must also follow the procedure laid down in the Mental Health Review Tribunal Rules 1983 and where the Rules are silent on a point of procedure the tribunal must follow the rules of natural justice. The function of a tribunal is to review the justification for the patient's continued detention or guardianship at the time of the hearing. It has no power to consider the validity of the admission that gave rise to the liability to be detained.

Part VI (Sections 80–92) relates to the removal and return of patients within the United Kingdom or abroad

Part VII (Sections 93–113) relates to the management of property and affairs of patients

The powers of the judge or Master of the Court of Protection are exercisable when the court is satisfied, after considering medical evidence, that a person is incapable, by reason of mental disorder, of managing and administering his property and affairs. Invoking the jurisdiction of the Court of Protection in respect of the property and affairs of patients has the effect of suspending their ability to act for themselves in all areas within its jurisdiction, even if they actually had the capacity to do so in some respects or from time to time (see Law Commission reports (Law Commission 1992, 1993)). The Court of Protection does not have jurisdiction over the management or care of the patient's person or where the patient should live.

Guidance to receivers who have been appointed by the Court of Protection is in a Handbook for receivers published by the Public Trust Office (Public Trust Office 1993). For information about the appointment of the Public Trustee as receiver under the Mental Health Act 1983, see Jones (1991). See also Managing other people's money (Letts 1990).

Part VII provisions include those relating to judges' functions, wills, power to appoint receivers, Lord Chancellor's Visitors, proceedings, procedures, appeals and enduring powers of attorney. See also the Court of Protection Rules 1984.

The Enduring Powers of Attorney Act 1985 enables donors to appoint an attorney to make legally binding decisions on their behalf and whose authority will not be revoked by donors' subsequent mental incapacity. In the event of the donor becoming mentally incapable, the attorney must apply to the Court of Protection for the instrument to be registered. (See Court of Protection (Enduring Powers of Attorney) Rules 1986. See also Further reading.)

Part VIII (Sections 114–125) relates to miscellaneous functions of local authorities and the Secretary of State

Provisions include:

s.114 Appointment of approved social workers (see above).

s.115 s.115 provides approved social workers with **powers of entry and inspection of premises** where a patient is believed to be living.

Powers of entry and inspection of mental nursing homes and residential care homes are contained in the Registered Homes Act 1984, Nursing Homes and Mental Nursing Homes Regulations 1984, Registered Homes (Amendment) Act 1991 and the Community Care (Residential Accommodation) Act 1992.

s.117 Aftercare. This section applies to persons who are detained under s.3, admitted to hospital in pursuance of a hospital order, under s.37, hospital order patients subject to restriction orders under s.41, or persons transferred to the hospital in pursuance of a transfer direction under ss.47 or 48, and then cease to be detained and leave hospital.

Subsection (2) says:

> It shall be the duty of the District Health Authority and of the local social services authority to provide, in co-operation with relevant voluntary agencies, after-care services for any person to whom this section applies until such time as the District Health Authority and the local social services authority are satisfied that the person concerned is no longer in need of such services.

s.117 A duty to make aftercare arrangements. This section should be read in conjunction with Section 7 of the Disabled Persons (Services, Consultation and Representation) Act 1986, the care programme approach (CPA) guidance and the Mental Health (Patients in the Community) Act 1995. The CPA requires that everyone with serious mental health problems requiring care from specialist mental health services should have a document and assessment of a person's health and social care needs leading to the development of an agreed care plan. A key worker is identified to monitor the delivery of the care plan and ensure that there are regular reviews of the client's progress. To necessitate this the aftercare requirements of Section 117 should be fulfilled. They are: prior to discharge the hospital managers should send written notification of the date of discharge to the health authority and local social services authority for the area in which the patient is to reside. These two authorities are required to cooperate in assessing the client's need for services. These assessments must be made before the patient is discharged.

s.118. s.118 provides for a **Code of practice.**

s.119. s.119 provides for the **payment of medical practitioners appointed by the Secretary of State to carry out certain functions under the Act** and for them to have access to detained patients cared for in mental nursing homes and to their records.

s.120. s.120 places duties relating to the **general protection of detained patients** on the Secretary of State who has directed the Mental Health Act Commission to carry out these duties on their behalf.

s.121 Mental Health Act Commission. This section provides for the continuance of the Commission and relates to its functions. The Regulations and Order concerning the functions, establishment and constitution of the Commission are the Mental Health Act Commission Regulations (1983) and the Mental Health Act Commission (Establishment and Constitution) Order 1983.

The Commission's functions are quite separate from those of MHRTs, which determine whether a patient should continue to be detained. The Commission has no power to discharge a patient.

s.123. s.123 provides for **transfers to and from special hospitals.**

s.125 Inquiries. The Secretary of State may cause an inquiry to be held in any case where he or she

thinks it advisable to do so in connection with any matter arising under the Act.

Part IX (Sections 126–130) relates to offences against patients

Part X (Sections 131–149) miscellaneous and supplementary

The miscellaneous provisions section includes a number of very important provisions including the following:

s.131 Informal admission of patients

(1) Nothing in this Act shall be construed as preventing a patient who requires treatment for mental disorder from being admitted to any hospital or mental nursing home in pursuance of arrangements made in that behalf and without any application, order or direction rendering him liable to be detained under this Act, or from remaining in any hospital or mental nursing home in pursuance of such arrangements after he has ceased to be so liable to be detained.

This section provides that patients can either enter hospital for treatment for mental disorder on an informal basis, or remain in hospital on an informal basis once the authority for their original detention has come to an end. There are no special formalities that need to be observed for an informal patient to be admitted to a psychiatric hospital and, subject to s.5, informal patients can leave hospital when they like. With the exception of s.57 provisions, informal patients are not subject to the Part IV consent to treatment provisions. Nor are they entitled to compulsory aftercare services.

Jones (1991) points out that there is no legally established mechanism for reviewing either the reasons for informal patients' admission to hospital or the justification for their continued hospitalization. Once informal patients have been admitted to hospital, no person or body is placed under any legal obligation to inform them of their legal status and of the fact that they are free to leave hospital whenever they wish. Paragraph 14.1 of the Code of practice (DOH & Welsh

Office 1993) states that 'it should be made clear to informal patients that they are allowed to leave hospital at any time'. The admission is informal, and not voluntary. It is not necessary for patients to express their consent to the admission and it is possible to admit patients on an informal basis as long as they are not indicating either verbally or through their actions that they object to the admission. Paragraph 2.7 of the Code of practice says:

> Where admission to hospital is considered necessary and the patient is willing to be admitted informally this should in general be arranged. Compulsory admission should, however, be considered where the patient's current medical state, together with reliable evidence of past experience, indicates a strong likelihood that he will change his mind about informal admission prior to his actual admission to hospital with a resulting risk to his health or safety or to the safety of others.

In addition, many old people with some degree of senile dementia live in local authority, voluntary or private residential care homes or nursing homes. Many others are living in their own or relatives' homes.

s.132 s.132 places a **duty upon hospital managers to provide information to detained patients** and their relatives to try to ensure that they understand which section of the Act authorizes the patient's detention and the effects of that section and their right to apply to MHRTs if applicable. Section 132 also places a further duty on hospital managers to ensure that patients understand the means by which their detention can be ended and the various safeguards from which they benefit, including those concerning consent to treatment, the Code of practice, the Mental Health Act Commission, patients' correspondence and legal aid schemes, which could help them obtain representation for a court appeal or MHRT.

s.133. s.133 sets out the **duty of managers to inform the nearest relative of discharge.**

s.135 Warrant to search for and remove patients. This section provides for a magistrate to issue a warrant authorizing police officers to enter private premises, using force if necessary, to remove a mentally disordered person liable to be detained or not. In the latter case, Subs. (1) provides for this, if it appears to a justice of the peace, on information on oath laid by an approved social worker, that there is reasonable cause to suspect that people believed to be suffering from mental disorder have been, or are being, ill treated, neglected or kept otherwise than under proper control, or being unable to care for themself, are living alone in any such place. In the execution of a warrant under Subs.(1), the constable must be accompanied by an approved social worker and a registered medical practitioner. A patient may be detained in a 'place of safety' for up to 72 hours. In this section 'place of safety' includes residential accommodation provided by a local social services authority under Part III of the National Assistance Act 1948, a hospital as defined by the Mental Health Act, a police station, a mental nursing home or residential home for mentally disordered persons or any other suitable place whose occupier is willing temporarily to receive the patient. Under the Police and Criminal Evidence Act 1984 a police officer may enter and search any premises without a warrant under this section if this is required to save life or limb or prevent serious damage to property. Persons removed to a police station as a place of safety under this section are protected by the PACE Codes of practice (HO PACE 1991).

Local social services authorities have a duty to provide temporary protection for the property of persons admitted to hospital or to accommodation provided under Part III of the National Assistance Act 1948.

s.136 Mentally disordered persons found in public places. Subsection (1) says:

> If a constable finds in a place to which the public have access a person who appears to him to be suffering from mental disorder and to be in immediate need of care or control, the constable may, if he thinks it necessary to do so in the interests of that person or for the protection of other persons, remove that person to a place of safety within the meaning of section 135 above.

People can be detained in a place of safety for up to 72 hours so that they can be examined by a doctor and interviewed by an approved social worker in order that suitable arrangements can be made for treatment or care. A person does not have to commit an offence before the police can use their power to remove but, Jones (1991) submits, in most cases the behaviour of the persons removed would have justified their being charged with an offence against public order. See Chapter 10 of the DOH/WO Code of practice (DOH & Welsh Office 1993) and the Police and Criminal Evidence Act Codes of practice (HO PACE 1991).

s.137 Provisions as to custody, conveyance and detention. This section specifies the circumstances whereby a person is deemed to be in legal custody and provides that anyone who is required or authorized to detain or convey a person who is in legal custody shall have the powers of a constable when so acting.

Of the **Schedules to the Act,** Schedule 1 relates to application of certain provisions to patients subject to hospital and guardianship orders and Schedule 2 to MHRTs.

MENTAL HEALTH PROCEDURAL PRACTICE

Care programme approach

Introduced in 1991, this is intended to be the cornerstone of the government's mental health policy. This process applies to all people experiencing serious mental health problems who are clients of mental health services, whether on an informal or formal basis. The care programme approach (CPA) consists of four stages, which should be applied to all clients in all cases. They are:

◆ a systematic assessment of the health and social care needs
◆ development of a care plan that meets the assessed need; this care plan should actively involve all relevant care agencies and the client in its formulation
◆ identification of a key worker who should monitor the delivery of care in line with the care plan

◆ review of the client's progress and amendment of the care plan as appropriate.

The CPA approach is aimed at ensuring that key principles of good practice are delivered. These include systematic multidisciplinary assessment, planning, monitoring and reviewing a care plan, the inclusion of users and carers in the formulation and delivery of care and identification of a lead person or key worker. All of this is undertaken within a framework that is flexible and responsive to the client's changing needs.

Supervision registers

Since April 1994, mental health care providers have been required to maintain a supervision register as part of the CPA. A patient may be placed on the register by the responsible consultant psychiatrist if the patient:

◆ has a severe mental illness
◆ is a patient of specialist psychiatric services
◆ may pose a significant risk of committing serious violence or suicide or severe self-neglect.

All patients placed on the register should be subject to a care plan that aims to reduce risk and is subject to regular review whilst contact is maintained by a key worker. The register is a means to ensure that the highest priority is given to those patients so registered in accessing resources to facilitate care. Information listed on the register should include the person's full name, address, date of birth, etc., information as to the person's status under the Mental Health Act, type of risk posed to self and others and a record of violent or self-destructive behaviour, name and contact details of the key worker and other professionals involved along with date of last and next review. Removal from the register can occur only when the person has been assessed as no longer posing a significant risk to themself or others.

Sex Offenders Act 1997

Under this legislation those who are detained under the 1983 Mental Health Act (or criminal law) and have a conviction for a sexual offence against either an adult or a child must inform the police of their whereabouts within 7 days of their arrival in any given area. People who are subject to this legislation and detained under the Mental Health Act should be informed of this legal requirement.

Children and Young Persons Act 1933

This legislation identifies a list of offences against children. A child is defined by the 1989 Children Act as anyone under the age of 18. This list is updated in line with any new legislation relating to serious crimes against children. The list includes such crimes as murder, manslaughter, assault, rape, abduction, procurement for purposes of intercourse and other areas of sexual and/or physical abuse. The Children and Young Persons Act 1933 identifies those people so convicted of such crimes as posing a significant danger to children. This group of people are termed Schedule One Offenders. It is the responsibility of service providers to identify Schedule One Offenders in their care, to ensure that these people pose no danger to children by either restricting or denying access to children or monitoring closely any contact permitted to occur. In the planning of discharge, care providers have a duty to notify the local social services department of the address of future residence. The conditions applying to Schedule One are intended to apply for the duration of the offender's lifespan.

OTHER STATUTORY SOCIAL SERVICES

Local authorities have statutory responsibility for providing social services for mentally disordered people of all ages in their area. As well as aiding their rehabilitation and preventing recurrence of mental disorder, social services can help prevent other vulnerable people from becoming mentally ill by supporting them in times of extra stress. Powers and duties of local authority social services authorities are listed in Schedule 1 to the Local Authority Social Services Act 1970 and the Local

Authority Social Services (Designation of Functions) Order 1989. People who suffer from mental disorder and learning disabilities come within the definition of 'disabled person' in s.29 of the National Assistance Act 1948, which is also the definition used in the Disabled Persons (Services, Consultation and Representation) Act 1986 and the National Health Service and Community Care Act 1990.

In order to understand the statutory provisions, a number of Acts need to be read together. The National Health Service and Community Care Act 1990 does not consolidate social welfare legislation by replacing earlier relevant statutes. Many of the 1990 Act's community care provisions are based on earlier statutes, which still remain in force as amended by subsequent legislation.

Part III of the National Health Service and Community Care Act 1990 relates to community care in England and Wales. Sections 42–45 relate to the provision of accommodation and welfare services and ss.46–50 to general provisions concerning community care services.

Section 46 provides for local authority plans for community care services and says in this section:

> 'community care services' means services which a local authority may provide or arrange to be provided under any of the following provisions;
> (a) Part III of the National Assistance Act 1948;
> (b) Section 45 of the Health Services and Public Health Act 1968;
> (c) Section 21 of and Schedule 8 to the National Health Service Act 1977; and
> (d) Section 117 of the Mental Health Act 1983.

The above provisions, together with s.2 of the Chronically Sick and Disabled Persons Act 1970, s.4 of the Disabled Persons (Services, Consultation and Representation) Act 1986, s.47 of the 1990 Act and the various relevant directions issued by the Secretary of State, provide the basic legal framework under which local authorities provide care in the community.

The 1990 Act provides for the government to make specific grants to local authorities for mental illness social services. However, the government wishes local authorities to arrange that community care be increasingly provided by the voluntary and especially the private sectors.

The Department of Health has produced much guidance arising from the 1990 Act.

Part I of the Health and Social Services and Social Security Adjudications Act 1983 also relates to community care, s.1 providing for joint financing and Part VIII permitting local authorities to make charges for certain social services.

Collecting and disseminating information

The Chronically Sick and Disabled Persons Act 1970 s.1, as amended by the Disabled Persons (Services, Consultation and Representation) Act 1986 s.9, requires every social services authority to gather information on how many disabled persons are living in its area and inform itself as to how it should plan to meet their needs. It also places a duty on the local authority to publish general information about its services for disabled persons and ensure that anyone who uses these is given information about other relevant services. The National Health Service and Community Care Act 1990 emphasizes the publication of information about the assessment process, the availability of services and access to the complaints procedure.

Assessment of needs

See Chronically Sick and Disabled Persons Act 1970 s.1; Disabled Persons (Services, Consultation and Representation) Act 1986 s.4(a) and (b), s.8; Children Act 1989 s.17 and Schedule 2 Part I; National Health Service and Community Care Act 1990 s.47. Section 4 of the 1986 Act relates to services under the 1970 Act and provides that, when requested to do so by disabled persons, their authorized representative, or any person who provides care for them in the circumstances mentioned in s.8, a local authority shall decide whether the needs of the disabled person call for the provision by the authority of any services in accordance with s.2(1) of the 1970 Act. Section 4 places a clear duty on local social services authorities to decide, when requested to do so, whether

the needs of a disabled person require the provision of welfare services under s.2 of the 1970 Act. The provision in the 1986 Act relating to the authorized representative is not in force. See also DHSS Circular no. LAC(87)6 (DHSS 1987). Section 8 of the 1986 Act relates to the duty of the local authority, when assessing the needs of a disabled person who receives a substantial amount of regular care from a person other than an employee of the statutory social services, to have regard to the carer's ability to continue to provide that care. It also requires the local authority to provide an interpretation service if the carer is unable to communicate effectively by reason of mental or physical incapacity and, in determining whether such a service is required, the local authority must take into account any views expressed by the carer. Although Subs. (1) relating to carers is in force, Subs. (2) relating to communication is not. Paragraph 6 of DHSS Circular no. LAC(87)6 (DHSS 1987) says, although the section places no specific requirement on the local authority to provide services or support for the carer, authorities will no doubt continue as part of normal good practice to have regard to the possible need for such services and to the desirability of enabling the disabled person to continue living at home for as long as possible if this is what that person wishes.

Section 47 of the National Health Service and Community Care Act 1990 provides for assessment of needs for community care services. The local authority must assess both the needs of the local population and the social care needs of individuals. After assessing individual needs, local authorities must arrange appropriate packages of care which may include a range of options. Services provided should reflect the client's choice.

Section 17 of the Children Act 1989 relates to the provision of services for children in need, their families and others.

The provision of services in the community

These are provided under the National Assistance Act 1948 s.29 as extended by s.2 of the Chronically Sick and Disabled Persons Act 1970, the Disabled Persons (Services, Consultation and Representation)

Act 1986 and the National Health Service and Community Care Act 1990 Part III. Section 29 as amended states in Subs. (1) that a local authority may, with the approval of the Secretary of State, and to such extent as he or she may direct in relation to persons ordinarily resident in the area of the local authority, make arrangements for promoting the welfare of persons to whom this section applies—that is, persons who are blind, deaf or dumb, or who suffer from mental disorder of any description and other persons who are substantially and permanently handicapped by illness, injury or congenital deformity or such other disabilities as may be prescribed by the Minister. Section 29(4) lists the types of arrangement that may be made under Subs. (1). Section 2 of the 1970 Act extends s.29 of the 1948 Act and places a duty on local authorities to make arrangements for all or any of the matters specified.

The National Health Service Act 1977 ss.3, 21(1)(b) and Schedule 8 para. 2(1) are also relevant. Section 21(1) states that the services described in Schedule 8 in relation to care of mothers and young children, prevention, care and aftercare and home help and laundry facilities are functions exercisable by local social services authorities, and that Schedule 8 has effect accordingly. The Schedule requires that local social services authorities provide necessary home help and laundry facilities for persons handicapped as a result of having suffered from illness or by congenital deformity. Local authority social services also have responsibility under Schedule 8 to provide day services for adults with mental handicap. The Schedule also provides that local social services authorities may, with the Secretary of State's approval and direction, provide preventive services, care and aftercare for persons suffering from mental disorder and who are received into guardianship. Under ss.3 and 21 respectively health services and social services may provide aftercare services for mentally ill and mentally handicapped persons discharged from hospital.

Provision of residential accommodation

The National Assistance Act 1948 s.21 enables local authorities to provide residential accommodation for sick, handicapped or elderly people and they must provide it to the extent that the Secretary of State has directed in DHSS Circular no. 13/74 (DHSS 1974). Accommodation is also provided in voluntary and private residential homes. See also the 1990 Act and the Community Care (Residential Accommodation) Act 1992. Under the 1990 Act local authorities are responsible for assessing individual needs for residential services and for paying fees for residents according to their assessments.

Registration of residential care homes

Local authorities are responsible for registering and inspecting residential care homes. See Registered Homes Act 1984, s.48 of the National Health Service and Community Care Act 1990, Registered Homes (Amendment) Act 1991 and Community Care (Residential Accommodation) Act 1992.

Compulsory admission into residential care

See National Assistance Act 1948 s.47 and National Assistance (Amendment) Act 1951.

Protection of property

See National Assistance Act 1948 s.48(1) above.

Sheltered employment

The Disabled Persons (Employment) Act 1958 s.3 empowers local authorities to make arrangements for the provision of facilities for enabling disabled persons to be employed or work under special conditions, including sheltered employment.

Welfare of old people generally

The Health Services and Public Health Act 1968 s.45 relates to the promotion by local authorities of the welfare of old people generally.

Social work support in health settings

Local authority social services authorities provide social work support for the health service.

Housing

Part III of the Housing Act 1985 relates to housing the homeless and s.72 deals with cooperation between housing and social services authorities. Although local authority housing departments have primary responsibility for the homeless, s.72 attempts to ensure the cooperation of social services. Section 59 says a person has priority need if *inter alia* that person or anyone who lives or might reasonably be expected to live with him or her is especially vulnerable because of age, disability or other special reasons.

Access to personal files

The Access to Personal Files Act 1987 provides access for individuals to information about themselves maintained by certain authorities and allows them to obtain copies of, and require amendment of such information.

OTHER STATUTORY SERVICES FOR PERSONS WITH MENTAL DISORDER

Health services

Both specialist and generic medical services are provided under NHS legislation. Hospitals and local authorities are required to cooperate when mentally disordered people are discharged from hospital, as seen above. Local authority social services authorities provide social work support to the NHS.

Employment

The Department of Employment has primary responsibility for assisting disabled people find work under the Disabled Persons (Employment) Act 1944. See also local authorities' powers in relation to sheltered and other employment under the Disabled Persons (Employment) Act 1958.

Social security and welfare rights and benefits

People with mental health problems often face particular difficulties in claiming social security benefits (see Grimshaw 1993–94). See Social Security Acts 1975, 1986 and 1990.

For further law relating to people with learning disabilities see Wright (1992). Workers with mentally disordered people also need to know about legislation relating to antidiscrimination and substance misuse.

CHILDREN AND YOUNG PEOPLE

The DOH Code of practice (DOH & Welsh Office 1993) applies to all patients including those under 18 years. Chapter 30 gives guidance of particular importance to children and young people.

There is no minimum age limit for admission to hospital under the Act. Jones (1991) submits there is nothing in the Act that prevents a child being compulsorily admitted to hospital under Part II. Provisions in the Mental Health Act specifically relating to children and young people include the following.

s.131(2) Informal admission of patients

Paragraph 30.7 of the Code (DOH & Welsh Office 1993) provides guidance applicable to young people not detained under the Act in relation to consent to medical treatment.

Children in 'secure accommodation'

The Children (Secure Accommodation) Regulations 1991 provide that s.25 of the Children Act 1989, which sets restrictions on the use of secure accommodation for children, does not apply to a child who is detained under any provision of the Mental Health Act.

Confidentiality

Paragraph 30.11 of the Code (DOH & Welsh Office 1993) says young people's legal rights to confidentiality should be strictly observed.

Placement

Paragraph 30.12 of the Code maintains the principle that it is preferable for children and young people admitted to hospital to be accommodated with others of their own age group in children's wards or adolescent units, separate from adults. Under ss.85 and 86 of the Children Act 1989 the local social services authority must be notified if a child either is, or is intended to be, accommodated by a health or local education authority, or in a residential, nursing or mental nursing home, for more than 3 months.

Complaints

Paragraph 30.13 of the Code (DOH & Welsh Office 1993) says children and young people in hospital (both as informal and detained patients) and their parents or guardians should have ready access to existing complaints procedures, which should be drawn to their attention on their admission to hospital. Certain children are also entitled to use the Children Act complaints procedure established in accordance with the Representations Procedure (Children) Regulations 1991.

The Mental Health Act Commission is concerned about children with mental disorders who are outside the control of the Mental Health Act, 1983 (e.g. re. levels of dosage).

Other statutory social services for children and young people

The Children Act 1989 contains most of the other current legislative provisions relating to children except children in court proceedings or adoption. To some extent, the whole Children Act is relevant to mentally disordered children, but Part III of the Act makes special provision for 'children in need', which term includes 'disabled children'.

Section 17(10) states:

for the purposes of this Part a child shall be taken to be in need if
(a) he is unlikely to achieve or maintain, or to have the opportunity of achieving or maintaining, a reasonable standard of health or development without the provision for him of services by a local authority under this Part;
(b) his health or development is likely to be significantly impaired, or further impaired, without the provision for him of such services;

or

(c) he is disabled...

Section 17(11) states:

For the purposes of this Part, a child is disabled if he is blind, deaf or dumb or suffers from mental disorder of any kind or is substantially and permanently handicapped by illness, injury or congenital deformity or such other disability as may be prescribed; and in this Part 'development' means physical, intellectual, emotional, social or behavioural development; and 'health' means physical or mental health.

Section 17(1) states:

It shall be the general duty of every local authority ...
(a) to safeguard and promote the welfare of children within their area who are in need; and
(b) so far as is consistent with that duty, to promote the upbringing of such children by their families, by providing a range and level of services appropriate to those children's needs.

Section 17(2) states:

For the purpose principally of facilitating the discharge of their general duty under this section, every local authority shall have the specific duties and powers set out in Part I of Schedule 2.

This deals with local authority support for children and families including provision of services for families. This Schedule has the force of law and imposes on local authorities the following duties and powers:

1. identification of children in need and provision of information

2. maintenance of a register of disabled children
3. assessment of children's needs
4. prevention of neglect and abuse
5. provision of accommodation in order to protect the child (i.e. a local authority may assist another person obtain alternative accommodation away from the child's home in order to protect the child)
6. provision for disabled children
7. provision to reduce need for care proceedings, etc.
8. provision for children living with their families
9. family centres
10. maintenance of the family home
11. duty to consider racial groups to which children in need belong.

As seen above, s.17(11) states 'health' means physical or mental health. Many of the legislative provisions of the Children Act are preventive measures which, if skilfully applied, can help prevent mental disorder and preserve the mental health of both children and their families.

It is not possible here to describe or even list all the relevant provisions of the wide-ranging Children Act. Detailed regulations and guidance have been prepared by the government, including a document on children with disabilities (DOH 1991).

Other statutory services for children with mental disorder

Education

The Education Act 1981 places a duty on the local education authority to educate children in accordance with the assessment of their special educational needs. Sections 5 and 6 of the Disabled Persons (Services, Consultation and Representation) Act 1986 provide for the referral to local authority social services of disabled persons leaving special education.

Health services

Under NHS legislation, both generic and specialist medical services are provided for mentally disordered people of all ages.

Child guidance

Child guidance services are provided by local education authorities or social services.

Leisure and support services

Mentally disordered children and young people are entitled to use these as are others.

It needs to be borne in mind that children are often helped most by support of their families and therefore knowledge of legislation relating to adults as above is often needed by those working with children and young people.

RIGHTS AND DUTIES AS CITIZENS UNDER OTHER LEGISLATION

Marriage

A marriage can be void if either party did not give valid consent because of 'unsoundness of mind' or at the time of the marriage was suffering from a mental disorder within the meaning of the Mental Health Act 1983 which was of such a kind or to such an extent as to make the person unfit for marriage (Matrimonial Causes Act 1973). Any party to a marriage must be capable of giving valid consent, understand the nature and purport of the marriage, and freely give consent to it. Anyone who does not believe the patient capable of giving valid consent can object to the marriage. The marriage of patients detained under the Mental Health Act is provided for under s.1 of the Marriage Act 1983 and some such marriages have taken place out of hospital. Guidance on the procedure is in DHSS Circular no. HC(84)12/LAC(84)9 (DHSS 1984b), which points out that many patients detained under the Mental Health Act 1983 are capable of understanding the nature and purport of marriage and can consent to it.

Voting

The voting rights of informal patients are contained

in the Representation of the People Act 1983. Informal mental patients may have their names placed on the Register of Electors if they have made a valid declaration under s.7(4) of that Act (see DHSS Circular no. HC(83)14 (DHSS 1983b)). Households are asked to include on their electoral registration form people who normally live in the household but are temporarily away as voluntary patients in psychiatric hospitals. Patients who are detained in a hospital or mental nursing home are not entitled to have their names placed on the Register.

Serving on juries

Mentally disordered people ineligible to serve on juries fall into three categories:

1. any person under guardianship
2. any person who has been determined by a judge to be incapable of managing his property and affairs
3. anyone who suffers or has suffered from mental illness, psychopathic disorder, mental handicap or severe mental handicap and because of this is either resident in a hospital or similar institution or regularly attends for treatment by a medical practitioner.

The definitions of mental handicap and severe mental handicap for this purpose are the same as the definitions of mental impairment and severe mental impairment in the Mental Health Act, but without the reference to abnormally aggressive or seriously irresponsible conduct. The list of those ineligible does not include people living in the community and not receiving regular medical treatment (see Juries Act 1974).

Driving licences

An applicant for a driving licence must disclose any prescribed disability. See Hoggett (1990) and up to date driving licence application forms.

Contracts

A contract entered into by a mentally incapacitated person not subject to the jurisdiction of the Court of Protection is binding unless it can be proved that the other party knew of the incapacity. The main exceptions are contracts for 'necessaries' (see also Part VII of the Act and Law Commission Reports (Law Commission 1992 and 1993)).

Wills

A testator must be of sound mind, memory and understanding. The Court of Protection is empowered to make statutory wills on behalf of mentally incapable people (see Part VII of the Act and Law Commission Reports (Law Commission 1992 and 1993)). Rules of the Supreme Court 1965 and County Courts Rules 1981 contain special provisions governing the participation of people under a legal disability in legal proceedings.

Workers and volunteers in citizen advocacy schemes enable people with mental health problems obtain their legal rights as citizens.

RECURRENT THEMES

There are a number of themes that recur throughout all the above legislation, Memoranda, Circulars and Codes of practice. Paragraph 1.3 of the DOH Code of practice (DOH & Welsh Office 1993) sets out a number of broad principles to be applied when working under the Mental Health Act. These are also relevant to the other legislation and guidance outlined above. They include:

Respect for and consideration of individual qualities and diverse backgrounds—social, cultural, ethnic and religious

Section 13(2) of the Mental Health Act 1983, for example, says patients are to be interviewed 'in a suitable manner'. However, Barnes (1990) discusses the apparent unequal application of the law relating to assessment for compulsory detention, when racist and sexist attitudes seem to affect outcomes. Workers need to remember, too, that mental disorder is only one aspect of an individual's personality.

Treatment or care in the least controlled and segregated facilities practicable

The principle of 'the least restrictive alternative' is relevant at all stages of a patient's 'career', with the emphasis first on care in the community, then informal admission, the least restriction if admitted, and discharge and aftercare as soon as possible thereafter. This principle applies to children as well as adults and to those involved in criminal proceedings.

The promotion of self-determination and personal responsibility

The provisions refer at times to the involvement of patients. Often this can be through advocacy schemes. Vulnerable people will need to be listened to and given information so that they can make informed choices. They need to be empowered so that the care packages provided for them under recent legislation reflect their real needs.

Legal rights to be drawn to the patient's attention

The legal rights include those relating to consent to treatment, MHRTs, the Mental Health Act Commission and complaints procedures. The manager has a duty under s.132 to inform detained patients of their legal position and rights, both orally and in writing.

Concern for relatives and other carers and emphasis on partnership with them

Sometimes there is conflict between the patient's rights and avoiding risk to the health or safety of the patient or to others. In such complex cases, it is especially important for the professionals involved to understand the relevant law.

Prevention

The risks can often be reduced by early and skilful use of preventive measures to support those who are especially vulnerable.

Interprofessional cooperation

This is another recurrent theme. Paragraphs 2.28–2.29 of the DOH Code of practice (DOH & Welsh Office 1993) offer guidance when there are disagreements between professionals.

Access to information

Access to information is stressed in most of the relevant legislative provisions including the National Health Service and Community Care Act 1990.

All the above sounds fine, but lack of resources often prevents some of the potentially most useful legislative provisions either being implemented at all or being as effective as they might be. Pressure needs to be maintained to remedy this and remind those responsible that The health of the nation (DOH 1992b) includes mental health as one of its targets.

NEW DEVELOPMENTS

In late 1998 the government announced its intention to review the 1983 Mental Health Act. The then Health Secretary, Frank Dobson said, in announcing the review, 'The law on mental health is based on the needs and therapies of a bygone age. Its revision in 1983 merely tinkered with the problem'. The proposed legislation will ensure English mental health law complies with the European Convention on Human Rights, to which the UK is now a signatory.

This review will cover such areas as compliance orders and community treatment orders to provide a legal framework to ensure patients deemed to present a risk or be at risk get supervised care. This may provide for the extension of sectioning or other legal powers to certain categories of nurses. Furthermore the question of treatability under Sections 3 and 37 is likely to be removed in cases where potential patients are deemed to pose a significant risk to either themselves or others. Any new powers are expected to be in balance with additional rights of assessment and independent review.

In line with this review and the findings of the Fallon Inquiry into the Personality Disorder Unit at Ashworth Hospital, the position with regard to hospital orders for patients with a diagnosed personality disorder is to be clarified. This clarification will seek to resolve the conflict surrounding the issues of resistance to treatment and security as a form of treatment. The findings of the inquiry may provoke the formulation of a legal framework in which hybrid hospital orders are used to enforce defined treatment underpinned by security for that minority of individuals with severe personality disorder.

SUMMARY

The 1983 Mental Health Act is the most important piece of legislation currently on the statute book affecting the care of the mentally ill in England and Wales; it is mirrored by similar legislation in both Scotland and Northern Ireland. However, similar to all legislation, it is a product of its time. It has been subject to some tinkering, particularly in 1995, and is due for a complete overhaul. It has sought to provide an opportunity to combine the need to provide protection for the individual and general public and ensure the that the liberty of the individual is protected. Central to its operation is the concept of 'enabling'—that is, the Act in its construction facilitates the movement from one power to another, or from one section to another. In doing this it facilitates clinical intervention. The amending legislation of 1995 provided additional powers in order to ensure that clients did not become lost to the system on discharge and established the concept of legal enforced clinical supervision on discharge to those individuals detained under treatment orders.

As is the case with all legislation, mental health law is subject to legal challenge, amendment and replacement. The reader would be well advised to monitor such changes through the various professional journals and via Nigel Turner's Hyperguide to the Mental Health Act at:

http://www.hyperguide.co.uk/mha/index.htm

FURTHER READING

Children's Legal Centre 1991 The mental health handbook. The Children's Legal Centre, 20 Compton Terrace, London N1 2UN

Cretney S M 1991 Enduring powers of attorney, 3rd edn. Jordan, Bristol

Cretney S, Davis G, Kerridge R, Borkowski A 1991 Enduring powers of attorney. Lord Chancellor's Department, London

Department of Health 1989 An introduction to the Children Act 1989. HMSO, London

Jones R M 1993 Encyclopedia of social services and child care law. Sweet & Maxwell, London

REFERENCES

Barnes M 1990 Assessing for compulsory detention. Applying the social perspective. In: Cohen J, Ramon S (eds) Social work and the Mental Health Act 1983 (England and Wales). British Association of Social Workers, Birmingham

CCETSW (Central Council for Education and Training in Social Work) 1992 Paper 19.27 A double challenge. working with people who have both learning difficulties and a mental illness. Report of a joint CCETSW/Royal College of Psychiatrists Symposium. CCETSW, London

CCETSW (Central Council for Education and Training in Social Work) 1993 Paper 19.19 Requirements and guidance for the training of social workers to be considered for approval in England and Wales under the Mental Health Act 1983. CCETSW, London

DOH (Department of Health) 1991 Children with disabilities: guidance. Department of Health, London

DOH (Department of Health) 1992a Letter. Mental Health Act 1983: Code of practice and attached proposed amendments. Department of Health, London

DOH (Department of Health) 1992b The health of the nation: a strategy for health in England (Cm. 1986). HMSO, London

DOH (Department of Health) 1993a Circular no. LAC(93)19

DOH (Department of Health) 1993b Mental Health Act 1983: Code of practice revision and attached further proposed amendments. Department of Health, London

DOH & Welsh Office 1992 Letter. Mental Health Act 1983. Code of practice issued under Section 118. Department of Health and Welsh Office, London

DOH & Welsh Office 1993 Mental Health Act 1983. Code of Practice, 2nd edn. HMSO, London

DHSS 1974 Circular No. 13/74

DHSS 1983a Mental Health Act 1983 memorandum on Parts I to VI, VIII and X. HMSO, London

DHSS 1983b Circular no. HC(83)14

DHSS 1984a Circular no. DDL(84)4

DHSS 1984b Circular no. HC(84)12/LAC(84)9

DHSS 1986 Circular no. LAC(86)15/WO circular No. 51(86)

DHSS 1987 Circular no. LAC(87)6

Grimshaw C 1993–94 A to Z of welfare benefits for people with a mental health problem: a practical guide for service users. Mind, London

Hoggett B 1990 Mental health law, 3rd edn. Sweet & Maxwell, London

HO 1990 Provision for mentally disordered offenders. Circular no. 66/90. HMSO, London

HO PACE 1991 Codes of practice of Police and Criminal Evidence Act 1984, 2nd edn. HMSO, London

Jones R M 1991 Mental Health Act manual, 3rd edn. Sweet & Maxwell, London

Law Commission 1992 Consultation paper no. 128. Mentally incapacitated adults and decision-making: a new jurisdiction. HMSO, London

Law Commission 1993 Consultation paper no. 130. Mentally incapacitated and other vulnerable adults: public law protection. HMSO, London

Letts P 1990 Managing other people's money. Age Concern, London

Public Trust Office 1993 Handbook for receivers. Protection Division of the Public Trust Office, Stewart House, 24 Kingsway, London WC2B 6JX

Wright E E 1992 The law relating to people with mental handicap. In: Thompson T, Mathias P (eds) Standards and mental handicap. Keys to competence. Baillière Tindall, London

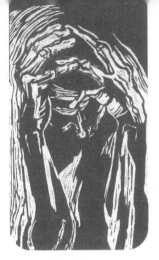

Glossary

Accountability Liability; being answerable for one's own actions; the need to explain and justify decisions taken or activities performed, as the best course available within prevailing circumstances. Accountability is awarded in an authority to act, and requires detailed knowledge of the proposed course of action, the alternatives available, the potential implications and repercussions of each, to be weighed in reaching a conclusion.

Acute confusional state A sudden and rapid onset of confusion, of an alarmingly high level, usually a symptom of an acute physical illness. The duration can be short and the cause can be treated.

Affect A subjective interpretation of the feelings accompanying an idea or image. Similar in meaning to 'mood', it can be defined as a state of emotional tone or feeling which can fluctuate between range of depression and elation.

Affective disorder Disorder of mood including the commoner disturbances in emotional equilibrium which may form part of an overall clinical picture in mental disorder; depression, anxiety, incongruity and blunting of affect, la belle indifference, lability, hostility, depersonalization. There may be difficulty in differentiating the symptoms of major affective disorders from environmental causation or organic illness, therefore careful assessment and history taking are particularly important.

Alma Ata The city which was the venue for 1978 World Health Organization International Conference on Primary Care.

Alzheimer's disease Causes of dementia due to an acceleration of the general loss of branch cells beyond the normal level. Occurs in 20% of people over the age 80. A progressive and global disorder commoner in women.

Arbitrary inference This is a type of error in logic as identified by Beck; it is characterized by the individual jumping to a conclusion on the basis of little objective evidence; it may also occur when there is contrary evidence.

Assessment Involves acquiring information about a person or situation that may include a description of the person's wants, needs, wishes and ambitions. Part of a larger procedure and service to support planning towards goals that have been separately identified.

Asylum Latin meaning 'sanctuary', a place of refuge for debtors and fugitives from the law or other persecutors: a term used historically in relation to institutions providing relief for the 'unfortunates' of society—the blind and the mentally ill, for example.

Attention The focusing of information-collecting apparatus upon selected aspects of the environment; conscious awareness of relevant stimuli accompanied by a central nervous system readiness to respond.

Audit Commission An independent organization set up by the government to review all aspects of the work of local government and, since the introduction of the NHS and Community Care Act 1990, also the work of the NHS. Pays particular attention to issues of quality, efficiency, effectiveness, and value for money.

Automatic thoughts As described by Beck these are contained in a stream of thoughts which is usually going on in an individual's head. They affect the person's feeling and inform their behaviour, but often occur without the person being aware of them. It is only when individuals are asked to focus in on their unreported thoughts that they become aware of them.

Basal ganglia Subcortical masses of grey matter embedded in each cerebral hemisphere, comprising the corpus striatum (caudate and lentiform nuclei), amygdaloid body and claustrum. Other structures have also been considered to be part of the basal ganglia.

Behaviour Campbell defines it as 'the manner in which anything acts or operates'—observable performance or overt activity; general reaction to internal or external motivating stimuli.

Behavioural therapy A therapeutic approach based on the experimental work describing classical and operant conditioning. It emphasizes the central role of reinforcement in establishing and maintaining both adaptive and maladaptive behaviour. The focus of the therapy is the observable behaviour. It utilizes a non-mediational model in arriving at a formulation of a problem.

Care management A process introduced in the NHS and Community Care Act (1990) that provides a consistent approach for matching individual needs to services (rather than the other way around). The process depends upon the holistic assessment of individual needs and the appointment of a care manager who is responsible for the design and costing of a care package that will be systematically evaluated in respect of its effectiveness in meeting the identified needs of the client concerned.

Carer Refers to a person who participates in recognized care (formally or informally), in relation to an individual experiencing a mental health problem.

Catastrophizing This is often a feature of the cognitive style of anxious people. It is seen in the person who typically anticipates the worse possible outcome of events.

Cerebellum The part of the mesencephalon situated on the back of the brainstem, to which it is attached by three cerebellar peduncles on each side; it consists of a median lobe (vermis) and two lateral lobes (the hemispheres).

Cerebral cortex The convoluted layer of grey matter covering the cerebral hemispheres, which governs thought, reasoning, memory, sensation, and voluntary movement.

Chronic confusional state A slow and insidious onset of confusion that is likely to go unnoticed. A symptom of chronic physical illness such as thyroid hormone deficiency. May occur over a period of years but with treatment it can be reversed.

Circadian rhythm An innate cyclical pattern of activity or behaviour that operates on the timing associated with a lunar day.

Classical conditioning The early work of Pavlov exemplifies this process of learning, which is the encouragement of new behaviour by modifying the stimulus–response association.

Client The lay but equal partner within a professional consultation; a seeker of professional guidance and specialist skills.

Client-centred therapy An approach to therapy that considers clients as best able to deal with their difficulties. It is non-directive with the therapist offering non-judgmental support in the hope that given such support individuals will be able to work out and resolve their difficulties. There is no attempt by the therapist to interpret the nature of the problem for the client (see Unconditional positive regard). It requires skilled practitioners who are able to provide observation and feedback associated with therapeutic interventions. Sometimes called Rogerian therapy where lay counsellors are trained in the Rogerarian humanistic approach of recognizing the client's capacity for growth and self-regulation.

Code of practice This was required under Section 118 of the Mental Health Act 1983. The Code offers a set of guidance notes intended, primarily, to accommodate the needs, rights and entitlements of mentally disordered persons who are detained under relevant Mental Health Act legislation.

Cognition A generic term utilized to describe those mental processes involved within the collection and storage of information. This is a general term that is used to describe the mental and internal events cognitive psychology concerns itself with. It can be used to refer to mental images and symbols, which may be reported by individuals as their thoughts about an event.

Cognitive behavioural therapy An approach to therapy that utilizes techniques from both behavioural and cognitive perspectives in therapy. It emphasizes the importance of utilizing a mediational model in arriving at a formulation of a problem, but highlights the importance of using both aspects of operant and classical conditioning in enabling clients to overcome their difficulties (see Behavioural therapy and Cognitive restructuring).

Cognitive disorder Disorder associated with the way in which an individual perceives and interprets the world. The underlying thought processes are seen as instrumental in determining how people behave and their emotional reactions.

Cognitive distortion Associated with cognitive disorder. Psychological stress is seen as a result of dysfunctional cognitions in which perceptions are interpreted inappropriately in disabling ways. Therapeutic strategies associated with the above include:

◆ cognitive therapy
◆ rational emotive therapy
◆ personal construct therapy
◆ transactional analysis
◆ neurolinguistic programming (NLP).

Cognitive disturbance Self-defeating attitude or responses that may become habitual particularly when directed towards lowered self-esteem.

Cognitive psychology An approach in psychology that studies the internal mental processes. Behaviour is explained using a model that takes account of mental events (see Mediational model).

Cognitive restructuring A technique used in the practice of cognitive therapy that through a

process of challenging an individual's interpretations of an event attempts to enable the clients to reconsider their construction of the event and to think about it in a different kind of way, thereby encouraging a different affective response.

Community mental health teams These teams have developed in the United Kingdom over the past two decades and are to be found in most areas in recognition of the fact that most people with mental health needs live in the community. Teams are based according to historical and geographical factors. Teams generally include a community mental health nurse, a consultant psychiatrist, a specialist social worker, a clinical psychologist and other members of the health care team. The function of the team is to support people living in the community and their carers. This may be done directly or by facilitation through generic health and community services.

Competence The optimum levels of performance possible within ideal circumstances. Wood & Powers indicate that competence requires the availability of detailed accurate knowledge, plus experience in performance, plus flexibility to meet changing environmental conditions and the performer demonstrating an appropriate mood, attention and motivational levels.

Congenital hyperthyroidism A condition in the newborn that results in overactivity of the thyroid gland producing an excess of thyroid hormones. Results in anxiety, restlessness, increased pulse, sweating and protuberance of the eyes. People with Down's syndrome are thought to have a slightly higher incidence than normal.

Contract culture Shorthand term used to refer to the introduction of *purchasers* and *providers* in health and social services. Services are now delivered on the basis of contracts drawn up between two groups. An example is when a regional health authority sets a contract for the number of preregistration mental health students with a college of health. In this case the RHA is the purchaser and the college the provider. An alternative term for purchasers is *commissioning agents*.

Contractual cycle The timetable that purchasers and providers work to in reviewing existing, and setting new, contracts. Usually done every 12 months so there is an annual contractual cycle.

Dangerousness The probability that an individual will commit a violent act upon the person of another (or others) in the near or distant future, if afforded the opportunity to do so.

Demarcation When applied to professions and occupations, refers to the boundaries put around skills, tasks, activities that are felt to be unique, or exclusive, to a particular profession or occupation.

Dementia An organic mental disorder resulting in a lowering of the usual level of mental ability.

Depersonalization A characteristic of depression when individuals are aware of a change in self and may feel that they have become so different as to have become detached from their personality. They may describe the feeling as 'if in a dream' or 'like an automaton'. Mild depersonalization can occur in states of physical and mental fatigue.

Deviation Different from expected standards associated with a particular course or status; a movement away from the 'norm', which involves judgements being made in regard to the acceptable parameters of this 'norm' and which is often accompanied by a specific qualifying term, for example, a health deviation, sexual or social deviation.

Emotion An amalgamation of consciously perceived feelings and the objective manifestations accompanying such feelings, for example, physiological changes.

Empathy An accurate understanding or perception of another person's emotional state. It should not be confused with sympathy in which there is a sharing of the feeling of another person. Empathy is related to feeling for the other person; sympathy is related to feeling with the other person.

Errors in logic These refer to the way in which depressed people typically interpret events in the world. Beck noted a distinctive cognitive style in this group of people. He described this style and categorized several errors in logic.

Extrapyramidal system A functional, rather than anatomical, unit comprising the nuclei and fibres (excluding those of the pyramidal tract) involved in motor activities; they control and coordinate especially the postural, static, supporting, and locomotor mechanisms. It includes the corpus striatum, subthalamic nucleus, substantia nigra and red nucleus, along with their interconnections with the reticular formation, cerebellum and cerebrum; some authorities include the cerebellum and vestibular nuclei.

Family psychotherapy The application of psychotherapeutic techniques within a family context (see Personal psychotherapy).

Functional analysis This technique is aimed at establishing a relationship between the environment and behaviour. It involves collecting detailed information about both the client's behaviour and aspects of the environment so that an hypothesis may be made regarding aspects of the environment which may be cueing or reinforcing the behaviour.

Good subject effect This refers to the fact that individuals, when taking part in a psychology experiment, may try to guess the purpose of the experiment and give the answers they think the experimenter would like, rather than the answer they would give if they were not subject to this influence.

Health care 'Investigation, diagnosis, treatment, rehabilitation and continuing care', identified within Caring for people: community care in the next decade and beyond.

Health of the nation Government white paper published by the Department of Health in 1992 outlining strategy for health in England.

Health promotion The World Health Organization's definitions of health promotion: 'Health promotion is the process of enabling people to increase control over and to improve, their health'. There are seven major areas of health promotion activities: health education programmes (primary, secondary and tertiary); preventive health services; community-based work; organizational development; healthy public policies; environmental health measures; economic and regulatory activities.

Human information processing The general model used in cognitive psychology, which argues that cognitive processes occur in stages. These stages are often likened to computer programs in which there is an input of information followed by some internal processing of the input during which the message is coded. The input can then either be stored or used straightaway to guide and inform behaviour.

Hypothalamus The portion of the diencephalon lying beneath the thalamus at the base of the cerebrum, and forming the floor and part of the lateral wall of the third ventricle. Anatomically, it includes the optic chiasm, mamillary bodies, tuber cinereum, infundibulum, and hypophysis (pituitary gland), but for physiological purposes the hypophysis is considered a distinct structure. The hypothalamic nuclei activate, control and integrate many of the involuntary functions necessary for living. The various hypothalamic centres influence peripheral autonomic mechanisms, endocrine activity, and many somatic functions, e.g. a general regulation of water balance, body temperature, sleep, thirst, and hunger, and the development of secondary sexual characteristics.

Individual programme plan (IPP) A system for making plans for one person based on the strengths and needs of that person as an individual with the assistance of people who are well known to him/her. A meeting is held to formulate the IPP at which objectives are set to be achieved within a specific timespan. The person responsible for each need is identified. Any service deficits that prevent the need from being met are also identified and managers are informed. In this way service provision can be based on the needs of clients.

Individualized patient care Care focused upon the unique requirements of the individual in pursuit of a state of well-being, which includes the targeting of resources to that end.

Infradian rhythm An innate biological cycle which occurs on a schedule exceeding a lunar day —that is, monthly or annually.

Institution A designated establishment approved by a local health authority to receive and care for mentally ill people.

Institutionalization (i) Described by Martin (1955) as the loss of volition and individuality

apparent in many long term psychiatric patients. Often used in conjunction with the term 'institutional neurosis' coined by Russell Barton in 1959. This describes the constellation of adverse effects of protracted institutional living. (ii) The habituation of an individual to the patterns of behaviour and routines associated with, and expected in, an institution: this requirement to conform is associated with restrictions in personal freedom and choice, creating loss of individuality and the uniqueness of the person.

Joint training Training programmes where staff from different occupations train together, such as nurses and social workers, and obtain joint qualifications approved by the professional bodies. This can be at either the pre- or postregistration levels of training. If staff from different occupations train together but do not receive the qualification of the other profession this is referred to as *shared training* or *shared learning*. In such circumstances, students from different occupations may cover only part of a course together whereas with joint training the whole course has to be covered.

La belle indifference A term sometimes applied to an apparent lack of concern commonly associated with symptoms of hysteria. Its presence may indicate removal of anxiety by hysterical mechanisms. If anxiety is not completely removed emotional detachment or disassociation may result.

Labelling Grouping according to general or specific characteristics: categorization. Within a sociological perspective, labelling has been considered as one of the methods by which individuals who are 'different' or who fail to conform to societal norms and expectations are segregated from that society. A special status—criminal, schizophrenic, prostitute—is awarded by an authoritative body and this label generates a stigma and often weighty moral condemnation. Pickerill asserts that differentness has been recognized and responded to prior to the award of the official label and that the latter may merely confirm society's view.

Lability A rapid change in mood that can occur especially in elderly people with a mental disorder.

Language A system of symbolic communication by which thought and activity are made available to conscious awareness and which provides the basic vehicle used to both structure experiences and share these structures with others. Language similarly provides facility for a shared conjecture about the non-immediate world.

The Law of Effect As described by Thorndike this law demonstrates how if an event results in 'good' consequences it is likely to be repeated, but if the results are 'bad' then there is less likelihood of it being repeated and the relationship between stimulus and response is unlikely to be maintained.

Limbic system A system of brain structures common to the brains of all mammals, comprising the phylogenetically old cortex (archipallium and paleopallium) and its primarily related nuclei. It is associated with olfaction, autonomic functions, and certain aspects of emotion and behaviour.

Mediational model A way of explaining behaviour that takes account of cognitive factors. It was proposed as a result of experimental work done by Tolman, who although a behaviourist he argued for the recognition of mediating factors in the establishment and maintenance of behaviour (see Stimulus response model).

Memory Encoding, storage and retrieval of mental representations relating to current experiences for use at a later juncture.

Mental disorder A temporary imbalance within the citizen who retains the rights of citizenship; the imbalance may be recognized by various forms of malfunction in behaviour.

Mental health A term used in a broad, general sense to imply some optimum level of psychosocial functioning.

Mental Health Act Commission Is a body of 90 persons appointed by the Secretary of State to work on a part-time basis. Members are lawyers, doctors, nurses, social workers, psychologists and lay persons. Their remit is to care for the rights of patients detained in hospitals and nursing homes, within the meaning of the 1983 Mental Health Act.

Mental health nurse An appropriately qualified and experienced nurse who practises by virtue of their qualification in the maintenance and promotion of mental health and the treatment of mental illness.

Mental health nursing The identification of those positive characteristics of mental health still intact within an individual undergoing an illness event and the development of nursing strategies to strengthen the positive aspects of the individual whilst treating out the disordered behaviours.

Metaparadigms Concepts fundamental to an understanding—in the discipline of nursing these are human being; society; health/ill health; nursing.

Mood A general overview of predominant feelings: includes past and current affective experiences.

Multi-infarct dementia The second most common cause of dementia. Patchy loss of brain cells occurs owing to an impoverished blood supply to parts of the brain because of the thickening and narrowing of the arteries. Occurs in 55% of all cases of dementia. A progressive but intermittent disorder.

Needs Things that can be identified or assigned. They are presented as statements of fact which can be deduced by someone else.

Non-institutional An establishment that is outside of the local health authority provision for the care of mentally ill persons.

Nursing model A way of representing concepts and relationships which feature in the act of nursing.

Nursing process A systematic approach to providing nursing care, including the collection of data indicative of health/ill health; nursing diagnosis; care planning, in agreement with the patient; marshalling of required resources and delivery of care; evaluation of the nursing care delivered against specified outcomes.

Operant conditioning After the work of Skinner there was a recognition that if an organism emits a behaviour and this behaviour is reinforced then the behaviour is likely to be emitted again. The behaviour is seen to have an effect on the environment and depending on this consequent effect the behaviour may or may not be reinforced.

Optimum health The concept associated with the desirable state of mental and physical well-being. WHO defines health as a state of 'ideal physical, psychological and social wellbeing and not merely the absence of disease'.

Overgeneralization This error in logic is exemplified by the individual who, on the basis of the outcome of one incident assumes all other similar incidents will have the same results.

Paradoxical intention A technique used in a range of psychotherapies in which individuals are goaded into doing what they most fear. It is argued that the use of humour is important in this approach. It is a technique that should be used only by those who are trained in its use.

Patient A passive recipient and focus of professional illness-orientated, nursing, medical and paramedical personnel.

Perception The organization and interpretation of stimuli into meaningful knowledge.

Performance The levels of skilled activity observable within the realities imposed by everyday personal, professional and environmental constraints.

Personal construct theory Frames of reference which differ between individuals and professionals are included in the problems associated with using conceptual definitions interchangeably and sometimes wrongly. Of particular significance in this context is the way in which an individual may hold negative and distorted perceptions about their body or self-image. Factors which influence personal constructs include: internal such as how facts about one's self as a person are perceived; and external such as the reactions one individual experiences from the people with whom they are in contact. The self-construct is made up of abstractions built upon the individual's own behaviour and subsequent observations together with other responses for attitudes and performance.

Personal psychotherapy Treatment of emotional or psychosomatic disorders based on the application of psychological knowledge rather than on

physical forms of treatment. Explores inner feelings and encourages the exploration of 'inner' coping strategies to deal with stress and life events.

Personalization As an error in logic this is seen in individuals who interpret the outcome of events by only making reference to themselves. They have a particularly egocentric view of the world and assume that all the negative events that befall them are in some way their fault. This cognitive style should not be confused with ideas of self-reference which are a symptom of psychosis.

Phenylketonuria A condition resulting in brain damage caused by a deficiency of an enzyme (phenylalanine hydroxylase). The disorder is routinely tested for in the UK and USA and early treatment results in normal development. Treatment is with a low phenylalanine diet.

Pineal gland A small, conical structure attached by a stalk to the posterior wall of the third ventricle of the cerebrum, believed by many to be an endocrine gland. In certain amphibians and reptiles the gland is thought to function as a light receptor. In most mammals, including humans, it appears to be the major or unique site of melatonin biosynthesis. The effect of melatonin on the body and the exact function of the pineal gland remain obscure.

Positivism A predisposition to focus and build on strengths and positive points rather than weaknesses and negative points. A philosophy of approaching situations positively, which encourages favourable attitudes, policies, solutions and self-images.

Psychiatric nursing An appropriately qualified and experienced person who has received preparation for ensuring that relevant care is provided for mentally ill persons, in all stages of the life cycle.

Psychiatry A branch of medicine that deals with the study, treatment and prevention of mental illness.

Psychological situation Rotter's term used to describe how an understanding of not only the physical setting in which an event occurs but also the person's interpretation of that situation.

Reality orientation A technique in which the repeated presentation of facts with positive reinforcement and encouragement is used to help dementia sufferers to make use of their remaining faculties: unlikely to help those suffering from severe dementia.

Reinforcement This term suffers from overuse to the point that it has almost lost its meaning. It stems from the original use in psychology as part of learning theory where it was used to describe something that has an effect of strengthening a bond of association which has developed between a stimulus and a response. It should *not* be used as synonymous with the term 'reward'.

Reinforcement value Rotter argued that humans attach different values to various activities and rewards and that this has an influence on the way people behave in response to stimuli.

Reminiscence therapy Stimulations of the memory to recall past and pleasant events which has the therapeutic value of helping elders to improve their confidence.

Responsibility An onus; an obligation; a duty one is charged with conducting.

Rogerarian therapy Therapeutic input based on the expert theorist Carl Rogers who expounded the view that the whole task of psychotherapy is the task of dealing with a failure of communication.

Role A conspicuous part played in life; a more or less prescribed pattern of activity with associated parameters: may be ascribed at birth—woman, son, queen—or may be acquired in relation to social function—teacher, student, Pope. The professional nurse assumes a variety of roles within care provision in negotiation with the client, his significant others and professional colleagues. Associated roles include care manager, care collaborator, interventionist, resource manager, health promoter, facilitator, researcher, adviser and energizer.

Schedules of reinforcement The delivery of reinforcement varies in time, an individual action can be reinforced immediately after it happens, after a given period of time, or at a time which is independent of the action. Depending on when the reinforcement is delivered there will be a different schedule of reinforcement. A schedule may be simple or compound, *intermittent reinforcement* is an example of a simple schedule. Under the condition of intermittent reinforcement an action is literally reinforced intermittently.

Secondary gains A gain derived from being ill. This is especially associated with the gains derived from avoidance of conflict and should be seen as a potential reinforcer not just for the victim of the illness, but also for those associated with the individual.

Security A developmental and existential requirement of the individual related to feelings of safety.

Selective abstraction This refers to a persistent error in logic that is demonstrated by the individual who takes details of events out of context and as a result misinterprets them.

Self-disclosure Part of a stage used in Rogerarian therapy where there is an increasing ownership of self-feelings. Eventually feelings are expressed or experienced with full immediacy and flow to full results. Any problems expressed are perceived as subjective and not as an object external to self and divorced from feelings. As counselling relationships develop clients feel more confident in disclosing more intimate details about themselves.

Self-instructional techniques A general term used to refer to a variety of techniques which employ self-talk. This is the process whereby individuals literally tell themselves what to do in a situation. It is based on the experimental work that demonstrates a guiding link between motoric behaviour and the emission of verbal self-instruction.

Sensory ganglia Any of the ganglia of the peripheral nervous system that transmit sensory impulses; also, the collective masses of nerve cell bodies in the brain subserving sensory functions.

Setting events Those events in the environment that prompt a response. They can be manipulated in order to alter behaviour, they may be equated with unconditioned stimuli in classical conditioning which through a process of association become conditioned stimuli. In operant conditioning they are assessed as antecedent behaviour, which prompts behaviour.

Shaping A technique widely used in behavioural therapy in which an individual is taught to perform new behaviours through a series of approximations to the required outcome.

Shared action planning A system based on the IPP approach, which emphasizes the importance of relationships and friendships as the core principle for the development of care plans. It ensures that service users share in all aspects of the process as joint decision makers. It involves goals, aims, assessment and provides strategies and actions to ensure that outcomes are evaluated in accordance with prescribed action plans.

Skill A learned or developed ability to perform to a prescribed standard.

Social care 'Help with personal and domestic tasks, such as cleaning, washing and preparing meals, with disablement equipment and home adaptations, transport, budgeting and other aspects of daily living' is the definition provided within Caring for people: community care in the next decade and beyond. Mental health care personnel, including nurses, encounter deficits in an individual's daily living skills as both a precipitating factor and a resultant feature of mental health problems. Currently, therefore 'social care' is an integral part of the mental health nurse's focus of attention.

Social cognitive theory An elaboration of learning theory which takes account of cognitive elements in the establishment, maintenance and exhibition of behaviours. It highlights the importance of anticipation of the value of reinforcement and the belief in one's ability to reproduce the behaviour.

Social psychiatry The practice of psychiatry based on a social model of mental health and illness. The model is one in which relationships and the context of the environment are viewed as crucial to mental well-being. The primary focus is on family and group relationships.

Social skills training Focused training aimed at generating and maintaining competent social skills which are culturally appropriate. Often includes the reinforcement of interpersonal interactions. The types of social reinforcer that may be used as part of a structured programme include attention, assertion, praise, approval, smiles and physical contact. It can be inferred that social behaviour involves complex cognitive, personal belief and emotional processes.

Standard questionnaires An assessment tool that has been developed in such a way as to ensure both validity and reliability. There are numerous commercially available assessment tools that may be used to assess a range of behaviours and cognitions.

Statutory bodies Bodies, e.g. United Kingdom Central Council for Nursing, Midwifery and Health Visiting and National Boards for Nursing, Midwifery and Health Visiting, set up by statute and responsible for the formal education for professional nursing practice. They are responsible for the standard, kind and content of practice and are accountable to the government and public.

Stimulus response model This model dis-regards the notion of an intervening variable in the acquisition and display of a behaviour. It is the model that is favoured by behaviourists who argue that observable behaviour is the only legitimate object of study and that it can be explained by a consideration of the establishment of the links made via association during the learning process (see Classical conditioning and Operant conditioning).

Systematic desensitization As described by Wolpe this refers to a method of treating phobias. It is based on the practice of pairing a feared object or situation with relaxation; the relaxation will have the effect of inhibiting the physiological response that leads to the experience of fear; in addition there will be an element of learning via classical conditioning in which the feared object becomes paired with the feeling of relaxation. The treatment of phobias is often done in a systematic way through a series of stages during which clients are exposed to the stimulus that is increasingly more fearful for them.

Therapeutic alliance Refers to the interpersonal process that is central to the practice of mental health nursing. It emphasizes the interpersonal interactions with individual groups coping with current or potential mental health problems.

Thinking The skill in manipulation of images and symbolic representations to arrive at strategies by which changes in status may be managed. This is achieved by the utilization of previous knowledge and current understanding of the presenting situation, and involves patterns of activity such as reasoning and problem solving in an attempt to make sense of data available.

Total institution A term introduced by Goffman in 1961 as part of his attempt to identify those institutional forces and practices that combine to erode individuality and self esteem.

Transactional analysis A term introduced by Eric Berne in the 1960s which broadened the humanistic approach to psychotherapy. The technique focuses on the interpersonal 'transactions' of the client. It is best viewed as a communication tool and therapeutic approach that helps the practitioners consider their own responses as well as those of the client.

Ultradian rhythm An innate cyclical activity which is seen to occur on a greater frequency than daily; that is, seen several times a day.

Unconditional positive regard As described by Rogers, this refers to a central element of the behaviour of a therapist involved in client-centred psychotherapy. He considers it to be vital in practice of psychotherapy. It describes an approach in which the client is not challenged in their revelations or attempts at resolution of their difficulties.

User An individual who requires access to the mental health services in relation to treatment for a mental health problem.

WHO targets for all by the year 2000 (TFA) Targets in support of the European Regional Strategy for Health for All.

Workforce planning The collection of statistics on all aspects of staffing services. This includes figures on recruitment, retention, qualifications, hours of work and the like. Used to be called *manpower planning* or *manpower studies*. A particular emphasis is placed upon projecting future workforce needs as services evolve.

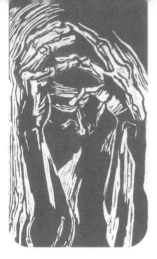

Index